MILADY'S STANDARD: Professional Barbering

Maura Scali-Sheahan

Endorsed by

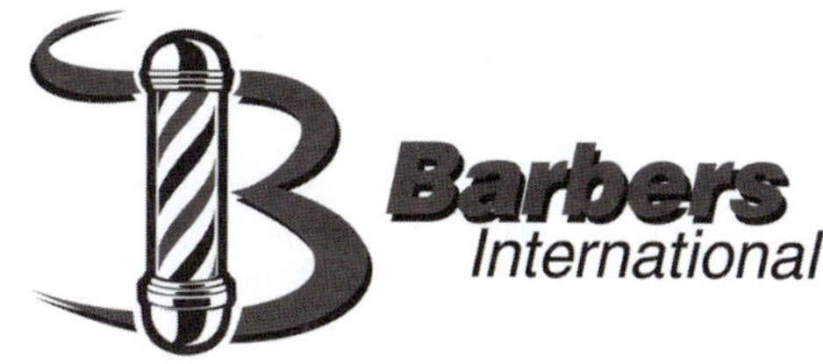

www.barbersinternational.com

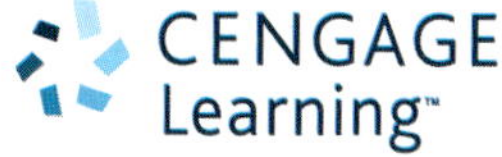

Australia • Brazil • Japan • Korea • Mexico • Singapore • Spain • United Kingdom • United States

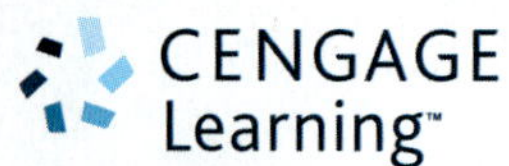

Milady's Standard: Professional Barbering
Maura Scali-Sheahan

President, Milady: Dawn Gerrain

Director of Editor: Sherry Gomoll

Acquisitions Editor: Brad Hanson

Developmental Editor: Jennifer Radalin

Editorial Assistant: Jessica Burns

Director of Production: Wendy A. Troeger

Production Manager: JP Henkel

Production Editor: Nina Tucciarelli

Production Assistant: Angela Iula

Director of Marketing: Wendy Mapstone

Channel Manager: Sandra Bruce

Library of Congress Control Number: 2005007287

ISBN-13: 978-1-4018-7395-0

ISBN-10: 1-4018-7395-2

Milady
Executive Woods
5 Maxwell Drive
Clifton Park, NY 12065
USA

Cengage Learning is a leading provider of customized learning solutions with office locations around the globe, including Singapore, the United Kingdom, Australia, Mexico, Brazil, and Japan. Locate your local office at: **international.cengage.com/region**

Cengage Learning products are represented in Canada by Nelson Education, Ltd.

For your course and learning solutions, visit **delmar.cengage.com**

Visit our corporate website at **cengage.com**

Notice to the Reader

Publisher does not warrant or guarantee any of the products described herein or perform any independent analysis in connection with any of the product information contained herein. Publisher does not assume, and expressly disclaims, any obligation to obtain and include information other than that provided to it by the manufacturer. The reader is expressly warned to consider and adopt all safety precautions that might be indicated by the activities described herein and to avoid all potential hazards. By following the instructions contained herein, the reader willingly assumes all risks in connection with such instructions. The publisher makes no representations or warranties of any kind, including but not limited to, the warranties of fitness for particular purpose or merchantability, nor are any such representations implied with respect to the material set forth herein, and the publisher takes no responsibility with respect to such material. The publisher shall not be liable for any special, consequential, or exemplary damages resulting, in whole or part, from the readers' use of, or reliance upon, this material.

Printed in the United States of America
6 7 8 9 10 11 12 11 10 09

PART 1

ORIENTATION TO BARBERING

PART 2

THE SCIENCE OF BARBERING

PART 3

PROFESSIONAL BARBERING

PART 4

ADVANCED BARBERING SERVICES

PART 5

THE BUSINESS OF BARBERING

PART 3

PROFESSIONAL BARBERING

PART 4

ADVANCED BARBERING SERVICES

PART 5

THE BUSINESS OF BARBERING

PROCEDURES

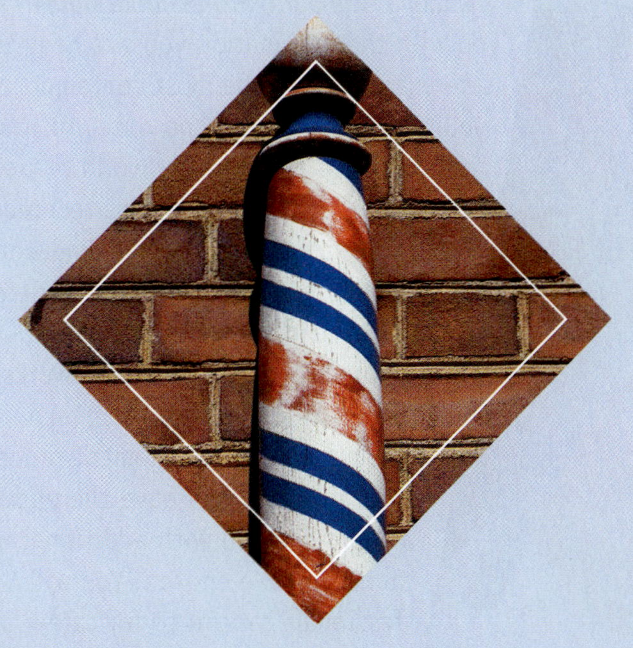

Preface

TO THE STUDENT

Congratulations! You have chosen a career filled with unlimited potential, one that can take you in many directions and holds the possibility to make you a confident, successful professional. As a barber, you will play a vital role in the lives of your clients. They will come to rely on you to provide them with ongoing service, enabling them to look and feel their best.

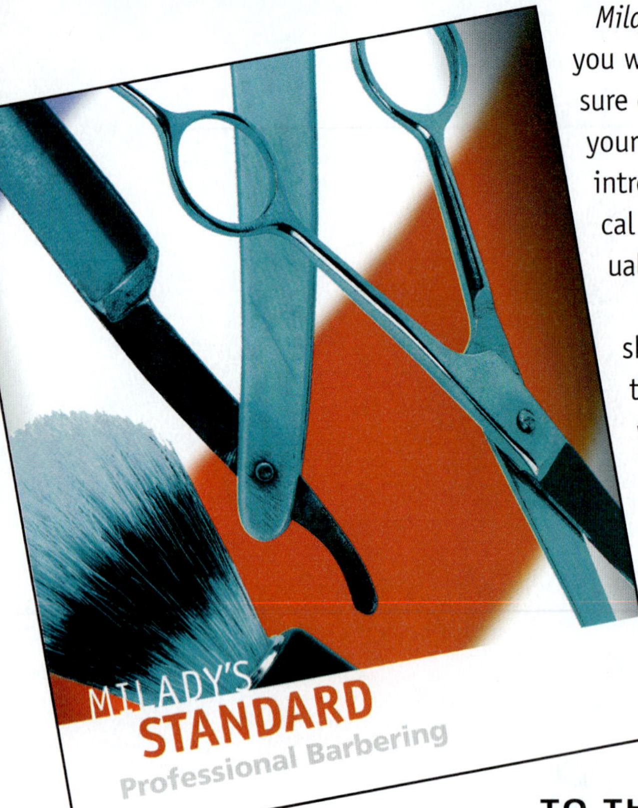

Milady's Standard: Professional Barbering was created to provide you with the information you will need to pass the state licensure exams as well the most contemporary techniques to ensure your success in school and once you're on the job. You will be introduced to a whole new world of creative expression, technical skills, and human relations techniques that will be continually enhanced as you spend time working in your profession.

You will learn from gifted instructors who will share their skills and experiences with you. You will meet other industry professionals at seminars, workshops, and conventions where you'll learn the latest techniques, specific product knowledge, and management procedures. All of the experiences in which you have the opportunity to participate will provide you with additional insights into the profession you have chosen. You will build a network of professionals to turn to for career advice, opportunity, and direction. Whatever direction you choose, we wish you a successful and enjoyable journey.

TO THE INSTRUCTOR

This edition of *Milady's Standard: Professional Barbering* was prepared with the help of many instructors and professionals. Milady surveyed 45 instructors during one focus group, held a second focus group made up of former students and users of the text, and received in-depth comments from 18 other experts to learn what needed to be changed, added, or deleted. Next, we consulted with educational experts to learn the best way to present the material, so that all types of learners could understand and process it. Finally, we sent the finished manuscripts to yet more subject-matter experts to ensure the accuracy and thoroughness of the material. What you hold in your hands is the result.

Milady's Standard: Professional Barbering contains new information on many subjects, including sanitation and infection control, hair and scalp disorders, hair replacement, and haircutting.

In response to the suggestions of the educators and professionals who reviewed the manuscript and to those submitted by students using this text, this edition includes dramatic changes, including full-color photos and illustrations, and many new chapters. Milady has also changed the design of the textbook and included new photography and illustrations to bring you the most valuable, effective educational material possible.

NEW ORGANIZATION AND CHAPTERS

The new text organization will help to present the material in a logical, sequential order. To help you locate information more easily, the chapters are now grouped into five main parts:

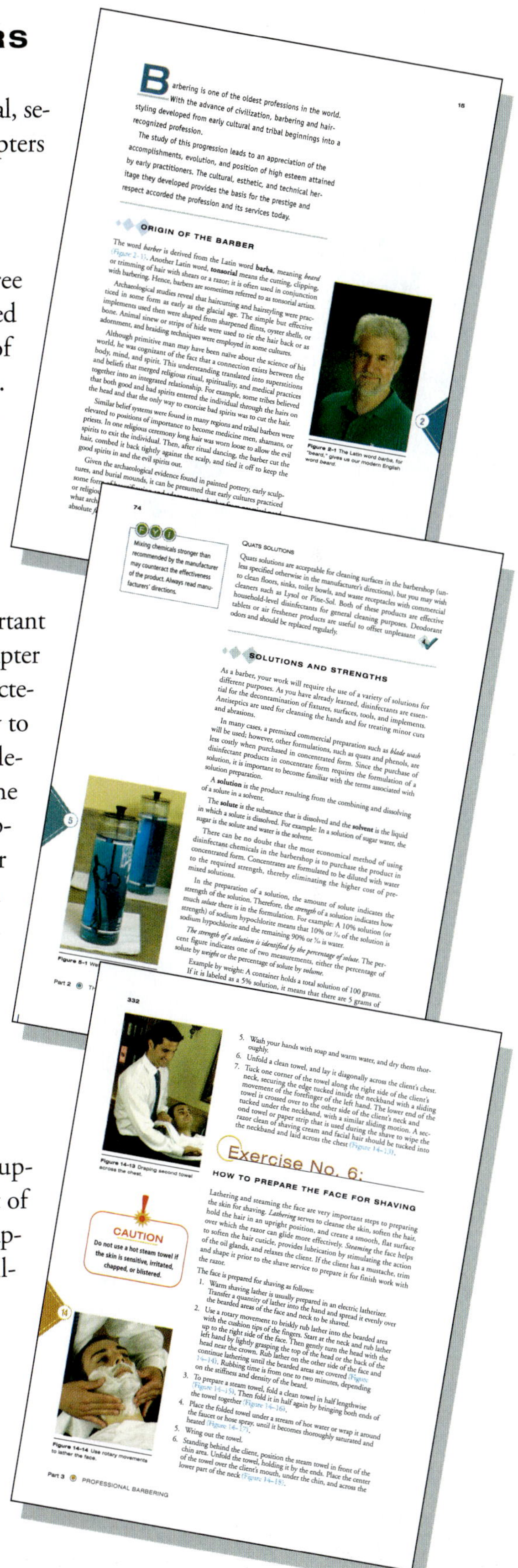

Part 1 - Orientation to Barbering consists of three chapters that cover the field of barbering and the personal skills needed to become successful. Chapter 1, Study Skills, focuses on the kind of techniques and habits needed to get the most out of your education. Chapter 2, The History of Barbering, outlines the origins of barbering and where it is going in the future. Chapter 3, Professional Image, stresses the importance of attitude, ethics, and health as well as outward appearance.

Part 2 - The Science of Barbering includes important information to keep barber and customer alike safe and healthy. Chapter 4, Bacteriology, contains current facts about infectious viruses and bacteria. Chapter 5, Infection Control and Safe Work Practices, tells how to prevent the spread of infection in the barbershop. Chapter 6, Implements, Tools, and Equipment, provides detailed information on the tools most used by barbers and how to care for them properly. Chapter 7, Anatomy and Physiology, Chapter 8, Chemistry, and Chapter 9, Electricity and Light Therapy, give essential scientific information that will affect how you work with clients and products. Chapters 10 and 11, Properties and Disorders of the Skin, and Properties and Disorders of the Hair and Scalp, provide the essential knowledge to recognize various disorders and those treatments that licensed barbers are qualified to offer their clients.

Part 3 - Professional Barbering offers new and updated material on every aspect of hair. From Chapter 12, Treatment of the Hair and Scalp, to Chapter 16, Men's Hairpieces, each of the chapters in this part offers step-by-step procedures accompanied by full-color photographs for accurate presentation of the material.

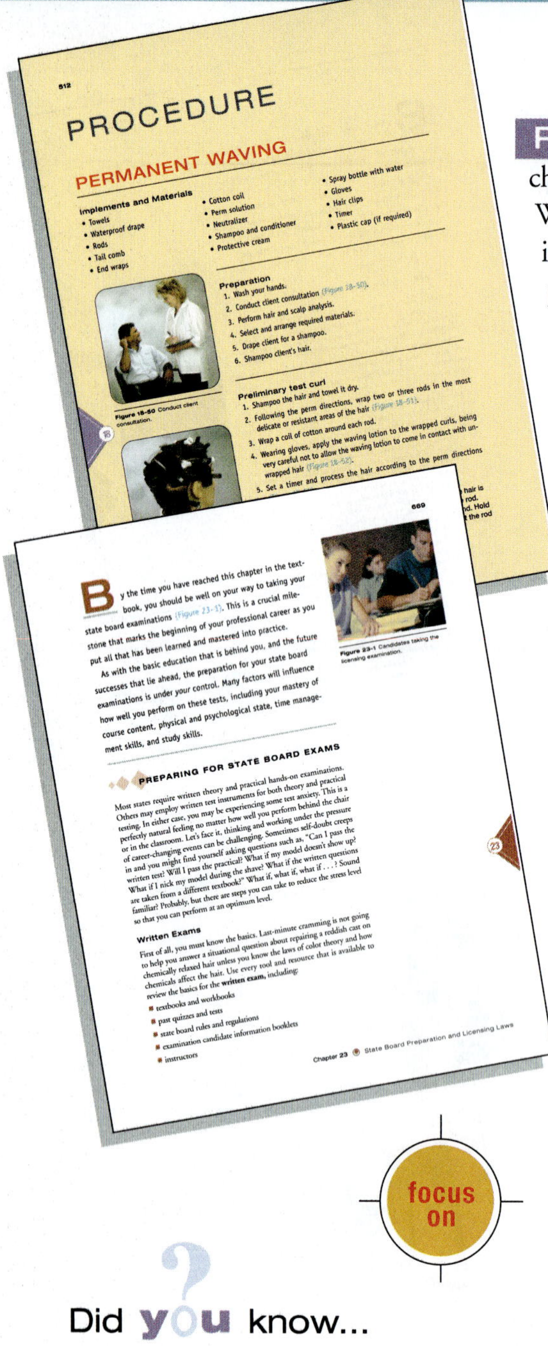
512

PROCEDURE

PERMANENT WAVING

Implements and Materials

- Towels
- Waterproof drape
- Rods
- Tail comb
- End wraps
- Cotton coil
- Perm solution
- Neutralizer
- Shampoo and conditioner
- Protective cream
- Spray bottle with water
- Gloves
- Hair clips
- Timer
- Plastic cap (if required)

Preparation

1. Wash your hands.
2. Conduct client consultation (Figure 18-50).
3. Perform hair and scalp analysis.
4. Select and arrange required materials.
5. Drape client for a shampoo.
6. Shampoo client's hair.

Figure 18-50 Conduct client consultation.

Preliminary test curl

1. Shampoo the hair and towel it dry.
2. Following the perm directions, wrap two or three rods in the most delicate or resistant areas of the hair (Figure 18-51).
3. Wrap a coil of cotton around each rod.
4. Wearing gloves, apply the waving lotion to the wrapped curls, being very careful not to allow the waving lotion to come in contact with unwrapped hair (Figure 18-52).
5. Set a timer and process the hair according to the perm directions

669

By the time you have reached this chapter in the textbook, you should be well on your way to taking your state board examinations (Figure 23-1). This is a crucial milestone that marks the beginning of your professional career as you put all that has been learned and mastered into practice.

As with the basic education that is behind you, and the future successes that lie ahead, the preparation for your state board examinations is under *your* control. Many factors will influence how well you perform on these tests, including your mastery of course content, physical and psychological state, time management skills, and study skills.

Figure 23-1 Candidates taking the licensing examination.

PREPARING FOR STATE BOARD EXAMS

Most states require written theory and practical hands-on examinations. Others may employ written test instruments for both theory and practical testing. In either case, you may be experiencing some test anxiety. This is a perfectly natural feeling no matter how well you perform behind the chair or in the classroom. Let's face it, thinking and working under the pressure of career-changing events can be challenging. Sometimes self-doubt creeps in and you might find yourself asking questions such as, "Can I pass the written test? Will I pass the practical? What if my model doesn't show up? What if I nick my model during the shave? What if the written questions are taken from a different textbook?" What if, what if, what if . . . ? Sound familiar? Probably, but there are steps you can take to reduce the stress level so that you can perform at an optimum level.

Written Exams

First of all, you must know the basics. Last-minute cramming is not going to help you answer a situational question about repairing a reddish cast on chemically relaxed hair unless you know the laws of color theory and how chemicals affect the hair. Use every tool and resource that is available to review the basics for the **written exam,** including:

- textbooks and workbooks
- past quizzes and tests
- state board rules and regulations
- examination candidate information booklets
- instructors

Chapter 23 State Board Preparation and Licensing Laws

Part 4 - Advanced Barbering Services contains four chapters devoted to additional services often found in the barber shop: Women's Haircutting and Styling, Chemical Texture Services, Haircoloring and Lightening, and Nails and Manicuring for those states requiring proficiency in these areas.

Part 5 - The Business of Barbering opens with the updated chapter, Barbershop Management, in which students are exposed to the ins and outs of owning and operating a barbershop. The Job Search offers tips on how to make the most of their first job, and the last chapter, State Board Preparation and Licensing Laws, provides students with some strategic methods to be used in preparation for the licensure examination and a general overview of barber licensing law.

ELEMENTS NEW TO THIS EDITION

As part of the comprehensive revision of this edition many new features have been added to help students master key concepts and techniques.

- Boxed features such as Focus On, Did You Know, FYI, Here's a Tip, and Caution provide hints, interesting information, and targeted skills, helping to sharpen skills and draw attention to special situations.
- Key Terms – The words students need to know in each chapter are given at the beginning in a list of key terms. The first time a word is used and defined in the text, the word appears in boldface. If the word is difficult to pronounce, a phonetic pronunciation appears after it in parentheses.
- Chapter Glossary – All key terms and their definitions are included in the glossary at the end of the chapter, as well as the Glossary/Index at the end of the text.
- Learning Objectives – each chapter begins with a list of learning objectives that highlight important information in the chapter.
- Review Questions – Each chapter ends with questions designed to test student's understanding of the information. The answers appear in the instructor's Course Management Guide.

focus on

Did you know...

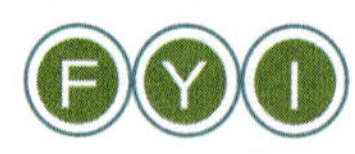

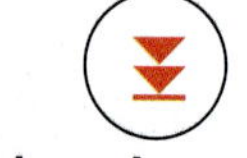

Here's a tip:

REMINDER

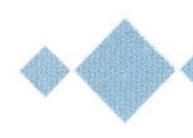

FRESH NEW DESIGN

The changes in this edition of *Milady's Standard: Professional Barbering* go far beyond the new content and features. New four-color art and photographs—over 1,000—enhance this book, along with a totally new text design that incorporates easy-to-read type and easy-to-follow layout.

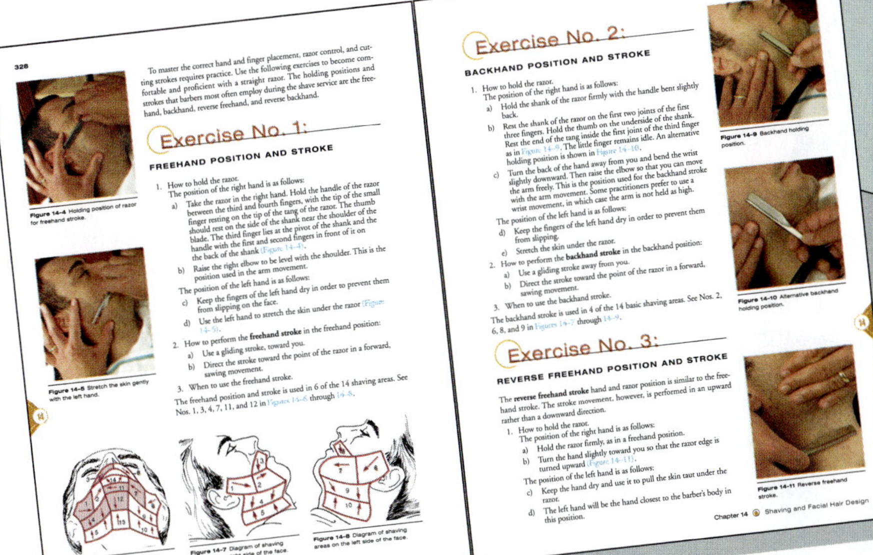

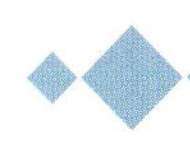

FRESH NEW ART

More than a thousand new full-color photographs and illustrations were created for this edition to complement the new text design. Photographs using mannequins and live models are included to illustrate styles and procedures. New structure graphics are used to show lines, forms, reference points, and more, ensuring comprehension of theory.

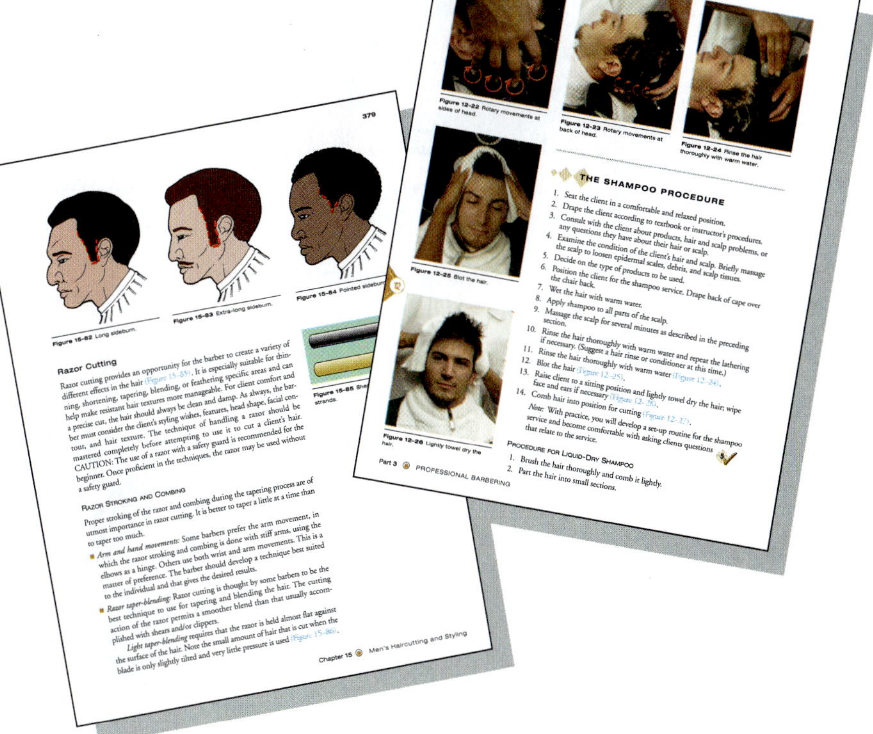

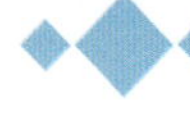

EXTENSIVE LEARNING/TEACHING PACKAGE

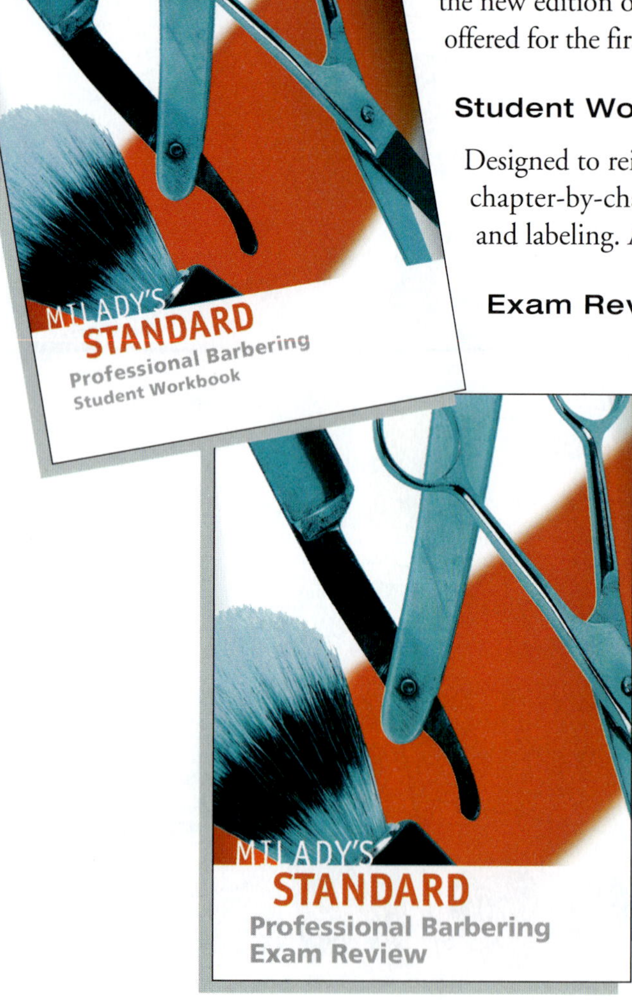

While *Milady's Standard: Professional Barbering* is the center of the curriculum, students and educators have a wide range of supplements from which to choose. All supplements have been revised and updated to complement the new edition of the textbook, and several new supplements are being offered for the first time with this edition.

Student Workbook

Designed to reinforce classroom and textbook learning, and contains chapter-by-chapter exercises including fill-in-the-blank, matching, and labeling. All are coordinated with the material from the text.

Exam Review

The Exam Review contains chapter-by-chapter questions and three sample state board examinations in a multiple-choice format to help students prepare for licensure. The questions are for study purposes only and are not the exact questions students will see on the licensure exam.

Student CD-ROM

The student CD-ROM is an interactive student product designed to reinforce classroom learning, stimulate the imagination, and aid in preparation for board exams. Featuring more than 30 video clips and graphic animations to demonstrate practices and procedures, this tool also contains a text test bank with 1,000 chapter-by-chapter or randomly accessed multiple-choice questions to help students study for the exam. There is also a game bank and a pronouncing glossary that pronounces and defines each term.

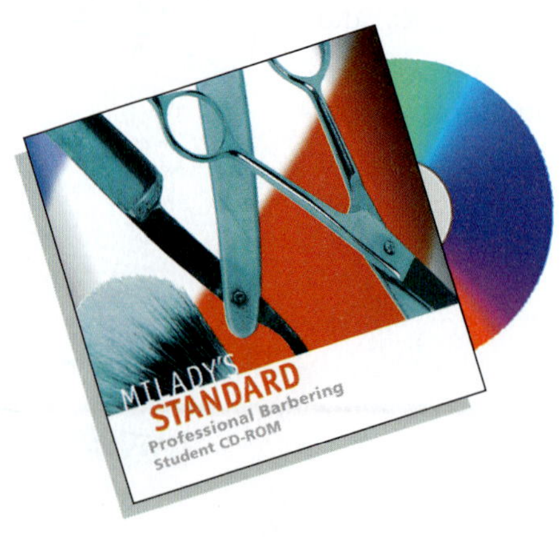

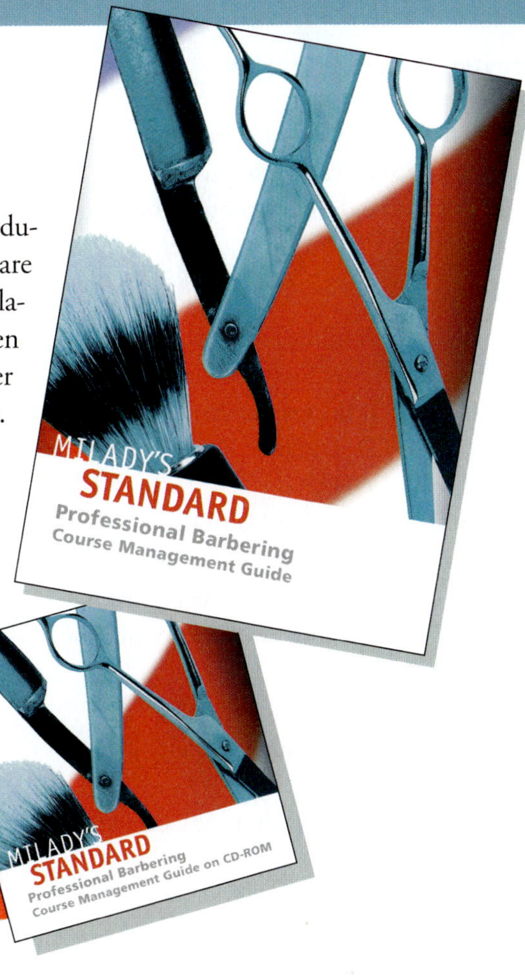

Instructor's Course Management Guide

The Course Management Guide contains all the materials educators need in one package. Included in this bound book are Lesson Plans, Chapter Tests, Transparency Masters, a Correlation Guide to help instructors find material that has been moved in the new edition of the textbook, and the answer keys to the Student Workbook and end-of-chapter exercises.

Instructor's Course Management Guide on CD-ROM

Everything found in the print version of the Course Management guide is contained on this easy-to-use CD-ROM. The print material is formatted in easy-to-print .PDF format so only select material need be printed and used at any given time. It also includes a computerized test bank containing multiple-choice questions that instructors can use to create random tests from a single chapter or the entire book. Answer keys are automatically created.

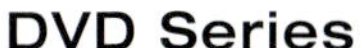

DVD Series

For the first time, Milady is offering a two-hour DVD series complete with all-new video content. The DVD set offers interactive content with features for classroom use that provide instructors with easy-search features and optional Spanish subtitles.

PowerPoint® Presentation

The new Instructor Support Slides use a PowerPoint® presentation making lesson planning simple yet incredibly effective. Complete with photos and art, this chapter-by-chapter CD-ROM has ready-to-use presentations that will help engage students' attention and keep their interest throughout. Instructors can use it as it is or adapt it to their own classrooms.

ACKNOWLEDGMENTS

The author and publisher wish to thank the professionals who took their valuable time to provide their insight and suggestions in the development of this book. We are indebted to them.

Reviewers:

Deborah Beatty, Columbus Technical College
Mary Bryant, New Tyler Barber College, Inc.
Forrest F. Green Jr., Michigan Barber School Inc.
Ray Grypp, Quad City Barber & Hairstyling College
Mary Lee Krantz, OSHA
Bennie Liburdi, Latham East Hair Design
O. D. Madison, Jr., Texas Barber College
Jonathan J. Manigo, USP Atlanta Penitentiary
La Nora Mattern, Xenon International School of Hair Design
Michael Mazza, Mike's Hairport
Phillip S. Mazza, Prince George's County Department of Corrections
Lonnie Morse, European Institute of Cosmetology, Oregon
Tena Northern, Academy of Hair Design
Sandra Peoples, T. H. Picken's Technical Center
Wendell Petersen, Tangle's Hairstyling
Jon Rogers, Santa Monica Community College
Sue Sansom, Arizona State N.I.C.
Zane Skerry, Massachusetts Barber Board

Focus Group Participants:

Emmitt Baker
Andre Cardona
Vedrick Dunbar
Nissey Edwards
Lontaze Maddox
Michael McDonald
Anetta Nadolna
Lavette Ray
Alex Washington
Carl J. Stillo, State Board Barber Examiner
Kenneth E. Kirkpatrick, Capitol Barbers, Minnesota State Barber Board
Charles Kirkpatrick, Arkadelphia Beauty College
Edwin C. Jeffers, Ohio Barber Board
Leroy Cain, Cain's Barber College Inc.
Curtis Park, River City Barbering
Nancy M. West, Casual Male Hair Styling
David Jones, Salon 106, Georgia State Board of Barbers
Ed Barnes, King's Row Hairstyling
Richard M. Brown, Hairworld Barber & Beauty Salon,
Bennie Lee Adkins, Philadelphia, Mississippi
Mike McBunch, The Hair Co
Leslie A. Thorson, Leslie's Barber & Styling
Janice Campbell, Consumer Member on Board
Van A. Heavrin, Disney Barber Shop
Frances L. Simpson, Hair Tech
Orin F. Burdette, Rehoboth Barber Shop, Inc.
Lee Roy Tucker, Tucker's Style Shop
Daniel Bryant, New Tyler Barber College Inc.
Donald Kay Baker, Chairman for the N.C.S.B.B.E., V.P. for N.A.B.B.A.
Vera Winfield, District of Columbia, Barker & Cosmetology Board
David H. Reed, Reed's Headquarters
Parsy L. Reed, Reed's Headquarters
Allan Nelson, The Barber Hut
Patrick Peralta, Nevada State Board of Cosmetology
Margie C. Sanchez, State of New Mexico Barber & Cosmetology Board
Claudia Montano, State of New Mexico
Donald S. Poulin,
Lee Cameroni, Pennsylvania State Barber Board
Shari D. Campbell, Kristi-Kuts
Sonoko Humphrey, Hair We Go Beauty Salon
James Spruill, Cutler Capers Beauty Supply
Theresa Iliff, MSP International Airport
Eva Sue Barne, Kings Row
Ray Schock, Mug & Brush Barber Shop
Larry M. Little, AR College of Barbering & Hair Design Inc.
Jerrel Dailey, Unique Barber Hairstyling
Charles Graf, Ohio State Barber Board
Nathaniel LaShore, Mr. N. Las Vegas Barber Shop
Helga LaShore, Mr. N. Las Vegas Barber Shop
Rocky McElvany, Oklahoma State Health Department
John E. Black, Belcaro Barber-Stylist
Larry W. Absten, West Virginia Board of Cosmetology & Barbering
William "Kirk" Kuykendall, Texas State Board of Barber Examiners

Special thanks to the following contributors for their support and assistance:

Ben Liburdi, Master Barber, Latham, New York, for use of his collection of antique and collectible barbering memorabilia.

Monica Cook, director, and staff and students of Jordan Lynn School for Appearance Enhancement, Schenectady, New York, for their help with mannequin preparation and model recommendations.

Peg Breen, Patti Golub, and staff and students of Capital Region Career and Technical School, Albany, New York, for use of their excellent facility for the photo shoot. Also to their barbering instructor and students for graciously participating as models and/or barbers for the photo shoot.

Vincenzo Federico, Master Barber, Vinny's Barber Shop, Colonie, New York, for stepping in at the last minute to assist with the photos.

Cory Cole, Master Barber, The Cole Group, Albany, New York, for assisting with the photo shoot.

Gregory Zorian, Jr., Master Barber, Gregory's Barbershop, Clifton Park, New York, for allowing us the use of his beautiful new location for photographs, as well as acting as a general subject-matter expert throughout the project.

Gregory Zorian III, Master Barber, Gregory's Barbershop for participating in the photo shoot.

Andis, Marvy Company, Wahl, and 44/20 for use of product photographs.

The Worshipful Company of Barbers, London, England, for use of image of the Holbein painting, King Henry VIII issuing charter to the Barber-Surgeon's company.

Guest Barbers

The author and editors would like to thank the following for their assistance:

Cory Cole, Master Barber
Vinny Federico, Master Barber
Laura Downs, Barber
Greg Zorian, Jr., Master Barber
Greg Zorian III, Master Barber
Helen Wos, Instructor/Barber
Lorilee Bird, Student Barber
Mark Blue, Student Barber
Christopher Morris, Student Barber
Kristen Santa Lucia, Student Barber

Models

Kevin Rivenburg
Jack Pendleton
Betty Dickson
Nick Laboda
Vishnu Persaud
Connor Gillivan
Ronald Vincent
Zachary James
Wayne Scace
Gerald O'Malley

PHOTOGRAPHY CREDITS

Chapter 1: chapter opener, Getty Images.

Chapter 2: chapter opener, Getty Images; Figures 2-2 and 2-5, Corbis; Figure 2-4 courtesy of the Worshipful Company of Barbers, London, UK; Figure 2-7 courtesy of William Marvy Company.

Chapter 3: Figure 3-10, Getty Images.

Chapter 4: chapter opener, Getty Images; Figure 4-6 courtesy of Robert A. Silverman, MD, Clinical Associate Professor, Department of Pediatrics, Georgetown University.

Chapter 5: Figures 5-1, 5-2, and 5-3 courtesy of William Marvy Company.

Chapter 6: chapter opener courtesy of William Marvy Company; Figures 6-20, 6-21, 6-22, 6-23, 6-24, 6-25, 6-26, 6-27 and 6-28, courtesy of the Andis Company; Figure 6-50 courtesy of Morris Flamingo, Inc./Campbell Lather King.

Chapter 7: chapter opener, Getty Images.

Chapter 8: chapter opener, Getty Images.

Chapter 9: chapter opener, Getty Images.

Chapter 10: chapter opener, Getty Images; Figures 10-6, 10-7, 10-10, 10-11, 10-13, 10-15, 10-16, 10-17, 10-18, 10-19, 10-20, 10-21, 10-23, 10-24, 10-25, reprinted with permission from the American Academy of Dermatology. All rights reserved. Figure 10-8 courtesy of Timothy Berger, MD, Associate Clinical Professor, University of California San Francisco. Figure 10-14, courtesy of the Centers for Disease Control and Prevention (CDC). Figures 10-12, 10-22, T. Fitzgerald, Color Atlas and Synopsis of Clinical Dermatology, 3E, 1996. Reprinted with permission of The McGraw-Hill Companies.

Chapter 11: chapter opener, Figures 11-2, 11-5a, 11-5b reprinted with permission of Clairol, Inc.; Figures 11-14, 11-16, and 11-19 courtesy of Robert

A. Silverman, MD, Clinical Associate Professor, Department of Pediatrics, Georgetown University; Figures 11-8, 11-12, and 11-14 courtesy of Pharmacia and Upjohn Company; Figures 11-15a & b photography courtesy of P & G Beauty. Figure 11-18, courtesy of Hogil Pharmaceutical Corporation; Figure 11-21 reprinted with permission from the American Academy of Dermatology. All rights reserved.

Chapter 15: Figure 15-60 and Figure 15-73 provided by Anetta Nadolna.

Chapter 17: Figures 17-2, 17-53, 17-65, 17-71, 17-76, photos used with permission of the authors, Martin Gannon and Richard Thompson, as featured in their book, Mahogany: Steps to Colouring and Finishing Hair. Copyright Martin Gannon and Richard Thompson. 1997. Figure 17-48, hair by Geri Mataya, makeup by Mary Klimek, photo by Jack Cutler. Figure 17-51 courtesy of Gebhart International, hair by Dennis & Syliva Gebhart, makeup by Rose Marie, production by Purely Visual, photo by Winterhalter. Figure 17-49, Getty Images. Figure 17-68, John Paul Mitchell Systems, The Relaxer Workshop, photo by Sean Cokes. Figure 17-70, Mario Tricoci Hair Salons & Day Spas, hair by Tricoci, makeup by Shawn Miselli. Figure 17-73, John Paul Mitchell Systems, hair by People and Schumacher, photo by Andreas Elsner. Figure 17-61, John Paul Mitchell Systems, hair by Jeanne Braa, photo by Albert Tolot.

Chapter 20: Figures 20-4 through 20-22, courtesy of Godfrey Mix, DPM, Sacramento, CA. Figure 20-17 courtesy of Orville J. Stone, MD, Dermatology Medical Group, Huntington Beach, CA.

Chapter 21: chapter opener, Figure 21-1, Getty Images.

Chapter 22: chapter opener, Getty Images.

Chapter 23: chapter opener, Figure 23-1, Getty Images. Figure 23-3 provided by Anetta Nadolna.

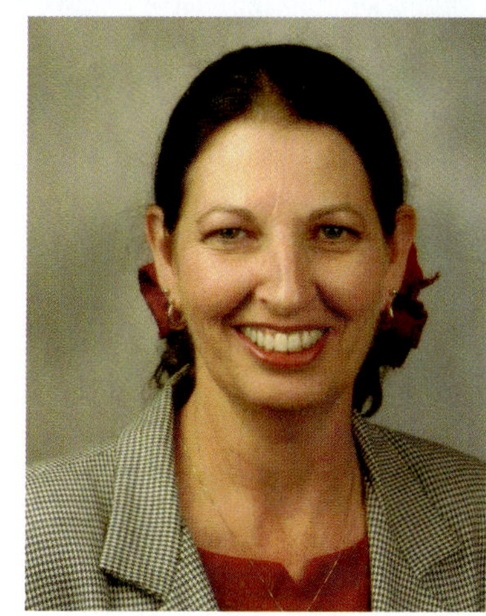

MAURA SCALI-SHEAHAN, Ed.D

Master Barber and Educator

Ms. Scali-Sheahan serves as an instructor for both vocational and teacher education courses at Florida Community College in Jacksonville, Florida. She has served on a variety of college councils and committees as well as the Illinois and Florida State Barber Boards.

Maura has been a presenter for The Career Institute since 2000. She developed a two-day seminar focused on the topic of student retention in schools based on *Milady's 9 Routes to Success* program and is dedicated to training educators in teaching methods and the design of instructional materials design. She is currently revising *Milady's Standard Professional Barbering* and its supplements for Thomson Delmar Learning.

In addition to full-time teaching at FCCJ and freelance writing for the industry, Maura is an adjunct instructor for Southern Illinois University's off-campus military programs. She has a Master's in Education with a specialization in Workforce Education, Training, and Development and a doctorate in Higher Education Leadership.

DEDICATION

A sincere thank you to the Thomson Delmar Learning and the Milady staff for their commitment to the enhanced quality and expansion of this textbook and its accompanying supplements . . .a new standard of excellence for instructional materials dedicated to the barbering profession has surely been achieved! It has been my pleasure, once again, to serve the barbering profession through the development of these materials.

This edition is dedicated to the educators, students, barbers, state board members, and industry professionals who continue to foster the art and science of barbering. May your commitment to our time-honored profession facilitate the achievement of your goals and professional success.

Sincerely,
Maura T. Scali-Sheahan
Jacksonville, Florida

part 1

ORIENTATION TO BARBERING

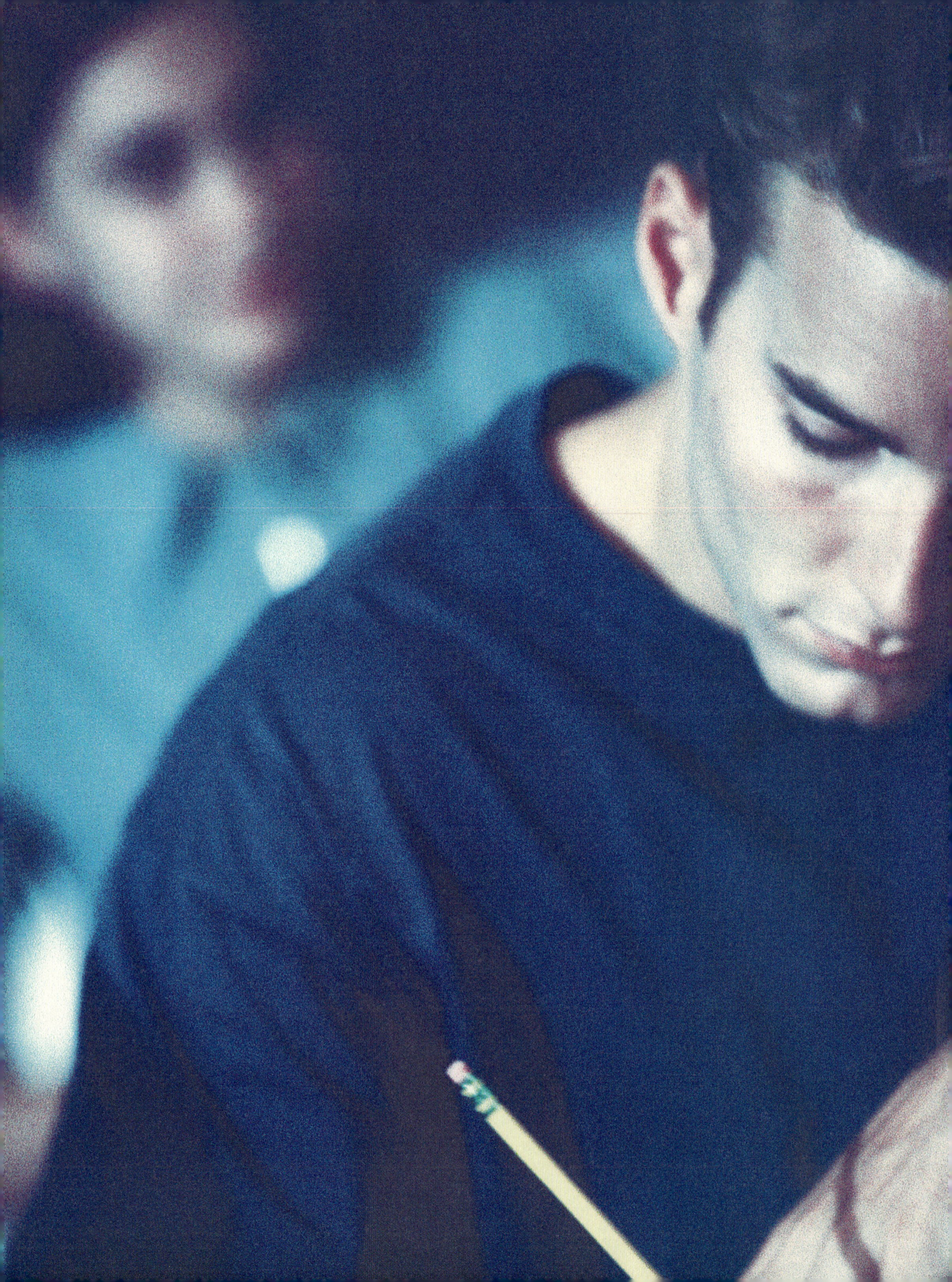

1 STUDY SKILLS

Chapter Outline

Learning Objectives

After completing this chapter, you should be able to:

1. Discuss methods that can be used to enhance short-term and long-term memory of new information.
2. Create a mind-map for a topic of study.
3. Identify your preferred learning style.

Key Terms

learning styles
pg. 7

mind-mapping
pg. 6

mnemonics
pg. 6

organization
pg. 6

repetition
pg. 5

Your orientation to the study of barbering begins with a review of the study skills you may have developed or forgotten over the years since your last school experience. For some of you, the barbering program you have begun may be your first postsecondary educational experience. For others, it might signal the preparation for a second or even third career after military service or years spent in other professions. Still others may be returning to barbering after an extended absence from the industry. Regardless of where you are coming from, you are now part of an exciting field, and effective study skills can help you to achieve your educational and professional goals within it.

One of the most important keys to your success as a student is your ability to learn and master new information. Some individuals learned effective study skills early on and have a relatively smooth time absorbing and understanding new information. Others may not have developed these skills and struggle with new learning situations. In either case, this chapter should help you develop new ways of receiving and processing information for the purpose of optimizing your educational experiences. As you develop your personal study skills, bear in mind that practice and a sense of discipline toward your studies *will help you to apply what is taught.*

STUDY SKILLS

Your personal study skills are highly individualized methods or tools that help you to absorb and retain new information. As such, they should help you to organize, store, and recall information. The following information-processing methods can be used to enhance and optimize the effort you put towards your studies:

- **Repetition:** Repetition improves your short-term memory. Whether you repeat information in your head, say it out loud, or write it down, repetition helps your short-term memory secure a firmer grasp on that information, making it easier to retrieve when needed.

- **Organization:** You can organize new information for both short-term and long-term memory use. To enhance your short-term memory, try categorizing the information into smaller segments. For example: The skin consists of three divisions. They are the epidermis, dermis, and adipose tissue. Contained within these divisions are eight layers of skin structures. Rather than trying to remember all eight layers, use the categories of the skin divisions to break the information down into three sections. Begin with the epidermis. Five of the eight layers start with the word *stratum,* which are found in the epidermis. The epidermis consists of five layers or *strata:* the stratum corneum, stratum lucidum, stratum granulosum, stratum spinosum, and stratum germinativum. Once you have mastered this information, you can move on to learning about the skin structures associated with the dermis and adipose tissue divisions. To promote better long-term memory, try to associate new information with prior knowledge through word association techniques. For example, based on what you now know about the epidermis, we will use word association techniques to remember the names and characteristics of two of the five layers:

Outermost layer: stratum *corn*eum—aka. *horny* layer; continually being shed; corn rhymes with horn.

Second layer: stratum *lucid*um—aka. clear layer; light penetrates through; lucid means clear; lucidum is a form of lucid and/or lucid is the root word of lucidum.

Similar word associations can be developed for the remaining layers of the epidermis as well. Create word associations that mean something to you so that you truly *learn* the material and aren't just memorizing it for the short term.

- **Mnemonics:** Yet another way to trigger your memory is through the use of mnemonics. Mnemonics can be acronyms, songs, rhymes, sentences, or any other device that helps you to recall information.
  - Using the first letters in a series of words creates acronyms. For example, try remembering the functions of the skin—sensation, heat regulation, absorption, protection, excretion, and secretion—through the word SHAPES. This is a particularly good acronym because skin also gives *shape* to the body.
  - Songs or rhymes don't have to be complicated. Something as simple as "keep the *air* and the *hair* moving when blow-drying" to prevent burning the client's scalp or "rock 'n' roll rodding creates a spiral perm" to illustrate a permanent-waving rodding technique can be effective reminders during application procedures. 1
- **Mind-mapping:** Mind-mapping is a fun and creative way to take notes or solve a problem. Write the main topic or problem in the center of a piece of paper. Jot down key words or ideas that come to mind and connect them to the main topic. Then, using the key words or ideas, create subconnections to other thoughts or information. Use color or symbols to highlight important information. See Figure 1–1. 2

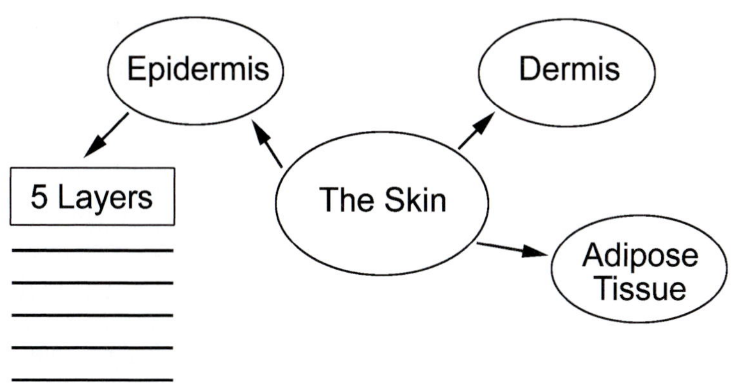

Figure 1–1 Mind-mapping.

LEARNING STYLES

One way to hone your study skills is to recognize that we all have different **learning styles** and that it helps to know what kind of learner you are. Knowing your particular learning style often makes it easier to organize new information because the methods used for retrieval and application are relevant and meaningful to you personally.

Learning styles are classifications that are used to identify the different ways in which people learn. Learning takes place through our individual *perceptions* of reality and the way in which we *process* information and experiences. Some individuals *feel* their way through new information or situations, while others *think* their way through. Therefore, perceptions of reality tend to be either more emotionally centered or more analytically based. When processing new information or experiences, some people watch and absorb while others act and do. When the two different ways of perceiving are combined with the two different ways of processing, four distinct learning styles emerge. Review the following learning style descriptions to determine the learning style that you think, or feel, is most applicable to you.

1. *Interactive learners.* Interactive learners (also known as imaginative or innovative learners) learn best by watching, listening, and sharing ideas. These are idea people who function best through social interaction and the opportunity to ask "why?" or "why not?" They tend to appreciate a learning environment that is interactive, supportive, sympathetic, and friendly. Interactive learners like to engage in classroom discussions and study well with a group of people.
2. *Reader/listener learners.* These individuals (also called analytic learners) are interested in facts and details. They learn best by thinking through the ideas or concepts that they have read or heard. Since the analytic learner's favorite question is "what?" they tend to work well in structured environments with instructors who answer their questions freely and keep them focused on the subject matter.
3. *Systematic learners.* The systematic learner (also known as commonsense learners) benefits more from new information when they can

connect it to real-life situations. They need to know how things work, enjoy practical applications, and tend to concentrate better when studying alone. The systematic learner's favorite question is "how?" and they favor a learning environment that challenges them to "check things out."

4. *Intuitive learners.* Intuitive learners (also called dynamic learners) like to learn through trial and error and self-discovery. They are open to possibilities, new ways of doing things, and tend to ask "what if?" Intuitive learners want to try out what they read about and actually experience what they study. Since they like variety, intuitive learners usually respond best to learning environments that facilitate the stimulation of ideas and the exploration of different ways to achieve the desired outcome.

Once you recognize your particular learning style, think about the ways in which those characteristics might be applied to your study habits to maximize your effectiveness as a student. Here are a few tips for classroom note-taking that have been designed around the four learning styles.

1. *Interactive learners:* Apply personal meaning to the topic. For example, ask yourself "why?" Why is the topic important and how does it relate to you and your future? Picture yourself in that future.
2. *Reader/listener learners:* List key words and facts. Analyze the concepts during study time for greater clarity and understanding as to *why* the facts are what they are. This understanding will help you to move more easily from Point A to Point B during practical applications.
3. *Systematic learners:* List key information—especially procedures—in an orderly fashion. You won't want to miss a step! Make notations along the margins that remind you to experiment with concepts that can be transitioned into practical applications.
4. *Intuitive learners:* Be open to accepting what is already known since doing so can eliminate some of the frustration associated with learning exclusively through the trial-and-error method. Pay attention to key concepts and list procedural steps when note-taking. When an idea comes to mind, note it in the margins for later exploration; if a topic triggers interest in another area, mark it for some independent study or experimentation. 3

DEVELOPING EFFECTIVE STUDY HABITS

An important part of developing effective study habits is knowing when, where, and how to study. Here are some pointers to keep in mind.

When

- Estimate how many hours of study you need.
- Plan your study time around the times of day when you are most energetic and motivated.
- Use "down" times, like riding on the bus, to study.

Where

- Select a quiet location where you will not be disturbed or interrupted.
- Study sitting in a chair or standing instead of lying down.
- Maintain a routine by studying in the same place whenever possible.

How

- Stay focused on your reason for studying by keeping your goals in mind.
- Resist distractions during study time.
- Be persistent, disciplined, and determined.
- Think about tackling the tougher chapters or topics first.
- Pace yourself with breaks, healthy snacks, and physical movement.

The development of good study habits is a skill that can be used beyond your barbering training and the classroom environment. It is a transferable skill that will be utilized throughout your lifetime as you grow to achieve your full personal and professional potential. For example, consider the ways in which effective study habits might help you begin the research needed to open a barbershop or to participate at a state board meeting. Each new life experience, information set, or professional challenge involves learning that will require study in some form. Effective study skills will help you to create your own "good luck" in your present and future endeavors.

chapter glossary

learning styles	classifications that are used to identify the different ways in which people learn
mind-mapping	a graphic representation of an idea or problem that helps to organize one's thoughts
mnemonics	any memorization device that helps a person to recall information
organization	a method used to store new information for short-term and long-term memory
repetition	repeatedly saying, writing, or otherwise reviewing new information until it is learned

chapter review questions

1. Identify the ability that is one of the most important keys to your success as a student.
2. Identify an organization method that can be used to enhance short-term memory.
3. Identify an organization method that can be used to enhance long-term memory.
4. Create a mind-map for this chapter.
5. Identify your preferred learning style.
6. Design a form or template for note-taking based on your preferred learning style.

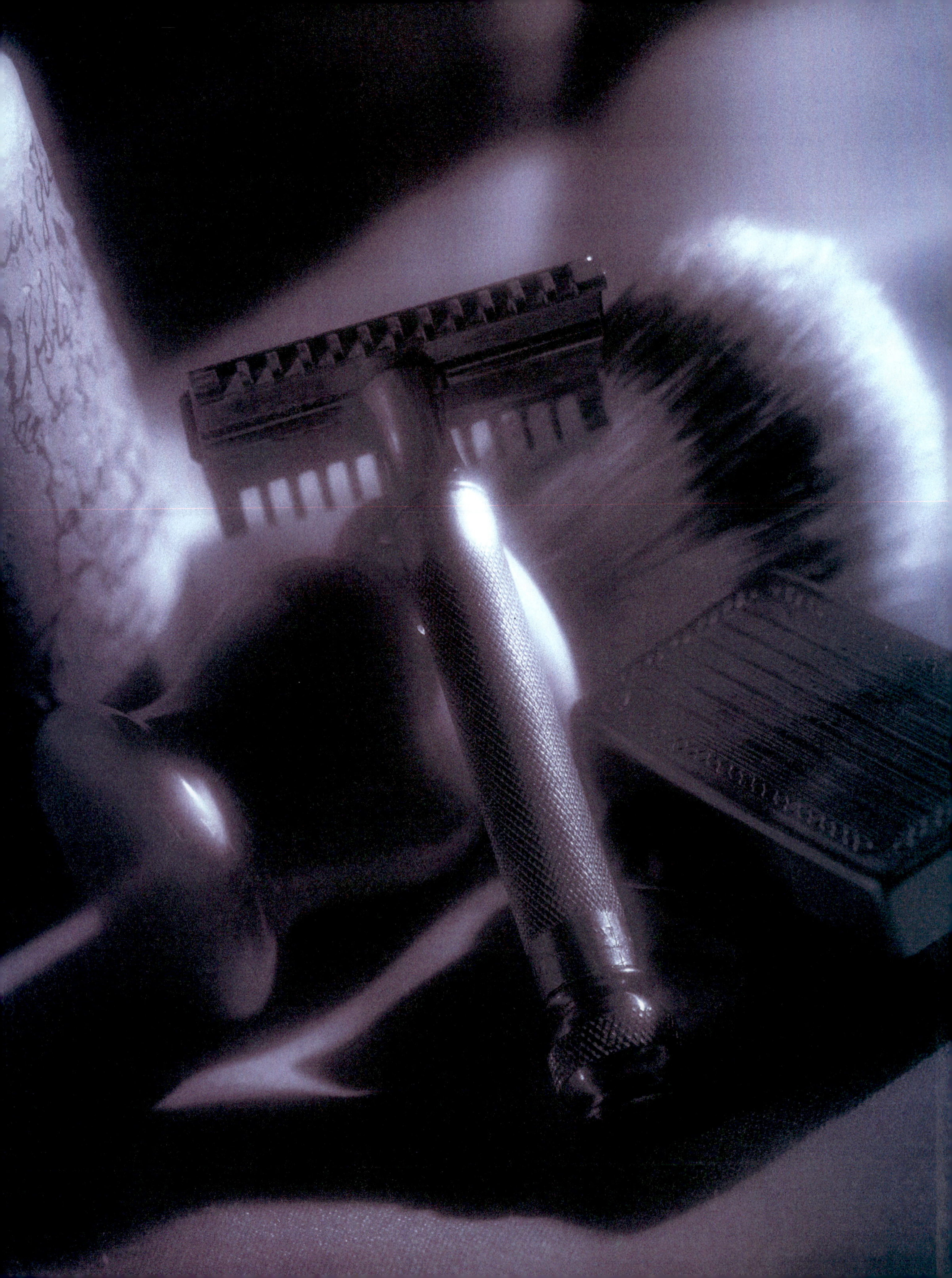

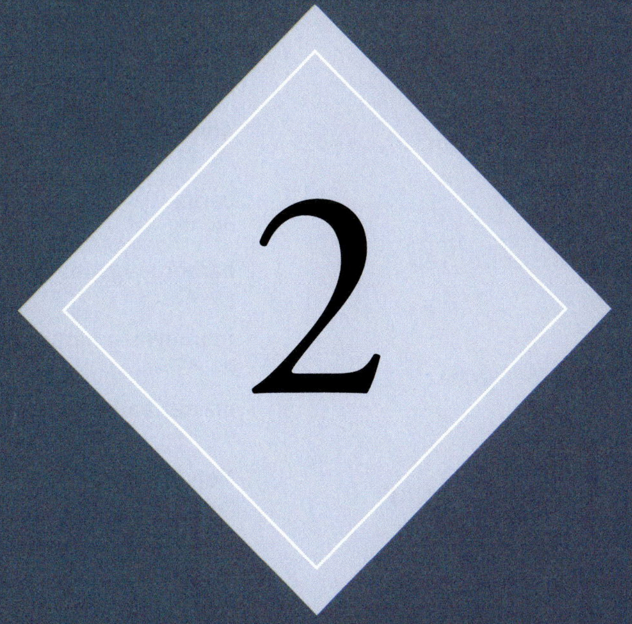

THE HISTORY OF BARBERING

Chapter Outline

Origin of the Barber • The Rise of the Barber-Surgeons
Modern Barbers and Barbering

Learning Objectives

After completing this chapter, you should be able to:

1. Define the origin of the word *barber.*
2. Demonstrate an understanding of the evolution of barbering.
3. Describe the barber-surgeons and their practices.
4. Explain the origin of the barber pole.
5. Identify and discuss organizations responsible for upgrading the barbering profession.
6. Explain the importance and function of state barber boards.

Key Terms

A.B. Moler
pg. 22

AMBBA
pg. 22

Ambroise Pare
pg. 21

barba
pg. 15

barber-surgeons
pg. 20

journeymen barber groups
pg. 22

master barber groups
pg. 22

Meryma'at
pg. 16

National Association of Barber Boards of America
pg. 22

Ticinius Mena
pg. 17

tonsorial
pg. 15

tonsure
pg. 17

Barbering is one of the oldest professions in the world. With the advance of civilization, barbering and hairstyling developed from early cultural and tribal beginnings into a recognized profession.

The study of this progression leads to an appreciation of the accomplishments, evolution, and position of high esteem attained by early practitioners. The cultural, esthetic, and technical heritage they developed provides the basis for the prestige and respect accorded the profession and its services today.

ORIGIN OF THE BARBER

The word *barber* is derived from the Latin word **barba**, meaning *beard* (Figure 2–1). Another Latin word, **tonsorial** means the cutting, clipping, or trimming of hair with shears or a razor; it is often used in conjunction with barbering. Hence, barbers are sometimes referred to as tonsorial artists.

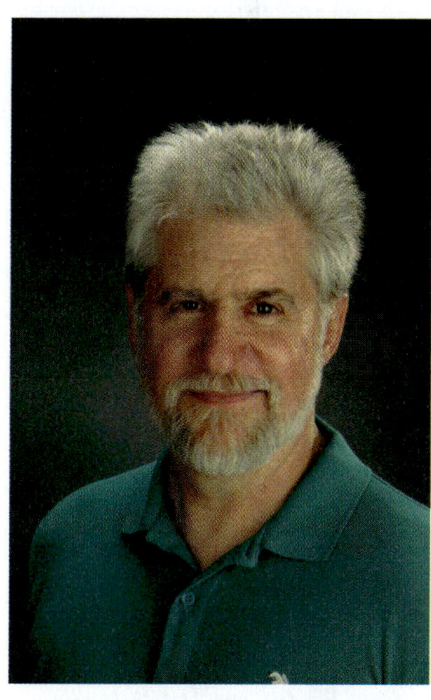

Figure 2-1 The Latin word *barba*, for "beard," gives us our modern English word *beard*.

Archaeological studies reveal that haircutting and hairstyling were practiced in some form as early as the glacial age. The simple but effective implements used then were shaped from sharpened flints, oyster shells, or bone. Animal sinew or strips of hide were used to tie the hair back or as adornment, and braiding techniques were employed in some cultures.

Although primitive man may have been naïve about the science of his world, he was cognizant of the fact that a connection exists between the body, mind, and spirit. This understanding translated into superstitions and beliefs that merged religious ritual, spirituality, and medical practices together into an integrated relationship. For example, some tribes believed that both good and bad spirits entered the individual through the hairs on the head and that the only way to exorcise bad spirits was to cut the hair.

Similar belief systems were found in many regions and tribal barbers were elevated to positions of importance to become medicine men, shamans, or priests. In one religious ceremony long hair was worn loose to allow the evil spirits to exit the individual. Then, after ritual dancing, the barber cut the hair, combed it back tightly against the scalp, and tied it off to keep the good spirits in and the evil spirits out.

Given the archaeological evidence found in painted pottery, early sculptures, and burial mounds, it can be presumed that early cultures practiced some form of beautification and adornment, whether from practical need or religious conviction. From a historical perspective, the division between what archaeological evidence leads us to *believe,* and what can be claimed as absolute *fact,* occurs with the rise of the Egyptians.

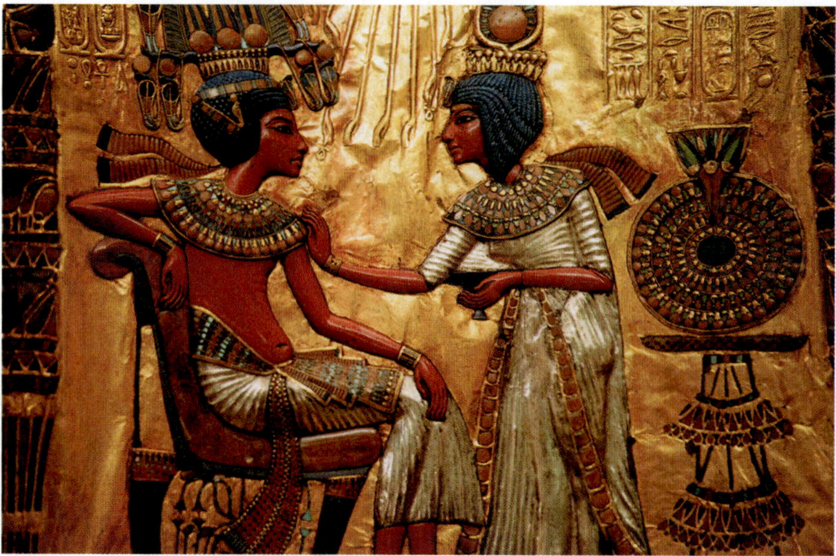

Figure 2–2 The Egyptians wore elaborate hairdos and makeup.

The Egyptian culture is credited with being the first to cultivate beauty in an extravagant fashion. Excavations from tombs have revealed such relics as combs, brushes, mirrors, cosmetics, and razors made of tempered copper and bronze. Coloring agents made from berries, bark, minerals, and other natural materials were used on the hair, skin, and nails. Eye paint was the most popular of all cosmetics and the use of henna as a coloring agent was first recorded in 1500 BC (Figure 2–2).

The use of barbers by Egyptian noblemen and priests 6,000 years ago is substantiated within Egypt's written records, art, and sculpture. The barber **Meryma'at** is one historical figure whose work was apparently held in such high esteem that his image was sculpted for posterity. Every third day, Meryma'at would shave the priests' entire bodies to ensure their purity before entering the temple. High-ranking men and women of Egypt had their heads shaved for comfort when wearing wigs and for the prevention of parasitic infestations.

In Africa, hair was groomed with intricately carved combs and ornamented with beads, clay, and colored bands (Figure 2–3). The Masai warriors wove their front hair into three sections of tiny braids and the rest of the hair into a queue down the back. Braiding was used extensively, with the intricate patterns frequently denoting status within the tribe.

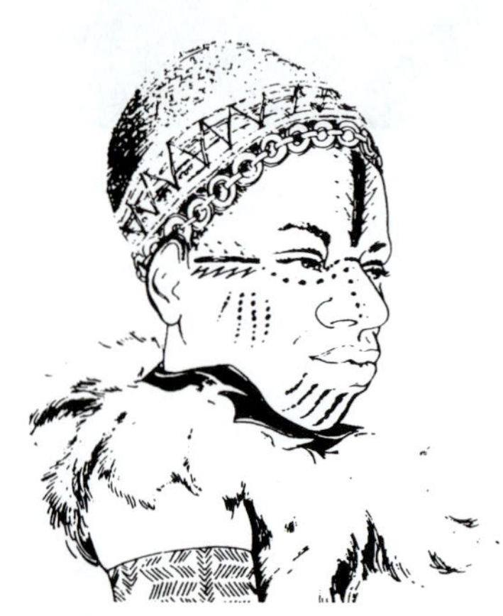

Figure 2–3 Africans groomed their hair with intricately carved combs and ornamental beads, clay, and colored bands.

According to biblical legend, Moses lived during the late thirteenth and early twelfth centuries BC. During Moses' lifetime, barbering services became available to the general population.

Later, during the Golden Age of Greece (500 BC), barbering and hairstyling became highly developed arts. More specifically, well-trimmed beards became status symbols and Greek men had them trimmed, curled, and scented on a regular basis. Due to the demand for their services, barbers rose in business prominence and barbershops evolved into local meeting places for social, political, and sporting conversation.

In the third century BC, Alexander the Great lost several battles to the Persians as a result of his warriors' beards. The Persians would grab the Macedonian warriors by their beards, dragging them to the ground where they were then speared. Alexander issued a decree that all soldiers were to be clean-shaven from that point on. Eventually, the general populace adopted the trend and, although beards lost favor, barbers were kept busy with performing shaves and haircuts.

Ticinius Mena of Sicily is credited with having brought shaving and barbering services to Rome in 296 BC. Men of Rome enjoyed tonsorial services such as shaves, haircutting and dressing, massage, and manicuring on a daily basis with a good portion of their day spent at the barber's. While the average citizen patronized the barbers' places of business, rich noblemen engaged private *tonsors* to take care of their hairdressing and shaving needs. The Romans expanded the concept of these personal services to include communal bathing and what became widely known as the Roman baths.

Clean-shaven faces were the trend until Hadrian came into power in 117 AD. Emperor Hadrian became a trendsetter as had others before him. In an attempt to hide some scars on his chin, he allowed his beard to grow. This resulted in the populace following his lead and the beard was again in fashion. 1

Customs and Traditions

In almost every early culture hairstyles indicated social status. Noblemen of ancient Gaul indicated their rank by wearing their hair long; this continued until Caesar made them cut it when he conquered them, as a sign of submission. In ancient Greece, boys would cut their hair upon reaching adolescence, while their Hindu counterparts would shave their heads. Following the invasion of China by the Manchu, Chinese men adopted the queue as a mark of dignity and manhood.

The ancient Britons were extremely proud of their long hair. Blond hair was brightened with washes composed of tallow, lime, and the extracts of certain vegetables. Darker hair was treated with dyes extracted and processed from plants, trees, and various soils. The Danes, Angles, and Normans dressed their hair for beautification, adornment, and ornamentation during battle with the Britons.

In ancient Rome, the color of a woman's hair indicated her class or rank. Noblewomen tinted their hair red; those of the middle class colored their hair blond; and poor women were compelled to dye their hair black. At various times in Roman history, slaves would be allowed to wear beards or not, depending on the dictates of the ruler.

In later centuries, religion, occupation, and politics also influenced the length and style of hair and the wearing of beards. Clergymen of the Middle Ages were distinguished by the **tonsure** (derived from the Latin *tondere*, "to shear"), a shaved patch on the crown of the head. During the seventh century, Celtic and Roman church leaders disagreed on the exact shape the tonsure should take. The circular tonsure, called the tonsure of St. Peter, left only a slight fringe of hair around the head and was preferred in Germany, Italy, and Spain. The Picts and Scots preferred a semicircular design, known as the tonsure of St. John. After much argument, the Pope eventually decreed that priests were to shave their beards and mustaches and adopt the tonsure of St. Peter.

Although the edicts of the church maintained some influence over priests and the general populace for several centuries, the wearing of beards and longer hairstyles had returned by the eleventh century. Priests curled or braided their hair and beards until Pope Gregory issued another decree requiring shaved faces and short hair. In 1972, the Roman Catholic Church finally abolished the practice of tonsure.

By the seventeenth century in England, political affiliation and religion could be indicated by the long, curling locks of the Royalist Anglican Cavaliers and the cropped hair of the Parliamentarian Puritan Roundheads. British barristers wore gray wigs while the various branches of the law and military wore specific styles according to their military corps.

Most rulers and monarchs become trendsetters by virtue of their position and power in society. Personal whim, taste, and even physical limitations could become the basis for changes in hairstyles and fashion. For example, when Francis I of France (in the sixteenth century) accidentally burned his hair with a torch, his loyal subjects had their hair, beards, and mustaches cut short.

During the reign of Louis XIV in the seventeenth century, noblemen wore wigs because the king, who was balding, did so. During the nineteenth century in France, men and women showed appreciation for antiquity by wearing variations of the "Caesar Cut," the style of the early Roman emperors.

The beliefs, rituals, and superstitions of early civilizations varied from one ethnic group to another, depending on the region and social interaction with other groups. There was a general belief among many groups that hair clippings could bewitch an individual. Hence, the privilege of haircutting was reserved for the priest, medicine man, or other spiritual leader of the tribe. According to the Greek philosopher and mathematician Pythagoras, the hair was the source of the brain's inspiration and cutting it decreased an individual's intellectual capacity. The Irish peasantry believed that if hair cuttings were burned or buried with the dead, no evil spirits would haunt the individual. Among some Native-American tribes it was believed that the hair and the body were so linked that anyone possessing a lock of hair of another might work his will on that individual.

The Beard and Shaving

The importance of the beard lies more in the past than the present. Nonetheless, it is interesting to note the various fashions and customs associated with it. Since the practice of shaving predates the written word, it is difficult to determine just when this form of hair removal began.

The excavation of early stone razors or scrapers from the Paleolithic period (40,000–10,000 BC) indicates that early man may have used these tools for hair removal as well as for the skinning of animals. By the time of the Neolithic period (8000–5000 BC) early man had created settlements and begun to farm and raise animals. Artwork of this period shows examples of clean-shaven men. The Egyptian pyramids of 7000 BC have yielded flint-bladed razors that were used by the ruling classes to shave their heads as well as their faces and by 4000 BC a form of tweezers was also used.

It stands to reason that the nomadic nature of many early groups would help to spread the practice of shaving throughout the rest of the continent. Mesopotamians of 3000 BC were shaving with obsidian blades and by 2800 BC the Sumerians were also clean-shaven. As evidenced by artwork of the period, we know that by 1000 BC Greek men were visiting the local barber for shaving services. Such shops became the gathering places where news was shared and camaraderie was found, not unlike some of the more traditional shops found today.

In early times, most groups considered the beard to be a sign of wisdom, strength, and manhood. In some cultures, it was thought of as almost sacred. Among Orthodox Jews, the beard was a symbol of religious devotion and to cut off one's beard was contrary to Mosaic law. In Rome, a young man's first shave on his twenty-second birthday constituted a rite of passage from boyhood to manhood and was celebrated with great festivity.

Certain rulers required that beards be removed. As previously mentioned, Alexander the Great ordered his soldiers to shave so their beards could not be seized in battle. Peter the Great encouraged shaving by imposing a tax on beards.

During the spread of Christianity, long hair came to be considered sinful and the clergy were directed to shave their beards. Although the shaving of the beard was forbidden among Orthodox Jews, the use of scissors to remove excess growth was permitted. The Muslims took great care in trimming their beards after prayer. The hair that was removed was saved and preserved so that it could be buried with its owner.

During the Middle Ages (476 to 1400 AD), three hairs from the king's beard were imbedded in the wax of the royal seal on a charter written in 1121. During the reign of Queen Elizabeth in England, it became fashionable to dye the beard and cut it into a variety of shapes. 2✓

THE RISE OF THE BARBER-SURGEONS

During the Middle Ages barbers not only practiced shaving, haircutting, and hairstyling but also entered the world of medicine where they figured prominently in the development of surgery as a recognized branch of medical practice. As the most learned and educated people of the Middle Ages (400–1500 AD), monks and priests became the physicians of the period. One of the most common treatments for curing a variety of illnesses was the practice of bloodletting and barbers were often enlisted to assist the clergy in this practice. In 1163, Pope Alexander III forbade the clergy to "draw blood or to act as physicians and surgeons" because it was contrary to Christian doctrine "for ministers of God to draw blood from the human body" (Moler, 1927). It was at this juncture in history that the barbers took over the duties previously performed by the clergy. They continued the practices of bloodletting, minor surgery, herbal remedies, and tooth pulling. For centuries, dentistry was performed only by barbers and for more than a thousand years they were known as **barber-surgeons**.

The barber-surgeons formed their first organization in France in 1096 AD. Soon after, the first school of surgery was established in Paris. During the 1100s, a guild of surgeons was organized from the barber-surgeon group that specialized in the study of medicine. To protect themselves, the Barbers' Company of London was formed during the thirteenth century with the objective of regulating the profession. The Barbers' Company was ruled by a master and consisted of two classes of barbers: those who practiced barbering and those who specialized in surgery.

Aside from the Barbers' Company, there was also a surgeon's guild in England. Although there is reason to believe that competition and antagonism existed between the two organizations, a parliamentary act united the two groups in 1450, but separated the practices of each profession. Barbers were limited to the practices of bloodletting, tooth-pulling, and the tonsorial services, and surgeons were forbidden to act as barbers.

In 1541, Henry VIII reunited the barbers and surgeons of London by granting a charter to the Company of Barber Surgeons. The Company commissioned Hans Holbein, a noted artist of the time, to commemorate the event (Figure 2–4).

2

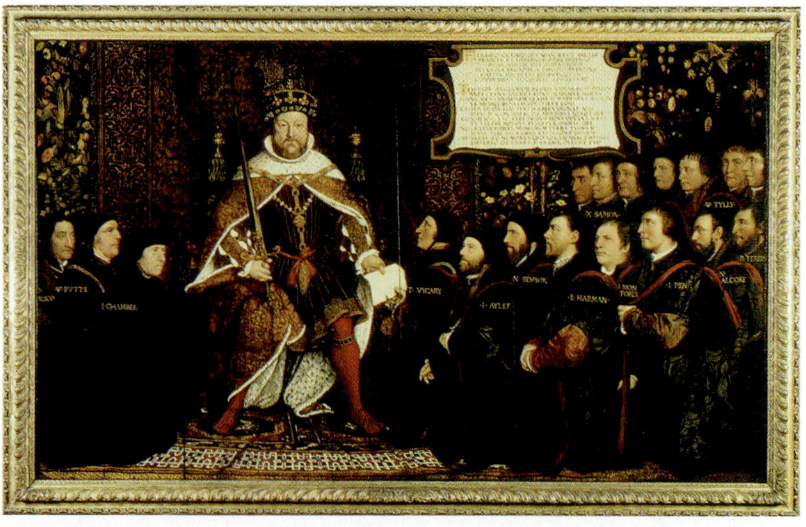

Figure 2–4 Hans Holbein painting. Henry VIII issuing a charter to the Company of Barber Surgeons.

With the advancement of medicine, the practice of bloodletting became all but obsolete. Although the barber-surgeons' medical practice dwindled in importance, they were still relied upon for dispensing medicinal herbs and pulling teeth. Finally, in 1745, a law was passed in England to separate the barbers from the surgeons and the alliance was completely dissolved.

Barber-surgeons had also flourished in France and Germany. The first barber-surgeons' corporation was formed in France in 1094. French barber-surgeons who were under the rule of the king's barber formed a guild in 1371 that lasted until about the time of the French Revolution. It is interesting to note that **Ambroise Pare**, who began his work as a barber-surgeon, is considered the greatest surgeon of the Renaissance and the father of modern surgery.

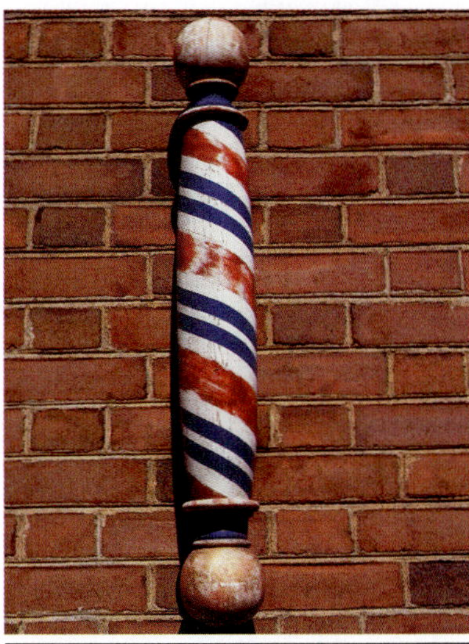

Figure 2-5 An example of the barber pole.

During the nineteenth century, wigs became so elaborate and fashionable that a separate corporation of barber-wigmakers was founded in France. Not until 1779 was a corporation formed in Prussia; this was disbanded in 1809 when new unions were started.

Many Europeans had become so dependent upon the services of the barber-surgeons that Dutch and Swedish settlers brought barber-surgeons with them to America to look after the well-being of the colonists.

The Barber Pole

The symbol of the barber-surgeon evolved from the technical procedure of bloodletting. The pole is thought to represent the staff that the patient would hold tightly in order for the veins in the arm to stand out during bloodletting. The bottom end-cap of modern barber poles represents the basin used as a vessel to either catch the blood (during bloodletting) or lather the face for shaving. The white bandages used to stop the bleeding were hung on the staff to dry. The stained bandages would then twist around the pole in the breeze, forming a red-and-white pattern. One interpretation of the colors of the barber pole is that red represented the blood, blue the veins, and white the bandages. Another interpretation explains that when the Barber Surgeon's Company in England was formed, barbers were required to use blue-and-white poles and the surgeons used the red-and-white ones. It is also thought that that the red, white, and blue poles displayed in the United States originated in deference to the nation's flag. Modern barbers have retained the barber pole as the foremost symbol of the business and profession of barbering (Figure 2–5).

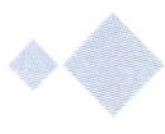

MODERN BARBERS AND BARBERING

By the nineteenth century, barbering was completely separated from religion and medicine and began to emerge as an independent profession. During the late 1800s, the profession's structure changed and it began to follow new directions. The formation of employer organizations known as **master barber groups**, and employee organizations known as **journeymen barber groups**, were the first steps toward upgrading and regulating the profession. During this era, the emergence and growth of these organizations helped to establish precedents and standards that have become part of the history of barbering.

The Journeymen Barbers' Union was formed at its first convention in Buffalo, New York, in 1887 and was affiliated with the American Federation of Labor. In 1893, **A. B. Moler** established America's first barber school in Chicago, Illinois. In the same year, he published the first barbering textbook, *The Moler Manual of Barbering*.

Minnesota was the first state to pass a barber-licensing law. This legislation, passed in 1897, set standards for sanitation, and the minimum education and technical requirements for barbers in that state.

In 1924, the Associated Master Barbers of America was organized in Chicago, Illinois. The name was changed in 1941 to the Associated Master Barbers and Beauticians of America (**AMBBA**). This association represented shop and salon owners and managers.

By 1925, the Associated Master Barbers and Beauticians of America established the National Educational Council, with the goal of standardizing and upgrading barber training. The council was successful in the standardizing of barber schools and barber instructor training, the establishment of a curriculum, and the promulgation of legislation necessary for the passage of state licensing laws.

The National Association of Barber Schools was formed in 1927. In cooperation with the Associated Master Barbers and Beauticians of America, it worked to develop a program standardizing the operation of barber schools.

By 1929, the National Association of State Board of Barber Examiners was organized in St. Paul, Minnesota. Its purpose was to standardize the qualifications required for barber examination applicants and the methods of evaluation to be used. The Associated Master Barbers and Beauticians of America also adopted a Barber Code of Ethics, to promote professionalism and responsibility in the trade (Figure 2–6). 5

Since 1929, all states, with the exception of several counties in Alabama, have passed laws regulating the practice of barbering and hairstyling. The state boards are primarily concerned with the maintenance of high educational standards in order to assure competent and skilled service. Today's state barber boards meet up to twice a year as members of the **National Association of Barber Boards of America**, whose mission, as printed on their Web site (www.nationalbarberboards.com), reads as follows:

Whereas,

- The National Association of Barber Boards of America represents 200,000 and the icon of the independent business person.
- The tonsorial arts have been a tradition in the United States of America since its inception.

Code of Ethics

A statement of the responsibility of this shop to its patrons.

We recognize the fact that you are entitled to every possible protection against infection and contagion while in this establishment, and we endeavor to discharge this responsibility by scrupulous adherence to all sanitary precautions.

We believe that you are entitled to the same courteous, careful and conscientious treatment from every practitioner in this establishment, whether you wish all of the services we have to offer or only one, and we sincerely try to carry out this principle.

The preparations dispensed in this establishment and sold for home use are all standard merchandise of the highest quality, bearing the original manufacturer's label.

We consider it our professional duty to suggest and explain to our patrons such services and applications as we think may be needed in any particular case. However, we do not mean to be offensive, overbearing or insistent, and will at all times respect the wishes of our patrons.

We regard the cosmetics for sale in our shop as legitimate aids to the preservation and beautification of hair and the proper care of the skin and scalp.

We feel that we owe the responsibilities enumerated above to every patron of this establishment, regardless of the frequency of his, or her, visits, and the owner would appreciate having called to his attention any lapse on his or her part or on the part of any of our co-workers.

Figure 2–6 Barber Code of Ethics.

- The time honored tradition of the neighbor barbershop continues to grow and prosper.
- The National Association of Barber Boards of America declares a week in September as National Barber Week in recognition of the contributions of the barbers to the fabric of our society.

Objectives:

1. To promote the exchange of information between state barber boards and state agencies examining licensing and regulating the barber industry.
2. To develop standards and procedures for examining barbers.
3. To develop standards for licensing and policing the barber industry.
4. To develop curriculum for educating barbers.
5. To promote continuous education in the barber industry.
6. To develop and promote procedures for insuring that the consumer is informed and protected.

In this chapter we have seen the progression of barbering from early man to today's regulatory agencies. As a profession, barbering has risen from tribal beginnings to carry the practice of haircutting, styling, and shaving to all parts of the world. Barbers have served as surgeons, dentists, and wigmakers. They have adapted to the eras into which they were born using the tools at hand. From the hand clippers of the 1890s to the variety of high-quality electrical tools available today, barbers have had to adapt to trends, politics, and technological advances to maintain the profession and their livelihoods (Figure 2–7). Some of these changes were challenging, as in the case of a king who dictated that wigs must be worn, while other changes

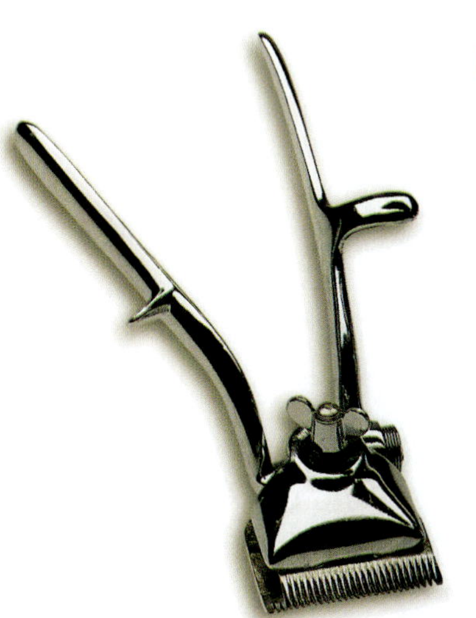

Figure 2–7 Barbers have adapted to the eras into which they were born using the tools at hand.

have served the profession in a beneficial way. Some of the changes that have improved the practice of barbering within the last century include:

1. The implementation of regulatory and educational standards.
2. Improved sanitation practices in the barbershop.
3. The availability and use of better implements and tools.
4. The availability and use of electrical appliances in the shop.
5. The study of anatomy dealing with those parts of the head, face, and neck serviced by the barber.
6. The study of products and preparations used in facial, scalp, and hair treatments.

The enforcement of state barber laws, the advancement of the industry, and the protection of the health, safety, and welfare of the public in the performance of barbering services must rest with today's barbers, schools, shops, associations, and state boards. As a student of barbering, you are now a member of this profession with its long and established history. Along with that membership comes a responsibility to maintain and enhance standards, continue the quest for knowledge, and to perfect the technical and social skills so necessary to this profession.

spotlight on

The Ed Jeffers Barber Museum

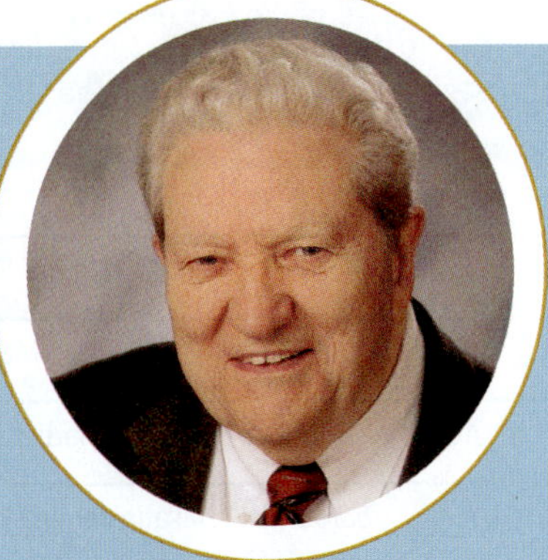

The Ed Jeffers Barber Museum is located in Canal Winchester, Ohio, and is open to the public by appointment. A virtual tour is available on http://www.edjeffersbarbermuseum.com.

Entering the Ed Jeffers Barber Museum is like taking a step back in time. The first thing that catches the eye is the number and variety of barber poles, including a one-of-a-kind antique red and white barber pole that must stand over 6 feet tall. Beautiful oak barber stations with red plush-upholstered seats invite one to sit down and relax while having a good old-fashioned "shave and a haircut."

The Ed Jeffers Barber Museum was started in Canal Winchester in 1988 with fewer than a dozen pieces. Today it has grown to several thousand individual artifacts from as early as the 1700s. Housed in over 3,500 square feet, the museum was created to preserve the roots and document the progression of the barbering profession. "It's important to know where we've come from and how we've progressed, in order to know where we're going," said museum founder Ed Jeffers in a brief interview.

Since its beginning, the museum has welcomed visitors from more than 44 states and 10 countries. It has been featured on television shows on the Discovery Channel and the Family Channel, as well as on television in Japan. The museum has also been featured in journals such as *Smithsonian* magazine and on the front page of the *Wall Street Journal* (July 30, 1999).

Jeffers was able to collect rare items from all over the country due to the positions he has held and currently holds. A barber for over 45 years, he has been a member of the Ohio State Barber Board for over 35 years and an officer with the National Association of Barber Boards of America for over 30 years.

chapter glossary

A. B. Moler	he wrote the first barbering textbook; opened the first barber school in Chicago in 1893
AMBBA	Associated Master Barbers and Beauticians of America
Ambroise Pare	French barber-surgeon who became known as the father of surgery
barba	Latin, for beard
barber-surgeons	early practitioners who cut hair, shaved, performed bloodletting and dentistry
journeymen barber groups	barber employee unions
master barber groups	employers' union
Meryma'at	Egyptian barber commemorated as a statue
National Association of Barber Boards of America	the association of the state barber boards
Ticinius Mena	Sicilian credited with bringing barbering and shaving to Rome in 296 BC
tonsorial	the cutting, clipping, or trimming of hair with shears or a razor
tonsure	a shaved patch on the head

chapter review questions

1. Identify the origin of the word *barber*.
2. Identify the name of the Egyptian barber commemorated in a sculpture.
3. Name the country that was one of the first to develop barbering as an art.
4. Name the person credited with bringing barbering and shaving to Rome.
5. Explain the duties of Egyptian barbers associated with the priests of that culture.
6. List the human characteristics sometimes associated with the wearing of a beard.
7. Explain the duties of the barber-surgeons.
8. Describe the barber's sign used by the barber-surgeons.
9. Explain the origin of the modern barber pole.
10. Identify the ethnic groups that brought the barber-surgeons to America.
11. Identify the name of the employer organizations.
12. Identify the name of the employee organizations.
13. Identify the year that A. B. Moler opened the first barber school in America.
14. Name the author of the first barbering textbook.
15. Identify the name of the first state to pass a barber license law and the year in which it was passed.
16. Explain the primary function of state barber boards.
17. Identify the organization under which state barber boards function nationally.

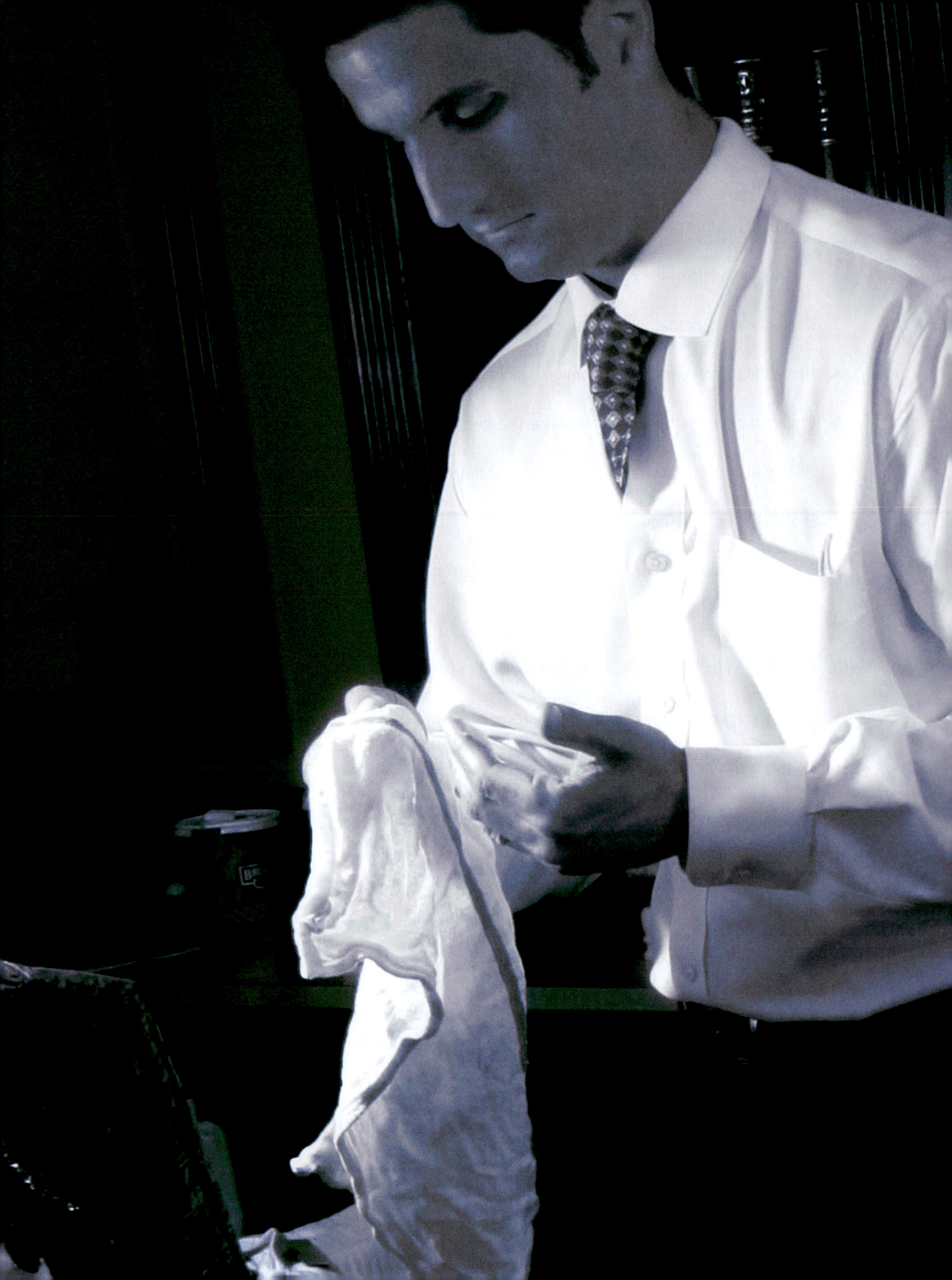

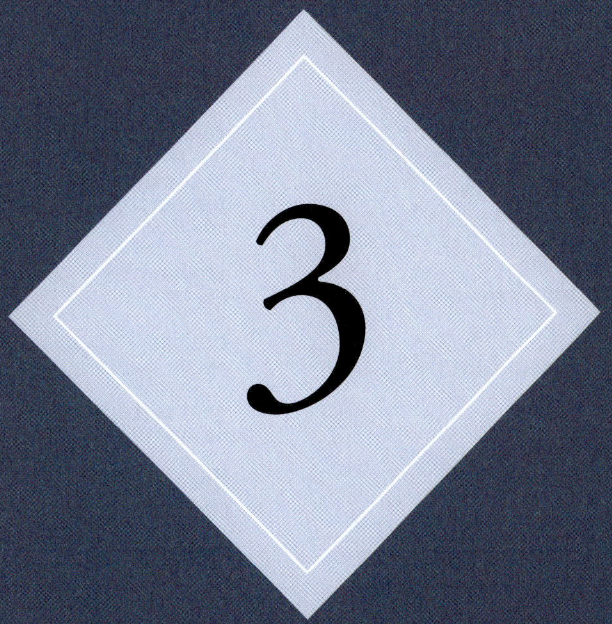

PROFESSIONAL IMAGE

Chapter Outline

Your Professional Image • Human Relations
The Psychology of Success • Guidelines for Student Success

Learning Objectives

After completing this chapter, you should be able to:

1. Define professional image.
2. Discuss the ways in which life skills, values, and beliefs influence your professional image.
3. Explain the relationship between personality and attitudes and the demonstration of professional behavior.
4. List the guidelines to maintaining personal and professional health.
5. Demonstrate an understanding of effective human relations and communication skills.
6. List the qualities of professional ethics.
7. Discuss the basic principles of personal and professional success.
8. Explain the concepts of motivation and self-management.
9. Create short-term and long-term goals.
10. Discuss time-management skills.

Key Terms

attitude
pg. 33

beliefs
pg. 32

compartmentalization
pg. 41

diplomacy
pg. 33

ergonomics
pg. 36

ethics
pg. 39

goal setting
pg. 43

life skills
pg. 31

motivation
pg. 42

personal hygiene
pg. 34

personality
pg. 33

professional image
pg. 31

rapport
pg. 37

receptivity
pg. 34

self-management
pg. 42

values
pg. 32

Did you know that you are a very unique and complex individual? Indeed, we are all unique and complex due to both the many similarities and differences that make each of us who we are. In this chapter, we are going to explore a variety of factors that originate from our innermost selves—factors that have the ability to influence and impact our professional image.

YOUR PROFESSIONAL IMAGE

The *image* you project to others is a reflection of you as an individual. Your personality, attitude, abilities, appearance, and moral character all help to create emotional and mental pictures in the hearts and minds of every person you interact with in daily life. This image is the *impression* you project to others in your personal and professional lives. And, although your personal image may differ somewhat from your professional image, the values and beliefs that guide you in both capacities stem from the inner source of the real and authentic you.

In this chapter, we define your **professional image** as the impression that you project as a person engaged in the profession of barbering. Your professional image consists of the outward appearance, attitude, and conduct that you exhibit in the workplace. In addition, it reflects your prior learning and life experiences or life skills that continually add to your total professional development. Ultimately, the professional image you project to coworkers and clients will influence and impact your present and future successes (Figure 3–1). 1

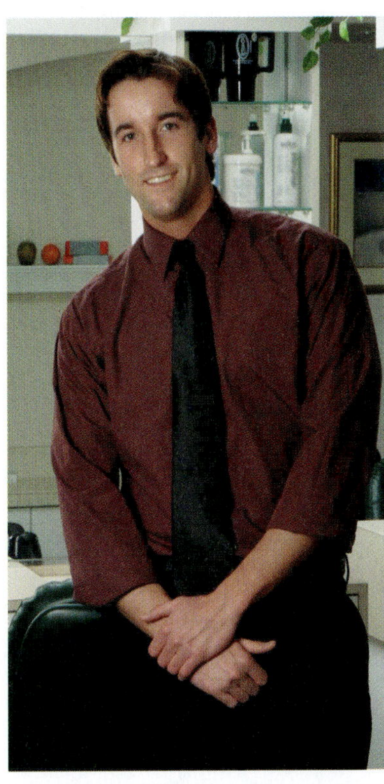

Figure 3-1 Project a professional image.

3

Life Skills

We begin our discussion of your professional image with some insights into what are known as **life skills**. This is an important basis from which to begin because life skills are the tools and guidelines that prepare you for living as a mature adult in a challenging and often complicated world. Life skills provide the foundation that will help you to face life's difficulties, successfully manage situations you find challenging, and empower you to reach your full personal and professional potential.

Life skills are developed through learning and experience. As such, many life skills are learned or experienced through our parents and families. Being considerate of others' feelings or valuing honesty are life skills that many of us have been taught from an early age. Other life skills, such as patience or adaptability, may have been learned from actual experiences or situations that required the application of these particular skills in order to complete the experience or handle the situation. In either scenario, once a life skill has been learned and practiced, it can become part of our personal foundation so that we are better prepared to successfully manage future life experiences.

While there are many life skills that can provide us with a solid foundation from which to support our personal and professional journeys through life, some of the most important are:

- A genuine concern and caring for other people.
- An ability to adapt to different situations.
- The development and achievement of goals.
- Persistence and a "can-do" attitude.
- Follow-through and the completion of jobs, tasks, and commitments.
- The development and use of common sense.
- The establishment of positive and healthy relationships.
- Approaching everything with a strong sense of responsibility and a positive attitude.
- Feeling good about yourself.
- Being cooperative.
- Being organized.
- Maintaining a sense of humor.
- Being patient with yourself and others.
- Being honest and trustworthy.
- Striving for excellence.

You are now at the beginning of your barbering education and training. Each student embarks upon this training with a set of life skills based on prior learning environments and opportunities that should grow and expand with new experiences. New experiences can be used as stepping-stones toward the development and enhancement of your personal and professional life skills. The attitude with which each individual meets and learns from each new experience originates from personal values and beliefs.

- *Values.* The deepest feelings and thoughts we have about ourselves and about life. **Values** consist of what we think, how we feel, and how we act based on what we think and feel. For example, let's say you value loyalty. You *think* it is important in a friendship and expect it in your relationships. One day you overhear a friend sharing with someone else something you've said to him or her in confidence and you *feel* hurt and betrayed. The way in which you react to the situation is an *action* that is taken in response to what you are *thinking* and *feeling.*
- *Beliefs.* Specific attitudes that occur as a result of our values and have a strong influence on how we act or behave in situations are **beliefs**. For example, if you value responsibility, you probably take on more than your share of commitments to family, school, workplace, or community. This example shows us the link between a positive belief and a resulting positive behavior; however, beliefs can be negative in nature as well.

When you tell yourself, or others, that you can't do something, you are setting yourself up for a negative self-fulfilling prophecy that comes true simply because you *think* it will come true. Conversely, you can use a positive self-fulfilling prophecy to inspire change, action, and a commitment to your goals by substituting "I can" for "I can't." Changing your beliefs will change your behavior and focusing on *what is* rather than *what is not* is a much more positive approach to attaining your goals. 2

Personality

Your **personality** plays an important role in both your personal and professional life. Personality can be defined as the outward reflection of inner feelings, thoughts, attitudes, and values. It is expressed through your voice, speech, and choice of words, as well as through your facial expressions, gestures, actions, posture, clothing, grooming, and environment. Your personality defines who you are and distinguishes you from others, making you the unique individual that you are. In the people-oriented profession of barbering, your personality becomes one of the most important demonstrations of your particular style of professionalism. In this section we will explore the many personal characteristics that are expressed through one's personality.

Attitude

There is an old adage that says, "The only difference between a good day and a bad day is your **attitude**." That is an effective reminder that we are in control of our attitudes and the outlook we have on life at any given point. Although one's attitude stems from innate values and beliefs, the adage also reminds us that an attitude does not have to be stagnant or "written in stone." Rather, attitudes can be altered or changed if we remain open-minded to new insights. This ongoing process is called attitude development and it can expand with each new life experience.

Although there are times when our attitudes may be influenced by friends, family, or circumstance, the extent to which we allow others or situations to *change* our attitude is really up to us. We can assume positive, negative, or neutral attitudes, but we also have to live with the consequences of our reactions. We also need to remember that attitude is one of the most obvious and apparent aspects of personality. It is there for all to see in both personal and professional life. Review the following aspects of a well-developed attitude to determine how you might enhance your own attitude development.

- *Diplomacy.* **Diplomacy** is the art of being tactful, and being tactful means being straightforward but not critical.
- *Emotional stability.* Learn to control your emotions. Do not reveal negative emotions such as anger, envy, and dislike. An even-tempered person is usually treated with respect.
- *Sensitivity.* Your personality shines the most when you show concern for the feelings of others. Sensitivity is a combination of understanding,

empathy, and acceptance that leads to being compassionate and responsive to other people.

- *Receptivity.* **Receptivity** means being interested in other people and to be responsive to their ideas, feelings, and opinions.
- *Courtesy.* Courtesy and good manners reflect your thoughtfulness toward others. Good manners are expressed by treating others with respect, exercising care of other people's property, being tolerant and understanding of others' shortcomings and efforts, and being considerate of those with whom you work. Courtesy is one of the most important keys to a successful career. 3✓

Personal and Professional Health

In accordance with the general concepts of a profession that helps others to look their best, barbers should strive to reflect their own best image. An important aspect of this representation is the barber's personal health and physical appearance. To achieve success in this area, it is helpful to follow a set of guidelines that help to maintain both a healthy body and mind.

- *Hygiene.* Hygiene is the branch of applied science concerned with healthful living; its main purpose is to preserve health.
- *Personal Hygiene.* **Personal hygiene** is the daily maintenance of cleanliness and healthfulness through certain sanitary practices. These include daily bathing or showering, shaving, the use of deodorant or antiperspirant, teeth brushing and flossing, the use of mouthwash, and clean, well-groomed hair and nails (Figure 3–2).

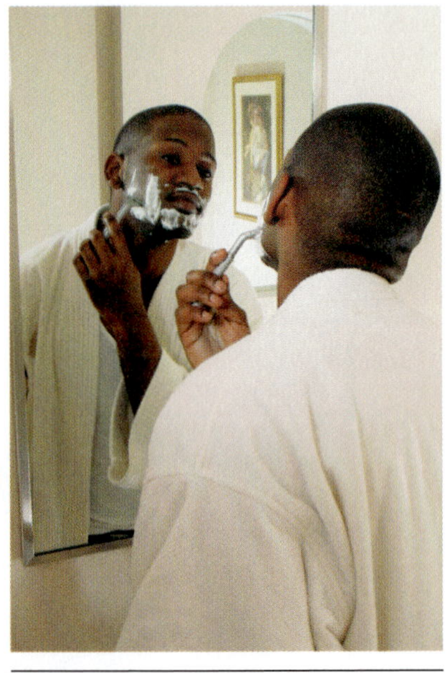

Figure 3-2 Practice personal hygiene every day.

3

- *Personal Grooming.* Personal grooming is an extension of personal hygiene. A well-groomed barber is one of the best advertisements for the barbershop or salon. If you present a poised and attractive image, your clients will have confidence in you as a professional. Many shop owners and managers consider appearance, personality, and poise to be as important as technical knowledge and manual skills. While some barbershops do not require standard uniforms, they may have a specific dress code. For example, some shops require that personnel wear a barbering smock, jacket, or even a tie. Select your outfits so that you reflect the image of the shop and dress for success. Clothes should be clean and pressed. Shoes should be polished and kept in good repair. Excessive jewelry should be avoided but a wristwatch will help you to maintain your schedule.
- *Rest and Relaxation.* Adequate sleep is essential for good health because without it you cannot function efficiently. The body needs to be allowed to recover from the fatigue of the day's activities and should be replenished with a good night's sleep. Body tissues and organs are rebuilt and renewed during the sleeping process. The amount of sleep needed to feel refreshed varies from person to person. Some people function well with six hours of sleep while others need eight hours. According to medical professionals an average of seven or eight hours of sleep each night is

recommended. Relaxation is important as a change of pace from day-to-day routine. Going to a movie or a museum, reading a book, watching television, or dancing are ways to "get away from it all." When you return to work, you will feel refreshed and eager to attend to your duties.

- *Nutrition.* What you eat affects your health, appearance, personality, and performance on the job. The nutrients in food supply the body with energy and ensure that the body functions properly. A balanced diet should include foods containing a variety of important vitamins and minerals. Drink plenty of water daily. Try to avoid sugar, salt, caffeine, and fatty or highly refined and processed foods.
- *Exercise.* Exercise and recreation in the form of walking, dancing, sports, and gym activities tend to develop the muscles and help to keep the body fit. A couple of the benefits resulting from regular physical activity are:
  1. An improvement in the proper functioning of organs.
  2. An improvement in blood circulation and an increased supply of oxygen.
- *Stress Management and a Healthy Lifestyle.* Stress is defined as the inability to cope with a real or imagined threat that results in a series of mental and physical responses or adaptations. The way in which individuals perform under stressful situations depends on their personality type, temperament, physical health, and coping skills. Practice stress management through a combination of rest, relaxation, exercise, and daily routines that provide you with time to calm the body and its systems. To maintain a healthy lifestyle, avoid substances that can have a negative effect on health, such as tobacco, alcohol, and drugs. Live a life of moderation in which work and activities are balanced so that you can achieve a sense of harmony in your life.
- *Healthy Thoughts.* The body and mind operate as a unit; therefore thoughts and emotions can influence the body's activities. A thought may either stimulate or depress the way the body functions. Strong emotions such as worry and fear have a harmful effect on the heart, arteries, and glands. Depression weakens the functioning of the body's organs, thereby lowering resistance to disease.
- *Posture.* Your posture is an aspect of your physical presentation that is important to your professional image. Good posture presents your personal appearance to its best advantage, helps to create an image of confidence, and lessens fatigue and the possibility of other physical problems (Figure 3–3).

  Working as a barber, you will spend most of your time in a standing position. Your arms will often be raised in a position that is almost equal to the height of your shoulders. These repetitive motions can create physical stress in the hands, wrist, arm, shoulder, and lower back areas that may require physical or movement therapies to maintain proper body alignment. You can, however, help to alleviate some of these possible conditions by being consciously aware of your standing posture and by practicing some of the following guidelines (Figure 3–4).

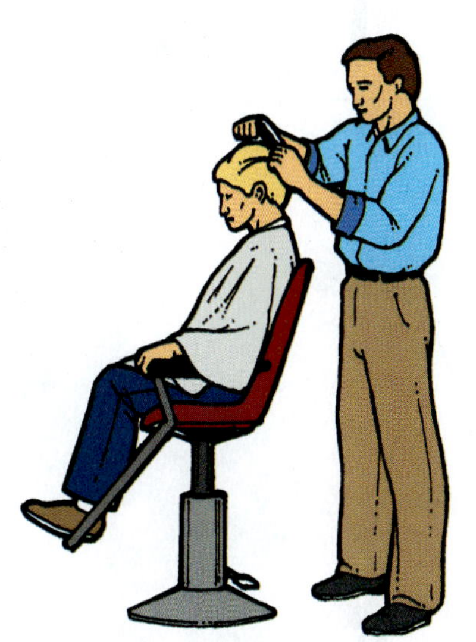

Figure 3–3 Good posture is essential.

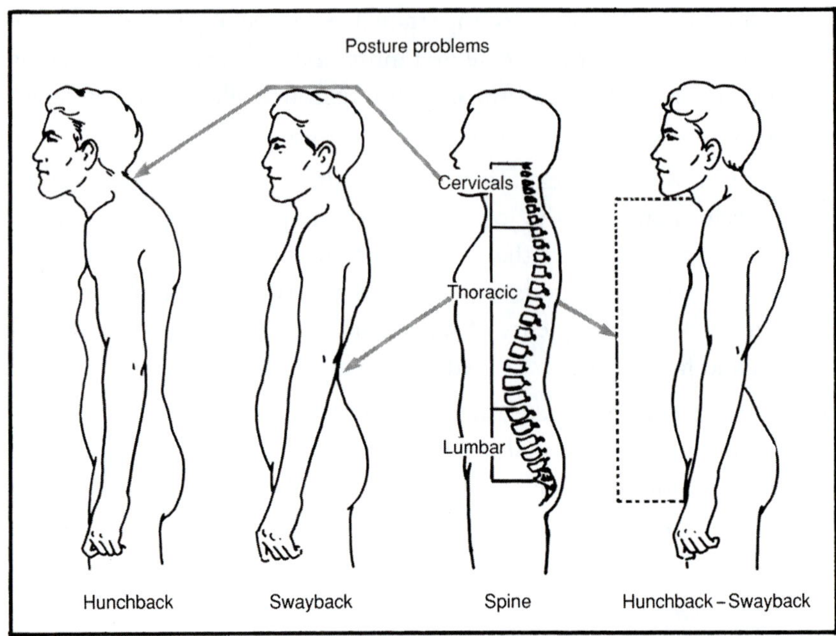

Figure 3-4 Posture problems.

1. Keep your head up and chin parallel to the floor.
2. Keep the neck elongated and balanced above the shoulders.
3. Lift your upper body so that your chest is up and out—do not slouch.
4. Hold your shoulders level and relaxed.
5. Stand with your spine straight.
6. Pull in your abdomen so it is flat.

Just as there is a mechanically correct posture for standing, there is also a correct sitting posture. Use the following guidelines to learn to sit correctly in a balanced position (Figures 3–5 and 3–6).

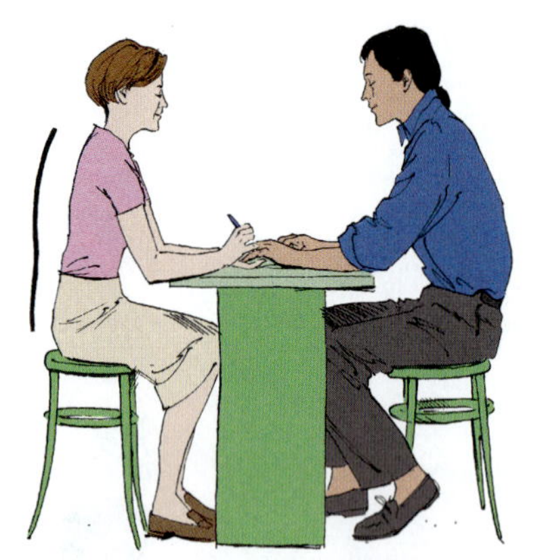

Figure 3-5 Good sitting posture.

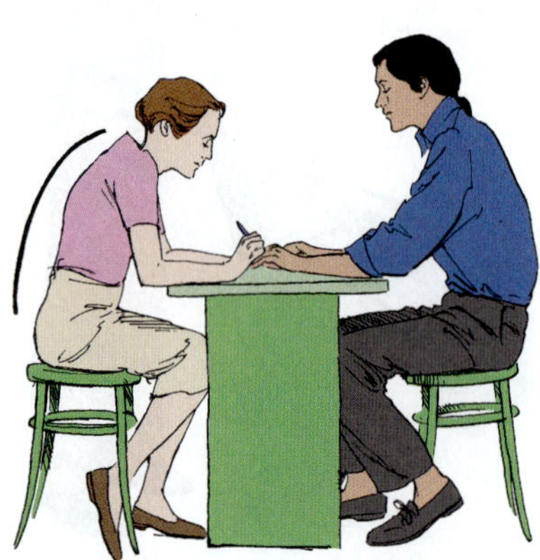

Figure 3-6 Poor sitting posture.

1. Keep your hips level and horizontal, not forward or backward.
2. Flex your knees slightly and position them over your feet.
3. Lower your body smoothly into a chair, keeping your back straight.
4. Keep the soles of your feet on the floor directly under your knees.
5. Have the seat of the chair even with your knees. This will allow the upper and lower legs to form a 90-degree angle at the knees.
6. Rest the weight of your torso on the thigh bones, not on the end of the spine.
7. Keep your torso erect.
8. Make sure your desk is at the correct height so that the upper and lower parts of your arm form a right angle when you are writing.

- *Ergonomics.* **Ergonomics** is the study of human characteristics for the specific work environment. As previously mentioned, barbers are particularly susceptible to problems of the hands, wrists, arms, shoulders, neck, back, feet, and legs. Prevention is the key to alleviating these problems by fitting your work to your body and not your body to your work (Figure 3–7). Practice some of the following suggestions to fit your work to your body more effectively.

1. Do not grip or squeeze tools and implements too tightly.
2. Do not bend the wrist up or down constantly when cutting the hair or using a blow-dryer.
3. Try to position your arms at less than a 60-degree angle when holding your arms away from your body while working.
4. Avoid bending or twisting your body.
5. Wear appropriate and supportive shoes or footwear.
6. Adjust the height of the chair so that the client's head is at a comfortable working level.
7. Tilt the client's head as necessary for better access during hair services.
8. Keep your wrists in a straight or neutral position as much as possible.
9. Keep tools and implements sharpened and well lubricated. 

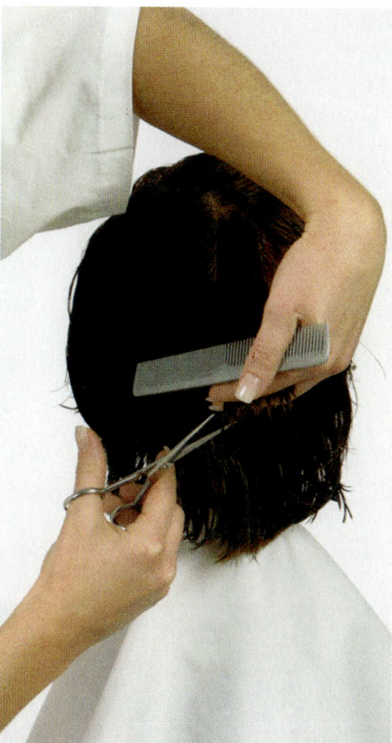

Figure 3–7 Improper haircutting position.

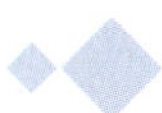

HUMAN RELATIONS

Human relations is the psychology of getting along well with others. Effective human relations skills help you to build rapport with clients and coworkers. **Rapport** may be defined as a close and empathetic relationship that establishes agreement and harmony between individuals. Your professional attitude is expressed by your self-esteem, confidence, and the respect you show others. Good habits and practices acquired during your education lay the foundation for a successful career in barbering. The following guidelines for good human relations will help you to gain confidence, deal courteously with others, and become a successful professional.

- Always greet a client by name, using a pleasant tone of voice. Address clients by their last name as in "Mr. Jones" or "Mrs. Smith" unless the client prefers first names or it is customary to use first names in the barbershop.
- Be alert to the client's mood. Some clients prefer quiet and relaxation; others like to talk. Be a good listener and confine the conversation to the client's needs. Never gossip or tell off-color stories.
- Topics of conversation should be carefully chosen. Friendly relations are achieved through pleasant conversations. Let the client guide the topic of conversation. In a business setting it is best to avoid such controversial topics as religion and politics, personal problems, or issues relating to other people. Never discuss other clients or coworkers, and always maintain an ethical standard of confidentiality.

- Make a good impression by looking the part of the successful barber, and by speaking and acting in a professional manner at all times.
- Cultivate self-confidence, and project a pleasing personality.
- Show interest in the client's personal preferences and give the client undivided attention.
- Use tact and diplomacy when dealing with problems you may encounter. Deal with all disputes and differences in private. Take care of all problems promptly and to the client's satisfaction.
- Be capable and efficient.
- Be punctual. Arrive at work on time and keep appointments on schedule. Plan each day's schedule so that you manage your time effectively.

In addition to basic human relations skills, barbering students need to cultivate other aspects of a professional image that impact their success in the profession. Some desirable qualities for effective client relations are:

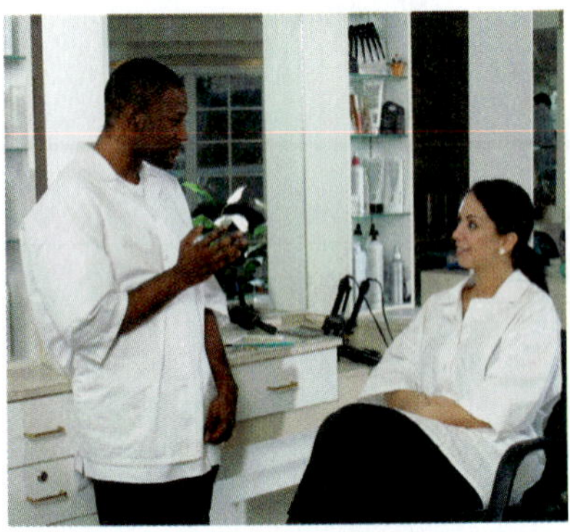

Figure 3-8 Being receptive is a good personal skill.

- *Talk less, listen more.* There is an old saying that we were given two ears and one mouth for a reason. When you practice good listening skills, you are fully attentive to what the other person is saying. If there is something that you don't understand, ask questions to gain understanding (Figure 3–8).
- *Emotional control.* Learn to control your emotions. Try to respond rather than to react. Do not reveal negative emotions such as anger, envy, and dislike through gestures, facial expressions, or conversation. An even-tempered person is usually treated with respect.
- *Positive approach.* Be pleasant and gracious. Be ready with a smile of greeting and a word of welcome for each client and coworker. A good sense of humor is also important in maintaining a positive attitude. A sense of humor enriches your life and cushions the disappointments. When you are able to laugh at yourself, you will have gained the ability to accept and deal positively with difficult situations.
- *Good manners.* Good manners reflect your thoughtfulness toward others. Treating others with respect, exercising care of other people's property, being tolerant and understanding of their shortcomings and efforts, and being considerate of those with whom you work, all express good manners. As previously mentioned, courtesy is one of the most important keys to a successful career.
- *Mannerisms.* Gum chewing and nervous habits, such as tapping your foot or playing with your hair, detract from the effectiveness of your image. Yawning, coughing, and sneezing should be concealed with your hand in front of your mouth. Control negative body language—sarcastic or disapproving facial grimaces, for example. Exhibiting pleasant mannerisms and attractive gestures and actions should be your goal at all times.

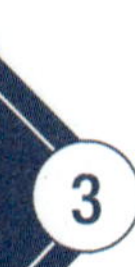

Effective Communication Skills

Effective communication is one of the barber's most important human relations skills. Communication includes listening skills, voice, speech, and conversational ability—all of which are necessary to forming satisfying relationships with customers (Figure 3–9).

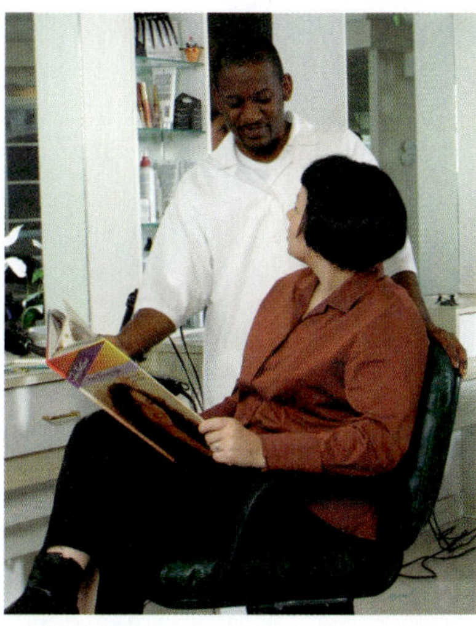

Figure 3-9 Communication is part of building relationships.

Communication is the act of transmitting information in the form of symbols, gestures, or behaviors to express an idea or concept so that it is clearly understood. When you communicate, you participate in sending and receiving messages and establishing relationships. When communicating with clients, there are several steps you can take to ascertain their service expectations.

- *Organize your thoughts.* What question or information do you want your client to understand? For example, a client with medium-length hair that covers the top part of the ears, says he want a trim. You will need to determine just what the client's definition of a trim is and may ask if he wants the tops of his ears covered or not.
- *Clarify.* The next step is to clarify what the client is telling you. In the preceding scenario, let's say the client's response to the question is that he wants his hair "over the ears." This answer still does not provide you with the information you will need to proceed with the haircut. Why? Because you now have to clarify what the client's definition of "over the ears" means to him. Does it mean covering the tops of the ears, or does it mean above and/or around the ears?
- *Repeat.* Once you have an understanding of the client's definition of "over the ears," repeat back to the client your interpretation of what you think he told you. This communication step will provide you with further clarification and the opportunity to make other interpretation changes or to reach an understanding of the client's expectations.

There are many ways in which effective communication skills can impact your professional success. Review the following barbershop or salon activities that will benefit from effective communication skills.

- Making contacts and networking.
- Meeting and greeting clients.
- Understanding a client's service needs, likes, dislikes, and desires.
- Self-promotion and building a clientele.
- Selling services and products.
- Telephone conversations and appointment bookings.
- Conversation and interaction with the shop or salon staff, clients, and vendors.

Professional Ethics

Ethics are the principles and standards of good character, proper conduct, and moral judgment. The governing board or commission of a particular occupation often creates a *Code of Ethics,* which specifically relates to the characteristics of that profession. In barbering, for example, state boards set the ethical standards that all barbers who work in that state must follow.

3

Ethics, however, goes beyond a set of rules and regulations. In barbering, ethics is also a code of conduct, which is expressed through your personality, human relations skills, and professional image.

Ethical conduct helps to build the client's confidence in you. Having clients speak well of you is the best form of advertising and helps to build a successful business. All professional barbers should practice the following rules of ethics.

1. Give courteous and friendly service to all clients. Treat everyone honestly and fairly; do not show favoritism.
2. Be courteous and show respect for the feelings, beliefs, and rights of others.
3. Keep your word. Be responsible and fulfill your obligations.
4. Build your reputation by setting an example of good conduct and behavior.
5. Be loyal to your employer, managers, and associates.
6. Obey all provisions of the laws relating to barbers in your state.
7. Practice the highest standards of sanitation to protect your health and the health of your coworkers and clients.
8. Believe in your chosen profession. Practice it faithfully and sincerely.
9. Do not try to sell clients a product or service they do not need or want.
10. As a student, be loyal and cooperative with school personnel and fellow students. Comply with all school policies and procedures.

Questionable practices, extravagant claims, and unfulfilled promises violate the rules of ethical conduct and cast an unfavorable light on barbers. Unethical practices affect the student, practicing barbers, the school, barbershops or salons, and the entire industry. 6

3

THE PSYCHOLOGY OF SUCCESS

Defining *success* is a highly individualized and personal matter. For some, money is the measure of their success; for others, career satisfaction or helping others makes them feel successful and fulfilled. Regardless of your personal definition of success, there are some basic principles that form the foundation of personal and professional success.

- *Build self-esteem.* Self-esteem is based on inner strength and begins with trusting in your ability to reach your goals. It is a form of self-belief that helps you to feel good about yourself and what you can accomplish.
- *Visualize.* Visualize yourself in whatever scenario is relevant to the situation or environment that requires your attention. Picture yourself as a confident and competent person who earns the trust and respect of the others involved in the scenario. The more you practice visualization techniques, the more easily you can turn possibilities and dreams into realities.

- *Build on your strengths.* Spend time doing whatever it is that helps you maintain a positive self-image. Use personal-interest areas to provide incremental challenges that help you to build on strengths and expand your success-building options (Figure 3–10).
- *Be kind to yourself.* Put a stop to self-critical and negative thoughts that can work against you. If you make a mistake, tell yourself that it is okay and you will do your best next time.
- *Define success for yourself.* Be a success in your own eyes and do not depend on other people's definition of success. What is right for others may not be right for you.
- *Practice new behaviors.* Practicing new behaviors that are not a part of your regular lifestyle can help you to develop personally and professionally. For example, if you are nervous about speaking in front of your classmates, practice! Take advantage of every opportunity to hone your speaking skills and create a stepping-stone path to success that will make it easier for you each time you engage in the activity. Remember that creating success is a skill that can be learned, so don't be afraid to try new things.
- *Keep your personal life separate from your work or school life.* Another aspect of success psychology is the ability to keep your personal and professional lives separate. While we all have responsibilities and concerns that impact our multidimensional lives, it is important to know when, where, and to what extent it is permissible to talk about personal issues. In the work and school environments, the answer is almost never. People who talk about themselves (or others) at work or school can negatively impact and undermine the professional atmosphere that is an important aspect of work and learning environments. In the barbershop or salon, clients should not be subjected to comments about coworkers, personal opinions, or complaints. Clients patronize a barbershop to receive personal services and should be treated with the utmost professionalism. If you find it difficult to keep your personal life out of these environments, try an exercise known as **compartmentalization**. Imagine that you have two filing cabinets; one is labeled Personal and the other, Professional. Visualize yourself locking the Personal file cabinet before leaving for work or school and opening the Professional cabinet when you arrive at your destination. This exercise helps you to store things away in the different compartments of the mind—and it works.
- *Keep your energy up.* Successful people know how to pace themselves. Get enough rest, exercise, eat a nutritious diet, and spend time with family and friends. Successful people know that having a clear head, a fit body, and the ability to refuel and recharge are important conditions to maintaining a successful lifestyle.
- *Respect others.* Make a point of relating to everyone you know with a conscious feeling of respect. This includes using good manners with others: use words like *please, thank you,* and *excuse me.* Avoid interrupting or speaking when someone else is talking. Be respectful of others and they will be respectful you.

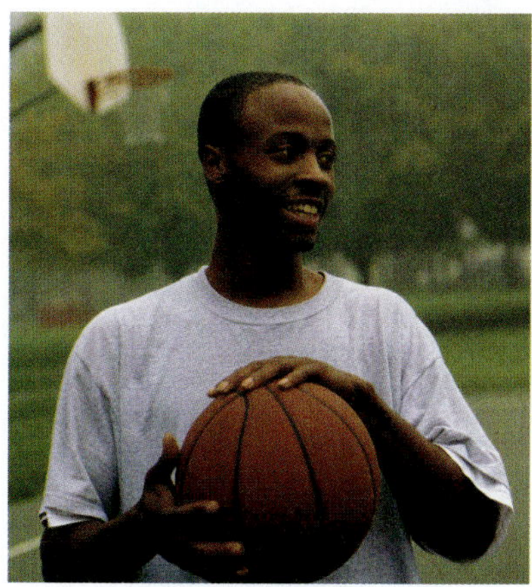

Figure 3–10 Recreational activities help you build on strengths and maintain a positive self-image.

3

- *Stay productive.* The three habits that can keep you from maintaining peak performance are procrastination, perfectionism, and the lack of a game plan. Work on eliminating these troublesome habits and you will see an almost instant improvement in your ability to achieve your goals.
- *Remind yourself.* Success is a choice . . . and it is your choice. 

Motivation and Self-Management

Motivation originates from a desire for change and serves as the ignition for success. **Self-management** is the fuel that will keep you going on the long ride to your destination. It is important to feel motivated, especially when you are a student. The best motivation for learning comes from an inner (intrinsic) desire to know more about a particular interest or subject matter. If you have always been interested in the profession of barbering, then you are likely to be interested in the material you will be studying in barbering school. If your motivation stems from some external (extrinsic) source such as parents or friends, you may not complete your studies because you will need more than a push from others to make a career for yourself. You need to feel a sense of excitement and a good reason that begins *within you* for staying the course. No one should have to motivate you to study other than yourself. *You are in charge of managing your own life and learning.*

While motivation propels you to do something and may originate from within you instinctually, self-management is a well-thought-out process for the long term. For example, since you want to be a licensed barber you are motivated to the extent that you enrolled in a barbering program to reach that goal. But that is just the beginning, isn't it? You've probably already used some self-management skills to arrange your schedule, financing, transportation, or the like to begin this program. Now you will have to use other self-management skills to apply yourself to your studies and to complete the program. 8

3

Access Your Creative Capabilities

In most conversations, when we use the word *creative* we think of particular talents or abilities in the arts such as painting, singing, acting, or even hairstyling. But being creative or having a sense of creativity is not limited to these artistic expressions. Creativity also functions as an unlimited inner resource of ideas and solutions for the many challenges we face in our lives and can be accessed by each of us to find new ways of thinking and problem solving. To enhance your creativity skills, keep the following guidelines in mind.

- *Stop criticizing yourself.* Criticism blocks the creative mind from exploring ideas and discovering solutions to challenges.
- *Refrain from asking others what to do.* In one sense, this can be a way of hoping that others will motivate you instead of you finding the motivation from within. This does not rule out the importance of mentors or of what can be learned from others, but being able to tap into your own creativity is the best way to manage your own success.

- *Change your vocabulary.* Build a positive vocabulary of active problem-solving words such as *explore, analyze, determine, judge, assess,* and so on.
- *Ask for help when you need it.* Being creative does not mean doing everything by yourself. The best self-managers ask for help, utilizing family, friends, peers, coaches, and mentors to stimulate their creativity. Sometimes creativity is best stimulated in an environment in which people work together, brainstorm, and pool their ideas.

Goal Setting

What are you working toward at this time in your life? What do you dream about doing? Turning dreams into reality is what **goal setting** is all about. Picture a goal in your mind. Is it working in a barbershop or salon, or do you see yourself owning your own business? Do you think you have the drive and desire to make your dreams happen? If so, do you also have a realistic plan for reaching your goals? Goal setting helps you decide what you want out of life and when you know what your goal is, you can map the best route for getting to your destination. Setting goals is like bringing a map along on a road trip to somewhere you've never been before.

There are two types of goals: short term and long term. *Short-term goals* usually refer to those goals you wish to accomplish within a year or less. *Long-term goals* are measured in longer segments of time such as 5 years, 10 years, or even longer. Both require careful thought and planning.

Goal setting is a process. The first step is to identify both your short-term and long-term goals. Then write them down! Seeing your goals in written form will help you to focus on them so that you can develop a plan for achieving them. As you develop your plan keep the following in mind:

- Express your goals in a positive way and be specific.
- Make your goals measurable and set deadlines for accomplishing each one.
- Plan for your goals and make a list of the tasks that need to be completed. Check off each item on the list as it is accomplished.

Remember, the important elements of goal setting are to have a plan, to reexamine it often so that you can make sure you are on track, and to be flexible to changes that may have to be made along the way. 9

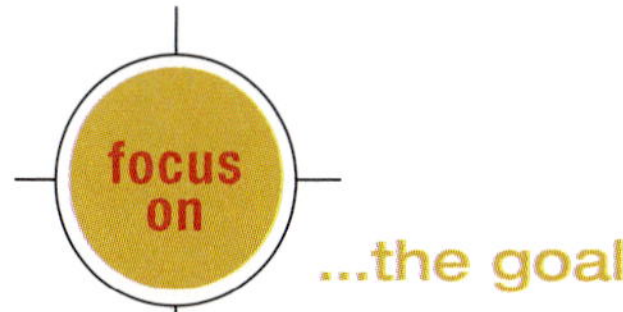

Try this visualization exercise: Visualize your short- and long-term goals along a pathway of stepping-stones. Your ultimate goal is at the far end of the pathway and each stone represents the successful completion of a step that you will have to take toward attaining your goal. Map out realistic short- and long-term goals. Use checkpoints along the way so that you know when you are close to achieving a goal and when you have arrived. Then celebrate the accomplishment!

Time Management

One way to reach your goals more effectively is to manage your time as efficiently as you can. According to time management experts, everyone has an "inner organizer" and can learn to manage their time more efficiently. Here are some tips from the experts.

- Learn to prioritize by listing tasks in an order of most to least important.
- Schedule in blocks of unstructured time for flexibility.
- Stress is counterproductive so pace yourself and don't take on more than you can handle.
- Learn problem-solving techniques to save time when seeking solutions.

- Take time out when you need to reenergize.
- Carry a notepad with you to record great ideas or reminders.
- Make daily, weekly, and monthly schedules.
- Identify your peak-energy and low-energy times of the day and plan accordingly.
- Utilize to-do lists.
- Make time management a habit.
- Reward yourself for work well done.

GUIDELINES FOR STUDENT SUCCESS

1. Participate in the classroom in a courteous manner.
2. School regulations are important—obey them all.
3. Turn off pagers and cell phones. Personal calls interfere with teaching and learning.
4. Be careful with all school equipment and supplies.
5. Be clean and well groomed at all times.
6. Cooperate with teachers and school personnel.
7. Use notebooks and workbooks as important review aids.
8. Avoid loafing as it makes a poor impression on others and wastes valuable learning time.
9. Be courteous and considerate at all times.
10. Be tactful and polite to clients.
11. Observe safety rules and prevent accidents.
12. Develop a pleasing personality.
13. Think and act positively.
14. Attend trade shows and conventions to increase knowledge.
15. Stay on task and carefully complete all homework assignments.
16. Keep clothes and uniforms spotlessly clean.
17. Follow teachers' instructions and techniques.
18. Show clients that you are interested and sincere.
19. Maintain good attendance.
20. Ask for clarification of anything you do not understand.
21. Bathe daily and use a deodorant.
22. Develop and exhibit good manners at all times.
23. Be respectful to teachers and supervisors.
24. Develop good work habits essential to success.
25. Comply with state board laws, rules, and regulations that govern the profession. These regulations are designed to contribute to the health, safety, and welfare of the public and the community.

chapter glossary

attitude	a manner of acting, posturing, feeling, or thinking that shows a person's mood, disposition, mind-set, or opinion
beliefs	specific attitudes that occur as a result of our values
compartmentalization	the capacity to keep different aspects of your mental activity separate so you can achieve greater self-control
diplomacy	the art of being tactful
ergonomics	the study of human characteristics related to the specific work environment
ethics	principles of good character, proper conduct, and moral judgment, expressed through personality, human relations skills, and professional image
goal setting	the identification of short- and long-term goals
life skills	tools and guidelines that prepare you for living as an adult in a challenging world
motivation	a desire for change
personal hygiene	the daily maintenance of cleanliness and healthfulness through certain sanitary practices
personality	the outward expression of inner feelings, thoughts, attitudes, and values as expressed through voice, gestures, posture, clothing, grooming, and environment
professional image	the impression projected by a person in any profession, consisting of outward appearance and conduct exhibited in the workplace
rapport	a close and empathetic relationship that establishes agreement and harmony between individuals
receptivity	the extent to which one is interested in and responsive to others' ideas, feelings, and opinions
self-management	the ongoing process of planning, organizing, and managing one's life
values	the deepest feelings and thoughts we have about ourselves and about life

chapter review questions

1. Define professional image. What personal elements does a professional image consist of?
2. Define life skills. List five life skills that you would like to enhance for your own professional growth.
3. Identify and list five values that are the most important to you personally.
4. Explain one way in which attitudes can be altered or changed.
5. List nine basic requirements for personal and professional health.
6. Define ergonomics.
7. Define human relations and list five desirable qualities for effective client relations.
8. Define rapport.
9. List three communication steps that will help to determine a client's service expectations.
10. Define professional ethics. Identify three actions that violate the rules of ethical conduct and cast an unfavorable light on barbers.
11. Explain the vision of professional success you have for yourself.
12. Identify where the best motivation for learning originates.
13. List a minimum of three short-term goals and three long-term goals that you have developed for yourself.
14. Explain the primary purpose of state board laws, rules, and regulations.

part

2

THE SCIENCE OF BARBERING

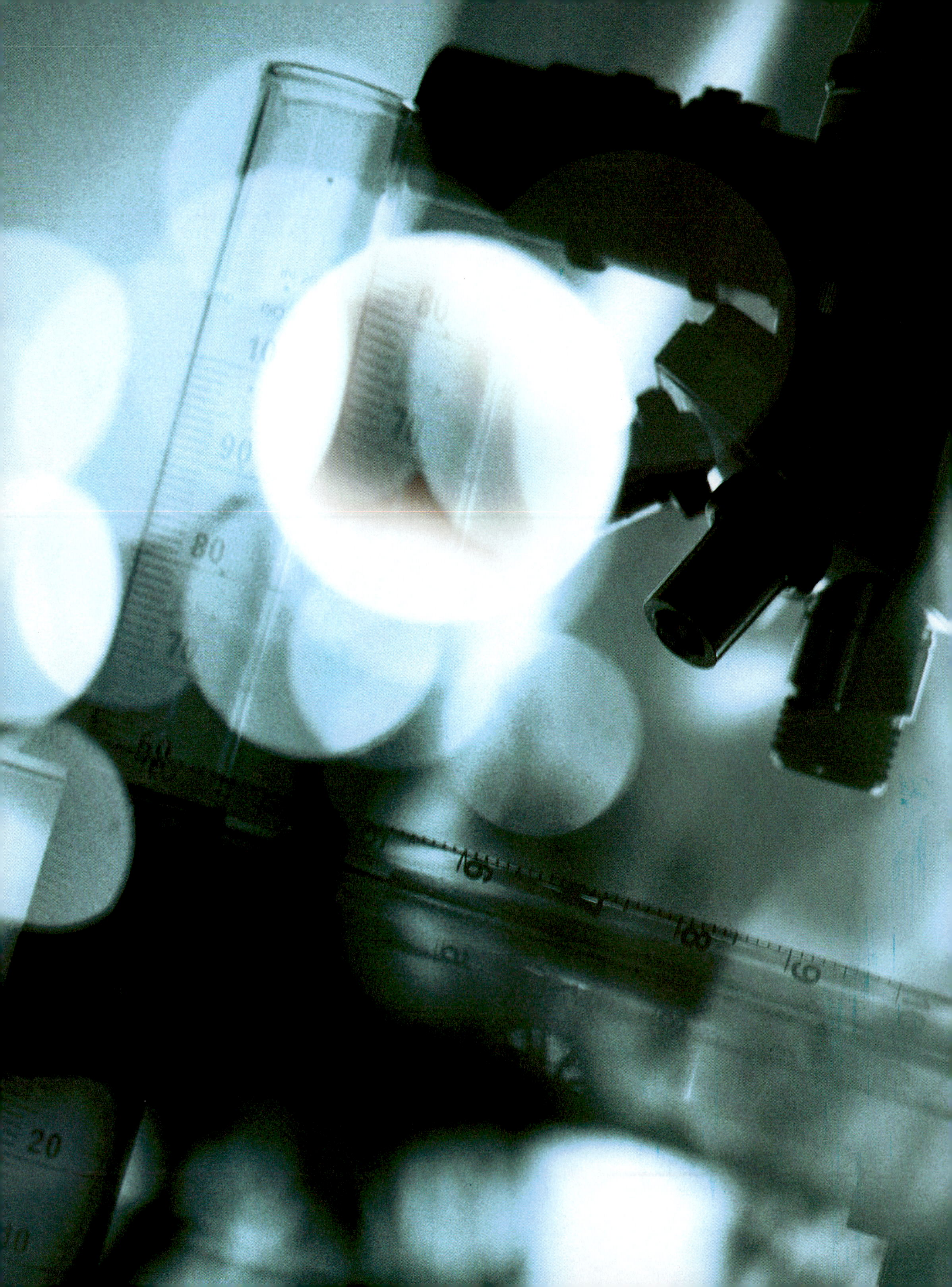

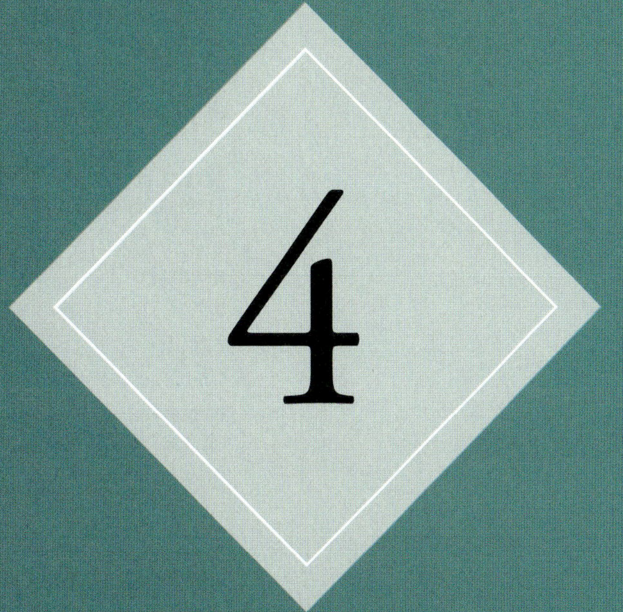

BACTERIOLOGY

Chapter Outline

Learning Objectives

After completing this chapter, you should be able to:

1. List the classifications and types of bacteria.
2. Describe the growth and reproduction of bacteria.
3. Explain the relationship of bacteria to the spread of disease.
4. Discuss hepatitis transmission and prevention.
5. Discuss HIV/AIDS transmission and prevention.

Key Terms

Each year, the barbering industry services hundreds of thousands of clients. That means that barbers and their clients are exposed to billions of bacteria, germs, and viruses that can result in illness and infection. To limit the exposure and spread of disease, state barber boards and health departments require that sanitary measures be applied while barbering professionals are serving the public.

As a professional barber, it is your responsibility to ensure that your clients receive their services in a safe and sanitary environment. In this chapter, you will learn the nature of various organisms, their relationship to disease, and how their spread can be prevented in the school and barbershop. An understanding of these topics will help you to safeguard your health and the health of your clients; it is important to realize that contagious diseases, skin infections, and blood poisoning can be caused by the transmission of infectious material from one individual to another or through the use of unsanitary tools and implements. It is imperative that safe and sanitary work practices become a part of your daily routine. We begin our discussion of infection control with an overview of one-celled microorganisms known as bacteria.

BACTERIOLOGY

Bacteriology (bac-ter-i-OL-o-gy) is the science that deals with the study of microorganisms (my-kroh-OR-gan-iz-ums) called bacteria.

Bacteria (bac-TER-i-a), also known as germs or microbes, are minute, one-celled microorganisms that exist almost everywhere: on the skin; in water, air, decayed matter, and bodily secretions; on the clothing; and beneath the nails. Bacteria can only be seen with the aid of a microscope and are so small that 1,500 rod-shaped bacteria barely reach across the head of a pin.

Types of Bacteria

The hundreds of different kinds of bacteria are classified into two general types depending on whether they consist of beneficial or harmless qualities (nonpathogenic) or harmful or disease-producing characteristics (pathogenic).

1. **Nonpathogenic** (non-path-uh-JEN-ik) organisms make up the majority of bacteria. They can be beneficial or harmless and perform many useful functions such as decomposing refuse and improving the fertility of the soil. Saprophytes (SAH-pruh-fyts) are a type of nonpathogenic bacteria that live on dead matter and do not produce disease. In the human body, nonpathogenic bacteria help to metabolize food, protect against infectious microorganisms, and stimulate the immune response.
2. **Pathogenic** (path-uh-JEN-ik) organisms, although in the minority, are harmful and cause considerable damage by invading plant or human tissues. Pathogenic bacteria produce disease. To this group belong the *parasites,* which require living matter for their growth and survival.

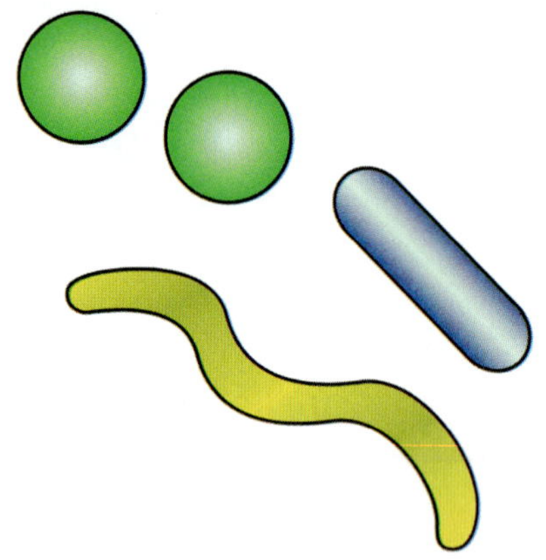

Figure 4-1 Shapes of pathogenic bacteria.

Classifications of Pathogenic Bacteria

Bacteria have distinct shapes that help to identify them. Pathogenic (harmful) bacteria are classified as cocci, bacilli, or spirilla (Figure 4–1).

1. **Cocci** are round-shaped organisms that appear singly or in the following groups (Figure 4–2):
    a) **Staphylococci**: Pus-forming organisms that grow in bunches or clusters. They cause abscesses, pustules, pimples, and boils.
    b) **Streptococci**: Pus-forming organisms that grow in chains. They cause infections such as strep throat, tonsillitis, lung and throat diseases, and blood poisoning.
    c) **Diplococci**: They grow in pairs and cause pneumonia and gonorrhea.

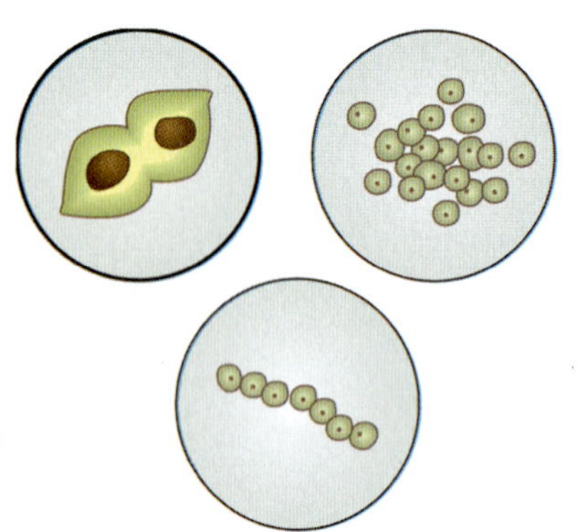

Figure 4-2 Forms of cocci (round).

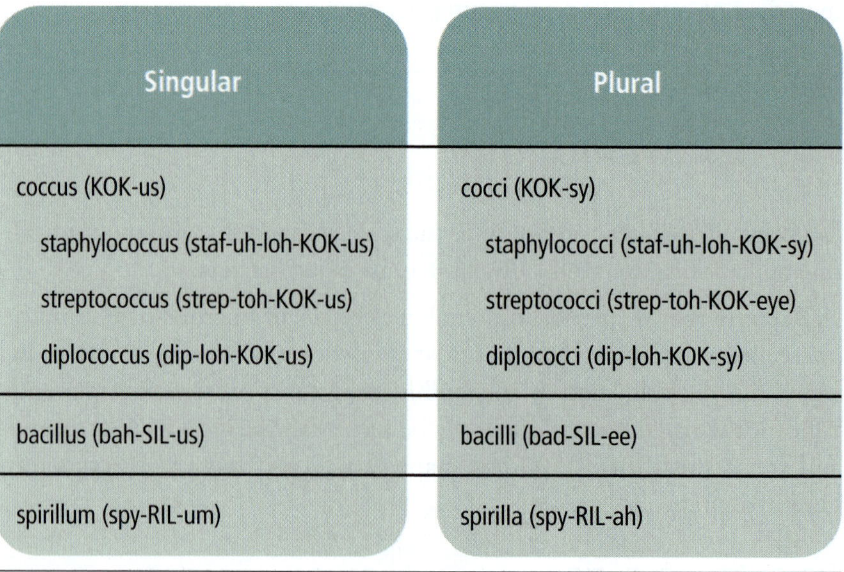

Singular	Plural
coccus (KOK-us)	cocci (KOK-sy)
staphylococcus (staf-uh-loh-KOK-us)	staphylococci (staf-uh-loh-KOK-sy)
streptococcus (strep-toh-KOK-us)	streptococci (strep-toh-KOK-eye)
diplococcus (dip-loh-KOK-us)	diplococci (dip-loh-KOK-sy)
bacillus (bah-SIL-us)	bacilli (bad-SIL-ee)
spirillum (spy-RIL-um)	spirilla (spy-RIL-ah)

Table 4-1 Pronunciations of Terms Relating to Pathogenic Bacteria

4

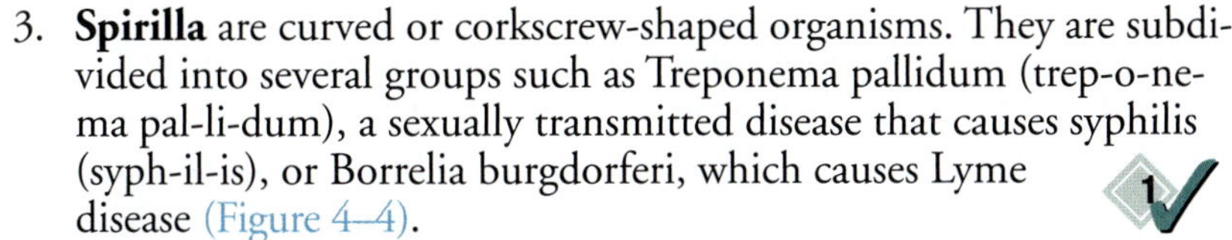

2. **Bacilli** are short, rod-shaped organisms. They are the most common bacteria and produce diseases such as tetanus (lockjaw), typhoid fever, tuberculosis, and diphtheria (Figure 4–3).
3. **Spirilla** are curved or corkscrew-shaped organisms. They are subdivided into several groups such as Treponema pallidum (trep-o-ne-ma pal-li-dum), a sexually transmitted disease that causes syphilis (syph-il-is), or Borrelia burgdorferi, which causes Lyme disease (Figure 4–4).

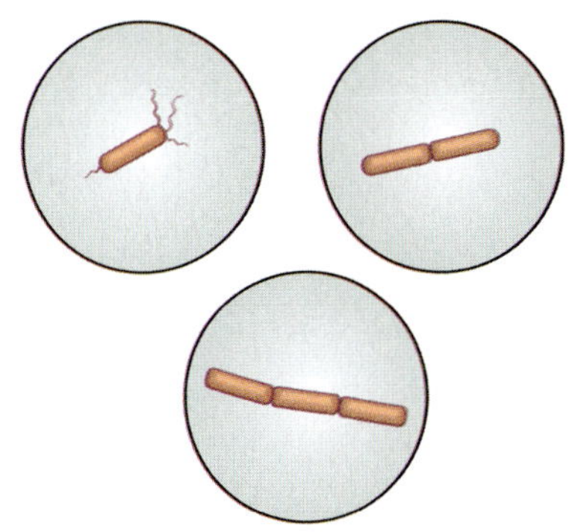

Figure 4-3 Forms of bacilli bacteria.

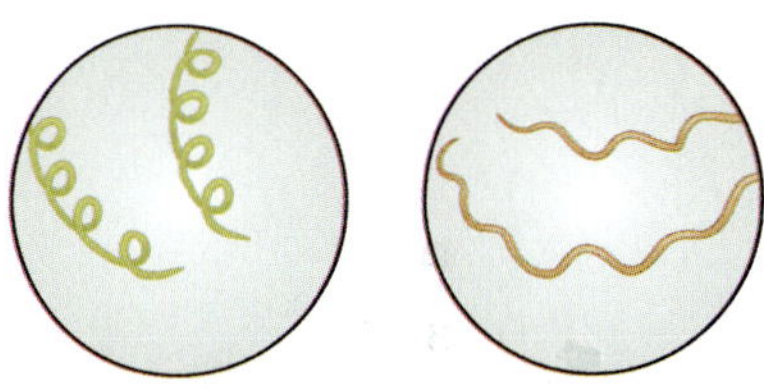

Figure 4-4 Forms of spirilla bacteria.

Movement of Bacteria

Cocci rarely show active motility (self-movement). They are transmitted in the air, in dust, or within the substance in which they settle. Bacilli and spirilla are both motile and use hairlike projections, known as **flagella** (fla-GEL-la) or cilia (CIL-i-a), to move about. A whiplike motion of these hairs propels the bacteria in liquid.

Bacterial Growth and Reproduction

Bacteria generally consist of an outer cell wall and internal protoplasm (see Chapter 7). They manufacture their own food from the surrounding environment, give off waste products, and grow and reproduce. Bacteria have two distinct phases in their life cycle: the **active** or **vegetative stage**, and the **inactive** or **spore-forming stage**.

Active or Vegetative Stage

During the active or vegetative stage, bacteria grow and reproduce. These microorganisms multiply best in warm, dark, damp, and dirty places where sufficient food is present. When conditions are favorable, bacteria grow and reproduce. As food is absorbed, the bacterial cells grow in size. When the maximum growth is reached, the cells divide into two new cells. This division is called **mitosis** (mi-TO-sis) and the cells that are formed are called daughter cells. As mitosis occurs, one bacterium can create as many as 16 million germs in a 12-hour period. When favorable conditions cease to exist, bacteria either die or become inactive.

Inactive or Spore-Forming Stage

Some bacteria can lie dormant. during their inactive stage. Certain bacteria, such as the anthrax and tetanus bacilli, may survive the inactive stage by forming spherical spores that have tough outer coverings to withstand periods of famine, dryness, and unsuitable temperature. In this stage, spores can be blown about in the dust and are not harmed by disinfectants, heat, or cold. When favorable conditions are restored, the spores change into the active form and again start to grow and reproduce.

Bacterial Infections

Pathogenic bacteria become a menace to health when they invade the body. An **infection** occurs if the body is unable to cope with the bacteria and their harmful toxins. There can be no disease without the presence of pathogenic bacteria.

The presence of **pus** is a sign of infection. Pus is a fluid that contains white blood cells, dead and living bacteria, waste matter, tissue elements, and body cells. A **local infection** is indicated by a lesion containing pus and usually appears in a particular area of the body. Infected scrapes or cuts, pimples, and boils are examples of *localized* infections. Staphylococci (*staph*) are among the most common pus-forming human bacteria and are carried by approximately one-third of the population. Staph can be picked up from surfaces such as doorknobs and countertops but is more frequently transferred through skin-to-skin contact or through unclean implements. Antibiotics once controlled these bacteria, but certain strains of staph are now resistant to the drugs. A **general infection** results when the bloodstream carries the bacteria and their toxins to all parts of the body, as in blood poisoning or syphilis. Barbers can help to limit the spread of staph and other diseases by practicing effective sanitation procedures in the barbershop.

When a disease spreads from one person to another by contact, it is considered to be **contagious** or communicable. If a disease simultaneously attacks a large number of people living in a particular area or locality, it is called an epidemic.

Some of the more contagious diseases or disorders that will prevent a barber from servicing clients are tuberculosis, the common cold, ringworm, scabies, head lice, and viral infections. The chief sources of contagion are unclean hands or implements, open sores, pus, oral or nasal discharges, and the common use of drinking cups and towels. Uncovered coughing or sneezing and spitting in public also spread germs. The spread of infection can be prevented and controlled through conscientious personal hygiene, effective sanitation procedures, and public sanitation.

Viruses

A **virus** is a submicroscopic structure so small that it can pass through a porcelain filter. Viruses are capable of infecting almost all plants and animals, including bacteria, and cause common colds, respiratory and gastrointestinal infections, influenza, measles, mumps, chicken pox, smallpox, rabies, yellow fever, hepatitis, polio, and HIV, which causes AIDS.

Viruses live only by penetrating cells and becoming a part of them. Bacteria are organisms that can live on their own. It is for this reason that bacterial infections can usually be treated with specific antibiotics. Generally, viruses are resistant to antibiotics and are hard to kill without harming the body in the process. Although vaccinations can prevent certain viruses from penetrating cells, vaccinations are not available for all virus types.

BLOODBORNE PATHOGENS

Disease-producing bacteria or viruses that are carried through the body in blood or body fluids, such as hepatitis and HIV, are called **bloodborne pathogens.** Blood-to-blood contact might occur if you accidentally cut a client who is HIV-positive or infected with hepatitis and you continue to use the implement without disinfecting it and then puncture your skin or cut another client with the contaminated tool. Similarly, if you are shaving a client's face or neck with a razor or clipper blades, body fluid can be picked up from a blemish or open sore, making transmission possible.

How Pathogens Enter the Body

Pathogenic bacteria or viruses may enter the body by way of:

1. A break in the skin, such as a cut, pimple, or scratch.
2. The mouth (contaminated food or water).
3. The nose (breathing).
4. The eyes or ears.
5. Unprotected sex.

The body fights infection by means of its defensive forces, which include:

1. The unbroken skin, the body's first line of defense.
2. Body secretions such as perspiration and digestive juices.
3. White blood cells, which destroy bacteria.
4. Antitoxins, which counteract the toxins produced by bacteria and viruses.

Infections created by pathogenic bacteria or viruses can be prevented and controlled through personal hygiene and public sanitation.

Sepsis is the poisoned state caused by the absorption of pathogenic microorganisms and their products into the bloodstream. It is because of the possibility of poisoning due to pathogenic bacteria that barber schools and shops must maintain high standards of cleanliness and sanitation in order to achieve an environment that is as **aseptic** (free of disease germs) as possible.

Symptoms are signs of disease. **Subjective symptoms**, such as itching, burning, or pain, can be felt by the person. **Objective symptoms** like pimples, boils, or inflammation can be observed.

Table 4–2 lists general terms and definitions associated with diseases and disorders.

Term	Definition
acute disease	disease having a rapid onset, severe symptoms, and a short course or duration
allergy	reaction due to extreme sensitivity to certain foods, chemicals, or other normally harmless substances
aseptic	freedom from disease germs
chronic disease	disease of long duration, usually mild but recurring
congenital disease	disease that exists at birth
contagious disease	disease that is communicable or transmittable by contact
contraindication	any condition or disease that makes an indicated treatment or medication inadvisable
diagnosis	determination of the nature of a disease from its symptoms
disease	abnormal condition of all or part of the body, organ, or mind that makes it incapable of carrying on normal function
epidemic	appearance of a disease that simultaneously attacks a large number of persons living in a particular locality
etiology	study of the causes of disease and their mode of operation
infectious disease	disease caused by pathogenic microorganisms or viruses that are easily spread
inflammation	condition of some part of the body as a protective response to injury, irritation, or infection, characterized by redness, heat, pain, and swelling
objective symptoms	symptoms that are visible, such as pimples, pustules, or inflammation
occupational disease	illness resulting from conditions associated with employment, such as coming in contact with certain chemicals or tints
parasitic disease	disease caused by vegetable or animal parasites, such as pediculosis and ringworm
pathogenic disease	disease produced by disease-causing bacteria, such as staphylococcus and streptococcus (pus-forming bacteria), or viruses
pathology	science that investigates modifications of the functions and changes in structure caused by disease
prognosis	foretelling of probable course of a disease
seasonal disease	disease influenced by the weather
sepsis	the poisoned state caused by the absorption of pathogenic microorganisms and their products into the bloodstream
subjective symptoms	symptoms that can be felt, such as itching, burning, or pain
systemic disease	disease that affects the body generally, often due to under- or overfunctioning of the internal glands
venereal disease	contagious disease commonly acquired by contact with an infected person during sexual intercourse, characterized by sores and rashes on the skin

Table 4-2 General Terms Relating to Disease

PARASITES

Parasites are plant or animal organisms that live on another living organism, drawing their nourishment from the host organism without giving anything in return.

Plant (vegetable) parasites or **fungi** (FUN-jy), such as molds, mildews, rusts, and yeasts, can produce contagious skin diseases such as ringworm or favus (FAY-vus). Nail fungus can be contracted through improperly disinfected implements or through moisture trapped under nail enhancements. Nail fungus is chronic and usually localized but can be spread to other nails and from client to client if implements are not disinfected before and after each use. Generally, treatment is applied directly to the affected area; however, serious cases require a physician's care (Figure 4–5).

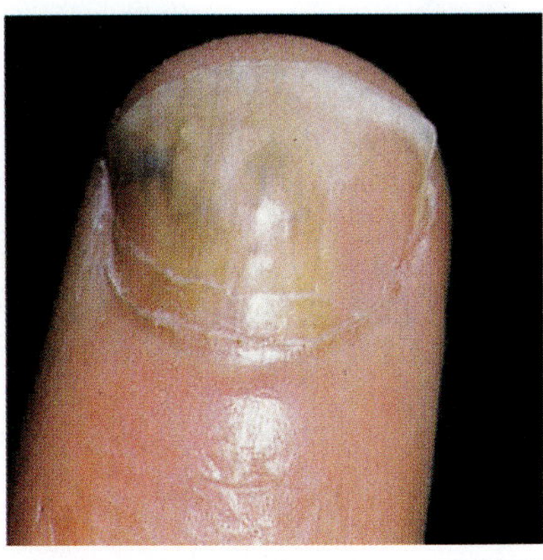

Figure 4-5 Nail fungus.

Animal parasites are also responsible for contagious diseases and conditions. Itch mites can burrow under the skin causing itching and inflammation. This contagious disorder is known as **scabies** (SKAY-beez) and is pictured in Figure 4–6. **Pediculosis** (puh-dik-yuh-LOH-sis) is the technical term for an infestation caused by the head or body louse (Figure 4–7). Neither of these disorders should be treated in the barbershop or school. Clients should be referred to a physician and any tools, equipment, or seating they may have come into contact with should be thoroughly decontaminated with disinfects and pesticides.

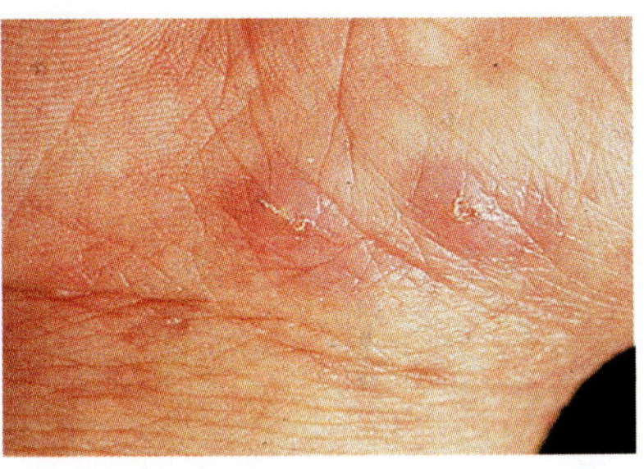

Figure 4-6 Scabies.

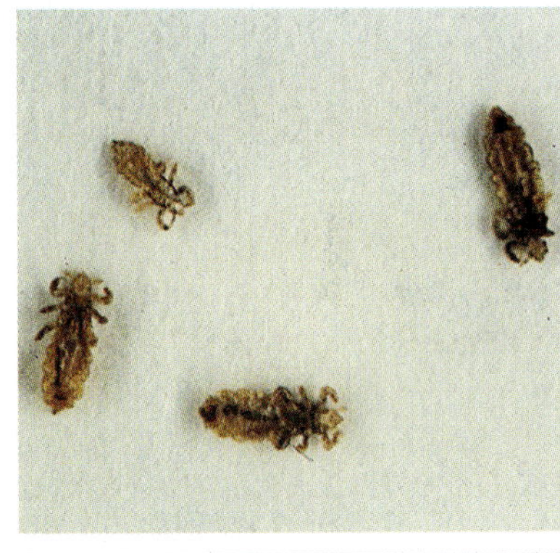

Figures 4-7 Head lice.

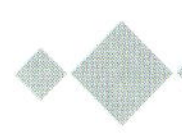

IMMUNITY

Immunity is the ability of the body to resist invasion by bacteria and to destroy bacteria once they have entered the body. Immunity against disease may be natural or acquired and is a sign of good health. **Natural immunity** is the natural resistance to disease that is partially inherited and partially developed through hygienic living. **Acquired immunity** is developed after the body has overcome a disease or through inoculations, such as vaccinations.

A **human disease carrier** is a person who is immune to a disease, but harbors germs that can infect other people. Typhoid (TY-phoid) fever and diphtheria (diph-THER-i-a) may be transmitted in this manner.

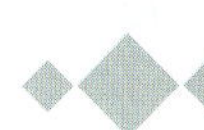

HEPATITIS

Hepatitis is a disease marked by inflammation of the liver. Although it is a bloodborne virus similar to HIV in transmission, it is more easily contracted than HIV because it is present in all body fluids. There are three types of hepatitis that are of concern to barbers.

1. *Hepatitis A Virus* (HAV). This flu-like illness usually lasts about three weeks with symptoms that include jaundice (yellowing of the skin or eyes), fatigue, nausea, fever, abdominal pain, and loss of appetite. The disease is spread through close household contact such as poor sanitation, poor personal hygiene; common bathroom use; contaminated foods and liquids; and sexual contact. Although a person who has recovered from HAV will not get it again, a vaccine is also available to prevent contraction of the disease.
2. *Hepatitis B Virus* (HBV). This form of hepatitis is a serious disease that accumulates in the blood and can cause lifelong hepatitis infection, cirrhosis of the liver, liver failure, liver cancer, and death. Although the disease can mirror flu-like symptoms, about half the people infected with the disease may not show symptoms. The disease can be transmitted through blood products and saliva, sexual contact, or parenteral exposure (piercing mucous membranes or the skin barrier) to blood or blood products. A vaccine is available.
3. *Hepatitis C Virus* (HCV). Hepatitis C can progress slowly and may include symptoms of fatigue and abdominal pain. The disease is transferred through parenteral contact, sexual activity with infected partners, blood transfusions with HCV-contaminated blood, and illegal drug injections. No vaccine is available. 4

HIV/AIDS

A discussion of HIV/AIDS should begin with an understanding of the terms associated with the subject. The most common terms used in conjunction with this topic are:

- human immunodeficiency virus (HIV)
- acquired immunodeficiency syndrome (AIDS)
- AIDS-related complex (ARC)
- Sexually transmitted disease (STD)

4

The **human immunodeficiency virus** (HIV) is the virus that causes AIDS (**acquired immunodeficiency syndrome**). AIDS is the onset of life-threatening illnesses that compromise the immune system as a result of HIV infection and disease.

HIV is passed from person to person through body fluids such as blood, breast milk, semen, and vaginal secretions. The most common methods of transferring the virus are through sexual contact with an infected person, the use of or sharing of dirty hypodermic needles for intravenous drug use, the transfusion of infected blood, and from mother to child during pregnancy and birth.

A person can be infected with HIV for up to 11 years without having symptoms and, if not tested, may not realize that they are infecting other people. Unlike most other viruses, HIV is not transferred through casual contact with an infected person, sneezing, or coughing because it is not an airborne virus; nor is it transmitted by holding hands, hugging, or sharing household items like telephones or toilet seats. It can, however, enter the bloodstream though cuts and sores and may be transmitted in the barbershop by improperly sanitized sharp implements. For example, if you were to cut a client infected with HIV or full-blown AIDS you might transfer blood to a haircutting implement, razor, manicuring implement, etc. Then, if you cut another client and transfer the infected blood to the second client through the wound, that client also risks being infected.

Although the human immunodeficiency virus may lie dormant in an infected person's system for 10 years or more, it can also mature into a fatal disease in 2 to 10 years. Testing for the virus may be performed on an anonymous basis and should be sought if an individual has engaged in any behavior that puts them at risk of being infected.

The immune system works to defend the body against infection. Especially important in this process are the following body parts and systems: the bone marrow, where lymphocytes (B and T cells) are manufactured; the thymus gland, where T cells mature; the lymphoreticular system, which provides storage sites for mature B and T cells; and the bloodstream, which contains cellular elements of the immune system.

Leukocytes, or white blood cells, are divided into two categories, lymphocytes and phagocytic cells. T-4 cells, a type of lymphocyte, trigger appropriate responses from other specialized white blood cells, such as activating the cells to produce the antibodies.

Remember that a virus is the smallest disease-producing microorganism. Consisting of genes surrounded by a protein layer, a virus is able to reproduce within the body by utilizing specific body cells.

One of the most difficult aspects of treating HIV infection is that HIV is a retrovirus. This means that the virus uses the reproductive processes of the host cell (to which it becomes attached) to duplicate itself.

When HIV enters the bloodstream, it searches for a CD4 molecule to which it can attach itself. CD4 molecules are present on T-helper cells (among others), and very often the virus attaches itself to this specific cell. Once attached, these cells are considered target cells. The virus then sheds its outer covering of protein and enters the target cell through the area of attachment. The T cell signals the B cells to produce antibodies, while the HIV begins to convert RNA into viral DNA. Once converted, the altered DNA has the ability to pass into the nucleus of the target cell, where duplication begins. The newly formed viral process begins again, leaving the destroyed T cell in its wake. This lowers the strength of the immune system, with the result that the body becomes susceptible to opportunistic diseases, which can eventually cause death.

HIV is considered to be a weak virus when compared to other viruses such as polio; however, unlike polio, which has characteristics that respond to treatment, once HIV locks into the T cell in the bloodstream, it is nearly impossible to destroy. HIV is not thought to survive in open environments, especially when subjected to cold surfaces, drying, or ultraviolet light, and can be killed through the use of household bleach or hospital-grade disinfectants. The virus cannot live in food or drink. Coughing and sneezing will not transmit HIV because it is not an airborne virus. There should be no risk from handling the linens of HIV or AIDS-infected persons as long as universal precautions are followed and there is no direct contact with the blood or bodily fluids.

The Stages of HIV/AIDS

Once HIV has entered the bloodstream and the immune response begins, antibodies will normally be produced within a range of two weeks to six months. The production of the antibodies is known as seroconversion. At this point, HIV can be passed along to others.

The symptom stages are as follows:

Stage 1—HIV infection: no physical indications of illness; antibodies to virus may be present.

Stage 2—ARC: chronic fatigue; unexplained chills, fever, or night sweats; 10 percent or greater weight loss without dieting; skin disorders; enlarged liver and/or spleen; swollen lymph glands; chronic diarrhea.

Stage 3—AIDS: all of the above symptoms, as well as hair loss; skin and other cancers; pneumonia and other infections; and nerve and brain damage. Individuals in the final stage of HIV infection (full-blown AIDS) usually exhibit the most severe characteristics of the disease.

Preventing HIV/AIDS

To date, there is no vaccine to prevent HIV infection, nor is there a cure for AIDS. Early intervention is the key to obtaining whatever treatments are available that may be beneficial in improving the immune response and the delay of the progression of the disease.

Those individuals who are at risk of contracting HIV/AIDS may be helped by eliminating all known causes of immune system suppression and by utilizing any and all therapies that stimulate immune system function. The correct diet, including vitamin, mineral, and herbal supplements; exercise; a healthy environment; and a proper mental attitude all contribute to the well-being of the immune system.

In many states, professionals are currently required to attend an HIV/AIDS education course prior to licensure and license renewal, and in some cases, HIV/AIDS instruction has been added to school curriculum requirements. Strict adherence to precautionary and sanitary measures in the workplace assists in the protection of the health, safety, and welfare of professionals and their clients. Universal precautions will be discussed in

Chapter 5 and should be followed at all times.

The following suggestions may also serve as helpful reminders to student barbers:

- Avoid accidents and practice all safety precautions applicable to the shop or school.
- Wash hands with an antibacterial soap before and after servicing each client.
- Always sanitize tools and implements before and after each client.
- Sanitize equipment, such as headrests; chair backs; armrests; and facial, massage and manicure tables, before and after client services.
- Use disposable gloves whenever possible.
- If you cut, nick, or scrape yourself, treat the wound immediately and cover it.
- If you cut, nick, or scrape a client, apply gloves and treat wound to the extent of your state board allowances and limitations.
- Avoid exposure and contact with another person's bodily fluids, especially blood.
- Attend available seminars and classes that provide updates on HIV/AIDS research.
- If you feel there is any chance that you have contracted HIV, or if you simply wish to ease your mind, have an HIV antibody test performed. Keep in mind your responsibility to others and to yourself to minimize the risk of spreading this fatal disease.

As you will also learn in Chapter 5, bacteria may be destroyed through the use of disinfectants; intense heat such as boiling, steaming, baking, or burning; and ultraviolet rays. 5

spotlight on

Dianna Chute Kenneally

Dianna Chute Kenneally is a Senior Hair Scientist at P&G Beauty in Cincinnati, Ohio. She has 21 years experience in research and has been developing hair care products for the past 12 years. She has a degree in chemical engineering from Case Western Reserve University and a business degree from Xavier University. Most recently, Kenneally worked with Milady to bring the latest scientific and medical findings about hair and dandruff care products to barbers and cosmetologists.

It seems I've always been interested in a career in science. My father was a chemical engineer during the heyday of the space race. My parents encouraged my sisters and I to pursue our interests in science, where opportunities for women were growing by leaps and bounds. During college I spent several summers working for chemical and consumer goods companies. That is when I realized the tremendous role chemistry plays in consumer products—things we all use. I knew then that I wanted to work on products that made people's lives a little better everyday and have some fun in the process. P&G Beauty has been the perfect fit for me. I have had the opportunity to work directly with stylists, barbers, dermatologists, and consumers while researching new high-tech hair care formulas and products.

What an amazing time to be a hair care scientist! The past 20 years have seen rapid technological innovation, particularly in shampoo formulations. Prior to 1987, shampoos had to strike a balance between good cleaning ability and overdrying hair. The introduction of Pert Plus, the first 2-in-1 shampoo containing silicone, started a revolution. Shampoos no longer had to compromise on cleaning ability to leave hair feeling smooth and soft. As manufacturers learned more about silicone they also learned how to deposit other beneficial ingredients, like volumizers, moisturizers, and fragrances, on the hair and scalp. Benefits such as shine and improved fullness can now be provided through shampoo. As a result of new technologies, anti-dandruff shampoos have also left behind the harsh and smelly formulas of the past. Modern anti-dandruff shampoos deliver active ingredients like pyrithione zinc to the scalp more efficiently, eliminate dandruff faster, and provide the same benefits to the hair and pleasant user experiences as cosmetic shampoos.

In the future, I believe hair care products will continue to become more specialized and efficacious. Consumers want products designed for their individual hair type and style—with no compromises. In particular, with the aging of the baby boomers you will see more clients concerned about thinning hair and loss of pigment and texture. Many scientists are looking at genetics for answers to prevent age-related hair changes. In the meantime, we will see more products utilizing advanced polymer and conditioner formulations designed to help improve the thickness and shine of aging hair and to protect color from fading.

chapter glossary

acquired immunodeficiency syndrome	AIDS is the onset of life-threatening illnesses that compromise the immune system as a result of HIV infection and disease
acquired immunity	an immunity that the body develops after it overcomes a disease or through inoculation
active stage (vegetative)	the stage in which bacteria grow and reproduce. Also known as the vegetative stage
aseptic	free of disease germs
bacilli	rod-shaped bacteria that produce diseases such as tetanus, typhoid fever, tuberculosis, and diphtheria
bacteria	one-celled microorganisms also known as germs or microbes
bloodborne pathogens	disease-causing bacteria or viruses that are carried through the body in the blood or body fluids
cocci	round-shaped bacteria that appear singly or in groups
contagious (communicable)	a disease that may be transmitted by contact
diplococci	round-shaped bacteria that cause diseases such as pneumonia
flagella	hairlike extensions that propel bacteria through liquid
fungi	plant parasites such as molds, mildew, yeasts, and rusts that can cause ringworm and favus
general infection	an infection that results when the bloodstream carries bacteria or viruses to all parts of the body
hepatitis	a bloodborne disease marked by inflammation of the liver
human disease carrier	a person who is immune to a disease, but harbors germs that can infect other people
human immunodeficiency virus	the virus that causes AIDS
immunity	the ability of the body to resist invasion by bacteria and to destroy bacteria once they have entered the body
inactive stage (spore-forming)	the stage in which certain bacteria can lie dormant until conditions are right for growth and reproduction
infection	the result when the body is unable to cope with the invasion of bacteria and their harmful toxins
local infection	an infection that is limited to a specific spot or area of the body
mitosis	the division of cells during reproduction
natural immunity	A natural resistance to disease that is partially inherited and partially developed
nonpathogenic	beneficial or harmless bacteria that perform many useful functions
objective symptoms	symptoms that can be seen
parasites	plant or animal organisms that live on other living organisms without giving anything in return
pathogenic	harmful, disease-producing bacteria

pediculosis	a contagious infestation caused by head or body louse
pus	a fluid that contains white blood cells, dead and living bacteria, waste matter, tissue elements, and body cells; is a sign of infection
scabies	a contagious disorder caused by the itch mite
sepsis	a poisoned state caused by the absorption of pathogenic microorganisms into the bloodstream
spirilla	curved or corkscrew-shaped bacteria that can cause syphilis and Lyme disease
staphylococci	pus-forming bacteria that cause abscesses, pustules, pimples, and boils
streptococci	pus-forming bacteria that cause infections such as strep throat, tonsillitis, lung and throat diseases, and blood poisoning
subjective symptoms	symptoms that can be felt or experienced
virus	an infectious agent that lives only by penetrating cells and becoming a part of them

chapter review questions

1. What are bacteria?
2. Name and describe the two main classifications of bacteria.
3. Name and describe three forms of pathogenic bacteria.
4. How do bacteria move about?
5. How do bacteria multiply?
6. Describe the active and inactive stages of bacteria.
7. Name the most common pus-forming human bacteria.
8. What is a contagious or communicable disease?
9. How can infections be controlled or prevented?
10. What are the differences between local and general infections?
11. What are the differences between bacteria and viruses?
12. What is the definition of a natural immunity? Acquired immunity?
13. Why is hepatitis more easily contracted than HIV?
14. Identify the virus that causes AIDS. Define AIDS.
15. What methods can be used to destroy bacteria?

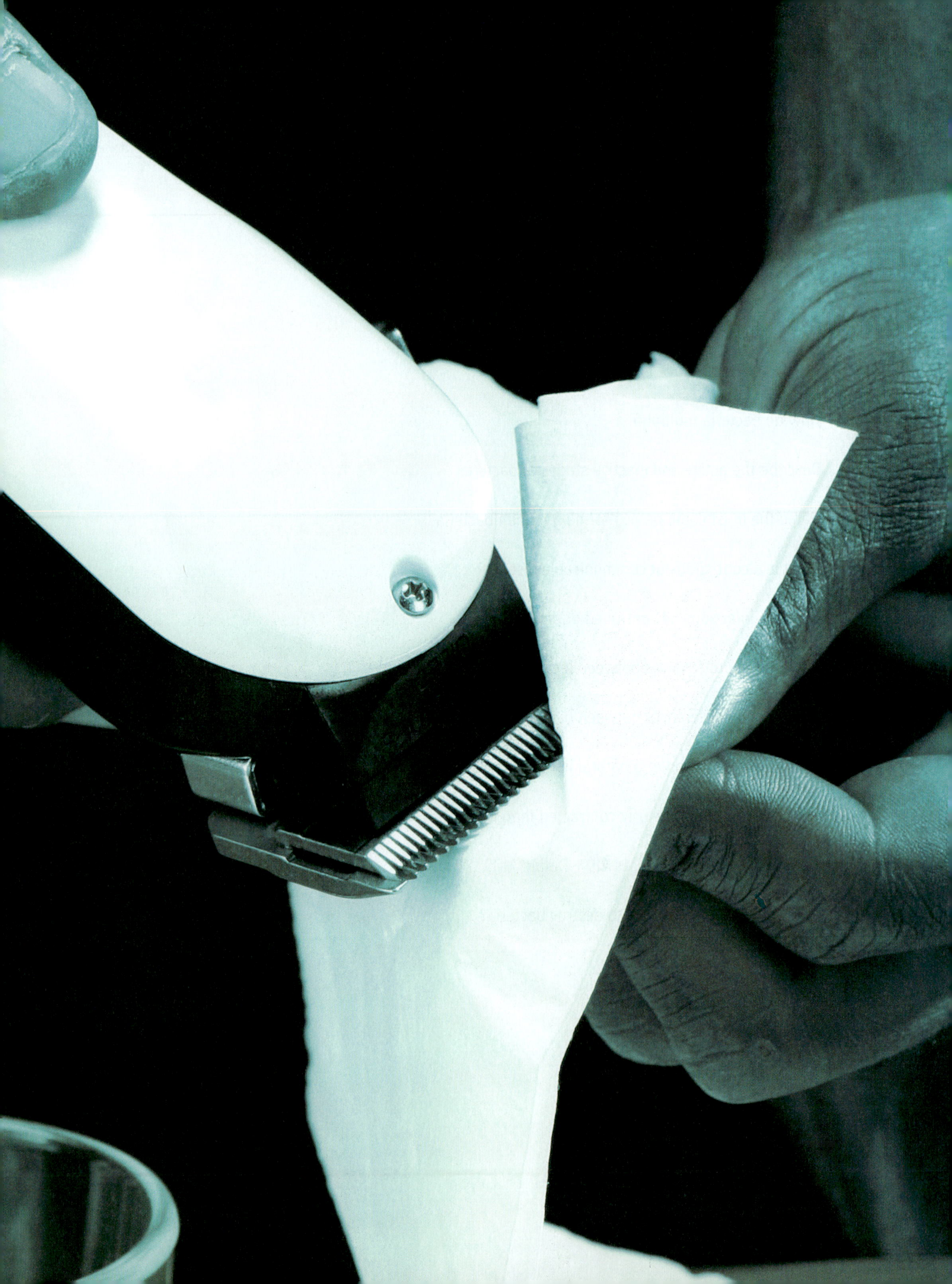

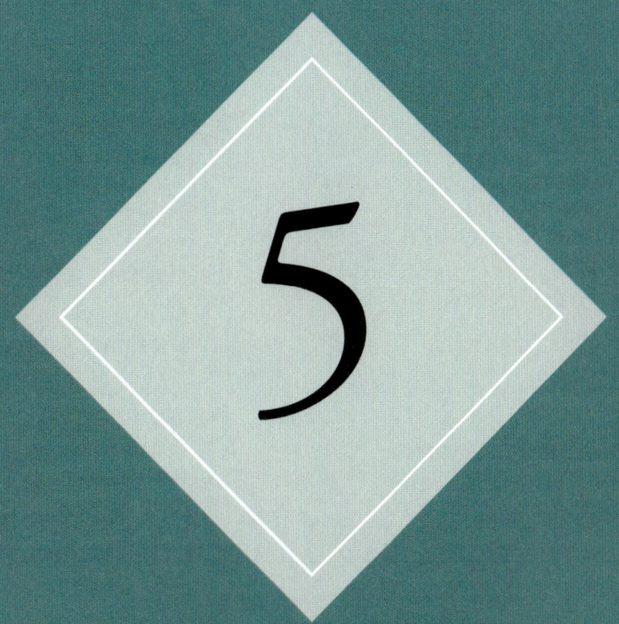

INFECTION CONTROL AND SAFE WORK PRACTICES

Chapter Outline

Principles of Prevention and Control • Levels of Prevention and Control
Solutions and Strengths • Sanitizers • Disinfection Procedures
Universal Precautions • OSHA • Public Sanitation
Safe Work Practices • Professional Responsibility

Learning Objectives

After completing this chapter, you should be able to:

1. Discuss the ways in which infectious materials may be transmitted in the barbershop.
2. Define decontamination.
3. List three levels of decontamination used for the prevention and control of pathogen transmittal.
4. Identify the chemical decontamination agents most commonly used in barbershops.
5. Demonstrate proper decontamination procedures for tools, equipment, and surfaces.
6. Discuss Universal Precautions and your responsibilities as a professional barber.

Key Terms

State barber boards and health departments require that sanitary measures be applied while serving the public. Contagious diseases, skin infections, and blood poisoning can be caused by the transmission of infectious material from one individual to another or through the use of unsanitized combs, clippers, razors, shears, or other barbering tools and implements. As a professional barber, it is your responsibility to employ sanitation methods that will help to safeguard your health and the health of your clients.

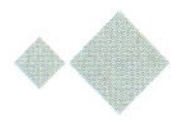

PRINCIPLES OF PREVENTION AND CONTROL

A client's first impression of the shop begins the moment they open the door, so a clean and sanitary environment should extend beyond each barber's immediate work area. All of the sights, sounds, smells, and general ambience of the barbershop meld together to form this impression regardless of how many times a client has visited the shop. In essence, this "first" impression happens over and over again because clients do not see you or the shop daily. A clean and orderly barbershop will help build client confidence and trust in you and your coworkers because it shows them that care is being taken to provide a safe and professional business environment.

Contamination

No matter how clean a surface looks, it is probably contaminated. Bacteria, viruses, and fungi act as contaminants and can be found almost anywhere. In the barbershop, these microorganisms can live on tools, implements, styling chairs, countertops, and even in the air; therefore, it is the barber's responsibility to control the spread of infection and disease through the use of effective sanitation methods.

Decontamination

It would be virtually impossible to keep the barbershop free from all contamination. However, there are methods available that will ensure an optimum level of cleanliness. The removal of pathogens and other substances from tools or surfaces is called **decontamination.**

Decontamination involves the use of *physical* or *chemical* means to remove, inactivate, or destroy pathogens to make an object safe for handling, use, or disposal. The three main levels of decontamination are sterilization, disinfection, and sanitation. State barber boards and health departments require only *disinfection* and *sanitation* procedures since these are the most efficient and effective methods for infection control in the barbershop environment. 

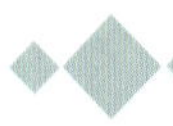

LEVELS OF PREVENTION AND CONTROL

Sterilization is the process of rendering an object germ-free by destroying all living organisms on a surface. Although it is the highest level of effective decontamination, it is not a practical option in the barbershop because the sterilization of metal implements would require either steaming in an autoclave or dry heat (in the form of baking) to be rendered truly *sterile*. These methods are too time-consuming and require expensive equipment.

Health departments and state barber boards recognize that it is virtually impossible to completely sterilize barbering tools and implements, therefore it is generally recognized that this equipment will be disinfected or sanitized rather than sterilized. Throughout the text, the terms *sanitize* or *sanitizing* is used to denote the act of thoroughly cleaning an item or surface with soap or detergents and water or as a required first step in the disinfection process. The terms *disinfect* or *disinfection* is used to indicate the process of thoroughly cleaning and disinfecting a tool or surface with chemical agents to achieve an optimum level of decontamination in the barbershop environment.

Disinfection is a higher level of decontamination than sanitation and second only to sterilization. Disinfection requires the use of chemical disinfectants to destroy most bacteria and some viruses.

Sanitation or sanitizing is the third or lowest level of decontamination and may be known as sanitation or sanitizing. To sanitize means to "significantly reduce the number of pathogens found on a surface." Barbering tools, implements, and other surfaces are sanitized or cleansed by washing with soaps or detergents and are disinfected through the application of chemical disinfectants. Hand washing or antiseptics applied on the skin are also forms of sanitation.

Prevention and Control Agents

The agents or methods used to decontaminate barbering tools and shop surfaces are either physical or chemical in nature. As will be seen, chemical agents are usually the more efficient and effective choice of professional barbers and regulatory agencies.

Physical Agents

Physical agents such as moist heat (boiling water), steaming (autoclave), and dry heat are rarely used in today's barbershops. Generally speaking, these methods are impractical, inefficient, and expensive in terms of time, convenience, and cost. The only physical methods still used routinely in barbershop sanitation procedures are the ultraviolet rays housed within an electric UV sanitizer. An ultraviolet-ray electric sanitizer will keep disinfected tools and implements sanitary until they are removed for use.

Chemical Agents

Chemical agents are the most effective sanitizing and disinfecting methods used in barbershops to destroy or check the spread of pathogenic bacteria. Within the chemical agents group are antiseptics and disinfectants. See Table 5-1 for a listing of these products.

Antiseptics are substances that *may* kill, retard, or prevent the growth of bacteria and can generally be used safely on the skin. Because they are weaker than disinfectants, antiseptics are not effective for use on implements and surfaces. Hydrogen peroxide is a good example of an antiseptic.

Disinfectants are the chemical agents used to destroy most bacteria and some viruses. They are used to disinfect and control microorganisms on hard, nonporous surfaces such as clipper blades, shears, and razors, but should *never be used on the skin, hair, or nails*. Any chemical agent or substance that is powerful enough to destroy pathogens can also damage skin. 3

Types of Chemical Disinfectants

There are many prepared chemical disinfectant products available for use in the barbershop. To perform the *optimum level* of disinfection, disinfectants must be effective against bacteria (bactericide), fungi (fungicide), viruses (virucide), tuberculosis (tuberculocidal), Pseudomonas (pseudomonacidal), HIV-1, and Hepatitis B. The ability to combat these organisms places this type of disinfectant into the **hospital-grade tuberculocidal disinfectant** group. The extent to which a disinfectant is effective against specific organisms and/or is considered an **EPA-registered disinfectant** is found on the product label. Consult your barber board or health department for a list of approved disinfectants in your state and consider the requirements of a good disinfectant as follows:

1. Convenient to prepare.
2. Quick acting.
3. Preferably odorless.
4. Noncorrosive.
5. Economical.
6. Nonirritating to the skin. (Caution: Most disinfectants will cause skin irritation at some point. Avoid prolonged contact.)

In addition to hospital-level disinfectants, other chemicals commonly used in the barbershop include sodium hypochlorite, quaternary ammonium compounds, phenols, alcohols, and prepared commercial products.

Sodium Hypochlorite

Sodium hypochlorite (common household bleach) compounds are frequently used to provide the disinfecting agent chlorine. One of the key advantages of chlorine is its ability to destroy viruses, so many prepared disinfectants contain sodium hypochlorite. A 10% solution is recommended with an immersion time of 10 minutes. (See formulation directions in Table 5–1.)

CAUTION

Disinfectants must be approved by the Environmental Protection Agency (EPA) and by each individual state. When choosing a disinfectant product, look for the EPA registration number on the label. This assures that the product is safe and effective. It should be noted that although disinfectants may be safe to use, they are still too harsh for human skin or eye contact. Always wear gloves and safety glasses to prevent accidental exposure.

CAUTION

In the past, fumigants in the form of formaldehyde vapors have been used in dry cabinet sanitizers to keep sanitized implements sanitary. Tablet or liquid formalin releases formaldehyde gas, which has since proven to be irritating to the eyes, nose, throat, and lungs. Formaldehyde can cause skin allergies and has long been suspected of being a cancer-causing agent. Although formalin is an effective disinfectant, it is not safe for shop or salon disinfection. Many states have prohibited the use of formalin; refer to your state board rules and regulations for specific or updated information.

Quaternary Ammonium Compounds

Quaternary Ammonium Compounds (quats) are effective disinfectants for sanitizing tools and may also be used to clean countertops. Quats are odorless, nontoxic, and fast acting, requiring a short disinfection time. Most quat solutions disinfect implements in 10–15 minutes, but the time will vary depending on the strength of the solution. Check the product label to make sure that it contains a rust inhibitor and avoid long-term immersion of implements. Leaving some tools in the solution too long may damage them. Traditionally, a 1:1000 solution has been used to sanitize implements with an immersion time of one to five minutes. Refer to your state barber board rules and regulations for their specific requirements and always follow the manufacturer's directions when preparing the solution.

Phenols

Phenols, like quats, have been used to disinfect implements for many years. Although caustic and toxic, phenols are relatively safe and extremely effective when used according to the directions. Care should be taken with rubber and plastic materials as they may become softened or discolored with continued phenol use. In addition, phenolic disinfectants can cause skin irritation, so avoid skin contact and wear protective gear. Concentrated phenols can seriously burn the skin and eyes, and are poisonous if ingested.

Did you know...

In states requiring hospital-level disinfection, the use of alcohol for decontamination purposes may be illegal since alcohol is not an EPA-registered disinfectant. To be safe, check with your state barber board or health department.

Alcohol

Alcohol is an organic compound. While there are many types of alcohols used in science and manufacturing, the two most common forms utilized by barbers are ethyl alcohol and isopropyl alcohol. In some states, it may be permissible to use 70% to 90% ethyl or isopropyl alcohol products to disinfect implements such as shears, razors, or the glass electrodes of high-frequency machines used for facial and scalp treatments. A 50–60% isopropyl alcohol may be used on the skin as an antiseptic and alcohol-based hand sanitizing gels may be used when water is not readily available.

Prepared commercial products

Prepared commercial products are available in a variety of formulations and may be purchased through barber supply and retail stores. Products such as Lysol or Pine-Sol are sufficient for the all-purpose cleaning of doorknobs, walls, and floors. Others, like Clippercide and Marvicide, are designed for the disinfection of clippers, trimmers, and metal implements. Current formulations of these products are effective against bacteria, fungi, and viruses and are usually available in liquid and spray formulas. As a cautionary note, commercially prepared products designed for use on clippers usually perform at least one of three functions: disinfection, lubrication, or cooling. While there are products that may accomplish all three tasks, others may perform only one, so read labels carefully before purchasing and know the intended function of the product.

Antiseptics

Name	Form	Solution Strength	Use (Follow manufacturer's directions)
Boric acid	Crystals	2–5%	Cleanse eyes and skin.
Hydrogen peroxide	Liquid	3–5%	Cleanse skin and minor cuts.
Isopropyl alcohol (Rubbing alcohol)	Liquid	50–60%	Skin, cuts. Not to be used if irritation is present.
Sodium hypochlorite	Crystals	.5%	Rinse the hands.
Styptic (alum)	Stick, powder, or liquid		Stops bleeding of nicks or slight cuts in the skin. Use powder or liquid form only. Apply with cotton swab and discard.
Tincture of iodine	Liquid	2%	Cleanse cuts and wounds.

Disinfectants

Name	Form	Solution Strength	Use (Follow manufacturer's directions)
Commercial products	Liquids, sprays	Per manufacturer	Disinfect and/or cool, and lubricate clippers, trimmers, etc. Apply for 3–10 minutes per manufacturer's directions.
Ethyl alcohol (Grain alcohol)	Liquid	70–90%	Immerse sharp cutting edges or glass electrodes for a minimum of 10 minutes.
Isopropyl alcohol (Rubbing alcohol)	Liquid	70–90%	Immerse sharp cutting edges or glass electrodes for a minimum of 10 minutes.
Phenols	Liquid	10%	Floors, sinks, etc.
Quats	Powder, tablet, or liquid	1:1000	Immerse for 5–20 minutes. Check with state barber board and manufacturer's directions.
Sodium hypochlorite	Liquid	10%	Immerse sharp cutting edges or glass electrodes for a minimum of 10 minutes.

Table 5-1 Antiseptic and Disinfectant Products Used in the Practice of Barbering

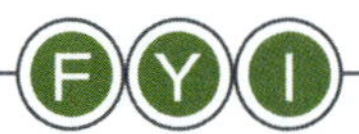

Mixing chemicals stronger than recommended by the manufacturer may counteract the effectiveness of the product. Always read manufacturers' directions.

QUATS SOLUTIONS

Quats solutions are acceptable for cleaning surfaces in the barbershop (unless specified otherwise in the manufacturer's directions), but you may wish to clean floors, sinks, toilet bowls, and waste receptacles with commercial cleaners such as Lysol or Pine-Sol. Both of these products are effective household-level disinfectants for general cleaning purposes. Deodorant tablets or air freshener products are useful to offset unpleasant odors and should be replaced regularly. 4

SOLUTIONS AND STRENGTHS

As a barber, your work will require the use of a variety of solutions for different purposes. As you have already learned, disinfectants are essential for the decontamination of fixtures, surfaces, tools, and implements. Antiseptics are used for cleansing the hands and for treating minor cuts and abrasions.

In many cases, a premixed commercial preparation such as *blade wash* will be used; however, other formulations, such as quats and phenols, are less costly when purchased in concentrated form. Since the purchase of disinfectant products in concentrate form requires the formulation of a solution, it is important to become familiar with the terms associated with solution preparation.

A **solution** is the product resulting from the combining and dissolving of a solute in a solvent.

The **solute** is the substance that is dissolved and the **solvent** is the liquid in which a solute is dissolved. For example: In a solution of sugar water, the sugar is the solute and water is the solvent.

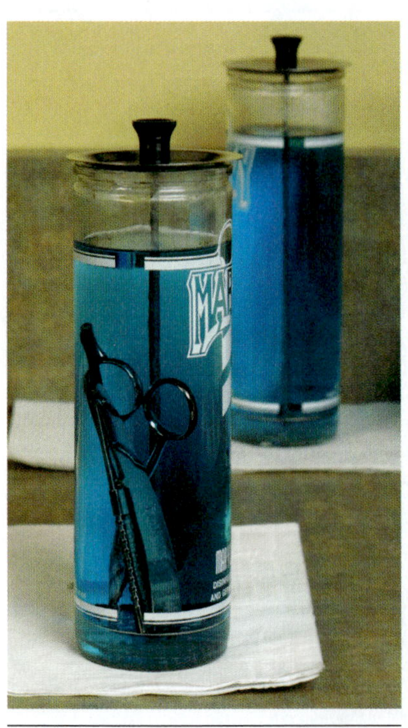

Figure 5-1 Wet sanitizer.

There can be no doubt that the most economical method of using disinfectant chemicals in the barbershop is to purchase the product in concentrated form. Concentrates are formulated to be diluted with water to the required strength, thereby eliminating the higher cost of premixed solutions.

In the preparation of a solution, the amount of solute indicates the strength of the solution. Therefore, the *strength* of a solution indicates how much *solute* there is in the formulation. For example: A 10% solution (or strength) of sodium hypochlorite means that 10% or $\frac{1}{10}$ of the solution is sodium hypochlorite and the remaining 90% or $\frac{9}{10}$ is water.

The strength of a solution is identified by the percentage of solute. The percent figure indicates one of two measurements, either the percentage of solute by *weight* or the percentage of solute by *volume.*

Example by weight: A container holds a total solution of 100 grams. If it is labeled as a 5% solution, it means that there are 5 grams of solute in the formulation.

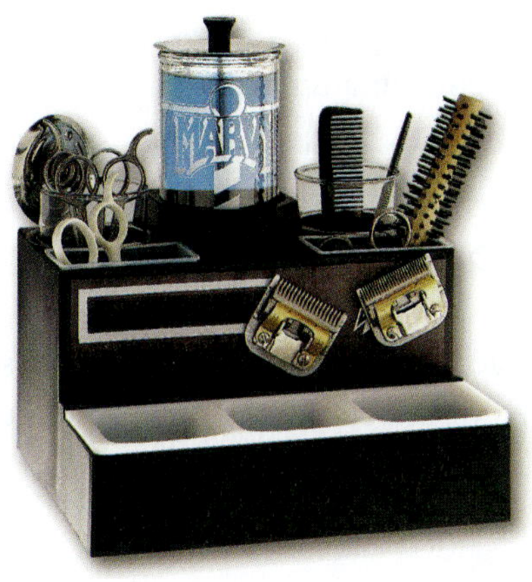

Figure 5–2 Wet sanitizer.

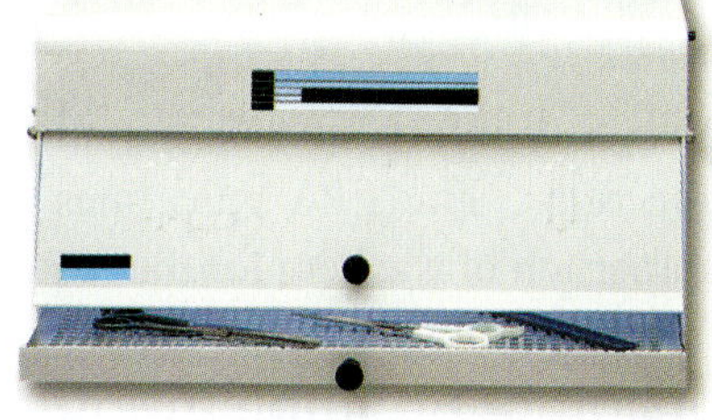

Figure 5–3 Ultraviolet-ray sanitizer.

Example by volume: A 1-gallon container contains a 20% by volume solution. This means that 20% of the solution is solute. Let's say you want to duplicate the formula. You would have to know the number of ounces of solute and solvent needed to mix the formula. There are 128 ounces in a gallon, therefore 20% or 25.6 ounces of solute and 80% or 102.4 ounces of solvent would be needed to duplicate the solution.

Because the percent figure measures either weight or volume, you need to pay attention when reading labels. Simply remember that, like strength, the percentage tells you how much solute there is in the solution. Now that you are familiar with the preparation of solutions, the next step is to discuss the various sanitizing units available for use in the barbershop.

SANITIZERS

A **wet sanitizer** is a covered receptacle large enough to hold a disinfectant solution in which objects can be completely immersed. Wet sanitizers are available in a variety of shapes and sizes so select the size most appropriate for the tools or implements that you will be disinfecting (Figures 5–1 and 5–2).

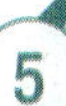

Ultraviolet-ray sanitizers are usually metal cabinets with ultraviolet lamps or bulbs that are used to store disinfected tools and implements. They are effective for keeping clean brushes, combs, and implements sanitary until ready for use, but they are not capable of sanitizing or decontaminating an object. Items must be thoroughly disinfected before being placed in the sanitizer. Follow the manufacturer's directions for proper use and check your state barber board regulations concerning the use of ultraviolet-ray cabinets (Figure 5–3).

A **dry or cabinet sanitizer** is an airtight cabinet containing an active fumigant such as formalin. This fumigant produces a formaldehyde vapor that destroys bacteria on tools and implements. Although dry sanitizers used to be a standard barbershop fixture for the disinfection and storage of tools, modern methods and products have replaced them. Today, barbers

CAUTION

Prior to using disinfectant solutions for metal tools and implements, make sure that the product contains a rust inhibitor such as *sodium nitrate*.

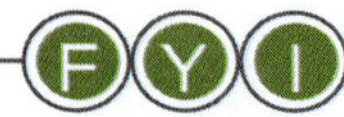

Tools and implements must be cleaned prior to disinfectant immersion to comply with decontamination rules and to avoid solution contamination.

The procedures for the immersion of implements into a chemical solution must conform to the state board of barbering regulations in your state.

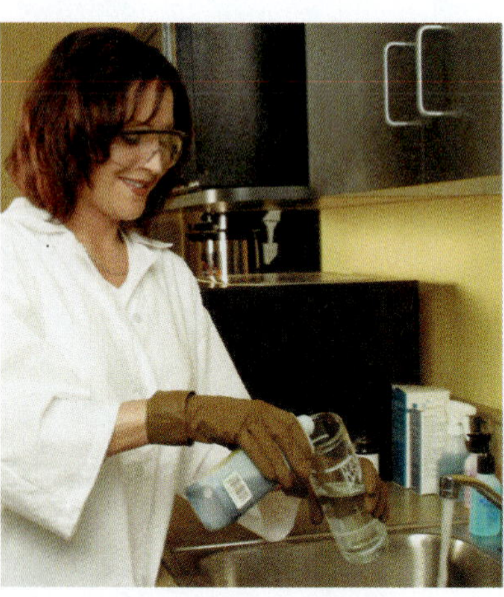

Figure 5-4 Read manufacturer's directions and mix accordingly.

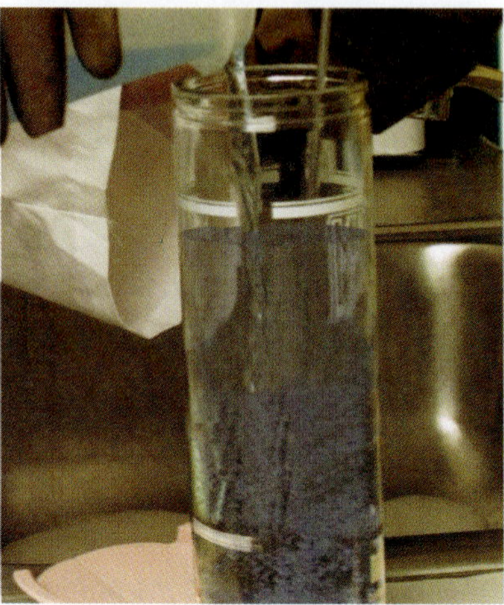

Figure 5-5 Carefully pour disinfectant into the water when preparing disinfectant solution.

may store their disinfected implements in closed plastic containers, plastic wrap, or "zip-lock" plastic bags to help prevent contamination.

DISINFECTION PROCEDURES

Always disinfect tools and implements according to the manufacturer's directions. The EPA guidelines for wet disinfectants require complete immersion of the item for the required amount of time.

Disinfecting Implements

Tools and implements must be disinfected. These include combs, brushes, clipper guards, shears, razors, and any other items that can be immersed in a disinfectant solution.

Quats Solution Disinfection

1. Read manufacturer's directions for quats or other disinfectant solution. Mix accordingly (Figures 5–4 and 5–5). To mix a 1:1000 quat solution, add 1¼ oz. quat solute to 1 gallon of water. Add the quats concentrate after filling the container with water to eliminate excessive suds formation.
2. Remove hair from combs, brushes, etc. (Figure 5–6).
3. Wash item(s) thoroughly with hot water and soap.
4. Rinse item(s) thoroughly and pat dry.
5. Place item(s) in the wet sanitizer containing the disinfectant solution, immersing completely. Disinfect for the recommended time (Figure 5–7).
6. Remove item(s) from the disinfectant and rinse thoroughly (Figure 5–8).
7. Dry item(s) with a clean towel.
8. Store item(s) in a dry cabinet sanitizer, UV sanitizer, or other clean covered container until needed.

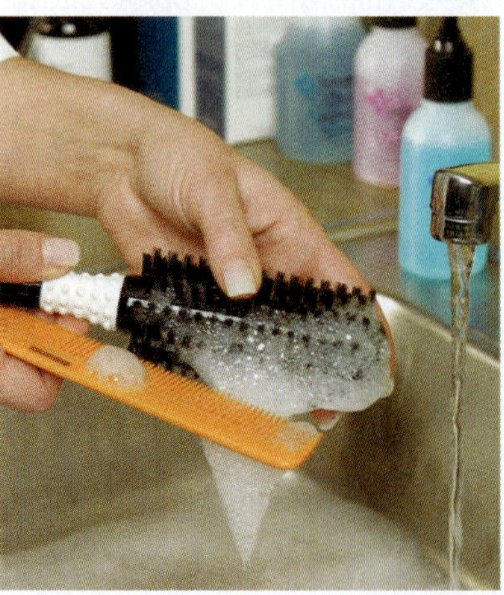

Figure 5-6 Remove hair from brushes and combs before disinfecting.

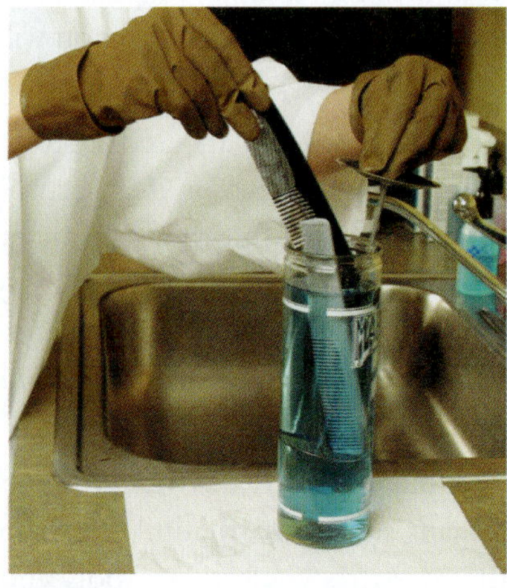

Figure 5-7 Immerse combs and brushes in disinfectant solution.

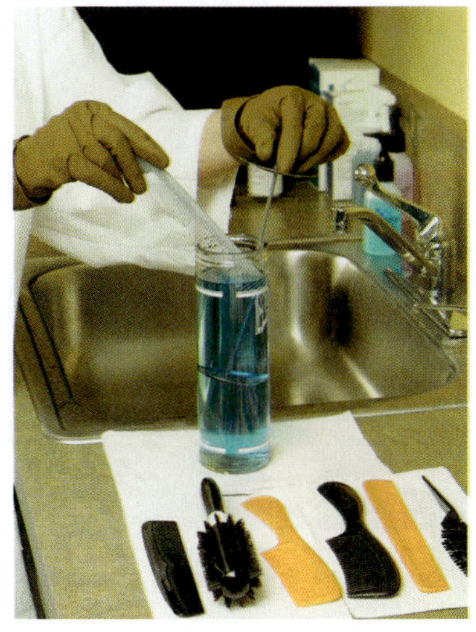

Figure 5-8 Remove implements, rinse, and dry thoroughly.

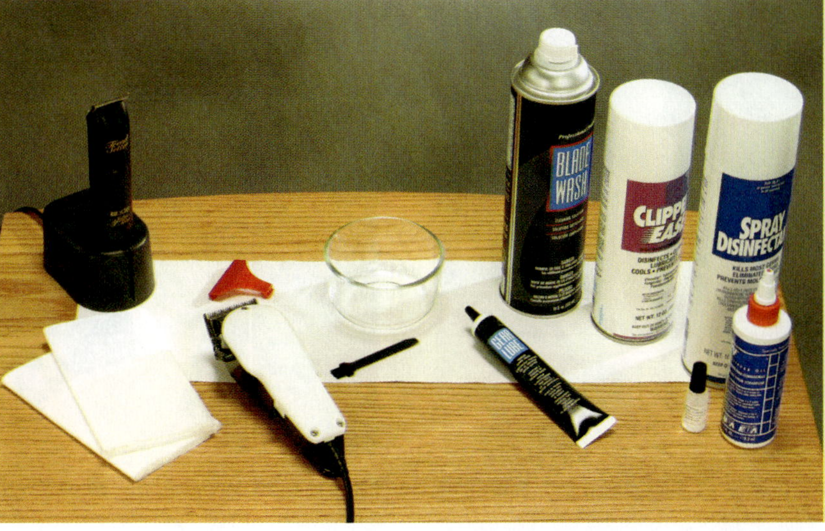

Figure 5-9 Arrange products, supplies, and tools on a clean, sanitized surface.

Alcohol Disinfection

To disinfect implements with fine cutting edges or electrodes, remove debris and particles and immerse them in 70% to 90% ethyl or isopropyl alcohol for the recommended amount of time. After disinfecting, dry tools and lubricate pivots or screws as needed; then place into a UV sanitizer or clean, closed container until needed for use. Check with state barber board law and regualtions regarding the use of alcohol a disinfectant to comply with established decontamination standards.

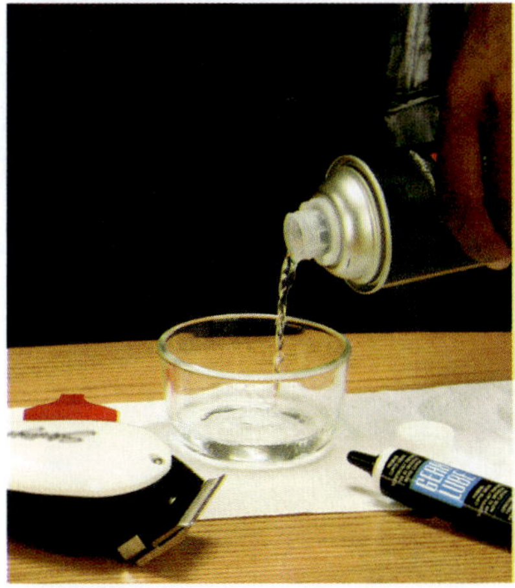

Figure 5-10 Pour blade wash into container.

Disinfecting Clippers and Outliners

The decontamination of electrical tools such as clippers and outliners requires a different approach than nonelectric tools and implements. Hair particles and bacteria become trapped between and behind clipper blades so thorough cleaning and disinfection of these tools is very important. Since they cannot be completely immersed in water-based disinfectants, and since most spray disinfectants alone are not sufficient for thorough disinfection, products containing a petroleum distillate, such as liquid blade washes, are the usual choice for the decontamination procedure.

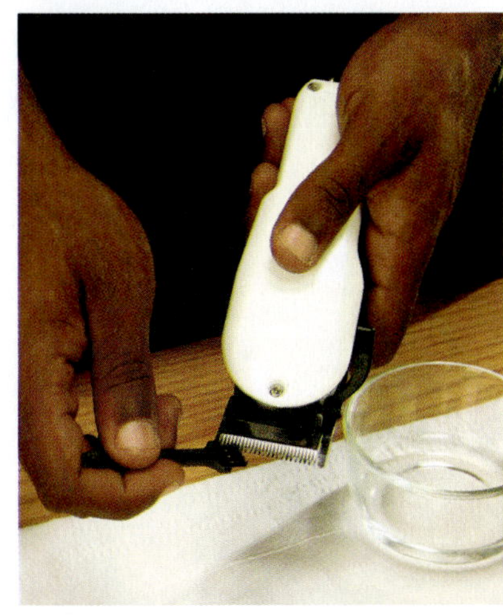

Figure 5-11 Remove hair particles from clipper blades.

Procedure for Disinfecting Clippers and Outliners

1. Arrange all supplies, products, and tools on a clean, sanitized surface (Figure 5–9).
2. Pour blade wash into a glass, plastic, or disposable container wide enough to accommodate the width of the clipper blades to a depth of approximately ½ inch (Figure 5–10).
3. Remove hair particles from clipper blades with a stiff brush (Figure 5–11).
4. Submerge only the cutting teeth of the clipper blades into the blade wash and turn the unit on. Run the blades in the solution until no hair particles are seen being dislodged from between the blades (Figure 5–12).

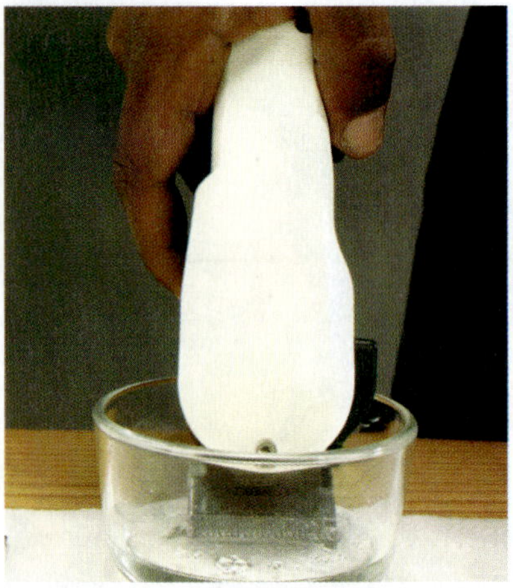

Figure 5-12 Submerge only the teeth of the clipper blades into blade wash.

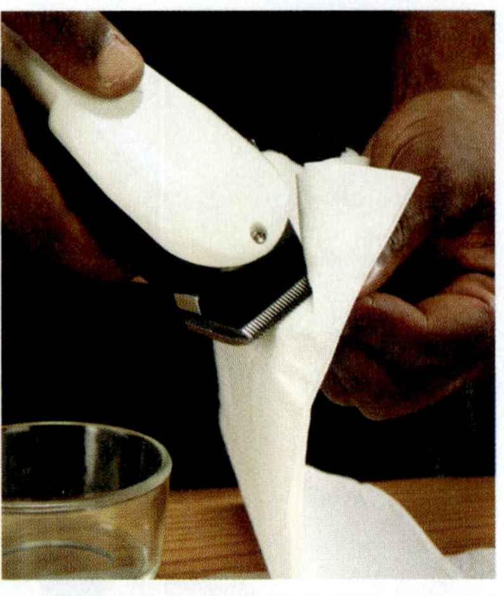

Figure 5-13 Wipe clipper blades with a clean, dry towel.

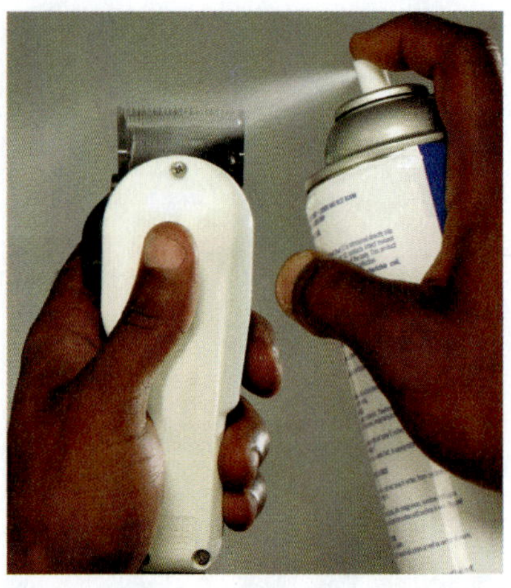

Figure 5-14 Spray clipper blades with lubricant.

5. Remove the clippers and wipe blades with a clean, dry towel (Figure 5–13).
6. Spray with a blade lubricant and/or spray clipper disinfectant. Grease/oil clipper parts as necessary (Figure 5–14).
7. Sanitize the conductor cord and store in a clean, closed container until needed for use.
8. Follow these procedures *before* and *after* servicing each client.

Note: Detachable clipper blades may be removed from the clipper, brushed clean, and immersed in blade wash for the recommended soaking time.

Decontaminating Towels, Linens, and Capes

Clean towels and linens must be used for each client. All towels, linens, and capes that come into contact with a client's skin should be laundered with detergent and bleach according to label directions. It is advisable to maintain a sufficient supply of these items for use in the barbershop to avoid the spread of infectious agents and particles. Disposable towels or neckstrips should be used to keep capes from touching the client's skin. If the neckline of a cape comes in contact with the client's skin, do not use it again until it has been laundered.

Disinfecting Work Surfaces

Before and after each client, an EPA-registered, hospital-grade tuberculocidal disinfectant should be used on all work surfaces and equipment that come into contact with the client or the barber's tools. This includes station counter-tops, barber chairs, headrests, shampoo bowls, and other surfaces.

Hand Washing

Hand washing is one the most important and easiest ways to prevent spreading germs from one person to another. Thorough hand washing requires rubbing the hands and under the nails with warm, soapy water for at least 20 seconds and drying with a clean paper towel. Moisturizing lotions can help prevent dry skin that may otherwise occur as a result of repeated hand washing.

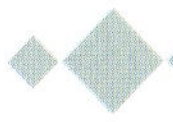

UNIVERSAL PRECAUTIONS

OSHA sets the standards that must be used in the industry for dealing with bloodborne pathogens. The standard prescribes the use of **Universal Precautions** as the approach to infection control (Table 5-2). Universal Precautions are a set of guidelines and controls, published by the Centers for Disease Control and Prevention (CDC), that require employers and employees to assume that all human blood and body fluids are infectious for HIV, HBV, and other bloodborne pathogens. Precautions include: hand washing; protective equipment such as gloves and goggles; injury prevention; and the proper handling and disposal of sharp implements (such as razor blades) and contaminated dressings or materials.

Item	Level of Decontamination	Procedure/Products
Any implement used to puncture or break the skin, or that which comes into contact with pus or other bodily fluids	Sterilization	Steam autoclave and dry heat. Dispose of all sharps in a sharps container.
Nonporous tools and implements (brushes, combs, razors, clipper guards) that have not come into contact with bodily fluids or blood	Disinfection	Completely immerse in an EPA-registered, hospital-grade bactericidal, pseudomonacidal, fungicidal, and virucidal disinfectant for amount of time specified by the manufacturer.
Nonporous tools and implements (brushes, combs, razors, clipper guards) that have come into contact with bodily fluids or blood	Disinfection	Completely immerse in an EPA-registered disinfectant with demonstrated efficacy against HIV-1/HBV or tuberculosis for amount of time specified by the manufacturer.
Nonporous tools and implements (brushes, combs, razors, clipper guards) that have come into contact with parasites such as head lice	Disinfection	Completely immerse in a Lysol solution (2 tablespoons in 1 quart water) for one hour.
Electrotherapy tools	Disinfection	Spray or wipe with an EPA-registered, hospital-grade disinfect specifically made for electrical equipment.
Countertops, shampoo bowls, sinks, floors, toilets, doorknobs, mirrors, etc.	Sanitation	Use EPA registered, cleaning product designed for surfaces.
Towels, linens, chair cloths, capes, etc.	Sanitation	Launder in hot water with detergent and bleach.
The barber's hands prior to and after each service	Sanitation	Wash with liquid antibacterial soap and warm water.

Table 5-2 Infection Prevention Guidelines

5

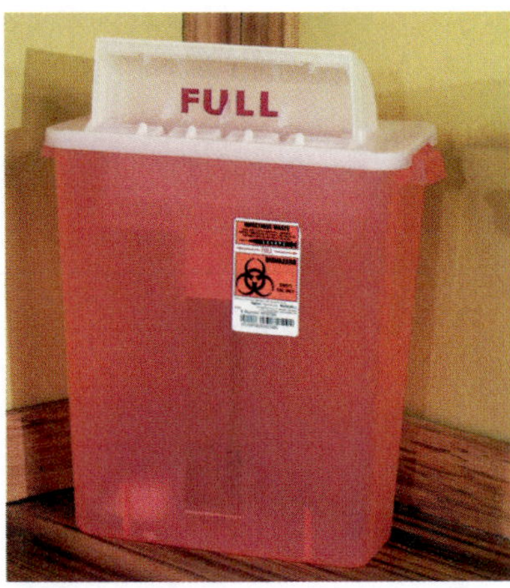

Figure 5-15 A sharps box.

Blood-spill Disinfection

Although the term "blood spill" may sound as though a significant amount of blood must be in evidence to be labeled as such, we use the term to denote any amount of bleeding that occurs as a result of an injury in the barbershop. Minor blood spills sometimes happen when the barber or client is accidentally cut with a sharp implement during a service procedure. When **blood-spill disinfection** is required the proper steps for protecting the health and safety of both individuals are as follows:

1. When a cut is sustained by the client, stop the service immediately and inform the client. Next, wash your hands, apply gloves, clean the injured area, and follow steps 2–8. If you sustain a cut, stop the service, check the client for the possible transmission of blood, wash your hands, and follow steps 2–8.
2. Apply antiseptic or styptic using a cotton swab. Do not contaminate the container.
3. Cover the injury with a Band-Aid or other appropriate dressing. Use a finger guard or gloves as necessary.
4. Disinfect the workstation as necessary.
5. Discard all disposable contaminated objects such as cotton, tissues, etc. by double-bagging. Use the appropriate biohazard sticker on a container for contaminated waste. Deposit sharp disposables in a sharps box (Figure 5–15).
6. When removing the gloves, peel one glove off from the wrist, allowing it to turn inside out and hold it in the gloved hand. Use the exposed hand to grasp a section of the inside of the second glove. When peeling off the second glove, stretch it over and around the first glove. Promptly dispose of the gloves in the appropriate biohazard container.
7. Wash your hands with soap and warm water before returning to the service.
8. All tools and implements that have come into contact with blood or body fluids must be disinfected by complete immersion in an EPA-registered, hospital-grade tuberculocidal disinfectant. Refer to Table 5–2 for other infection prevention guidelines.

Disinfecting Rules

1. Chemical solutions in sanitizers should be changed regularly. Change the solution when it becomes dirty, contaminated, or cloudy.
2. All metal implements should be disinfected, lubricated, and stored in airtight containers.
3. All items must be clean and free from hair and debris before being sanitized.
4. Sanitize electrical appliances by rubbing the surface with a cotton pad damped with 70% to 90% ethyl or isopropyl alcohol.
5. All cups, finger bowls, or similar objects must be disintected prior to being used for another client. Do not forget to disinfect such surfaces as headrests, shampoo bowl neck rests, and other equipment.

Decontamination Safety Precautions

1. Purchase chemicals in small quantities and store them in a cool, dry place as they can deteriorate when exposed to air, light, and heat.
2. Wear protective gloves, goggles, and aprons when mixing chemicals.
3. Carefully weigh, measure, and pour chemicals.
4. Keep all containers labeled, covered, and under lock and key.
5. Do not smell chemicals or solutions. Some have pungent odors and can irritate the nasal membranes.
6. Avoid spilling chemicals when diluting them.
7. Prevent burns by using forceps to insert or remove objects from heat sources.
8. Keep a complete first-aid kit on hand.
9. Maintain a complete MSDS record of all chemicals and products used in the barbershop.

OSHA

The Occupational Safety and Health Administration (**OSHA**) was created as a result of the Occupational Safety and Health Act of 1970 under the directive of the U.S. Department of Labor. OSHA's primary purpose is to regulate and enforce health and safety standards in the workplace.

The **Occupational Safety and Health Act**, which applies to almost every employer in the United States, including barbershops and styling salons, has significantly reduced personal injuries and illness due to the work environment. Two key functions of the act include: 1) the requirement of employers to furnish their employees with a working environment that is free from recognizable hazards and 2) the requirement of compliance with occupational safety and health standards as set forth by the act.

Of particular interest to barbers is the **Hazard Communication Rule**, which requires that chemical manufacturers and importers evaluate and identify possible health hazards associated with their products. Material Safety Data Sheets (**MSDS**) and required labeling are two important results of this rule. Additionally, the Hazard Communication Rule requires that this information be made available to workers through the Right-to-Know Law.

Material Safety Data Sheets

Material Safety Data Sheets provide vital information about products, ranging from ingredient content and associated hazards, to combustion levels and storage requirements. Barbershops and schools are required by law to maintain an MSDS for every product used on the premises (Figure 5–16).

An MSDS may be obtained from the product distributor or manufacturer when an order is placed but you must request it. Once received, the MSDS should be kept in a notebook or file in an organized format for easy

Material Safety Data Sheet
May be used to comply with
OSHAs Hazard Communication Standard,
29 CFR 1910.1200. Standard must be
consulted for specific requirements.

U.S. Department of Labor
Occupational Safety and Health Administration
(Non-Mandatory Form)
Form Approved
OMB No. 1218-0072

IDENTITY (As Used on Label and List)	Note: Blank spaces are not permitted. If any item is not applicable or no information is available, the space must be marked to indicate that.

Section I

Manufacturer s Name	Emergency Telephone Number
Address (Number, Street, City, State, and ZIP Code)	Telephone Number for information
	Date Prepared
	Signature of Preparer (optional)

Section II — Hazardous Ingredients/Identity Information

Hazardous Components (Specific Chemical Identity; Common Names(s))	OSHA PEL	ACGIH TLV	Other Limits Recommended	% (optional)

Section III — Physical/Chemical Characteristics

Boiling Point		Specific Gravity (H_2O - 1)	
Vapor Pressure (mm Hg.)		Melting Point	
Vapor Density (Air - 1))		Evaporation Rate (Butyl Acetate - 1)	

Solubility in Water

Appearance and Odor

Section IV — Fire and Explosion Hazard Data

Flash Point (Method Used)	Flammable Limits	LEL	UEL

Extinguishing Media

Special Fire Fighting Procedures

Unusual Fire and Explosion Hazards

(Reproduce locally) OSHA 174, Sept. 1985

Figure 5-16 A sample MSDS.

Material Safety Data Sheet (MSDS)

Section V — Reactivity Data

Stability	Unstable		Conditions to Avoid
	Stable		

Incompatibility (Materials to Avoid)

Hazardous Decomposition or Byproducts

Hazardous Polymerization	May Occur		Conditions to Avoid
	Will Not Occur		

Section VI — Health Hazard Data

Route(s) of Entry:	Inhalation?	Skin?	Ingestion?

Health Hazards (Acut and Chronic)

Carcenogenicity:	NTP?	IARC Monographs	OSHA Regulated?

Signs and Symptoms of Exposure

Medical Conditions
Generally Aggravated by Exposure

Emergency and First Aid Program

Section VII — Precautions for Safe Handling and Use

Steps to Be Taken in Case Material is Released or Spilled

Waste Disposal Method

Precautions to Be Taken in Handling and Storing

Other Precautions

Section VIII — Control Measures

Respiratory Protection (Specify Type)

Ventilation	Local Exhaust	Special
	Mechanical (General)	Other

Protective Gloves	Eye Protection

Other Protective Clothing or Equipment

Work/Hygienic Practices

Page 2

Figure 5-16 (continued)

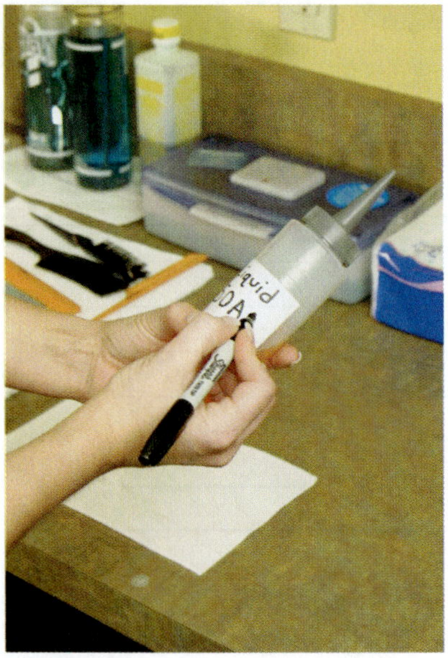

Figure 5–17 All containers should be labeled.

access. There are official guidelines for setting up an MSDS notebook that may be requested from your state's Department of Labor.

Labeling refers to the listing of ingredients on the packaging of a product and the appropriate hazard warning. When you think about the range of products used in the barbershop or styling salon, the importance of complying with this standard becomes obvious. Disinfectants, glass and surface cleaners, alcohols, and antiseptic solutions are just a few of the chemicals that can be found in the shop or salon environment. All products and containers are required to be labeled, even spray bottles filled with water (Figure 5–17). Through the efforts of OSHA, the law requires that chemical product labels contain the identity of the hazardous chemical(s) and the appropriate hazard warning. This information is required in order to provide the consumer with product knowledge, choices, and possible health warnings. It is one of the main reasons for always reading and following the directions provided by product manufacturers.

The standards set by OSHA are important to the barbering industry because of the nature of the chemicals used, some of which are combustible, caustic, or otherwise potentially harmful to the human body. All chemicals need to be mixed, stored, and disposed of properly. The requirements for the mixing and storing of chemical products are identified on the Material Safety Data Sheets; however the disposal of waste or outdated products requires more specific information. These procedures may be obtained from your local hazardous waste agency or office.

Federal law has provided the employer and employee certain guidelines for the promotion of *safe work practices*. The following general information has been provided to give barbering students a general understanding of certain federal requirements and their own inalienable rights.

Right-to-Know Law

The **Right-to-Know Law** requires that a Right-to-Know notice be posted in the work environment where toxic substances are present. (Obtainable through your state Department of Labor.) This notice advises the worker of specific rights under the Right-to-Know Law. The basic guidelines of federal legislation should define the employer's responsibilities and the worker's rights as outlined below:

Employer Responsibilities

1. Inform the worker of toxic substances in the workplace.
2. Maintain Material Safety Data Sheets and have them available upon request.
3. Provide education to the worker about the proper use of the substances and emergency procedures.
4. Notify the appropriate local agencies, such as the fire department and hazardous waste department, about the identity, characteristics, and location of the toxic substance(s).

Worker's Rights

1. Know the characteristics and location of toxic substances in the workplace.
2. Obtain relevant Material Safety Data Sheets.
3. May refuse to work with a listed toxic substance if not supplied with a copy of the MSDS.
4. Education and instruction (within first 30 days of employment) on the potentially adverse health effects of each toxic substance in the work environment and the appropriate emergency procedures.
5. Additional information from the Toxic Substances Information Center.
6. Protection from discharge, discrimination, or discipline for exercising your rights.

Cosmetics Labeling

The OSHA laws that require the labeling of hazardous chemical ingredients should not be confused with the U.S. Food and Drug Administration (FDA) labeling laws in regard to cosmetic preparations. "Cosmetic" preparations used in the barbershop include hair tonics, shampoos, conditioners, permanent wave solutions, hair color tints, chemical processors, hair sprays, gels, and many others. Most of us probably assume that these products have been proven safe and effective as it is obviously in the manufacturer's best interest to produce a reliable product. The potential consequences of lost sales or worse, consumer suits and court battles, are enough to keep manufacturers honest thereby providing some assurance that the products are safe to use in the barbershop. That said, however, it is important to realize that the FDA has rather limited authority over cosmetics in general.

Although the FDA enforces the Fair Packaging and Labeling Act of 1973, the agency regulates consumer cosmetic products only after they are released to the marketplace. The FDA does not review or approve cosmetic products before they are sold to the consumer. Nor does the FDA have the authority to require companies to safety test their products prior to marketing, mandate registration of the company, maintain ingredient data files, or report injuries associated with their product. Therefore, the responsibility of product safety rests with the manufacturer. If a new product is released and the safety of that product has not yet been substantiated, by law, the label must include the following: "Warning: The safety of this product has not been determined."

The FDA maintains a voluntary data collection program and through this information may monitor a company that conducts a product recall. Product recalls are voluntary actions on the part of cosmetic manufacturers. Occasionally, a product or product batch is found to be defective or harmful in some way and in most cases it is the manufacturer who will issue the recall. If complaints of adverse reactions to a product reach the FDA, they will provide follow-up investigations and inspections.

Once an investigation is warranted, the FDA is authorized to inspect manufacturing facilities, collect samples, and take legal action through the Department of Justice to remove misrepresented (improper labeling), harmful, or contaminated products from the market.

Although a cosmetic manufacturer may include almost any raw-material product in a cosmetic preparation, the FDA requires that the color additives used in cosmetics be tested for safety. In addition to maintaining a list of acceptable color additives and their purpose, the FDA also maintains a list of prohibited or restricted ingredients.

It is important for barbers to understand some of the regulations that apply to the manufacturing of consumer cosmetic products in order to provide a comparison when discussing "professional products." Consumer products are those that tend to be designated as "over-the-counter" preparations, meaning that they are available to and can be purchased by the general public at a retail store or outlet.

Professional products are those that are sold only to licensed barbers or other industry professionals. Product manufacturers do not have to adhere to the same labeling regulations for professional products as they do for retail products that are meant for use in the home. This is the reason why you may discover that some professional products do not contain a list of ingredients on the label. The lack of ingredient listing can present an obvious problem to the barber who has to choose a product for a client. Unless the ingredients are listed there is no way of knowing if the client may experience an allergic reaction to a product or whether the pH is appropriate for the hair or skin.

There are two courses of action that a barber can take if faced with either of these scenarios. Although manufacturers are not required to list professional product ingredients, labeling regulations mandate that the manufacturer's name, address, and warning statements be included on the label. Therefore, the barber may contact the company for necessary information. The second option is one you should already be prepared for. Remember those Material Safety Data Sheets? That's where you'll find the information needed to make a professional decision.

PUBLIC SANITATION

Public sanitation is the application of measures to promote public health and prevent the spread of infectious diseases. The importance of sanitation cannot be overemphasized. The barbering profession requires direct contact with clients' skin, scalp, and hair. Understanding sanitation and decontamination measures ensures the protection of the clients' health as well as your own.

Various government agencies protect community health by ensuring that food is wholesome, the water supply is untainted, and the refuse is disposed of properly. Barber boards and boards of health in each state have formulated sanitation regulations that all barbers must follow in the pursuit of their profession. The most basic sanitation regulations apply to air quality, water quality, and infectious diseases.

The air within a barbershop should be moist and fresh. Room temperature should be about 70 degrees Fahrenheit. The shop should be equipped with an exhaust fan or an air-conditioning unit. Air-conditioning is an advantage since it permits changes in the quality and quantity of air in the shop. The temperature and humidity of the air may also be regulated by means of air conditioning.

Water in the barbershop should be pure. Be aware that crystal-clear water still may be unsanitary if it contains pathogenic bacteria, which cannot be seen with the naked eye. Many municipal governments require water coolers in establishments that serve the general public.

A person ill with an infectious disease puts other people's health at risk. A barber with a cold or any other contagious disease should not serve clients. Likewise, clients suffering from infectious diseases should be tactfully encouraged to postpone their appointment until after they are well. This protects you and other clients being serviced.

Rules of Sanitation

1. Barbershops must be well lit, heated, and ventilated, in order to keep them clean and sanitary.
2. Walls, floors, and windows in the shop must be kept clean.
3. All barbering establishments must have hot and cold running water.
4. All plumbing fixtures should be properly installed.
5. The premises should be kept free of rodents and flies or other insects.
6. Dogs (with the exception of guide dogs), cats, birds, and other pets must not be permitted in a shop.
7. The barbershop should not be used for eating, or sleeping, or as living quarters. If square footage is sufficient, a small room at the back of the shop may be used by staff during their breaks. State boards and local building inspectors can provide standards and codes.
8. Clean and disinfect all implements as they are used and return them to their proper place.
9. Clean work areas, chairs, and mirrors.
10. Remove all hair and waste materials from the floor.
11. Rest rooms must be kept in a sanitary condition.
12. Each barber must be appropriately attired to work on clients.
13. Barbers must cleanse their hands thoroughly before and after serving a client.
14. Barbers must wash their hands after leaving the bathroom.
15. A freshly laundered towel or fresh paper towel must be used for each client. Towels ready for use must be stored in a clean, closed cabinet. All soiled linen towels and used paper towels must be disposed of properly. Keep dirty towels separate from clean towels.
16. Headrest coverings and neck strips or towels must be changed for each client.

- All tools and implements should be in good working condition. Replace damaged electrical cords, chipped clipper blades, cracked housings, broken shears, and other tools immediately. Never subject yourself or your client to the risks of faulty or broken equipment.
- Electrical cords deserve specific mention because they often become a safety hazard in the shop. Cords to clippers, trimmers, curling irons, and blow-dryers tend to become twisted and tangled during use. If the length of the cord is too long, it can get caught on the foot or arm rests of a hydraulic chair or even on the foot of a client! Some barbers replace the factory cord with a retractable cord device or purchase cordless trimmers, which eliminate the problem altogether. A well-planned workstation with sufficient and conveniently placed outlets can also help to minimize the "tangled cord syndrome."
- Do not overload electrical outlets.
- Barbering tools and implements are designed for specific purposes, so use the right tool for the job. Do not expect a trimmer to do the work of a clipper!

Equipment and Fixtures

- Keep all hydraulic chairs, headrests, shampoo chairs, heat lamps, and lighting fixtures in good working order. Tighten screws and bolts, grease or oil hinges, and service equipment mechanisms as needed.
- Dust and sanitize regularly to avoid buildup and to maintain sanitary conditions.
- Maintain lighting fixtures. Change bulbs when necessary to keep the workstation well lit.

Ventilation

- Proper ventilation and air circulation are extremely important in today's shop or salon. Fumes from chemical applications and nail care products require sophisticated filtration units that cleanse and detoxify the air. Once installed, air-filtration filters should be changed or cleaned regularly.
- Shops where full services such as chemical applications are not offered also require proper ventilation equipment. Particles from products such as talc, hair sprays, and disinfectants can be inhaled and may cause allergies or other health problems.

Attire

- Clothing should be comfortable and professional in appearance. Excessively baggy clothes can get in the way of your performance just as easily as tight clothing can restrict it.
- Wearing excessively long hair loose has been known to get caught in blow-dryer motor vents. Keep it pulled back or short enough to avoid entanglements.

- Necklaces should be of an appropriate length so as not to get caught on equipment or dangle in a client's face at the shampoo bowl or during a shave. Rings should not be worn on the index and middle fingers as they might interfere with haircutting accuracy. Watches should be waterproof and shock absorbent.
- Shoes should have nonskid rubber soles with good support.

Children

- Children can cause serious risk and injury to themselves in the shop environment. Being aware of their inquisitive natures and the speed with which they can move can help to prevent accidents from happening.
- Post notices in the reception area advising patrons that "Children are not to be left unattended."
- Do not allow children to play, climb, or spin on hydraulic chairs.
- Do not allow children to wander freely around the shop with access to workstations, storage areas, etc.
- When cutting a child's hair, try to anticipate their sudden moves. NEVER trust a young child to "hold their head still" while you approach their head area with shears or other tools. Instead, hold the child's head gently but firmly with one hand while cutting with the other. This technique is especially helpful when cutting around ears and at the nape. When trimming bangs or front hairlines, hold the hair between your fingers at a low elevation, cutting the hair on the inside of your palm, thereby putting the barrier of your fingers between the tool and the child's face.

Adult Clients

As barbers, many of the things we do to assure client comfort also fall under the category of safety precautions. In the following chapters you will learn the proper draping procedures and chemical application methods to ensure client safety and comfort from the standpoint of avoiding skin irritations, burns, wet or soiled clothing, etc.; however, there are also several commonsense services that should be performed. Using good manners and performing common courtesies will help you gain the reputation of being a safetyconscious and courteous barber.

- Assist clients (especially the elderly) in and out of hydraulic and shampoo chairs.
- Always lower the hydraulic chair to its lowest level and lock it in position so that it doesn't spin before inviting the client to be seated or leave the chair.
- Hold doors open for clients.
- Assist elderly clients in walking whenever necessary.
- Always support the back of the chair, and thus the client, when reclining or raising a chair back.

- Cushion the client's neck with a folded towel in the neck rest at the shampoo bowl. This is especially beneficial for clients with neck injuries such as whiplash.
- Support the client's head whenever appropriate at the shampoo bowl. Do not ask them to hold their head up for shampooing or rinsing. Instead, gently turn their head to the side for easier access to the back and nape areas.

Exits

- Exits should be well posted and identifiable. (Check with your local building inspection office for codes and requirements.)
- Employees should know where exits are located and how to evacuate the building quickly in case of fire or other emergencies.

Fire Extinguishers

- Fire extinguishers should be placed where they are readily accessible.
- All employees should be instructed in fire extinguisher use.
- It is a law that fire extinguishers be checked periodically. Be guided by the manufacturer's recommendations and state and local ordinances.

Chemicals

- Request an MSDS from your supplier(s) for all products purchased for the shop and maintain an MSDS notebook. Add to the notebook as new products are brought into the workplace.
- Take the time to study the MSDS from the manufacturer so that you will know how and where to store products and what procedures to follow in an emergency.
- There is a correct way to dispose of chemicals such as hair color tints, chemical relaxers, bleach, etc. Contact your local hazardous-waste department or agency for disposal guidelines.
- Never mix cleaning products together—especially bleach and ammonia.
- Never mix leftover chemicals together!
- Do not allow leftover chemicals to "stockpile." Dispose of products as often as necessary to maintain a safe environment.
- Check the inventory stock occasionally for plastic bottles with dents or bulges. This swelling of the container indicates that the contents are under pressure and could possibly explode.
- Wear goggles when pouring or mixing products. Add a lab apron and gloves when handling any caustic or skin-irritating material.
- Chemical spills require an absorbent material, such as sawdust, to clean up properly. Be guided by your local hazardous-waste agency.
- Every solution, liquid, cream, powder, paste, gel, etc., should be properly labeled. This requirement goes beyond labeled products purchased from

a supplier and includes spray bottles of water or setting lotions, sanitizing jars of alcohol, containers of blade wash, and any other substance used in the shop that is not contained within its original packaging.

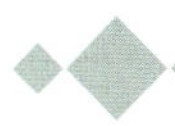

PROFESSIONAL RESPONSIBILITY

After studying this chapter, it should be clear that your responsibilities as a professional barber far exceed the requirement to perform a good haircut. This responsibility includes a certain awareness that can be developed and demonstrated from a sincere sense of caring when working with the public. It is this awareness or observation of the environment that helps you notice the "little things" that will make the barbershop safe for you and your clients. Responsible awareness also encourages you to do things the right way, rather than trying to take shortcuts.

Being prepared for emergencies is also a part of your professional responsibility. Every shop should have employee and clientele emergency information available near the telephone. An emergency phone number checklist should include the contact numbers for fire, police, and medical rescue departments; the nearest hospital emergency room; and taxis. Utility service companies, such as electricity, water, heat, air conditioning, etc., and landlord or custodial numbers are also helpful in an emergency or if something breaks down in the shop. Update this information on an annual basis and you will always be prepared.

As your sense of awareness increases and you begin to feel more comfortable and confident working with clients, the quality of your communication and human relations skills will increase as well. Subsequently, you will reap the benefits of a loyal clientele base. Behavior that stems from a knowledgeable and caring manner is what separates a true professional from a nonprofessional and being a *professional* is something you can take pride in.

chapter glossary

antiseptics	chemical agents that may kill, retard, or prevent the growth of bacteria; not classified as disinfectants
blood-spill disinfection	the procedures to follow when the barber or client sustains an injury that results in bleeding
decontamination	the removal of pathogens from tools, equipment, and surfaces
disinfectants	chemical agents used to destroy most bacteria and some viruses and to disinfect tools, implements, and surfaces
disinfection	second-highest level of decontamination used on hard, nonporous materials
dry or cabinet sanitizer	airtight cabinet containing an active fumigant used to store sanitized tools and implements
EPA-registered disinfectant	a product that has been approved by the Environmental Protection Agency as an effective disinfectant against certain disease-producing organisms
Hazard Communication Rule	requires that chemical manufacturers and importers evaluate and identify possible health hazards associated with their products
hospital-grade tuberculocidal disinfectant	disinfectants that are effective against bacteria, fungi, viruses, tuberculosis, Psuedomonas, HIV-1, and Hepatitis B and are registered with the EPA
MSDS	**(Material Safety Data Sheet)** provides product information as compiled by the manufacturer
Occupational Safety and Health Act	an act that led to the creation of OSHA, which regulates and enforces health and safety standards in the workplace
OSHA	Occupational Safety and Health Administration
public sanitation	the application of measures used to promote public health and prevent the spread of infectious diseases
Right-to-Know Law	requires employers to post notices where toxic substances are present in the workplace
safe work practices	the maintenance of sanitation standards and the application of safety precautions in the workplace environment
sanitation	the third or lowest level of decontamination; means to significantly reduce the number of pathogens found on a surface
solute	the substance that is dissolved in a solvent
solution	the product created from combining and dissolving a solute in a solvent
solvent	the liquid in which a solute is dissolved
sterilization	the process of rendering an object germ-free by destroying all living organisms on a surface
ultraviolet-ray sanitizer	sanitizer metal cabinets with ultraviolet lamps or bulbs used to store sanitized tools and implements
Universal Precautions	CDC guidelines and controls that require employers and employees to assume that all human blood and specified human body fluids are infectious for HIV, HBV, and other bloodborne pathogens
wet sanitizer	any covered receptacle large enough to permit the immersion of tools and implements into a disinfectant solution

chapter review questions

1. Identify two ways in which infectious materials may be transmitted in the barbershop.
2. Define decontamination. List and explain the three levels of decontamination.
3. List the chemical decontamination agents most commonly used in barbershops.
4. Explain the differences between solutes, solvents, and solutions.
5. Identify the two sanitizers most commonly used in barbershops.
6. List the steps used to disinfect implements and clippers, trimmers, or outliners.
7. List blood-spill disinfection procedures.
8. Explain what is meant by Universal Precautions.
9. List nine decontamination safety precautions.
10. Explain the purpose of an MSDS.
11. Explain the intent of the Right-to-Know Law.
12. List 11 safety-precaution areas that barbers should be aware of in the barbershop.

Learning Objectives

After completing this chapter, you should be able to:

1. **Identify the principal tools and implements used in the practice of barbering.**

2. **Identify the parts of shears, clippers, and razors.**

3. **Demonstrate the correct techniques for holding combs, shears, clippers, and razors.**

4. **Demonstrate honing and stropping techniques.**

Key Terms

blades
pg. 105

changeable-blade straight razor
pg. 108

comedone extractor
pg. 123

conventional straight razor
pg. 108

guards
pg. 106

high-frequency machine
pg. 123

hone
pg. 112

palming the shears
pg. 102

rotary motor clipper
pg. 104

Russian strop
pg. 114

serrated shears
pg. 102

set of the shears
pg. 102

shell strop
pg. 115

strop
pg. 112

taper comb
pg. 100

thermal
pg. 121

trimmers
pg. 105

All of the instruments and accessories used in the practice of barbering and barber-styling are considered to be the implements, tools, or equipment of the profession. In this chapter, nonmotorized items (combs, shears, etc.) are referred to as implements; electrically powered items (clippers, trimmers, etc.) as tools; and anything from barber chairs to steam towel cabinets are considered to be equipment.

Barbers should always use high-quality implements, tools, and equipment. When taken care of properly, well-tempered metal implements and electric tools will provide years of dependable service. Since a myriad of choices are available and may be confusing to the student, ask your instructor or a licensed barber to assist you in appropriate selections.

Although all of the implements and tools associated with barbering will probably be used at some time or another, the principal "tools of the trade" are combs, brushes, shears, clippers, trimmers, and razors. 1

COMBS

Combs are available in a variety of styles and sizes. The correct comb to use depends on the type of service to be performed and the individual preference of the barber. Combs are usually made of bone, plastic, or hard rubber. Since bone combs can be costly and plastic combs are not as durable as bone or rubber, most barbers prefer combs made of hard rubber.

The teeth of a comb may be fine (close together) or coarse (far apart). Fine-toothed combs may be used for general combing purposes, while wide-toothed combs are preferable for detangling or chemical processing. In either case, it is important that the teeth have rounded ends to avoid scratching or irritating a client's scalp. Some available comb styles are:

- The all-purpose comb, which may be used for general haircutting and styling. A popular size is 7¾ inches long (Figure 6–1).
- An all-purpose comb with a curved interior assists in lifting subsections and partings of hair while cutting. The usual size is 7½ inches long.

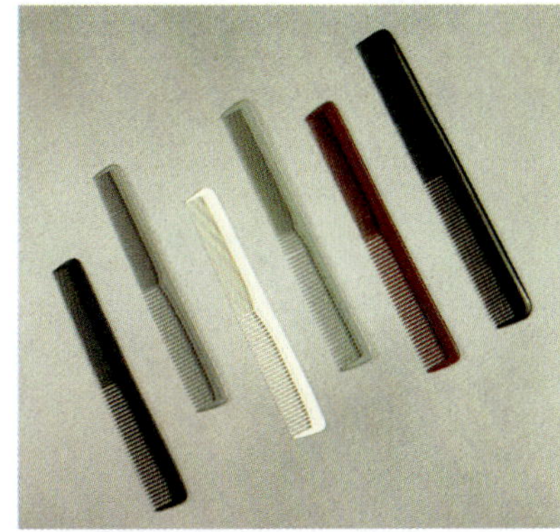

Figure 6–1 Assorted all-purpose combs.

6

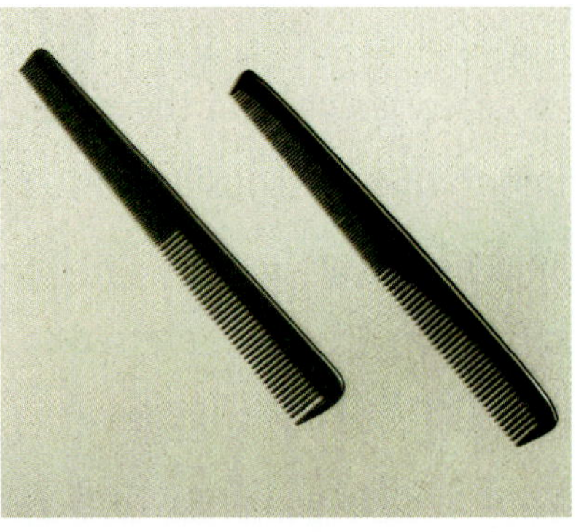

Figure 6-2 Taper combs.

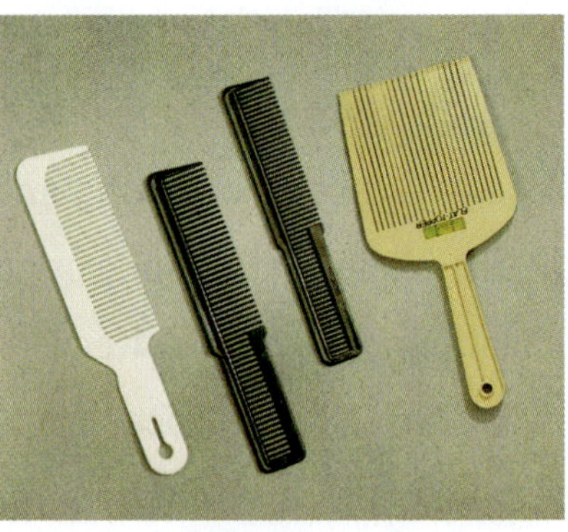

Figure 6-3 Flat-top combs.

Did you know...

Barbers can simplify their work when cutting hair by using light-colored combs on dark hair and dark-colored combs on light hair. This technique provides greater contrast between the comb and the hair, especially when employing the shear-over-comb method of cutting.

- A **taper comb** is used for cutting or trimming hair in those areas where a gradual blending of the hair is required. The tapered end is especially useful for mustache trims, tapering necklines, and blending around the ear areas. Taper combs are available with curved or straight interior sections as in Figure 6–2.
- A wide-toothed comb works best with clippers to achieve a flat-top style (Figure 6–3).
- Wide-toothed handle combs can be used to spread relaxer creams for chemical hair straightening or for detangling. They are also available with a curved interior (Figure 6–4).
- The tail comb is the best choice for sectioning long hair or when making partings to wrap on perm rods or rollers (Figure 6–5).
- The pick or Afro comb is usually the most efficient implement for combing through tight curl patterns or permanent waved hair (Figure 6–6).

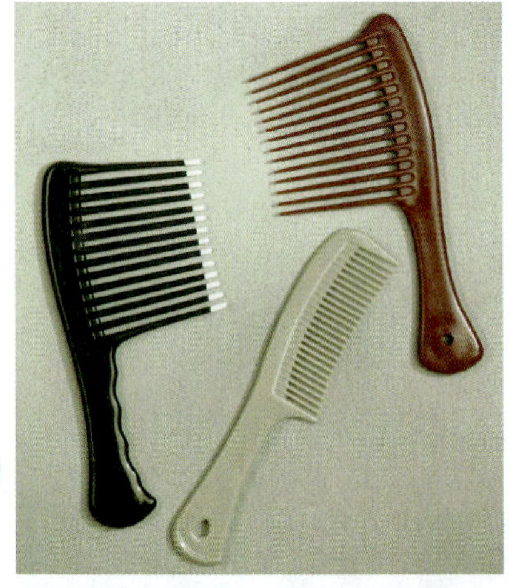

Figure 6-4 Wide-toothed combs.

Holding the Comb

The correct manner in which to hold the comb will be dictated by the type of comb used, the service being performed, and the dexterity and comfort of the barber. Figures 6–7 through 6–10 show correct and incorrect holding positions that are often used with an all-purpose comb. Be guided by your instructor and practice, practice, practice!

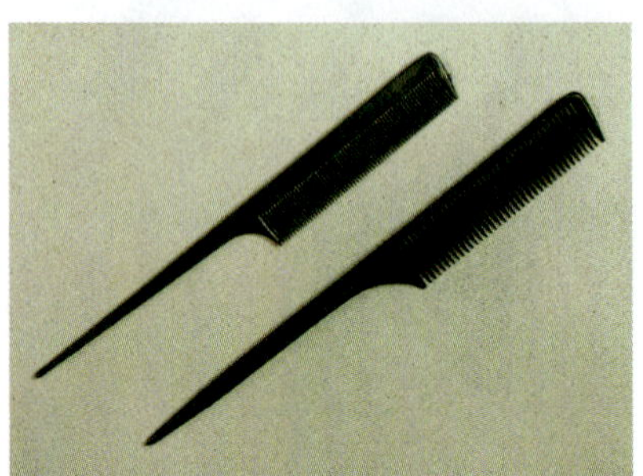

Figure 6-5 Tail combs.

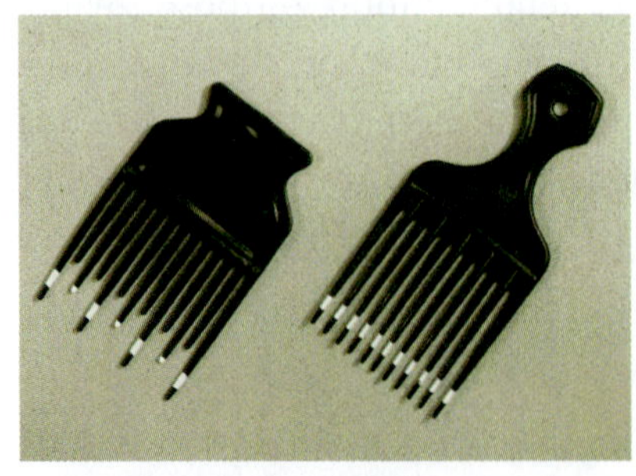

Figure 6-6 Pick or Afro combs.

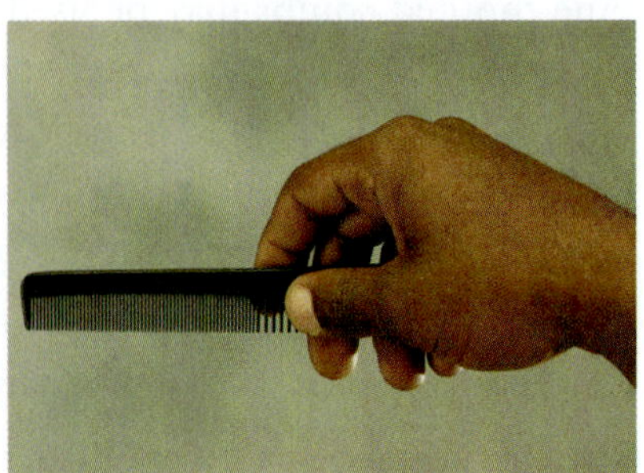

Figure 6-7 Proper comb-holding position.

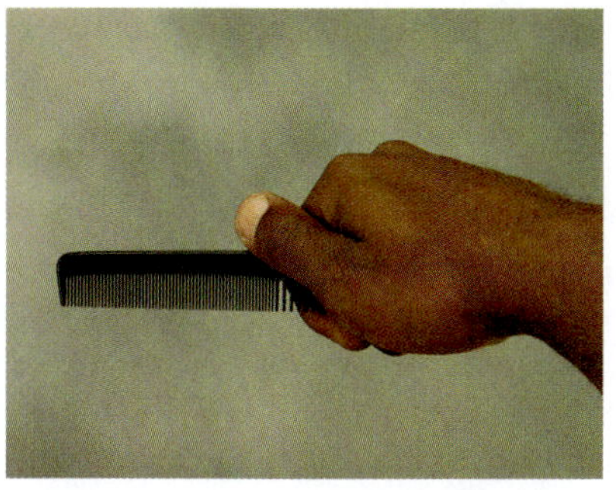

Figure 6-8 Improper comb-holding position.

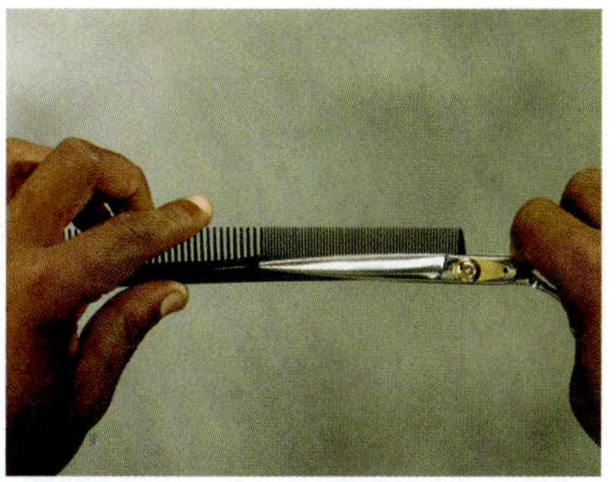

Figure 6-9 Proper holding position for shear-over-comb cutting.

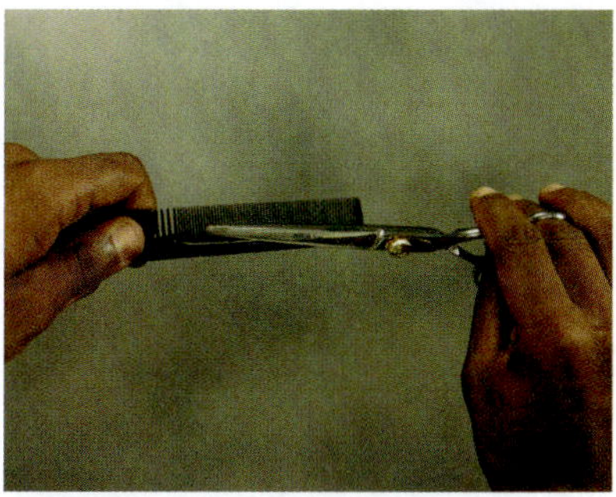

Figure 6-10 Improper holding position for shear-over-comb cutting.

Care of Combs

To keep combs in good condition, avoid exposing them to excessive or prolonged heat. Combs must be sanitized before and after each client has been served.

1. Remove or brush loose hairs from the comb.
2. Wash comb thoroughly with hot water and soap or detergent.
3. Rinse thoroughly and pat dry.
4. Place in a wet sanitizer with disinfectant for the recommended disinfection time.
5. Rinse comb, wipe dry, and place in a clean, closed container, dry sanitizer, or an ultraviolet-ray electrical sanitizer until needed.

Check your state board regulations concerning the use of fumigants in dry cabinet sanitizers.

HAIRCUTTING SHEARS

The two types of shears generally used by barbers and barber-stylists are the French style, which has a brace for the little finger, and the German type, which does not incorporate the finger brace into the design. Barbers typically choose the French design over the German type and both are now available in ergonomically designed styles (Figure 6–11). Haircutting shears with detachable blades have also become very popular. The old blades can be removed and replaced with new ones, thereby eliminating the need to send shears out to be sharpened.

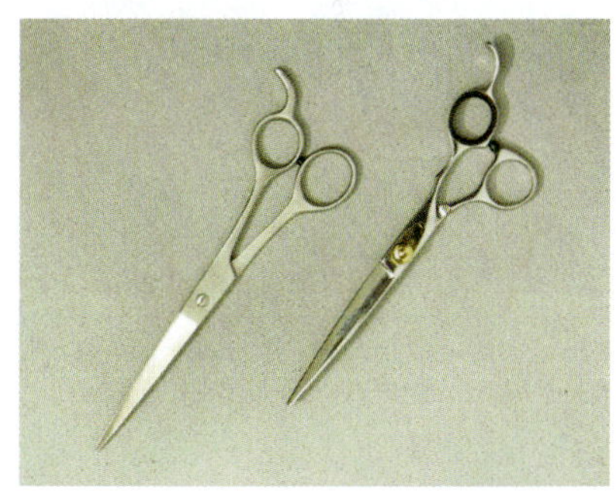

Figure 6-11 Haircutting shears.

Shear Facts

Shears are composed of two blades, one movable and the other stationary, fastened with a screw that acts as a pivot. Other parts of the shears are the cutting edges of the blades, two shanks, finger grip, finger brace, and thumb grip (Figure 6–12).

- *Size.* Shears are available in a variety of lengths, which are measured in inches and half inches. Most barbers prefer the 6½ to 7½ inch shears.
- *Grinds.* The grind of the shear refers to its cutting edge. The two main types of shear grinds are plain and corrugated. The plain grind is used most

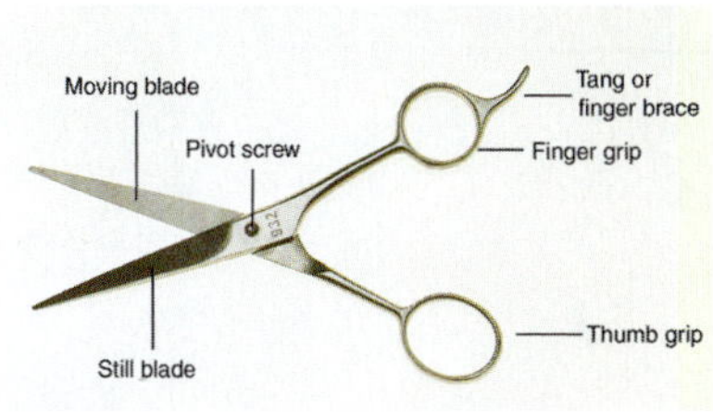

Figure 6-12 Parts of haircutting shears.

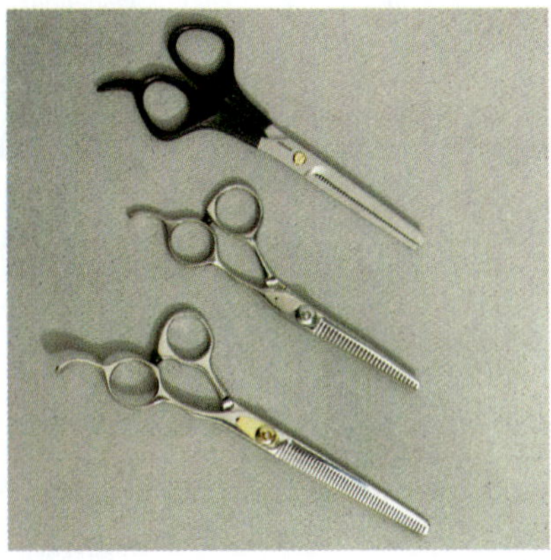

Figure 6–13 Thinning or texturizing shears.

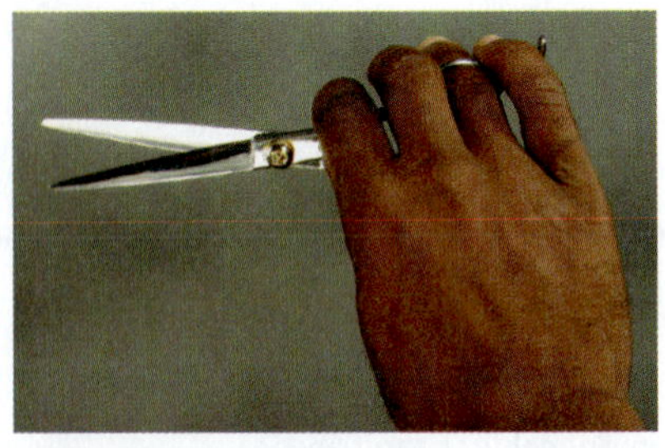

Figure 6–14 Correct finger placement and holding position of shears.

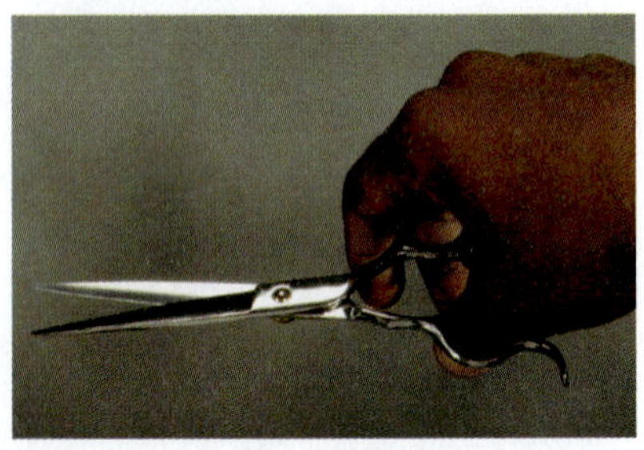

Figure 6–15 Incorrect finger placement and holding position of shears.

frequently and may be smooth (knife edge), medium, or coarse. The corrugated blade has imbrications or teeth, which assist the cutting process.

- *Set.* The **set of the shears** refers to the alignment of the blades. This alignment is just as important as the grind of the blades because even shears with the finest cutting edges will be inferior cutting tools if the blades are not set properly.

Thinning, or **serrated shears**, are used to reduce hair thickness or to create special texturizing effects. They may also be called texturizing shears. One type of thinning shear has notched teeth on the cutting edge of one blade, while the other blade has a straight cutting edge. The second type has overlapping notched teeth on the cutting edges of both blades (Figure 6–13).

Thinning shears also differ in respect to the number of notched teeth on the cutting blade. The greater the number of notched teeth, the finer the hair strands can be cut without noticeable cut marks. The most common type used is the single serrated blade having 30 to 32 notched teeth. Recent designs include a wider notching pattern, with indentations slightly recessed in the notching teeth in order to perform alternative texturizing techniques. Thinning shears are also available with detachable blades.

How to Hold Haircutting Shears

When picking up your shears in preparation for use, you will probably complete the following steps simultaneously.

1. Insert the ring finger into the finger grip of the still blade with the little finger resting on the finger brace. To ensure proper balance, brace the index finger on the shank of the still blade, approximately a half inch from the pivot screw.
2. Next, place the tip of your thumb into the thumb grip of the moving blade. The thumb grip should be positioned halfway between the end of your thumb and the first knuckle. Avoid allowing the thumb grip to slide below the first knuckle, as you will have less control of the cutting blade. See Figures 6–14 and 6–15 for correct and incorrect finger placement and holding positions of the shears.

Palming the Shears and Comb

The shears and comb should be held at all times during a haircut that requires these tools. For safety, shears need to be closed and resting in the palm while combing through the hair. This is called "**palming the shears**" and is achieved by slipping the thumb out of the thumb grip and simply pivoting the shear into the palm of the hand (Figure 6–16). With practice, palming will become a very natural motion. Thinning or texturizing shears should be held in the same manner as regular haircutting shears.

Once the shears are palmed, the process of combing through the hair is performed with the comb in the same hand as the shears (Figure 6–17). After the section of hair has been combed into position for cutting, the comb is transferred to the opposite hand and palmed (Figure 6–18).

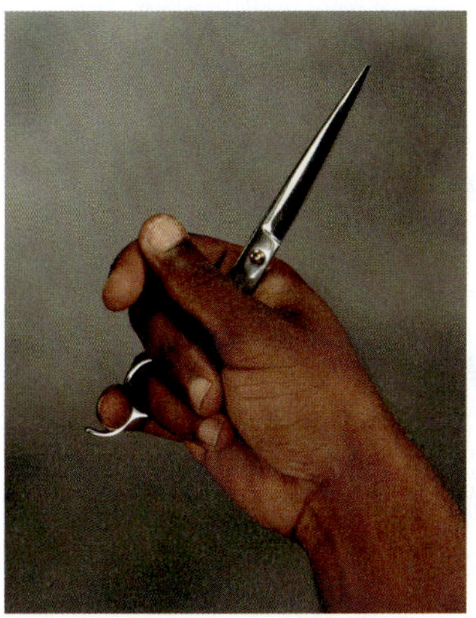

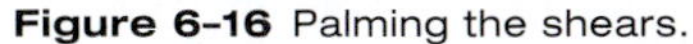

Figure 6-16 Palming the shears.

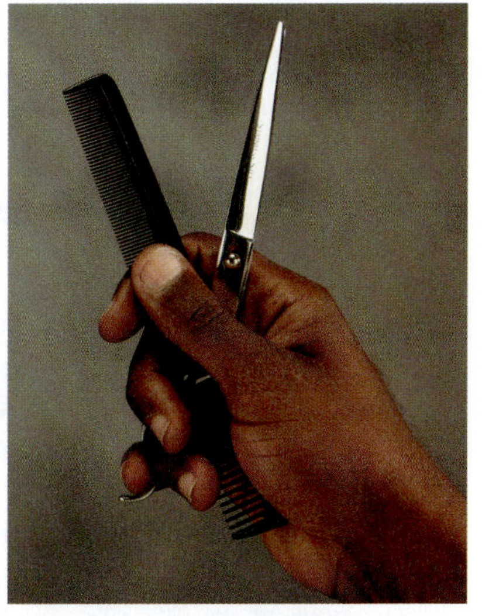

Figure 6-17 Holding the comb and shears.

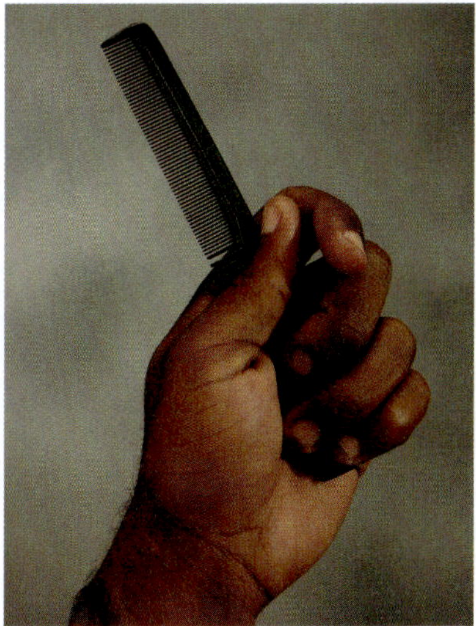

Figure 6-18 Palming the comb.

This allows the first two fingers of that hand to be free to maintain control of the hair and the shear hand free to cut the hair section (Figure 6–19).

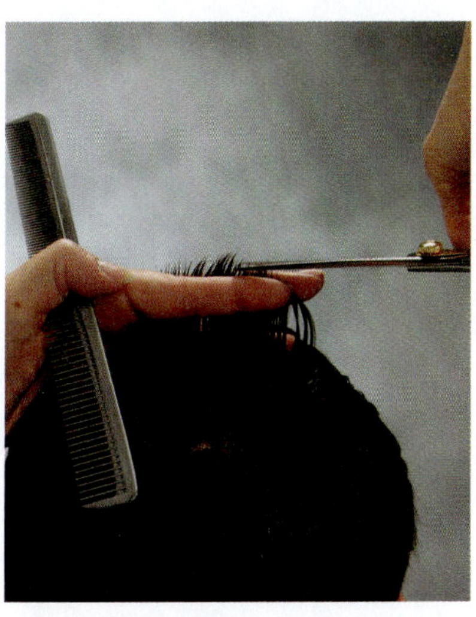

Figure 6-19 Correct palming of comb while cutting.

Care of Haircutting and Thinning Shears

1. Avoid dropping shears! Even one drop on a hard surface can ruin the set of the shears.
2. Protect shears in a leather sheath or holder when carrying them in a kit, bag, or case.
3. Never cut anything but hair with haircutting shears!
   NOTE: Use a less expensive shear on mannequin hair and save your finest tools for models and clients.
4. Disinfect shears after each use with 70% to 90% ethyl or isopropyl alcohol, or an appropriate disinfectant. Lubricate according to manufacturer's recommendations, applying the product to the pivot screw and the juncture of the blades to ensure smooth blade action. Wipe off excess product.
5. Place in a dry or ultraviolet sanitizer until needed for use.

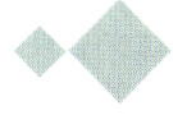

CLIPPERS AND TRIMMERS

Clippers and trimmers are two of the most important tools used in barbering. Clippers can be used for a variety of cutting techniques, from blending to texturizing. Trimmers, also referred to as edgers or outliners, are essential for finish and detail work.

Today's barber has a vast array of clipper styles from which to choose. Function, style, weight, contour, and speed are just some of the factors that should be considered when purchasing a clipper. For example, most clipper models are single speed but there are also two-speed models available. Some clippers utilize a detachable blade system, while others have a single

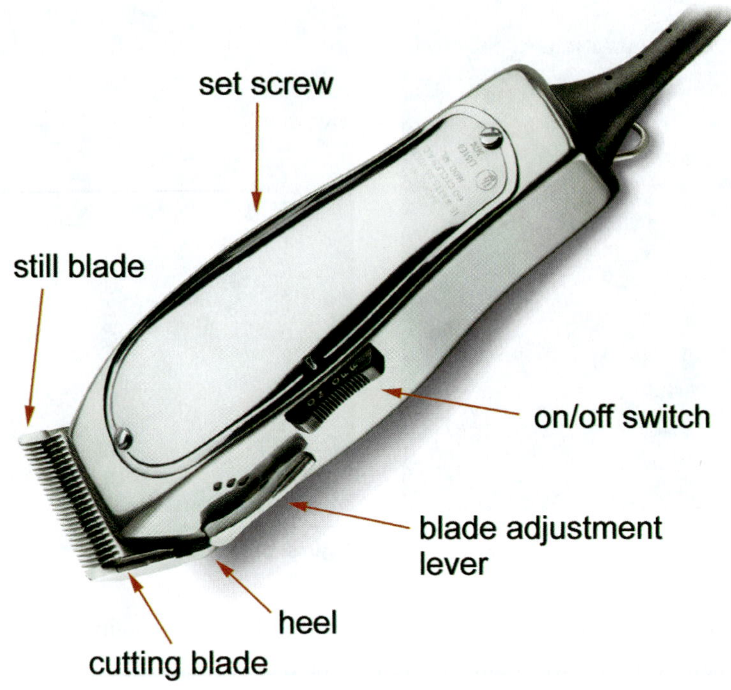

Figure 6–20 Visible parts of an electric clipper.

adjustable blade. Clippers with a single cutting head usually have a blade adjustment lever on the side of the unit and rely on clipper guards to vary the length of the hair being cut. Check with your local supplier for different models and styles.

Electric clippers are driven by one of three basic motor types: the rotary motor, pivot motor, and magnetic (vibratory) motor. The visible parts of an electric clipper are: the cutting blade, still blade, heel, switch, set or power screw, and conducting cord (Figure 6–20).

6

Rotary Motor Clippers

The **rotary** (or **universal**) **motor clipper** is capable of producing a powerful cutting action that is designed for the heavy-duty and continual use that is required in barbershops. These clippers have fewer moving parts, tend to require little maintenance, and run quieter than pivot or magnetic motor clippers. They can be used for wet or dry haircutting and have detachable cutting heads (clipper blades) that must be changed to achieve various hair lengths. If taken care of properly, these clippers can be used for many years with little or no repair (Figure 6–21).

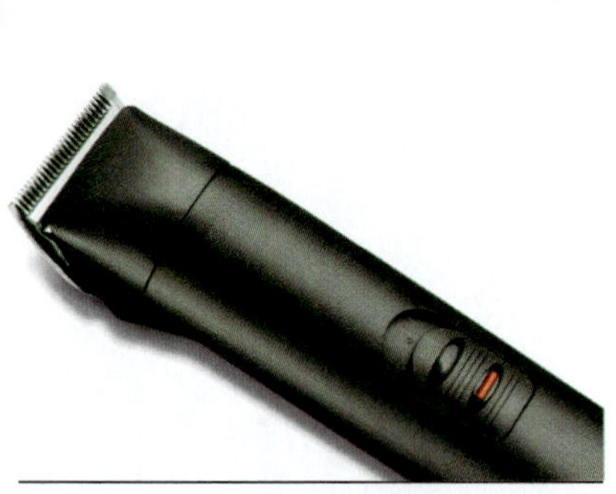

Figure 6–21 Rotary (universal) motor clippers.

Pivot Motor Clippers

Although the pivot motor clipper is not as powerful as a rotary motor clipper, it is twice as powerful as magnetic motor clippers. Pivot motor clippers produce twice the number of blade strokes because the blades are pulled both ways as opposed to the magnetic clipper, which pulls the blade in one direction. Like the rotary motor clipper, pivot motor clippers tend to require little maintenance and can be used for wet or dry haircutting. These clippers have an adjustable blade that is controlled by a lever on the side of the clipper and they are usually packaged with an assortment of attachable clipper guards or combs (Figure 6–22).

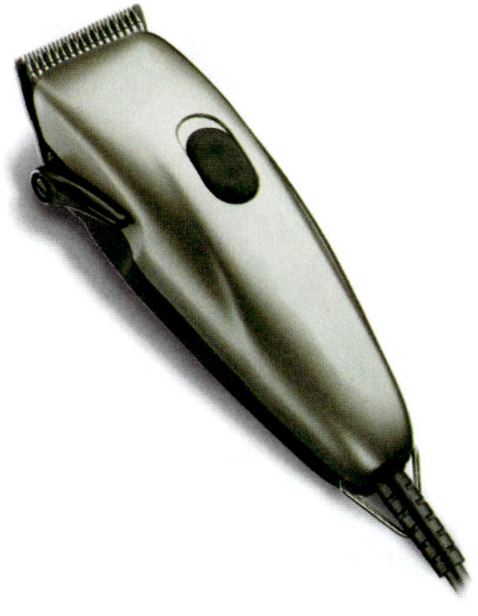

Figure 6-22 Pivot motor clippers.

Magnetic Clippers

Vibratory or magnetic clippers operate by means of an alternating spring and magnet mechanism (Figure 6–23). The magnetic motor pulls the blade in one direction and then retracts using the spring to return. These clippers run faster than the rotary motor type and usually have a single cutting head, which is adjustable for cutting a variety of hair lengths. New balding clipper models are now available with fine-toothed surgical blades for extra-close cutting. Comb attachments (guards) that leave the hair longer than the original cutting head (blades) snap or slide on for easy haircutting versatility.

An outliner, also known as a trimmer or edger, may utilize a magnetic or pivot motor. **Trimmers** have a very fine cutting head for outlining, arching, and design work. The cutting blade is usually available in two styles: a straight trimmer blade (Figure 6–24) and a T-shaped blade (Figure 6–25). The versatility and utility of the T-blade when trimming rounded or difficult areas makes it the number one choice of many barbers and stylists. The outliner is a very valuable implement for detail, precision design, and fine finish work on haircuts and facial hair trims.

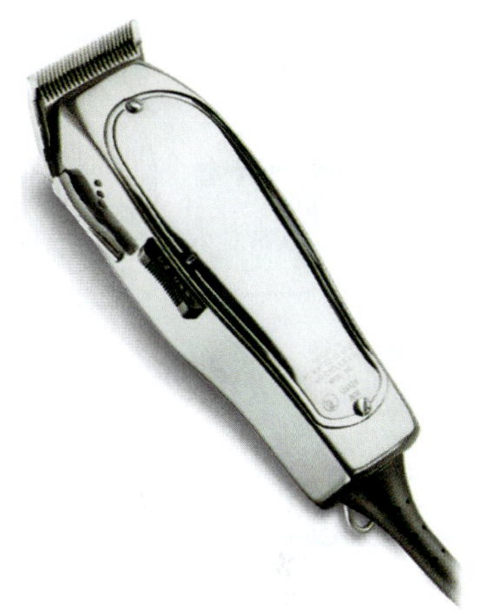

Figure 6-23 Magnetic motor clippers.

Cordless Clippers

A number of manufacturers have produced clippers and outliners that do not require an electric cord. These tools are designed to rest in a special unit that recharges their power. Cordless clippers are a very important innovation for barbers because they are easily maneuverable and portable (Figure 6–26).

Blades and Guards

Clipper **blades** are usually made of high-quality carbon steel and are available in a variety of styles and sizes. Some styles are intended for use with detachable blade clipper models, and others will serve as replacement

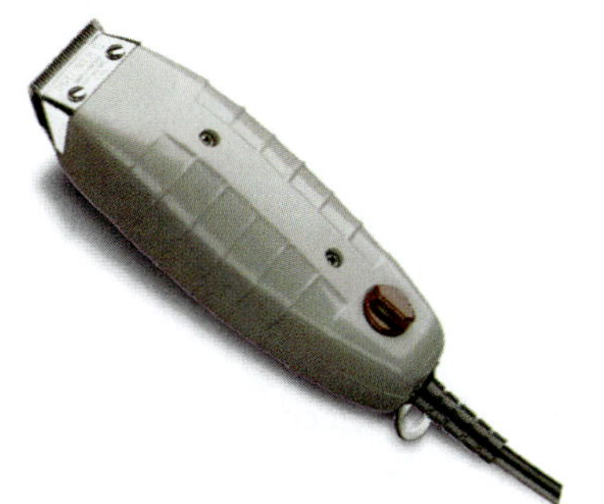

Figure 6-24 Straight-blade trimmer.

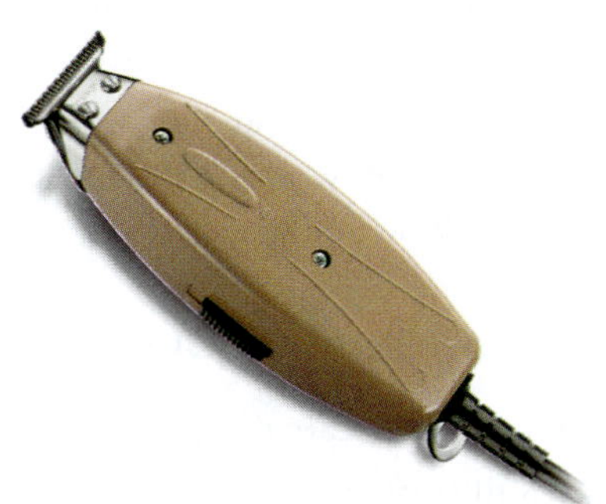

Figure 6-25 T-shaped blade trimmer.

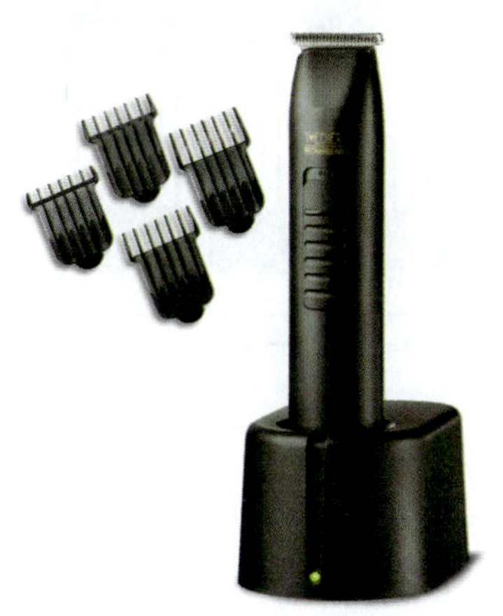

Figure 6-26 Cordless rechargeable outliner.

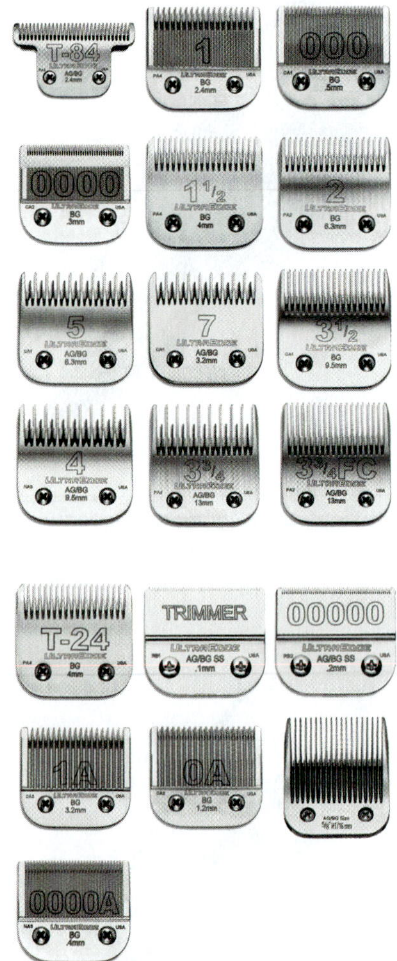

Figure 6-27 Clipper blades.

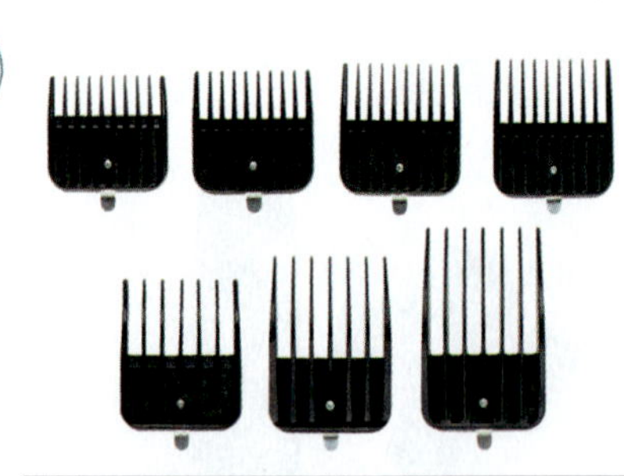

Figure 6-28 Clipper guards.

blades for certain clipper models. Blade sizes can also differ from one manufacturer to another and may not always indicate the same cutting length, so be careful when purchasing these items. Traditionally, the 0000 blade has produced the closest cut, but today's balding clipper blades may cut closer depending on the manufacturer. The size 3 clipper blade leaves the hair approximately 5/16 of an inch long. A good rule of thumb is to follow the manufacturer's recommendations for the style and size of clipper blades that are appropriate for their clipper models. Manufacturers are constantly improving their clipper blades to permit faster and more precise haircutting; be on the lookout for the newest in haircutting tools (Figure 6–27).

Clipper **guards**, also known as attachment combs, are most often made of plastic or hard rubber and can be used with most clipper models. The purpose of a clipper guard is to allow the hair to be left longer than what might be achieved from the size of the clipper blades alone. Like clipper blades, guards also help to ensure uniformity within the cut; however, since the guards do not do the actual cutting, they should not be confused with the clipper blades. Instead, guards are simply supplemental implements that the barber may use in the pursuit of versatile techniques and that can be added to his professional toolbox (Figure 6–28).

How to Hold Clippers

The technique used by a barber to hold the clippers is most often determined by the section of the head he or she is working on. Cutting the back section will necessitate holding the clippers differently than when cutting the top section. A general rule to follow is that the clipper should always be held in a manner that permits freedom of wrist movement. Three methods of holding clippers are explained below, but be guided by your instructor for alternative methods.

1. When the right-handed barber holds the clippers, the thumb is placed on top of the clipper with the fingers supporting it from the underside (Figure 6–29). This position is usually comfortable for tapering in the nape or side areas of a haircut or when the clipper is switched to the left hand while cutting hair sections from a different direction.
2. An alternative method is to place the thumb on the left side of the unit and the fingers on the right side, with the blades pointing up (Figure 6–30). Like the holding position in Figure 6–29, some may find this a comfortable position for tapering around the hairline.
3. Figure 6–31 shows an alternative underhand position that may be used when working the top section of a haircut from a side-view position.

Care of Electric Clippers

To take proper care of clippers and trimmers you will need a clipper brush with stiff bristles, a small container, blade wash, clipper oil, and lubricating or cooling sprays. **CAUTION**: While lubricating sprays may perform well as coolants, they may not contain sufficient oil for thorough lubrication.

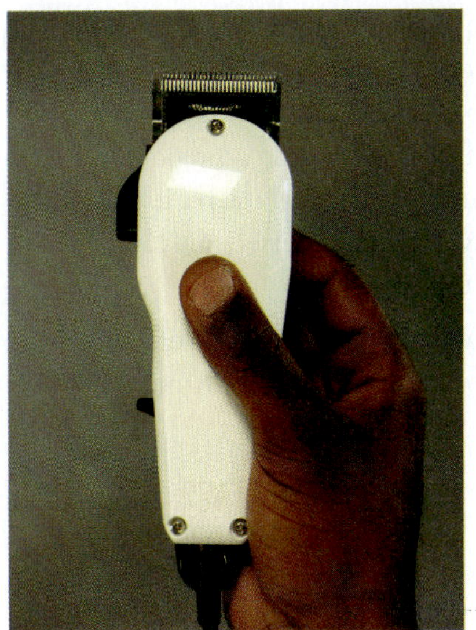

Figure 6-29 Clipper-holding position #1.

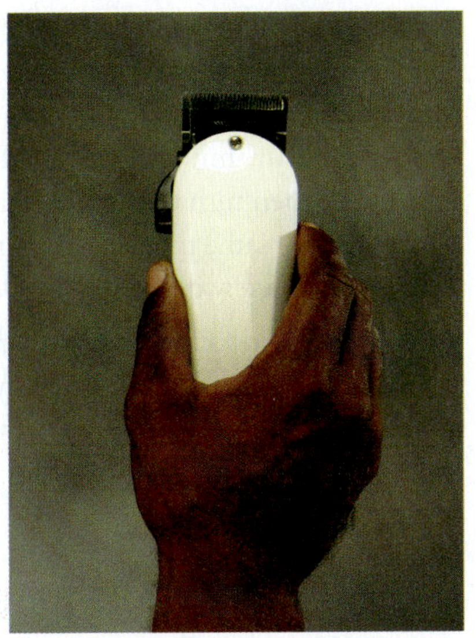

Figure 6-30 Clipper-holding position #2.

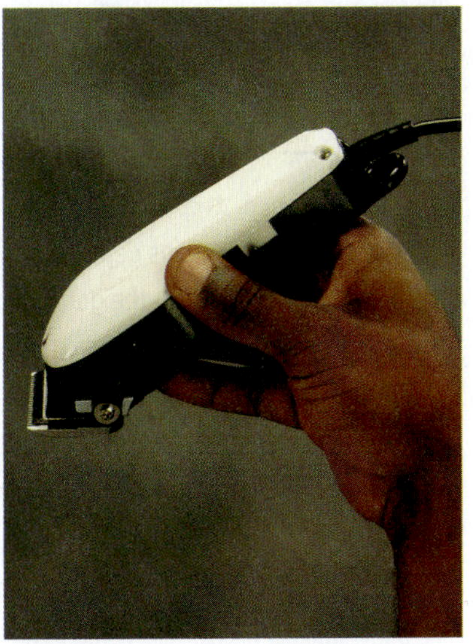

Figure 6-31 Clipper-holding position #3.

Since it is recommended that blades be oiled before, during, and after each use, it is very important to include these steps in your daily haircutting and clipper-maintenance routine. The following procedures outline some basic clipper-maintenance steps, but always read the manufacturers' directions for specific care of their tools. Your instructor may also guide you in the care of clippers and trimmers.

CAUTION

Never adjust clipper or trimmer blades flush to each other. Doing so can create a cutting edge that can lift the epidermal layers of the skin causing irritations, abrasions, cuts, and ingrown hairs. Blades should only be set as recommended by the manufacturer. The top or front blade should rest between 1/16 and 1/32 of an inch below the back blade depending on the tool. If a client requests a closer cut than what the clipper blade will produce, use balding clippers or a razor to shave the head.

General Maintenance Before, During, and After a Haircut

Hold the clippers with the blades pointed in a downward position. Use the clipper brush to remove hair particles. Immerse only the clipper blades in a shallow container of blade wash and turn the unit on. Run the clippers until all the hair embedded between the blades is removed. Make sure that the clippers remain in downward position so the blade wash does not accumulate in the motor. Turn the clippers off and wipe off excess blade wash. Again, while maintaining a downward position of the clippers, apply several drops of oil on the front and sides of the blades then wipe off excess oil with a soft cloth. Remember, even a minimal amount of oil in the motor may reduce the clippers' cutting ability.

Rotary motor clippers: To detach the cutting blade from the still blade, slide the still blade out from under the compression spring. The blades may be washed with hot water, reassembled, and a drop of oil placed in the two holes in the compression plate. Remove the nameplate and check the grease. The grease chamber should be kept about two-thirds full. If the gears should come out, be careful to reassemble them the same way as they were originally. Remove the carbon brush knobs and check the carbon brushes. If they are worn down, replace them with new brushes. Add a few drops of oil weekly to the *oiler* at the rear of the clippers. Clean the hair from the oil vents surrounding the switch to ensure proper ventilation.

When using clippers to cut the hair, the amount of hair that remains depends on whether the hair is cut with the grain or against the grain. For example, when using a 1" blade to cut with the grain, the approximate length of the hair that remains will be 1⅛" to 1⅜"; cutting against the grain will leave the hair from 1" to 1¼" long.

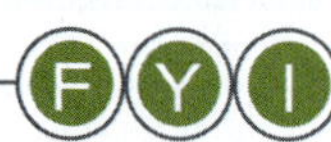

The position of the clipper blades relative to the skin and the hair's density and texture will determine the length of the hair that is left after cutting. Remember that angling the clipper blades toward the scalp or out toward the hair ends will produce different results.

Magnetic clippers: These do not require frequent internal greasing, although one or two drops of oil should be applied routinely between the blades. If vibratory clippers seem to be cutting exceptionally slow or are pulling the hair, immerse the blades in clipper oil or a prepared clipper cleaner and then turn the clippers on and off. This will clean the blades and oil them at the same time. Clippers may also be immersed in a cleaning solvent and then a few drops of oil added to the blades.

Properly cared for, electric clippers will last for years. Manufacturer's directions should be followed carefully to assure optimal performance and to maintain the validity of the warranty.

RAZORS

As the sharpest and closest cutting tool, razors are used for facial shaves, neck shaves, finish work around the sideburn and behind-the-ear areas, and haircutting. The razor of choice for professional barbering is the straight razor; safety razors should not be used to render professional services in the barbershop.

Straight Razors

There are two types of straight razors: the **changeable-blade straight razor** and the **conventional straight razor**, which requires honing and stropping to maintain its cutting edge. Both may be purchased with a razor guard. The razor guard is a razor attachment that is used in razor-cutting the hair (Chapter 15). The changeable-blade razor generally looks the same as the conventional straight razor and is used in the same manner. The benefits of using the changeable-blade straight razor are the easy replacement of blades from one client service to another and the maintenance of sanitation standards in the barbershop.

Selecting the right kind of razor is a matter of personal choice. The best guides for buying high-quality razors are as follows:

1. Consult with a reliable company representative or salesperson that can recommend the type of razor best suited to your work.
2. Consult with more experienced barbers about which razors they have found best for shaving and haircutting.
3. Experiment with a variety of razors to determine the most comfortable styles and types for your use.
4. Avoid judging a razor simply on color or design. Neither one of these characteristics provides a true indication of the razor's caliber as a cutting tool.

Structural Parts of a Straight Razor

The structural parts of both conventional and changeable-blade straight razors are the head, back, shoulder, tang, shank, heel, edge, point, blade, pivot, and handle (Figure 6–32).

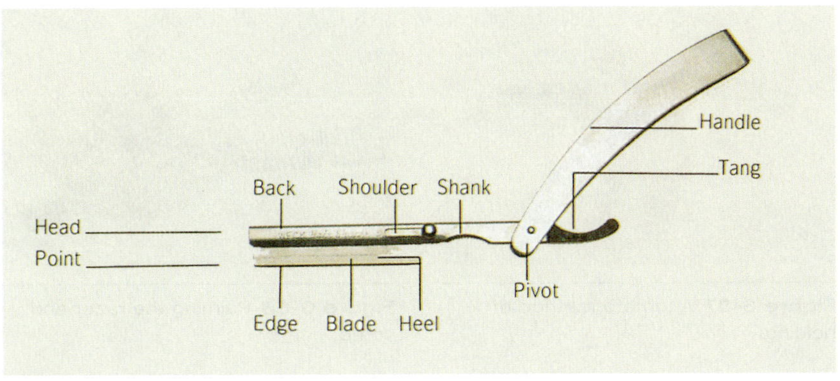

Figure 6-32 Parts of a razor.

Changeable-blade Straight Razor

The changeable- (or disposable-) blade straight razor is the most popular since it eliminates honing and stropping, saves time, is usually lighter, and uses a disposable blade, which helps to maintain sanitation standards. The razor is used without the guard for shaving, and with or without the guard for razor haircutting. Blades are available with a square point, rounded point, or a combination, with one end rounded and the other end squared (Figure 6–33).

2

Changing the Blade

Always follow the manufacturer's directions for inserting a new blade or removing an old blade from a changeable-blade razor. Some razor models are designed with a screw mechanism that releases the blade; others require a sliding motion for blade insertion and removal. The following guidelines explain the sliding motion method of blade replacement as illustrated in Figures 6–34 and 6–35.

1. Hold razor firmly above the joint of the handle and shank. Use the teeth of the razor guard to catch the blade and push it out of the

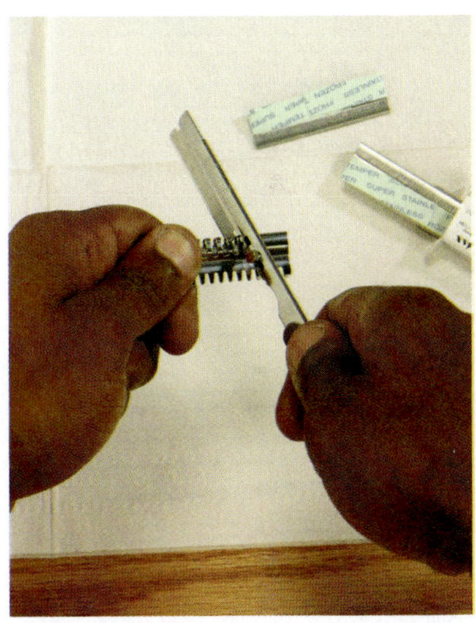

Figure 6-34 Removing the blade.

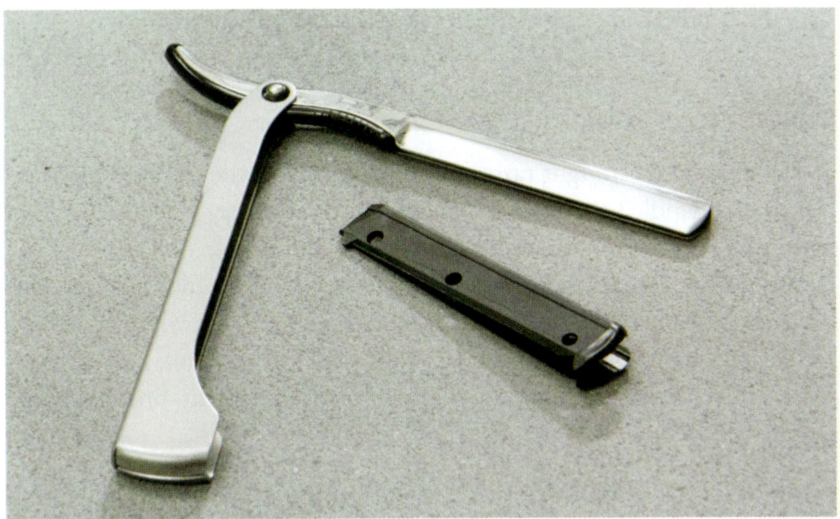

Figure 6-33 Changeable-blade razor.

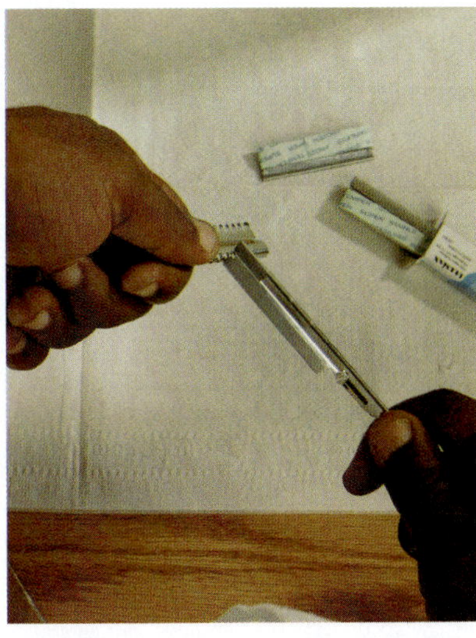

Figure 6-35 Correct blade insertion.

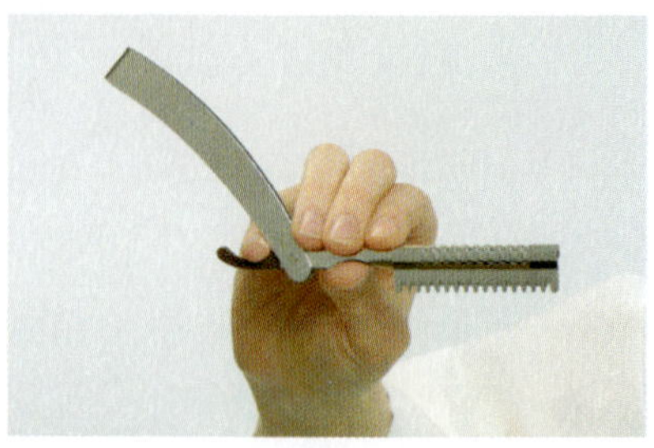

Figure 6-36 Holding razor properly.

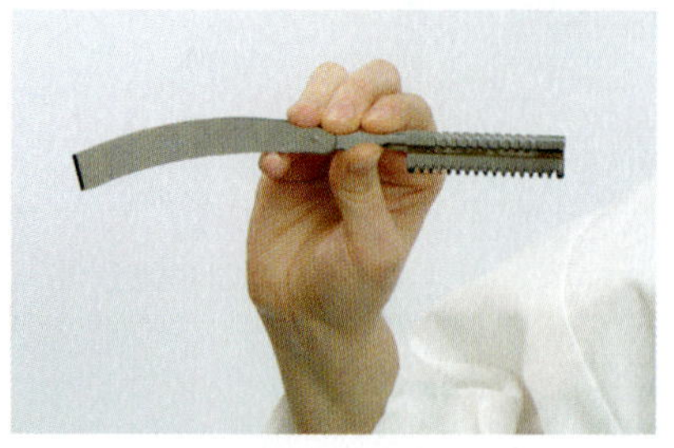

Figure 6-37 Alternate method of holding.

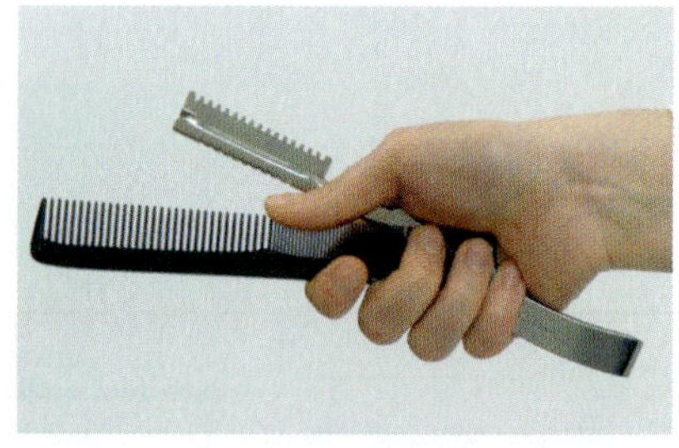

Figure 6-38 Palming the razor and comb.

razor. Always store used blades in a sharps container until ready for disposal (Figure 6–34).

2. To insert a new blade, position the end of the blade into the razor groove. Use the teeth of the razor guard to slide the blade in until it clicks into position (Figure 6–35).
   NOTE: Some razor blade packaging is designed to act as a blade dispenser. The razor groove is slid over the top of the blade from the side of the dispenser until the blade is in place.

Holding the Changeable-Blade Razor

There are several methods of holding the razor, depending on the service being performed. Specific techniques will be covered in the shaving and haircutting chapters; however, it is advisable for the students to practice and become familiar with the basic holding positions as follows:

1. The ball of the thumb supports the razor at the bottom of the shank between the blade and the pivot. The handle is angled up, allowing the little finger to rest on the tang. Place the index finger along the back of the razor for control with the two middle fingers resting comfortably along the top of the shank (Figure 6–36).
2. The razor is also held in a straightened position with the finger placement as shown in Figure 6–37. This holding technique may also be used during haircutting services.
3. To palm the razor, curl in the ring finger and little finger around the handle. Hold the comb between the thumb, index, and middle fingers (Figure 6–38).

3

Conventional Straight Razor

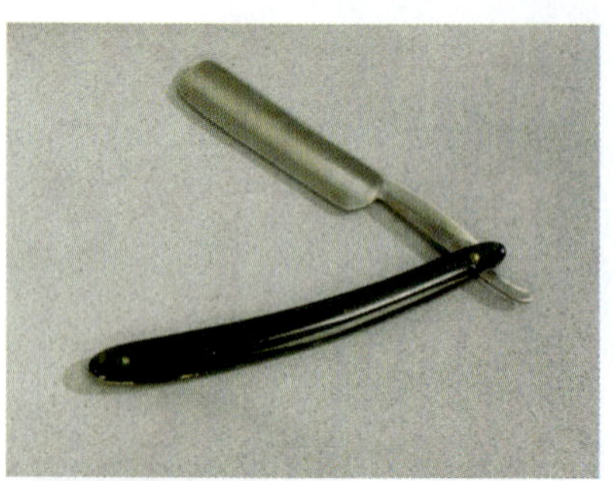

Figure 6-39 Conventional straight razor(s).

The conventional straight razor is composed of a hardened steel blade attached to a handle by means of a pivot. The handle may be constructed of hard rubber, plastic, bone, or new polymer materials and only the highest-quality conventional straight razor should be used. In order to determine the quality of the razor, the barber must consider the following factors: razor balance, temper, grind, finish, size, and style. In addition, barbers must master the techniques of honing and stropping in order to produce a fine cutting edge (Figure 6–39).

Straight Razor Balance

Razor balance refers to the weight and length of the blade relative to that of the handle. A straight razor is properly balanced when the weight of the blade and handle are equal. Proper balance of the razor allows for greater ease and safety in handling the razor during shaving. Opening the razor and resting it on the index finger at the pivot will test the balance of the razor. If the head of the razor moves up or down, the razor is not well balanced.

Razor Tempers

Tempering the razor involves a special heat treatment included in the manufacturing process. When a razor is properly tempered, it acquires the degree of hardness required for a good cutting edge. Razors can be purchased with a hard, soft, or medium temper. The barber should select the temper that produces the most satisfactory shaving results. While hard-tempered razors will hold an edge longer, they are difficult to sharpen; conversely, soft-tempered razors are easier to sharpen, but the sharp edge does not last long. For those reasons, many barbers prefer a medium-tempered razor.

Razor Grinds

The grind of a razor is the shape of the blade after it has been ground. There are two general types: the concave grind and the wedge grind.

Concave grind: The concave grind (often referred to as the hollow-ground razor) is available in a full concave, one-half concave, and one-quarter concave form. The back and edge of the razor looks hollow, being slightly thicker between the hollow part and the extreme edge. Many barbers prefer the hollow-ground razor since the resistance of the beard can be felt more easily thus alerting the barber to check the sharpness of the cutting edge. Although the one-half and one-quarter concave grinds are less hollow than the full concave, the outside dimensions of the blade appear the same.

Wedge grind: The wedge grind is neither hollow nor concave. Both sides of the blade form a sharp angle at the extreme edge of the razor. Most of the older razors were made with a wedge grind. Although learning how to sharpen a wedge grind may be a challenge, once mastered, this grind produces an excellent shave. It is especially preferred for men with coarse, heavy beards (Figure 6–40).

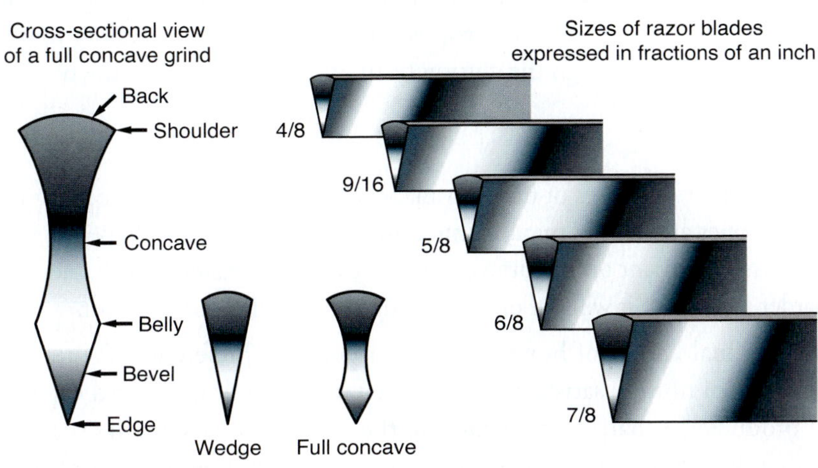

Figure 6-40 Razor grinds.

Razor Finish

The finish of a razor is the polish of its surface. This finish may be plain, crocus (polished steel), or metal-plated with nickel or silver. Of these types, the crocus finish is usually the choice of the discriminating barber. Although the crocus finish is more costly, it lasts longer and does not rust as easily as other finishes. Metal-plated razors are undesirable because the finish wears off quickly, which may hide poor-quality steel.

Razor Sizes

The size of the razor is measured by the length and width of the blade. The width of the razor is measured either in eighths or sixteenths of an inch, such as 4⁄8, 5⁄8, 6⁄8, 7⁄8 and 9⁄16. Two of the most common sizes are the 5⁄8 and 9⁄16 inch, with the 5⁄8 inch being the more popular.

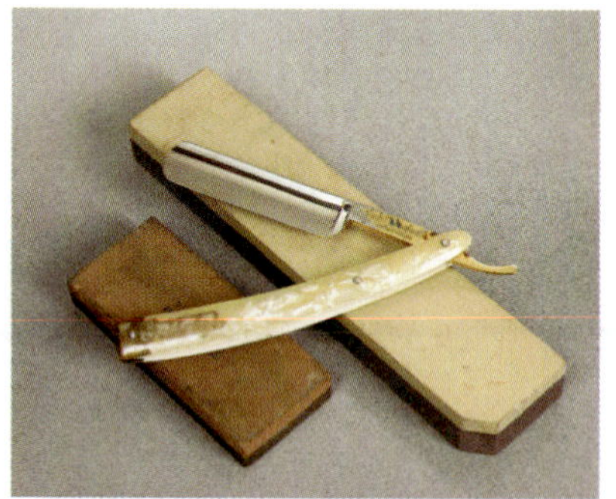

Figure 6-41 Hones with conventional straight razor.

Razor Styles

The style of a razor indicates its shape and design. Modern razors have such features as a back and edge that is straight and parallel to each other; a round heel; a square point; and a flat or slightly round handle. To prevent scratching the skin, the barber usually rounds off the square point of the razor slightly by drawing the point of the razor along the edge of the hone.

Razor Care

Razors will maintain their quality if care is taken to prevent corrosion of the extremely fine edge. After use, a razor should be cleaned, stropped, and a little oil applied to the cutting edge. Be careful not to drop the razor as doing so may damage the blade. When closing the razor, be careful that the cutting edge does not strike the handle. If the cutting edge strikes the handle when closing the razor, it may indicate that the handle is warped or that the pivot is too tightly riveted. The barber's tool kit should include several high-grade razors so that a damaged razor can be replaced immediately.

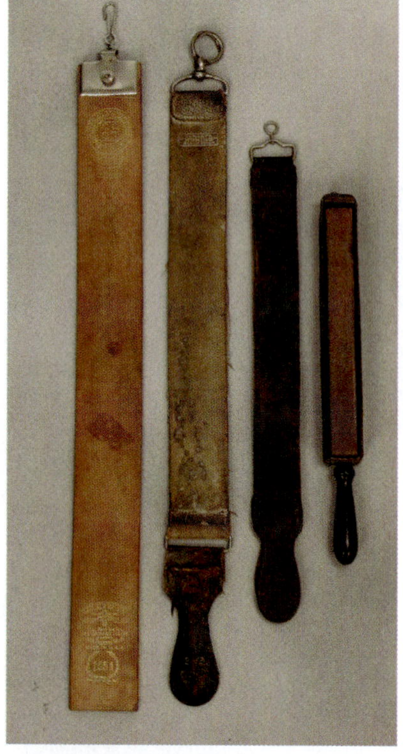

Figure 6-42 Strops.

Conventional Straight Razor Accessories

There are two vital accessories used with conventional straight razors: the hone and the strop. A **hone** is an abrasive material that has the ability to cut steel. It is used to grind the steel and impart an effective cutting edge to the razor's blade (Figure 6–41). A **strop** is a leather and canvas accessory that is used to smooth and align the cutting teeth of the razor edge (Figure 6–42).

Hones

There are various types of hones available for the purpose of sharpening razors. Hones are usually manufactured in a rectangular block shape for ease of blade placement on its surface. Since the abrasive material of the hone is harder than steel, it will cut or file the edge on the blade of the razor.

The final choice of hone is based on personal preference. Generally, any type of hone is satisfactory, provided it is used properly and capable of producing a sharp cutting edge on the razor. Students usually practice with a slow-cutting hone, while experienced practitioners generally prefer a faster-cutting hone. In selecting a hone, remember that the finer the abrasive, the slower its action. There are three main types of hones: natural, synthetic, and combination.

Natural hones are derived from natural rock deposits. Water or shaving lather is usually applied before use to facilitate movement of the razor's blade over the hone surface.

The *water hone* is a natural hone cut out of rock formations, usually imported from Germany. Accompanying the water hone is a small piece of slate of the same texture, called the rubber. When the rubber is applied over the hone, which is moistened with water, a proper cutting surface is created.

The water hone is primarily a slow-cutting hone. When used as directed by the manufacturer, a smooth and lasting edge will result. It is gray or brown in color. Of the two colors, the brown water hone is considered to be slightly superior, and also exerts a slightly faster cutting action. When honing, care should be taken not to work a bevel into the hone.

The *Belgian hone* is a natural hone cut from rock formations found in Belgium. It is a slow-cutting hone, but a little faster than the water hone, and can create a very sharp edge. Lather is generally applied to the hone to facilitate movement of the razor.

One type of Belgian hone consists of a light yellowish rock top glued on to the back of dark red slate. Its principal advantage is that it yields a keen cutting edge on the razor and can be used either wet or dry.

Synthetic hones, such as the Swaty hone and the carborundum (car-bor-un-dum) hone, are manufactured products. These hones may be used dry or lather may be applied before use. Because they cut faster than water hones, synthetic hones have the advantage of producing a keen cutting edge in less time. The carborundum hone is available in range of types from slow-cutting to fast-cutting. Many practitioners prefer the fast-cutting type because of its quick sharpening action, although care needs to be taken to avoid producing rough edges.

Combination hones consist of both a water hone and a synthetic hone. The synthetic side is a dark brown and is used first to develop a good cutting edge. To give the razor a finished edge, it is stroked over the side of the water hone.

Choosing a Hone

As with all the other barbering tools and implements, the type of hone used is a matter of personal choice. Most barbers use carborundum or combination hones, however, it is advisable to be familiar with the other types of hones and to understand the benefits of each.

The type of steel in a razor also makes some difference as to whether a good edge can be obtained with a particular type of hone. There are many other hones available in addition to the ones described that will give very satisfactory results. Be guided by your instructor and personal experimentation with different hones.

Care of Hones

Always clean the hone before using. Use water and a pumice stone to remove the tiny steel particles that accumulate on the surface of the hone. If a new hone is very rough, the same method can be used to work it into shape.

When wet honing is done, always wipe the hone dry after use. This aids the cleaning process and also wipes away the particles of steel that adhere to the cutting surface. Disinfect according to manufacturer's directions.

Strops

Unlike hones, which are designed to grind the edge of a razor, strops are intended to bring the razor to a smooth, whetted cutting edge. A good strop is made of durable and flexible material, has the proper thickness and texture, and shows a smooth, finished surface. Some barbers like a thin strop; others prefer a thick, heavy strop.

Most strops are made with two layers of material: one side of leather and the other side of canvas (see Figure 6–42). The leather side is made from cowhide, horsehide, or synthetic materials. Depending upon the material used and the style of construction, strops are categorized as follows: French or German, canvas, cowhide, horsehide, and imitation leather. The finer-quality strops are usually "broken in" by the manufacturer, requiring less "breaking in" by the barber.

The *French or German strop* is a combination strop with leather on one side and a finishing strop on the other. It is used by many barbers for styling razors and provides an all-in-one razor accessory.

The *canvas strop* is made of high-quality linen or silk, woven into a fine or coarse texture. A fine-textured linen strop is most desirable for putting a lasting edge on a razor. To obtain the best results, a new canvas strop should be thoroughly broken in. A daily hand-finish treatment will keep the strop surface smooth and in readiness for stropping. A canvas strop should be given the following treatment:

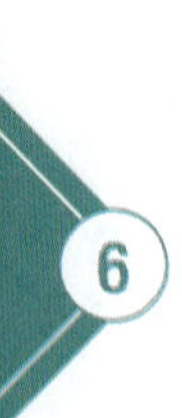

1. Attach the swivel end of the strop to a fixed point, such as a nail. (Most of the older barber chairs and some of the newer models have a metal loop attached to the arm of the chair for the purpose of stopping.)
2. Hold the other end tightly over a smooth and level surface.
3. Rub a bar of dry soap over the strop, working it well into the grain of the canvas.
4. Rub a smooth glass bottle over the strop several times, each time forcing the soap into the grain and also removing any excess soap.

The *cowhide strop* was originally imported from Russia. To this day it still bears the name **Russian strop**, even though it may be manufactured in this country. This name usually implies that the strop is made of cowhide and that the Russian method of tanning was employed. The cowhide or Russian strop is considered to be one of the best. When new, it requires a daily hand finish until it is thoroughly broken in. There are several ways to break in a Russian strop. A method frequently used is as follows:

1. Rub dry pumice stone over the strop in order to remove the outer nap and develop a smooth surface.
2. Rub stiff lather into the strop.
3. Rub dry pumice stone over the strop until smooth.
4. Clean off the strop.
5. Rub fresh, stiff lather into the strop.
6. Rub a smooth glass bottle over the strop several times until a smooth surface is developed.

Another method to break in a Russian strop is to omit the pumice stone. Instead, stiff lather is rubbed into the strop with the aid of a smooth glass bottle or with the palm of the hand.

Horsehide strops are divided into two main groups: the ordinary horsehide strop and the *shell.*

1. An ordinary horsehide strop is of medium grade, has a fine grain, and tends to be very smooth. In this condition it does not readily impart the proper edge to a razor. For this reason, it is not recommended for professional use. However, it is suitable for private use.
2. The second type of horsehide strop is called a shell or Russian **shell strop**. This is a high-quality strop taken from the muscular rump area of a horse. Although it is quite expensive, it makes one of the best strops for barbers and stylists. It tends to remain smooth and requires very little, if any, breaking in.

The *imitation leather strop* has not proven very satisfactory for use in the barbershop. Because of the availability of high-quality strops, it is wise to avoid strops made of imitation leather.

Strop Dressing

Strop dressing cleans the leather strop, preserves its finish, and also improves its draw and sharpening qualities. For proper use, apply a very small amount of dressing to the leather strop. Rub it into the pores well and remove any surplus. Always wait at least 24 hours between applications.

Honing and Stropping Procedures

Honing (hone-ing) is the process of sharpening a razor blade on a hone and the primary purpose is to obtain a perfect cutting edge on the razor. The blade is sharpened by honing the razor with *smooth, even strokes of equal number* and *pressure on both sides of the blade.* In addition, the *angle* at which the blade is stroked must be the same for both of its sides. Student barbers should use an old, damaged razor for practicing the honing process.

Honing the Razor

1. The first step in honing is to practice rolling the razor against the hone with no pressure. Use the fingers to turn the razor from one side to another without turning the wrist. Practice this rolling motion against the hone with no pressure until it is mastered. This will help to keep the razor in good condition and to maintain the equal pressure required in the honing process.

chapter review questions

1. List the principal tools and implements used in barbering.
2. What style comb is used for general cutting?
3. Name three services in which tapering combs may be used.
4. Identify the parts of haircutting shears.
5. What is the difference between German and French shears?
6. How are the lengths of shears usually measured? Which sizes are used most often?
7. Identify the two main types of shear grinds. Which type is used most frequently?
8. What are thinning shears used for?
9. List three types of clipper motors.
10. List the visible parts of electric clippers.
11. Identify the size of clipper blade that produces the shortest cut.
12. Name two types of straight razors.
13. List the 11 parts of a razor.
14. Explain the purpose of a hone.
15. List three types of hones.
16. Explain the movements used in honing.
17. Explain the purpose of a strop.
18. Name the type of strop that is considered to be the best for barbers.
19. Explain the movements used in stropping.
20. List some advantages of using an electric latherizer.

21. Identify the type of soap that is used in an electric latherizer.

22. List three methods of removing loose hair from the client's face and neck.

23. What does the word *thermal* mean?

24. Name the appliance that is used to heat thermal irons and pressing combs.

25. Explain the main function of the galvanic machine.

26. Identify two services that high-frequency machines might be used for.

27. What is the function of a comedone extractor?

28. What is the best type of chair for performing barbering services?

Muscle Structure

When a muscle contracts and shortens, one of its attachments usually remains fixed and the other one moves. A muscle has three parts: origin, belly, and insertion.

- The **origin of a muscle** refers to the more fixed attachment, such as muscles attached to bones or some other muscle. Muscles attached to bones are usually referred to as skeletal muscles.
- The **insertion of a muscle** refers to the more movable attachment, such as muscles attached to the movable muscle, to a movable bone, or to the skin. Pressure in massage is usually directed from the insertion to the origin.
- The **belly of a muscle** is the middle part of the muscle between the origin and the insertion.

Stimulation of Muscles

Muscular tissue can be stimulated by:

- massage (hand massage or electric vibrator).
- electric current (high-frequency or faradic current).
- light rays (infrared rays or ultraviolet rays).
- heat rays (heating lamps or heating caps).
- moist heat (steamers or moderately warm steam towels).
- nerve impulses (through the nervous system).
- chemicals (certain acids and salts).

Muscles of the Scalp, Face, and Neck

Barbers and stylists must be concerned with the voluntary muscles of the head, face, and neck. In order to perform grooming and professional services such as facial and scalp massage, it is essential to know the location of these muscles and the functions they control (Figure 7–9 and Figure 7–10).

Muscles of the Scalp

- **epicranius** (ep-ih-KRAY-nee-us) or occipito-frontalis: a broad muscle that covers the top of the skull and consists of two parts, the occipitalis and the frontalis.
- **occipitalis** (ahk-SIP-i-tahl-is): a muscle at the back part of the epicranius that draws the scalp backward.
- **frontalis** (frun-TAY-lus): the front portion of the epicranius that draws the scalp forward and causes wrinkles across the forehead.
- **aponeurosis** (ap-uh-noo-ROH-sus): a tendon that connects the occipitalis and the frontalis.

Muscles of the Eyebrows

- **orbicularis oculi** (or-bik-yuh-LAIR-is AHK-yuh-lye): completely surrounds the margin of the eye socket and closes the eyelid.

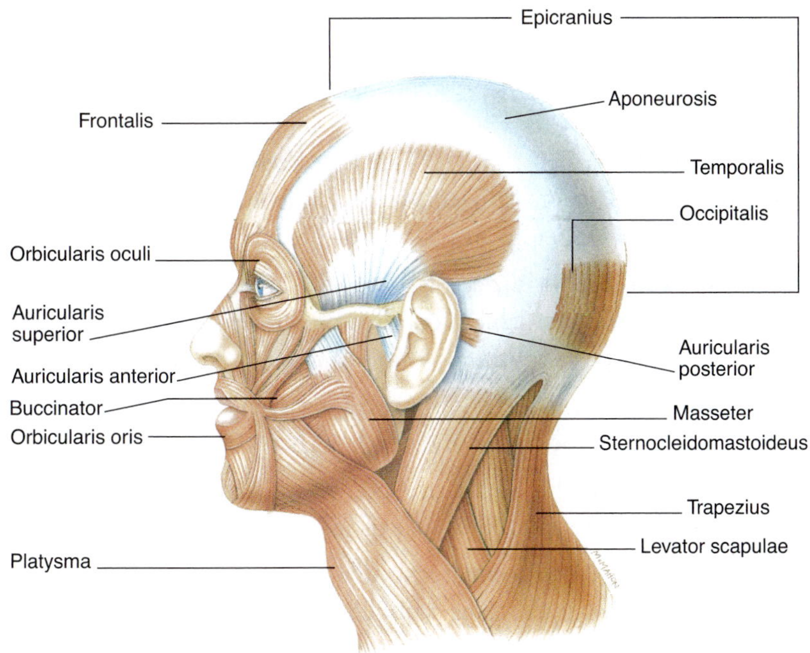

Figure 7-9 Muscles of the head, face, and neck.

- **corrugator** (KOR-oo-gay-tohr): muscle beneath the frontalis and orbicularis oculi that draws the eyebrows down and in. It produces vertical lines and causes frowning.

Muscles of the Nose

The **procerus** (proh-SEE-rus) covers the top of the nose, depresses the eyebrow, and causes wrinkles across the bridge of the nose. The other nasal

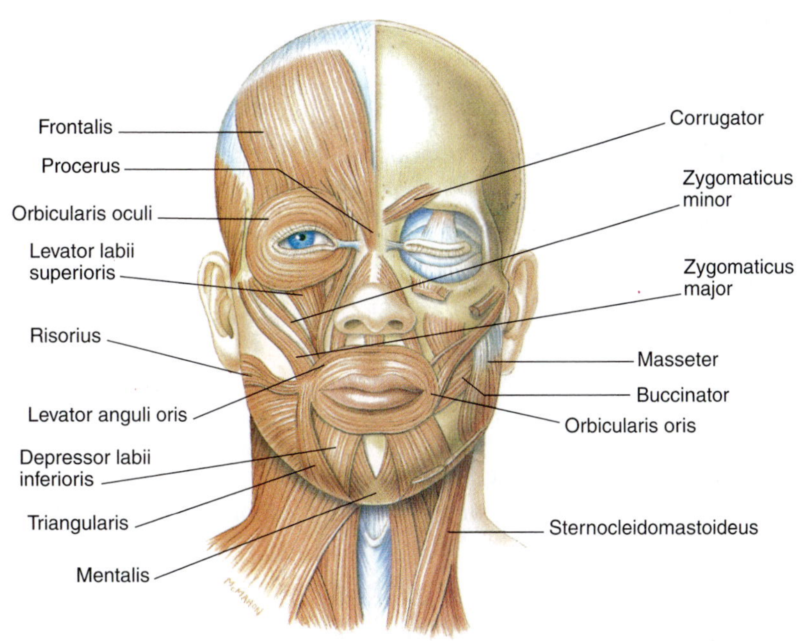

Figure 7-10 Muscles of the face.

muscles are small muscles around the nasal openings, which contract and expand the opening of the nostrils.

Muscles of the Mouth

- **levator labii superioris** (lih-VAYT-ur LAY-bee-eye soo-peer-ee-OR-is), also known as quadratus labii superioris: a muscle surrounding the upper lip. It elevates the upper lip and dilates the nostrils.
- **depressor labii inferioris** (dee-PRES-ur LAY-bee-eye in-FEER-ee-or-us), also known as quadratus labii inferioris: a muscle that surrounds the lower part of the lip, depressing the lower lip and drawing it a little to one side.
- **buccinator** (BUK-sih-nay-tur): muscle between the upper and lower jaws. It compresses the cheeks and expels air between the lips.
- **levator anguli oris** (lih-VAYT-ur ANG-yoo-ly OH-ris), also known as caninus (kay-NY-us): raises the angle of the mouth and draws it inward.
- **mentalis** (men-TAY-lis): situated at the tip of the chin. It raises and pushes up the lower lip, causing wrinkling of the chin.
- **orbicularis oris** (or-bik-yuh-LAIR-is OH-ris): forms a flat band around the upper and lower lips. It compresses, contracts, puckers, and wrinkles the lips.
- **risorius** (rih-ZOR-ee-us): extends from the masseter muscle to the angle of the mouth. It draws the corner of the mouth out and back.
- **zygomaticus** (zy-goh-MAT-ih-kus): extends from the zygomatic bone to the angle of the mouth. It elevates the lip.
- **triangularis** (try-ang-gyuh-LAY-rus): extends along the side of the chin and draws down the corner of the mouth.

Muscles of the Ear

- **auricularis** (aw-rik-yuh-LAIR-is) **superior**: muscle above the ear that draws the ear upward.
- **auricularis posterior**: muscle behind the ear that draws the ear backward.
- **auricularis anterior**: muscle in front of the ear that draws the ear forward.

7

Muscles of Mastication

The **masseter** (muh-SEE-tur) and the **temporalis** (tem-poh-RAY-lis) are muscles that coordinate in opening and closing the mouth, and are sometimes referred to as chewing muscles.

Muscles of the Neck

- **platysma** (plah-TIZ-muh): a broad muscle extending from the chest and shoulder muscles to the side of the chin and responsible for depressing the lower jaw and lip.
- **sternocleidomastoideus** (STUR-noh-KLEE-ih-doh-mas-TOYD-ee-us): extends from the collar and chest bones to the temporal bone in back of the ear that bends and rotates the head.

- **trapezius** (trah-PEE-zee-us): allows movement of the shoulders and covers the back of the neck. 

Muscles of the Hands

The hand is one of the most complex parts of the body, with many small muscles that overlap from joint to joint, providing flexibility and strength to open and close the hand and fingers. Important muscles to know include the:

- **abductor muscles**: muscles that separate the fingers.
- **adductor muscles**: muscles at the base of each finger that draw the fingers together.
- **opponent muscles**: muscles in the palm that act to bring the thumb toward the fingers.

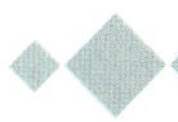

THE NERVOUS SYSTEM

Neurology is the study of the structure, function, and pathology of the nervous system. The nervous system is one of the most important systems of the body. It controls and coordinates the functions of all the other systems and makes them work harmoniously and efficiently. Every square inch of the human body is supplied with fine fibers known as nerves.

An understanding of how nerves work will help barbers to perform the massage services associated with shampoos, scalp treatments, and facials. It will also help to understand the effects that these treatments can have on the skin, scalp, and on the body as a whole.

Divisions of the Nervous System

The principal components of the nervous system are the brain, spinal cord, and the nerves themselves. The nervous system is divided into three main subdivisions: the cerebrospinal (ser-ree-bro-SPY-nahl), the peripheral (puh-RIF-uh-rul), and the autonomic (aw-toh-NAHM-ik) systems (Figure 7–11).

1. The cerebrospinal, or **central nervous system**, consists of the brain, cranial nerves, spinal cord, and spinal nerves. It controls consciousness and all mental activities, voluntary functions of the five senses, and voluntary muscle actions, including all body movements and facial expressions.
2. The **peripheral nervous system** is made up of sensory and motor nerve fibers that extend from the brain and spinal cord to all parts of the body. Their function is to carry impulses, or messages, to and from the central nervous system.
3. The **autonomic**, or sympathetic, **nervous system** is related structurally to the central nervous system, but its functions are independent of the will. This system is very important in the operation of internal body functions such as breathing, circulation, digestion, and glandular

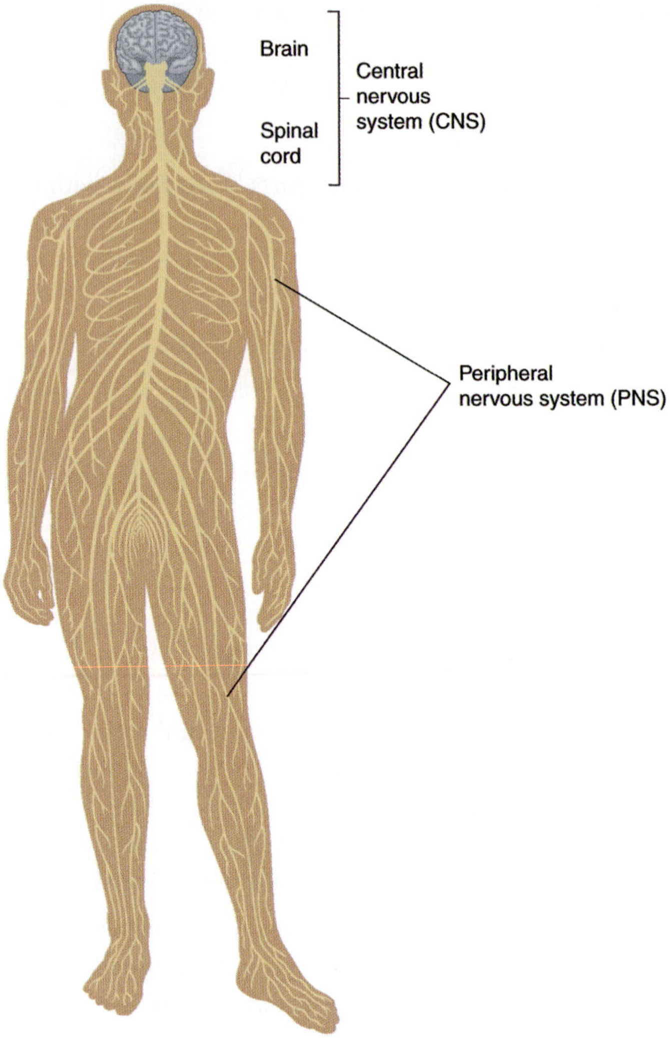

Figure 7-11 Principal parts of the nervous system.

7

activities. Its main purpose is to regulate these internal operations, keeping them in balance and working properly.

The Brain and Spinal Cord

The **brain** is the largest and most complex nerve tissue in the body. Weighing an average of 44 to 48 ounces, the brain is contained within the cranium and controls sensation, muscles, glandular activity, and the ability to think and feel. It sends and receives messages through 12 pairs of cranial nerves that originate in the brain and extend to various parts of the head, face, and neck.

The **spinal cord** is the portion of the central nervous system that originates in the brain, extends down to the lower extremity of the trunk, and is protected by the spinal column. Thirty-one pairs of spinal nerves that extend from the spinal cord are distributed to the muscles and skin of the trunk and limbs.

Nerve Structure and Function

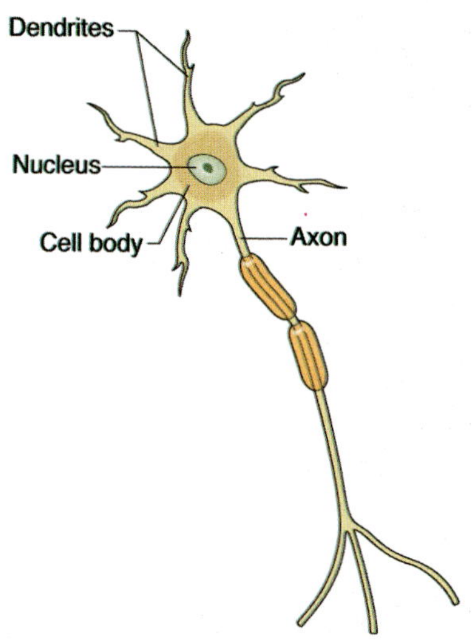

Figure 7–12 Nerve cell.

A neuron, or nerve cell, is the primary structural unit of the nervous system (Figure 7–12). It is composed of a cell body and nucleus with long and short fibers called cell processes. The short processes, called *dendrites*, carry impulses to the cell body. The longer processes, called *axons*, carry impulses away from the cell body to the muscles and organs. The cell body stores energy and food for the cell processes, which convey the nerve impulses throughout the body. Practically all of the axon nerve cells are contained in the brain and spinal cord.

Nerves are long, white cords made up of bundles of nerve fibers, held together by connective tissue, through which impulses are transmitted. Nerves have their origin in the brain and spinal cord, and distribute branches to all parts of the body to facilitate sensation and motion.

Nerve Stimulation

Stimulation to the nerves causes muscles to contract and expand. When heat is applied to the skin the underlying muscles relax; when cold is applied, contraction takes place. Nerve stimulation may be accomplished by any of the following:

- chemicals, such as certain salts or acids
- massage with the hands, massage tool, or an electric massager
- electric current such as Tesla high-frequency current
- light rays
- heat rays
- moist heat, such as warm steam towels

Types of Nerves

- **Sensory nerves**, also called *afferent* nerves, carry impulses or messages from sense organs to the brain, where sensations of touch, cold, heat, sight, hearing, taste, smell, and pain are experienced.
- **Motor nerves**, or *efferent* nerves, carry impulses from the brain to the muscles. The transmitted impulses produce movement.
- **Mixed nerves** contain both sensory and motor fibers and have the ability to send and receive messages.

Sensory nerves are situated near the surface of the skin. Motor nerves are in the muscles. As impulses pass from the sensory nerves to the brain and back over the motor nerves to the muscles, a complete circuit is established and movements of the muscle result.

A **reflex** is an automatic nerve reaction to a stimulus. It involves the movement of an impulse from a sensory receptor to the spinal cord and a responsive impulse to a muscle causing a reaction (for example, the quick removal of the hand from a hot object). Reflex action does not have to be learned.

Cranial Nerves

There are 12 pairs of cranial nerves. All are connected to a part of the brain surface. They emerge through openings on the sides and base of the cranium and reach various parts of the head, face, and neck. They are classified as motor, sensory, and mixed nerves, and contain both motor and sensory fibers.

The most important cranial nerves to consider when massaging the head, face, and neck are the fifth cranial, seventh cranial, and eleventh cranial nerves; and the cervical nerves, which are also involved in scalp and neck massage and originate in the spinal cord.

Fifth Cranial Nerve

The largest of the cranial nerves is the **fifth cranial nerve**, also known as the *trifacial* or *trigeminal* (try-JEM-in-ul) nerve. It is the chief sensory nerve of the face, and serves as the motor nerve of the muscles that control chewing. It consists of three branches: ophthalmic (ahf-THAL-mik), mandibular (man-DIB-yuh-lur), and maxillary (MAK-suh-lair-ee) (Figure 7–13).

The branches of the fifth cranial nerve that are affected by massage are the:

- **supraorbital** (soo-pruh-OR-bih-tul) **nerve**: affects the skin of the forehead, scalp, eyebrows, and upper eyelids.
- **supratrochlear** (soo-pruh-TRAHK-lee-ur) **nerve**: affects the skin between the eyes and upper sides of the nose.
- **infratrochlear** (in-frah-TRAHK-lee-ur) **nerve**: affects the membrane and skin of the nose.
- **nasal nerve**: affects the point and lower sides of the nose.
- **zygomatic** (zy-goh-MAT-ik) **nerve**: affects the skin of the temples, sides of the forehead, and upper part of the cheeks.

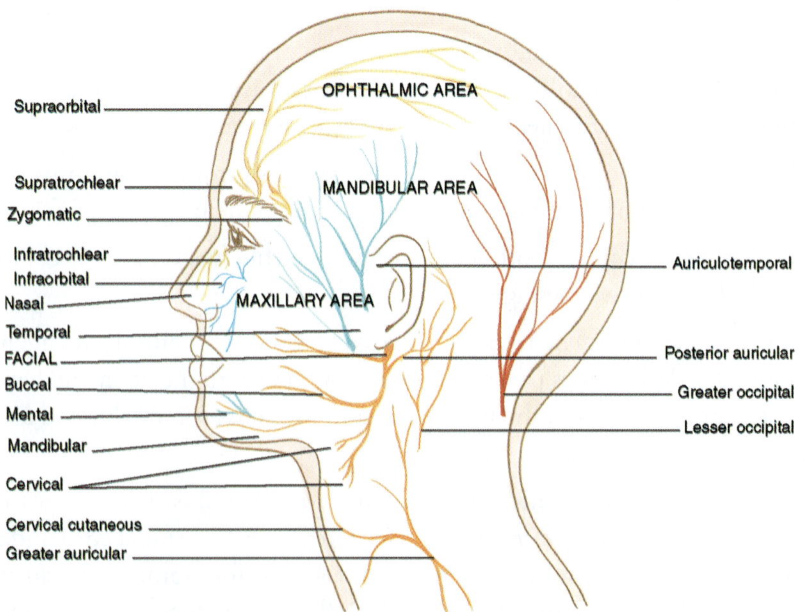

Figure 7-13 Nerves of the face and neck.

- **infraorbital** (in-frah-OR-bih-tul) **nerve**: affects the skin of the lower eyelids, sides of the nose, upper lip, and mouth.
- **auriculotemporal** (aw-RIK-yuh-loh-TEM-puh-rul) **nerve**: affects the external ear and the skin from above the temples to the top of the skull.
- **mental nerve**: affects the skin of the lower lip and chin.

Seventh Cranial Nerve

The **seventh cranial nerve** or facial nerve is the chief motor nerve of the face. It emerges near the lower part of the ear. Its divisions and their branches control all the muscles used for facial expression and extend to the muscles of the neck. The most important branches of the facial nerve are the:

- **posterior auricular nerve**: affects the muscles behind the ears at the base of the skull.
- **temporal nerve**: affects the muscles of the temples, sides of the forehead, eyebrows, eyelids, and upper part of the cheeks.
- **zygomatic nerve** (upper and lower): affects the muscles of the upper part of the cheeks.
- **buccal** (BUK-ul) **nerve**: affects the muscles of the mouth.
- **mandibular nerve**: affects the muscles of the chin and lower lip.
- **cervical nerve**: affects the sides of the neck.

Eleventh Cranial Nerve

The **eleventh cranial nerve** or *accessory nerve* is a spinal nerve branch that affects the muscles of the neck and back.

Cervical Nerves

The cervical or spinal nerves originate at the spinal cord. Their branches supply the muscles and scalp at the back of the head and neck, as follows:

- **greater occipital nerve**: located in the back of the head, affects the scalp as far up as the top of the head.
- **smaller** (lesser) **occipital nerve**: located at the base of the skull, affects the scalp and muscles of this region.
- **greater auricular nerve**: located at the side of the neck, affects the external ears and the areas in front and back of the ears.
- **cervical cutaneous nerve**: located at the side of the neck, affects the front and sides of the neck, as far down as the breastbone.

THE CIRCULATORY SYSTEM

The **circulatory system**, also referred to as the cardiovascular or vascular system, controls the steady circulation of the blood through the body by means of the heart and blood vessels. It is essential to proper circulation and the maintenance of good health. The vascular system is made up of two divisions.

1. The **blood vascular system** consists of the heart, arteries, capillaries, and veins for the circulation and distribution of blood throughout the body.
2. The *lymph vascular*, or lymphatic, system aids the blood vascular system and consists of lymph, glands, vessels (lymphatics), and other structures. Lymph is a clear yellowish fluid that circulates in the lymphatics of the body, helping to carry away waste and impurities from the cells, and is routed back into the circulatory system.

The Heart

The **heart** is a muscular, conical-shaped organ, about the size of a closed fist, that keeps the blood moving within the circulatory system (Figure 7–14). It weighs approximately 9 ounces and is located in the chest cavity where it is enclosed in a membrane, known as the **pericardium** (payr-ih-KAR-dee-um). The heartbeat is regulated by the vagus (tenth cranial nerve) and other nerves in the autonomic nervous system. The normal resting heartbeat of an adult is 72 to 80 times a minute.

The interior of the heart contains four chambers and four valves. The upper, thin-walled chambers are the right **atrium** (AY-tree-um) and left atrium. The lower, thick-walled chambers are the right **ventricle** (VEN-truh-kul) and left ventricle. Valves allow the blood to flow in only one direction. With each contraction and relaxation of the heart, the blood flows in, travels from the atria to the ventricles, and is then driven out to be distributed all over the body. The atrium is also called auricle.

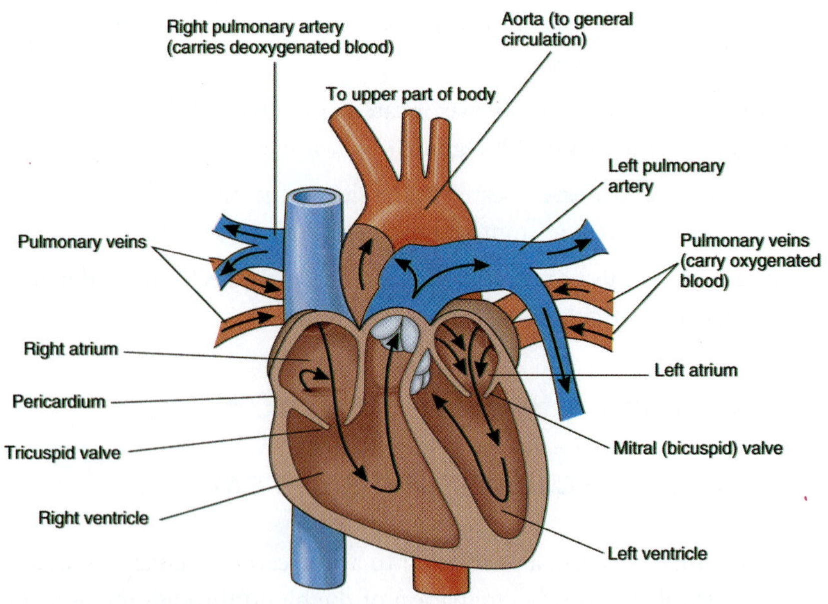

Figure 7–14 Anatomy of the heart.

Blood Vessels

The blood vessels are tubelike structures that include the arteries, capillaries, and veins. The function of these vessels is to transport blood to and from the heart, and to various tissues of the body.

- **Arteries** are thick-walled, muscular, and elastic tubes that carry pure blood from the heart to the capillaries. The largest artery in the body is the **aorta**.
- **Capillaries** are minute, thin-walled blood vessels that connect the smaller arteries with the veins. Through their walls, the tissues receive nourishment and eliminate waste products.
- **Veins** are thin-walled vessels that are less elastic than arteries. They contain cuplike valves to prevent backflow, and carry deoxygenated blood away from the capillaries back to the heart (Figure 7–15). Veins are located closer to the outer surface of the body than the arteries.

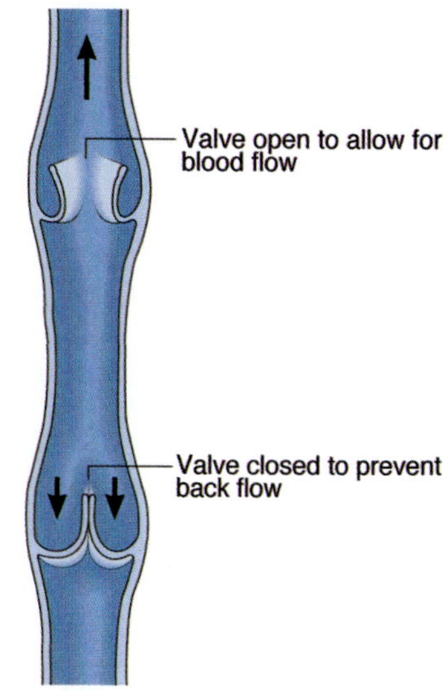

Figure 7-15 Valves in the veins.

Circulation of the Blood

The blood is in constant and continuous circulation from the moment it leaves the heart until it returns to the heart. There are two systems that control this circulation:

1. Pulmonary circulation is the blood circulation that goes from the heart to the lungs to be purified, and then returns to the heart.
2. General circulation is the blood circulation from the heart throughout the body and back again to the heart.

These two systems work in the following sequence:

1. Blood flows from the body into the right atrium.
2. From the right atrium, the blood flows through the tricuspid valve into the right ventricle.
3. The right ventricle pumps the blood to the lungs where it releases waste gases and receives oxygen. At this stage, blood is considered to be oxygen rich.
4. The oxygen-rich blood returns to the heart, entering the left atrium.
5. From the left atrium, the blood flows through the mitral valve into the left ventricle.
6. The blood then leaves the left ventricle and travels to all parts of the body.

The Blood

Blood is the nutritive fluid circulating through the circulatory system. It is a sticky, salty fluid, with a normal temperature of 98.6 degrees Fahrenheit, that makes up about one-twentieth of the body's weight. The average adult has 8 to 10 pints of blood that is bright red color in the arteries (except in the pulmonary artery) and dark red in the veins (except in the pulmonary vein). This color change occurs with the exchange of oxygen as the blood passes through the lungs and the exchange of oxygen for carbon dioxide as the blood circulates throughout the body.

Composition of Blood

The blood is composed of one-third cells in the form of red and white corpuscles and blood platelets, and two-thirds plasma.

- **Red blood cells**, also called *red corpuscles* or *erythrocytes* (ih-RITH-ruh-syts), are produced in the red bone marrow. They contain hemoglobin, a complex iron protein that gives blood its bright red color. The function of red blood cells is to carry oxygen to the body cells.
- **White blood cells**, also known as *corpuscles* or *leucocytes*, destroy disease-causing germs.
- **Platelets** are much smaller than the red blood cells. They contribute to the blood-clotting process that stops bleeding.
- **Plasma** is the fluid part of the blood in which the red and white blood cells and blood platelets flow. Strawlike in color, plasma is about 90 percent water. The main function of plasma is to carry food and secretions to the cells and to take carbon dioxide away from the cells.

Chief Functions of the Blood

Blood performs the following critical functions:

1. Carries water, oxygen, food, and secretions to body cells.
2. Carries carbon dioxide and waste products from the cells to be eliminated through the lungs, skin, kidneys, and large intestine.
3. Helps to equalize body temperature, thus protecting the body from extreme heat and cold.
4. Helps to protect the body from harmful bacteria and infections through the action of the white blood cells.
5. Through the clotting process, closes minute blood vessels that have been injured.

The Lymph Vascular System

The **lymph vascular system**, also called the lymphatic system, consists of lymph spaces, lymph vessels, lymph glands, and lacteals (LAK-teels) and acts as an aid to the blood system.

Lymph is a colorless, watery fluid that is derived from blood plasma, mainly by filtration through the capillary walls into the tissue spaces. By bathing all cells, the tissue fluid acts as a medium of exchange, trading its nutritive materials to the cells in return for the waste products of metabolism. This fluid is absorbed into the lymphatics or lymph capillaries to become lymph. It is then filtered and detoxified as it passes through the lymph nodes and eventually is reintroduced into the bloodstream.

The primary functions of the lymph vascular system are to:

1. Reach the parts of the body not reached by blood and to carry on an interchange with the blood.
2. Carry nourishment from the blood to the body cells.
3. Act as a defense against invading bacteria and toxins.

4. Remove waste material from the body cells to the blood.
5. Provide a suitable fluid environment for the cells.

Arteries of the Head, Face, and Neck

The **common carotid arteries** (kuh-RAHT-ud) are the main sources of the blood supply to the head, face, and neck (Figure 7–16). They are located on either side of the neck and each one is divided into an internal and external branch. The **internal carotid artery** supplies blood to the brain, eye sockets, eyelids, and forehead. The **external carotid artery** division supplies blood to the front parts of the head, face, and neck.

The external carotid artery subdivides into a number of branches providing a blood supply to the lower region of the face, mouth, and nose. The arterial branches that are most significant to barbers are the facial artery, superficial temporal artery, occipital artery, and the posterior auricular artery.

1. The **facial artery** or external maxillary supplies blood to the lower region of the face, mouth, and nose through the following branches:
   - **submental artery**: supplies the chin and lower lip.
   - **inferior labial artery**: supplies the lower lip.
   - **angular artery**: supplies the side of the nose.
   - **superior labial artery**: supplies the upper lip, and the septum and wings of the nose.
   - **infraorbital artery:** supplies the teeth, lower eyelid, eyes and upper lip.

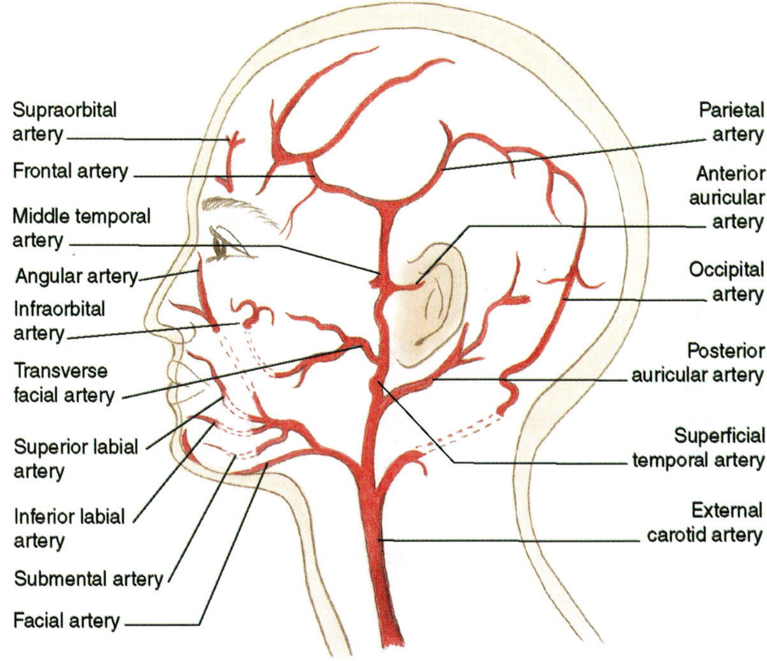

Figure 7-16 Arteries of the head, face, and neck.

2. The **superficial temporal artery** is a continuation of the external carotid artery, and supplies the muscles, skin, and scalp on the front, side, and top of the head. Some of its important branches are the:
   - **frontal artery**: supplies the forehead.
   - **parietal artery**: supplies the crown and sides of the head.
   - **transverse facial artery**: supplies the masseter.
   - **middle temporal artery**: supplies the temples and eyelids.
   - **anterior auricular artery**: which supplies the anterior part of the ear.
   - **supraorbital artery:** supplies the scalp and scalp muscle.
3. The **occipital artery** supplies the scalp and back of the head up to the crown. Its most important branch is the sterno-cleido-mastoid artery, which supplies the muscle of the same name.
4. The **posterior auricular artery** supplies the scalp, behind and above the ear. Its most important branch is the auricular artery, which supplies the skin in back of the ear.

Veins of the Head, Face, and Neck

The blood returning to the heart from the head, face, and neck flows on each side of the neck in two principal veins: the **internal jugular** and the **external jugular**. The most important veins are parallel to the arteries and take the same names as the arteries.

THE ENDOCRINE SYSTEM

The **endocrine system** consists of a group of specialized glands that affect the growth, development, sexual function, and health of the entire body. **Glands** are specialized organs that vary in size and function and have the ability to remove certain elements from the blood and to convert them into new compounds. There are two main types of glands.

- Exocrine glands, or duct glands, possess canals that lead from the gland to a particular part of the body. Sweat and oil glands of the skin and intestinal glands belong to this group.
- Endocrine glands, or ductless glands, release secretions called hormones directly into the bloodstream. This influences the welfare of the entire body since hormones such as insulin, adrenaline, and estrogen stimulate functional activity or secretion in other parts of the body.

THE DIGESTIVE SYSTEM

The **digestive system**, also known as the *gastrointestinal system*, is responsible for changing food into nutrients and waste. Digestive enzymes are chemicals that change certain kinds of food into a form that can be used by the body. When the food is in a soluble form, it is transported by the bloodstream and used by the body's cells and tissues. The entire digestive process takes about nine hours to complete.

THE EXCRETORY SYSTEM

The **excretory system** (EK-skre-tor-ee) is responsible for purifying the body by eliminating waste matter. The metabolism of body cells forms various toxic substances that, if retained, could poison the body. Each of the following organs plays a crucial role in the excretory system:

- The kidneys excrete urine.
- The liver discharges bile pigments.
- The skin eliminates perspiration.
- The large intestine evacuates decomposed and undigested food.
- The lungs exhale carbon dioxide.

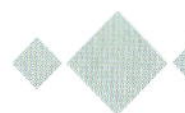

THE RESPIRATORY SYSTEM

The **respiratory system** enables breathing (respiration) and consists of the lungs and air passages (Figure 7–17). The **lungs** are spongy tissues composed of microscopic cells into which the inhaled air penetrates and is exchanged for carbon dioxide during one breathing cycle. The respiratory system is located within the chest cavity and is protected on both sides by the ribs. The **diaphragm** is a muscular partition that separates the thorax from the abdominal region and helps control breathing.

With each respiratory or breathing cycle an exchange of gases takes place. During inhalation oxygen is absorbed into the blood, while carbon dioxide is expelled during exhalation.

Oxygen is more essential than either food or water. Although a human being may live more than 60 days without food and a few days without water, life cannot continue without air for more than a few minutes.

The rate of breathing depends on the activity of the individual. Muscular activities and energy expenditures increase the body's demands for oxygen. As a result, the rate of breathing is increased. A person requires about three times as much oxygen when walking as when standing.

Nose breathing is healthier than mouth breathing because skin surface capillaries warm the air as the hairs that line the mucous membranes of the nasal passages catch airborne bacteria.

Abdominal breathing is of value in building health. Abdominal breathing means deep breathing, which brings the diaphragm into action.

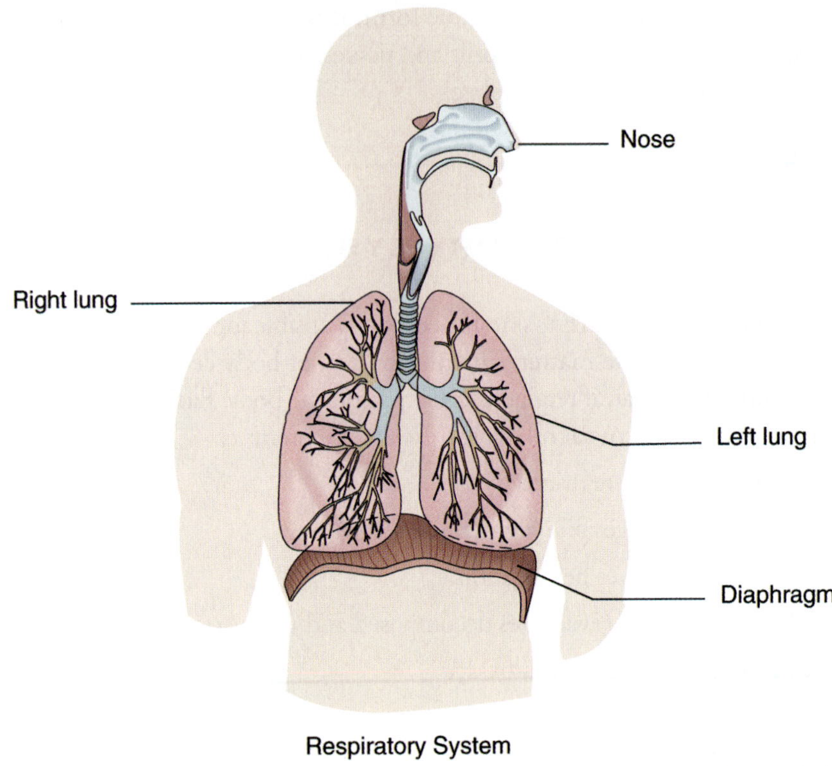

Figure 7–17 The respiratory system.

The greatest exchange of gases is accomplished with abdominal breathing. *Costal breathing* involves light, or shallow, breathing without action of the diaphragm.

THE INTEGUMENTARY SYSTEM

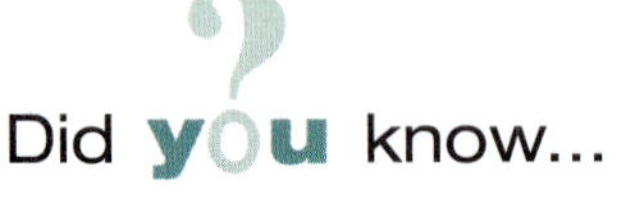

The skin is the body's largest organ.

The **integumentary system** consists of the skin and its various appendages, such as sweat and oil glands, hair, and nails, including sensory receptors. The histology of skin is discussed in detail in Chapter 10.

chapter glossary

abductor muscles	muscles that separate the fingers
adductor muscles	muscles at the base of each finger that draw the fingers together
anabolism	constructive metabolism; the process of building up larger molecules from smaller ones
anatomy	the science of the structure of organisms or of their parts
angular artery	supplies blood to the sides of the nose
anterior auricular artery	supplies blood to the front part of the ear
aorta	largest artery in the body
aponeurosis	tendon that connects the occipitalis and the frontalis
arteries	muscular, flexible tubes that carry oxygenated blood from the heart to the capillaries throughout the body
atrium	one of the two upper chambers of the heart through which blood is pumped to the ventricles
auricularis anterior	muscle in front of the ear that draws the ear forward
auricularis posterior	muscle behind the ear that draws the ear backward
auricularis superior	muscle above the ear that draws the ear upward
auriculotemporal nerve	nerve that affects the external ear and skin above the temple, up to the top of the skull
autonomic nervous system	the part of the nervous system that controls the involuntary muscles; regulates the action of the smooth muscles, glands, blood vessels, and heart
belly of a muscle	middle part of a muscle
blood	nutritive fluid circulating through the circulatory system that supplies oxygen and nutrients to cells and tissues, and removes carbon dioxide and waste from them
blood vascular system	group of structures (heart, veins, arteries, and capillaries) that distribute blood throughout the body
brain	largest and most complex nerve tissue; part of the central nervous system contained within the cranium
buccal nerve	nerve that affects the muscles of the mouth
buccinator	thin, flat muscle of the cheek between the upper and lower jaw
capillaries	thin-walled vessels that connect the smaller arteries to the veins
carpus	the wrist
catabolism	the phase of metabolism that breaks down complex compounds within the cells; releases energy to perform functions
cell membrane	part of the cell that encloses the protoplasm; permits soluble substances to enter and leave the cell
cell	basic unit of all living things

central nervous system	cerebrospinal nervous system consisting of the brain, spinal cord, spinal nerves, and cranial nerves
cervical cutaneous nerve	located at the side of the neck affecting the front and sides of the neck to the breastbone
cervical nerve	nerve that originates at the spinal cord affecting the scalp and back of the head and neck
cervical vertebrae	seven bones that form the top part of the spinal column in the neck region
circulatory system	controls the steady circulation of blood through the body by means of the heart and blood vessels
common carotid arteries	arteries that supply blood to the head, face, and neck
corrugator	facial muscle that draws eyebrows down and wrinkles the forehead vertically
cranium	oval, bony case that protects the brain
cytoplasm	all of the protoplasm of a cell except that in the nucleus
depressor labii inferioris	muscle surrounding the lower lip
diaphragm	muscular wall that separates the thorax from the abdominal region and helps control breathing
digestive system	the mouth, stomach, intestines, and salivary and gastric glands that change food into nutrients and wastes
eleventh cranial nerve	spinal nerve branch that affects the muscles of the neck and back
endocrine system	group of specialized glands that affect growth, development, sexual function, and general health
epicranius	broad muscle that covers the top of the skull; also know as occipito-frontalis
ethmoid bone	a light, spongy bone between the eye sockets forming part of the nasal cavities
excretory system	group of organs including the kidneys, liver, skin, large intestine, and lungs that purify the body by the elimination of waste matter
external carotid artery	supplies blood to the anterior parts of the scalp, face, neck, and side of the head
external jugular vein	vein located at the side of the neck that carries blood returning to the heart from the head, face, and neck
facial artery	supplies blood to the lower region of the face, mouth, and nose
facial bones	two nasal; two lacrimal; two zygomatic or malar; two maxillae; the mandible; two turbinal bones; two palatine; and the vomer
fifth cranial nerve	chief sensory nerve of the face; controls chewing
frontal artery	supplies blood to the forehead and upper eyelids
frontal bone	bone that forms the forehead
frontalis	anterior or front portion of the epicranium; muscle of the scalp
glands	specialized organs varying in size and function that have the ability to remove certain elements from the blood and to convert them into new compounds

greater auricular nerve	nerve at the sides of the neck affecting the face, ears, and neck
greater occipital nerve	located at the back of the head, affecting the scalp
gross anatomy	the study of large and easily observable structures on an organism as seen through visible inspection with the naked eye
heart	muscular cone-shaped organ that keeps blood moving through the circulatory system
histology	the study of the minute structure of various tissues and organs that make up the entire body of an organism
humerus	uppermost and largest bone in the arm
hyoid bone	U-shaped bone at the base of the tongue at the front part of the throat; also known as "Adam's apple"
indirect division	the method by which a mature cell reproduces in the body
inferior labial artery	supplies blood to the lower lip
infraorbital artery	supplies blood to the eye muscles
infraorbital nerve	affects the skin of the lower eyelid, side of the nose, upper lip, and mouth
infratrochlear nerve	affects the membrane and skin of the nose
insertion of a muscle	the more moveable attachment of a muscle to the skeleton
integumentary system	the skin at its appendages
internal carotid artery	supplies blood to the brain, eyes, eyelids, forehead, nose, and ear
internal jugular vein	located at the side of the neck; collects blood from the brain and parts of the face and neck
lacrimal bones	small bones located in the wall of the eye sockets
levator anguli oris	muscle that raises the angle of the mouth and draws it inward
levator labii superioris	muscle surrounding the upper lip
lungs	organs of respiration; spongy tissues composed of microscopic cells into which the inhaled air penetrates and is exchanged for carbon dioxide during one breathing cycle
lymph	clear yellowish fluid that circulates in the lymphatic system; carries waste and impurities from cells
lymph vascular system	acts as an aid to the blood system
mandible bone	lower jawbone
mandibular nerve	branch of the fifth cranial nerve that supplies the muscles and skin of the lower part of the face
masseter	one of the jaw muscles used in chewing
maxillary bones	bones of the upper jaw
mental nerve	affects the skin of the lower lip and chin

mentalis	muscle that elevates the lower lip and raises and wrinkles the skin of the chin
metabolism	a complex chemical process whereby cells are nourished and supplied with the energy needed to carry out their activities
metacarpus	bones of the palm of the hand
middle temporal artery	supplies blood to the temples
mitosis	cells dividing into two new cells (daughter cells)
mixed nerves	nerves that contain both sensory and motor nerve fibers; can send and receive messages
motor nerves	carry impulses from the brain to the muscles
muscular system	body system that covers, shapes, and supports the skeletal tissue
myology	study of the structure, functions, and diseases of the muscles
nasal bones	form the bridge of the nose
nasal nerve	affects the point and lower sides of the nose
nucleus	dense, active protoplasm found in the center of a cell; important to reproduction and metabolism
occipital artery	supplies the scalp and back of the head up to the crown
occipital bone	hindmost bone of the skull; located below the parietal bones
occipitalis	back of the epicranius; muscle that draws the scalp backward
opponent muscles	muscles in the palm that bring the thumb toward the fingers
orbicularis oculi	ring muscle of the eye socket
orbicularis oris	flat band around the upper and lower lips
organs	structures composed of specialized tissues performing specific functions
origin of a muscle	more fixed part of a muscle that does not move
parietal artery	supplies blood to the side and crown of the head
parietal bones	form the sides and top of the cranium
pericardium	membrane enclosing the heart
peripheral nervous system	connects the peripheral parts of the body to the central nervous system
phalanges	bone of the fingers or toes
physiology	study of the functions or activities performed by the body's structures
plasma	fluid part of blood and lymph

platelets	blood cells that aid in forming clots
platysma	muscle that extends from the chest and shoulder to the side of the chin; depresses lower jaw and lip
posterior auricular artery	supplies blood to the scalp, behind and above the ear
posterior auricular nerve	affects the muscles behind the ear at the base of the skull
procerus	muscle that covers the bridge of the nose, depresses eyebrows, and wrinkles the nose
radius	smaller bone in the forearm on the same side as the thumb
red blood cells	carry oxygen from the lungs to the body cells and transport carbon dioxide from the cells back to the lungs
reflex	automatic nerve reaction to a stimulus
respiratory system	consists of the lungs and air passages; enables breathing
risorius	muscle of the mouth that draws the corner of the mouth out and back as in grinning
sensory nerves	carry impulses or messages from the sense organs to the brain
seventh cranial nerve	chief motor nerve of the face
skeletal system	physical foundation of the body composed of bones and movable and immovable joints
smaller occipital nerve	affects the scalp and muscles behind the ear
sphenoid bone	connects all the bones of the cranium
spinal cord	the portion of the central nervous system that originates in the brain
sternocleidomastoideus	muscle of the neck that depresses and rotates the head
submental artery	supplies blood to the chin and lower lip
superficial temporal artery	supplies blood to the muscles of the front, sides, and top of the head
superior labial artery	supplies blood to the upper lip and region of the nose
supraorbital artery	supplies blood to the upper eyelid and forehead
supraorbital nerve	affects the skin of the forehead, scalp, eyebrows, and upper eyelids
supratrochlear nerve	affects the skin between the eyes and the upper side of the nose
systems	groups of body organs acting together to perform one or more functions
temporal bones	form the sides of the head in the ear region
temporal nerve	affects the muscles of the temple, side of the forehead, eyelid, eyebrow, and upper cheek
temporalis	muscle that aids in opening and closing the mouth and chewing

thorax	the chest
tissues	collection of similar cells that perform a particular function
transverse facial artery	supplies blood to the skin and the masseter
trapezius	muscle that covers the back of the neck, and upper and middle region of the back
triangularis	muscle that extend alongside the chin and pulls down the corner of the mouth
ulna	inner and larger bone of the forearm
veins	blood vessels that prevent backflow of the blood
ventricle	one of the two lower chambers of the heart
white blood cells	perform the function of destroying disease-causing germs
zygomatic bones	bones that form the prominence of the cheeks
zygomatic nerve	affects the skin of the temple, side of the forehead, and upper cheek
zygomaticus	muscle extending from the zygomatic bone to the angle of the mouth; elevates the lip as in laughing

chapter review questions

1. Define anatomy, physiology, and histology.
2. Identify the anatomical parts of the body that barbers will be most concerned with.
3. What is a cell?
4. Identify and describe the two phases of cell metabolism.
5. Define mitosis.
6. List five classifications of body tissues.
7. What is an organ?
8. List eight important organs of the body.
9. What are systems?
10. List 10 body systems.
11. List five primary functions of the bones.
12. Into how many parts is the skull divided? Name them.
13. How many bones are there in the cranium?
14. Identify the bone that joins all the cranial bones together.
15. How many bones are found in the face?
16. What is formed by the maxillae?
17. Identify the bony structure that is formed by the mandible.

18. Which bones form the prominence of the cheek?
19. Where is the hyoid bone located?
20. Define muscle.
21. Identify four important functions of the muscles.
22. List three kinds of muscular tissue.
23. Explain the difference between voluntary and involuntary muscles.
24. Define origin of muscle and insertion of muscle.
25. List and define the three main divisions of the nervous system.
26. List and define three types of nerves found in the human body.
27. Give an example of a nerve reflex.
28. Identify the two divisions of the circulatory system.
29. What is the function of the heart? What does it look like?
30. List three kinds of vessels found in the blood-vascular system.

31. What is the composition of the blood?
32. Explain the function of red blood cells.
33. Explain the function of white blood cells.
34. Identify and define the two main types of glands in the human body.

35. List the five important organs of the excretory system.

36. Describe a respiratory cycle.

37. Define the integumentary system.

38. List the appendages of the integumentary system.

- The *density* of a substance refers to its *weight* divided by its volume. For example, the volume of 1 cubic foot of water weighs 62.4 pounds. Therefore, its density is its weight (62.4 pounds) divided by its volume (1 cubic foot) which equals a density of 62.4 pounds per cubic foot. The degree of hardness of a substance can also relate to its density.
- *Melting* and *boiling points* are the degrees at which a substance will melt or boil.
- *Hardness* refers to a substance's ability to resist being deformed, such as by scratching or indentation.

Chemical properties are those characteristics that can only be determined with a chemical reaction and that cause a chemical change in the identity of the substance. Rusting iron and burning wood are examples of a change in chemical properties. In both these examples, the chemical reaction of oxidation creates a chemical change: iron is chemically changed to rust, and the wood is chemically changed to ash.

Physical and Chemical Changes of Matter

As can be seen from the discussion of the states of matter, matter can be changed in two different ways: physically and chemically.

- A **physical change** does not form a new substance; therefore there are no chemical reactions or new chemicals formed in the process (Figure 8–4). An example of physical change is ice melting to water. Temporary haircolor is another example of physical change because it physically adds color to the surface of the hair, but does not create a chemical change in the hair's structure or color.
- A **chemical change** occurs when there is a change in the chemical composition of a substance, as with the iron-to-rust example (Figure 8–5). Chemical changes in the hair can be created with permanent haircolor because the chemical reaction of oxidation takes place to develop the dye in the color. Oxidation creates chemical changes in the hair structure and in its color, forming new chemicals in the process.

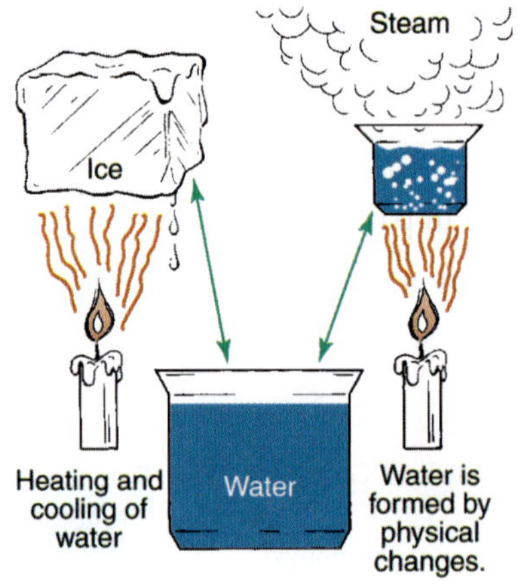

Figure 8–4 Physical changes.

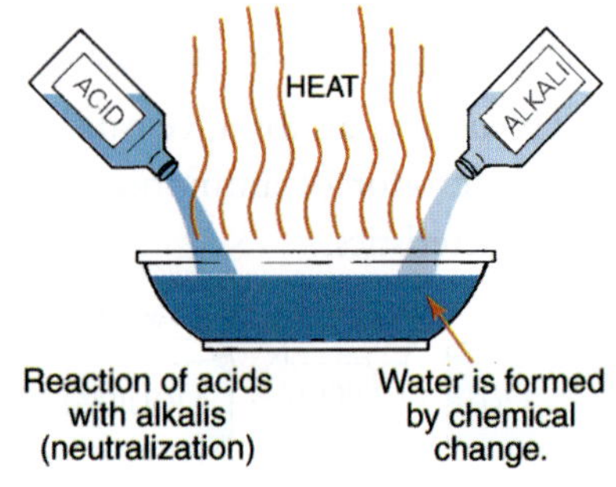

Figure 8–5 Chemical changes.

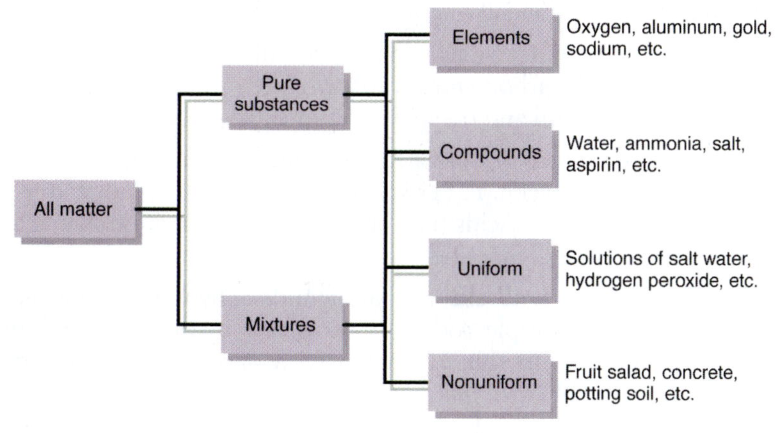

Figure 8-6 Pure substances and mixtures.

Pure Substances and Physical Mixtures

All matter can be classified as either a pure substance or a physical mixture (Figure 8–6). A **pure substance** is matter that has a fixed chemical composition, definite proportions, and distinct properties. Elements and compounds are pure substances.

Elemental molecules contain two or more atoms of the same element that unite chemically. Aluminum foil is an example of a pure substance; it is composed only of atoms of the element aluminum.

Chemical compounds are combinations of two or more atoms of different elements united chemically with fixed chemical composition, definite proportions, and distinct properties. Chemical compounds are the result of a chemical reaction. Water is a chemical compound consisting of two atoms of hydrogen and one atom of oxygen. Table 8–1 summarizes the differences between chemical compounds and physical mixtures.

Chemical Compounds	Physical Mixtures
Involve a chemical reaction	Do not involve a chemical reaction
Change the chemical properties	Change only the physical properties
Mixed in definite proportions	Mixed in any proportions
Water or salt are examples	Salt water is an example
Pure hydrogen peroxide	Solution of hydrogen peroxide

Table 8-1 Chemical Compounds and Physical Mixtures

8

Compounds can be divided into four classifications:

1. **Oxides** are compounds of any element combined with oxygen. For example, one part carbon and two parts oxygen equal carbon dioxide. One part carbon and one part oxygen equal carbon monoxide.
2. **Acids** are compounds of hydrogen, a nonmetal such as nitrogen, and, sometimes, oxygen. For example, hydrogen + sulphur + oxygen = sulphuric acid. Acids turn blue litmus paper red, providing a quick way to test a compound.
3. **Bases**, also known as **alkalis**, are compounds of hydrogen, a metal, and oxygen. For example, sodium + oxygen + hydrogen = sodium hydroxide, which is used in the manufacture of soap. Bases will turn red litmus paper blue.
4. **Salts** are compounds that are formed by the reaction of acids and bases, with water also produced by the reaction. Two common salts are sodium chloride (table salt), which contains sodium and chloride, and magnesium sulphate (Epsom salts), which contains magnesium, sulphur, hydrogen, and oxygen.

A **physical mixture** is a combination of two or more substances united physically in any proportions without a fixed composition. Pure air is a physical mixture of mostly nitrogen and oxygen gases. Concrete is another example because it is composed of sand, gravel, and cement. It is a mixture that has its own functions, yet does not lose the characteristics of the individual ingredients. 2

Did you know...

You can test water to determine whether or not it is soft water by using a soap solution. Use the following steps to test the water softness in your area.

1. Dissolve ¾ of an ounce of pure, powdered castile soap in a pint of distilled water.
2. Use a second pint bottle and fill it halfway with tap water.
3. Add about 7 drops (0.5 ml.) of the soap solution.
4. Shake the bottle vigorously. If lather forms at once and persists, the water is very soft.
5. If lather does not appear at once, add another 0.5 ml. of soap solution. Shake again. If an additional 0.5 ml. of the soap solution is needed to produce a good lather, the water is hard and should be softened for hair services in the barbershop.

THE CHEMISTRY OF WATER

Water (H_2O) is the most abundant and important of all chemicals, composing about 75 percent of the earth's surface and about 65 percent of the human body. Water is the universal solvent. Distilled or demineralized water is used as a nonconductor of electricity, while water containing certain mineral substances is known as an excellent conductor of electricity.

Water is purified through boiling, filtration, or distillation. Boiling water at 212 degrees Fahrenheit destroys most microbes and renders it suitable for drinking. During filtration, water passes through a porous substance, such as filter paper or charcoal, to remove organic material. Distillation is the process whereby water is heated to a vapor in a closed vessel. The vapors are captured and passed off through a tube into another vessel, where they are cooled and condensed to a liquid. This process purifies water used in the manufacturing of cosmetics.

Soft water is rainwater or chemically treated water that has low levels of mineral substances such as calcium and magnesium salts. Fewer amounts of such minerals in soft water allow for soaps and shampoos to lather freely. It is the best choice for use in the barbershop.

Hard water contains mineral substances, such as calcium and magnesium salts, that curdle or precipitate soap instead of permitting a permanent lather to form. Hard water may be softened by distillation or by the use of sodium carbonate (washing soda) or sodium phosphate.

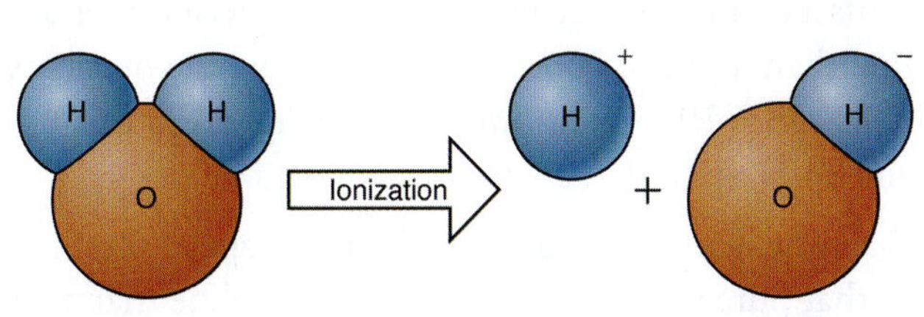

Figure 8–7 The ionization of water.

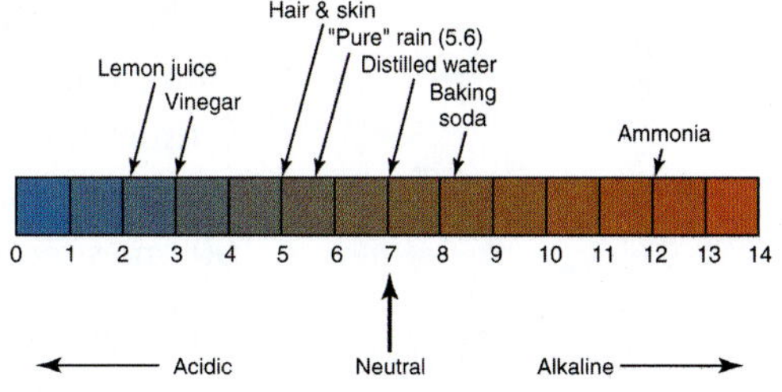

Figure 8–8 The pH scale (horizontal).

Water and pH

The letters **pH** denote **potential hydrogen**, the relative degree of acidity or alkalinity of a substance. The **pH scale** measures the concentration of hydrogen ions in acidic and alkaline solutions. Notice that pH is written with a small *p*, which represents quantity, and a capital *H*, which represents the hydrogen ion.

A basic understanding of ions is important to an understanding of pH. An **ion** is an atom or molecule that carries an electrical charge. **Ionization** is the separation of a substance into ions that have opposite electrical charges. A negatively charged ion is an anion, and a positively charged ion is a cation.

In pure water, some of the water molecules ionize naturally into hydrogen ions and hydroxide ions. The pH scale measures those ions. The hydrogen ion is acidic and the hydroxide ion is alkaline. The ionization of water is what makes pH possible because only aqueous (water) solutions have pH. Nonaqueous solutions, such as alcohol or oil, do not have pH. In pure water, every water molecule that ionizes produces one hydrogen ion and one hydroxide ion (Figure 8–7). Pure water contains the same number of hydrogen ions as hydroxide ions, which makes it neutral. Pure water is 50 percent acidic and 50 percent alkaline, as denoted by the number 7 on the pH scale (Figure 8–8).

The pH Scale

The pH values are arranged on a scale ranging from 0 to 14. A pH of 7 indicates a neutral solution, a pH below 7 indicates an acidic solution, and a pH above 7 indicates an alkaline solution (Figure 8–9).

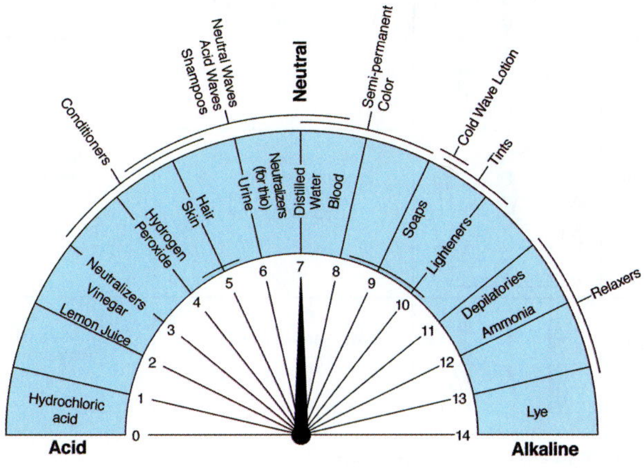

Figure 8–9 The pH scale.

8

The pH scale is a logarithmic scale, which means that a change of one whole number represents a tenfold change in pH. For example, a pH of 8 is 10 times more alkaline than a pH of 7. A change of two whole numbers indicates a change of 10 times 10, or a hundredfold change. A pH of 9 is 100 times more alkaline than a pH of 7.

The pH range of hair and skin is 4.5 to 5.5 with an average of 5 on the pH scale. That means that pure water is 100 times more alkaline than hair and skin, even though it has a neutral pH. Pure water can cause the hair to swell up to 20 percent.

Acids and Alkalis

All *acids* owe their chemical reactivity to the hydrogen ion (H^+). Acids have a pH below 7.0, taste sour, and turn litmus paper from blue to red. Acids contract and harden the hair (Figure 8–10). They also tighten the skin. Thioglycolic acid is an acid solution used in permanent waving.

All *alkalis* owe their chemical reactivity to the hydroxide (OH^-) ion. The terms *alkalis* and *bases* are interchangeable. Alkalis have a pH above 7.0, taste bitter, feel slippery on the skin, and turn litmus paper from red to blue. Alkalis soften and swell the hair (Figure 8–10). Sodium hydroxide (lye) is a very strong alkali used in chemical drain cleaners and chemical hair relaxers.

Solution	Effect on Hair		Important Features
Very Strong Acid (pH 0.0–1.0)		Dissolves hair completely.	Must not be applied to hair or scalp.
Strong to Mild Acid (pH 1.0–4.5)		Hair shrinks and hardens. Body is increased. Cuticle imbrications close up. Porosity is reduced. Sheen of hair is improved. Soap residues are removed. Neutralizes traces of alkalis.	Acid or cream rinses restore body to bleached, porous hair. Conditioners and fillers overcome the excess porosity of damaged hair. Special shampoos reduce tangling and matting of hair and prevent color loss. Hair creams increase sheen. Color rinses provide temporary effect. Neutralizers remove residual waving lotion.
Neutral (pH 4.5–5.5)		Hair is normal diameter. Texture and luster standard.	Neutral solutions are designed to prevent excess swelling of normal and damaged hair. Mild shampoos for normal cleaning and manageability of hair.
Mild Alkali (pH 5.5–10.0)		Hair swells. Porosity increases as imbrications open. Hair has a dry, drab appearance.	Tints and bleaches penetrate easier and chemical action increases. Cold wave solutions for resistant hair. Soap shampoos to overcome acidity of tap water. Activators for hydrogen peroxide.
Stronger Alkali (pH 10.0–14.0)		Dissolves hair completely.	Must not be applied to hair or scalp unless used as relaxers or depilatories.

Figure 8-10 The effect of pH on hair.

8

Acid-Alkali Neutralization Reactions

When acids and alkalis are mixed together in equal proportions, they neutralize each other to form water and a salt. For example, although hydrochloric acid is a strong acid and sodium hydroxide is a strong alkali, they will neutralize each other when mixed in equal amounts and form a solution of pure water and table salt. The neutralizing lotions in permanent waving products and the neutralizing shampoos associated with hydroxide hair relaxers work by creating the same type of acid-alkali neutralization reaction.

Oxidation-Reduction Reactions

Oxidation is a chemical reaction that combines an element or compound with oxygen to produce an oxide. When oxygen combines with another element, some heat is usually produced. Chemical reactions that are characterized by the giving off of heat are called *exothermic.* For example, exothermic permanent waving lotions produce heat because of an oxidation reaction. *Slow oxidation* occurs in oxidation haircolors and permanent wave neutralizers. When hydrogen peroxide is added to oxidation haircolors, there will be an increase in the temperature due to the process of oxidation. *Note:* To provide a frame of reference for slow oxidation, it might be helpful to know that *combustion* is a form of *rapid oxidation* reaction that produces a high quantity of heat and light. For instance, lighting a match is an example of rapid oxidation.

When oxygen is combined with a substance, the substance is *oxidized.* When oxygen is removed from a substance, the substance is *reduced.* Oxidizing agents are substances that release oxygen. Hydrogen peroxide is an oxidizing agent because it contains extra oxygen. When hydrogen peroxide is mixed with an oxidation haircolor, the haircolor gains oxygen. At the same time the hydrogen peroxide loses oxygen and is therefore reduced.

Oxidation and **reduction** always occur simultaneously and are referred to as **redox** reactions. In a redox reaction, the oxidizer is always reduced and the reducing agent is always oxidized.

Many oxidation reactions do not involve oxygen. Oxidation also results from the loss of hydrogen, and reduction is the result of the addition of hydrogen. Permanent waving is an example of this type of redox reaction. Permanent waving solution contains thioglycolate acid. The waving solution breaks the disulfide bonds in the hair through a reduction reaction that adds hydrogen ions to the hair. In this reaction, the hair is reduced and the perm solution is oxidized. After processing and rinsing, the neutralizer is used to oxidize the hair by removing the hydrogen that was previously added with the waving solution. When the hair has oxidized, the neutralizer will have been reduced in the process.

When performing chemical services, the term *oxidation* is used to define either the addition of oxygen or the loss of hydrogen. Conversely, the term *reduction* is used to define either the loss of oxygen or the addition of hydrogen. Refer to Chapters 18 and 19 for more detailed information about pH and the products used to effect chemical changes in the hair. 3

COSMETIC CHEMISTRY

Cosmetic chemistry is the scientific study of the cosmetic products used in the barbering and cosmetology industries. An understanding of the different types of products that are available will better equip barbers to service their clientele in the barbershop. The principal physical and chemical classifications of cosmetics are powders, solutions, suspensions, emulsions, soaps, and ointments.

Powders

Powders consist of a uniform mixture of insoluble substances, inorganic, organic, and colloidal, that have been properly blended, perfumed, and/or tinted.

Solutions

A solution is a mixture of two or more mixable substances that is made by dissolving a solid, liquid, or gaseous substance in another substance. A solute is any substance that is dissolved into a solvent to form a solution. A solvent is any substance, usually liquid, that dissolves the solute to form a solution. The components of a solution are illustrated in Figure 8–11. When a gas or a solid is dissolved in a liquid, the gas or solid is the solute and the liquid is the solvent.

Solutions are usually clear or transparent permanent mixtures of a solute and a solvent that do not separate upon standing. The particles in solutions are invisible to the naked eye. Salt water is a solution of a solid dissolved in a liquid. Water is the solvent that dissolves the salt and holds it in a solution. Air, salt water, and hydrogen peroxide are examples of solutions. Solutions

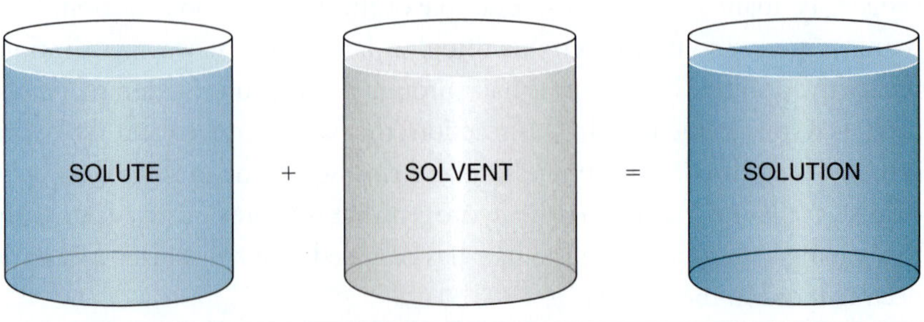

Figure 8-11 Components of a solution.

can also be prepared by dissolving a powdered solute in a warm solvent and stirring at the same time.

Water is a universal solvent. It is capable of dissolving more substances than any other liquid. Grain alcohol and glycerin are also used frequently as solvents. Water, glycerin, and alcohol readily mix with each other; therefore they are *miscible* (mixable). On the other hand, water and oil do not mix with each other; hence they are *immiscible* (unmixable).

The solute may be either a solid, liquid, or gas. For example, boric acid solution is a mixture of a solid in a liquid; glycerin and rose water is a mixture of two miscible liquids; ammonia water is a mixture of a gas in water.

NOTE: Solutions containing volatile substances such as ammonia and alcohol should be stored in a cool place to avoid evaporation.

Solutions may be classified as dilute, concentrated, or saturated solutions. A *dilute solution* contains a small quantity of the solute in proportion to the quantity of solvent. A *concentrated solution* contains a large quantity of the solute in proportion to the quantity of solvent. A *saturated solution* will not dissolve or take up more solute than it already holds at a given temperature.

Suspensions

Suspensions are uniform mixtures of two or more substances. The particles in suspensions can be seen with the naked eye because they are larger than the particles in solutions. Suspensions are not usually transparent, may be colored, and tend to separate over time. Many of the products used by barbers, such as hair tonics, are suspensions and should be shaken or mixed well before use. Salad dressing, calamine lotion, paint, and aerosol hair spray are also examples of suspensions.

Emulsions

Emulsions are suspensions (mixtures) of two immiscible liquids held together by an emulsifying agent. An emulsion is a suspension of one liquid dispersed in another. Although emulsions tend to separate over time, with proper formulation and storage an emulsion may remain stable for at least three years. Mayonnaise is an oil-in-water emulsion of two immiscible liquids. The egg yolk in mayonnaise emulsifies the oil droplets and disperses them uniformly in the water. Mayonnaise should not separate upon standing. Review Table 8–2 for a summary of the differences between solutions, suspensions, and emulsions.

Surfactants are substances that act as a bridge to allow oil and water to mix or emulsify. A surfactant molecule has two distinct parts: the head of the molecule is hydrophilic (water-loving) and the tail is lipophilic (oil-loving) (Figure 8–12). Since "like dissolves like," the hydrophilic head dissolves in water and the lipophilic tail dissolves in oil. Thus, the surfactant molecule dissolves in both water and oil and joins them together to form an emulsion. 4

Solutions	Suspensions	Emulsions
Miscible	Slightly miscible	Immiscible
No surfactant	No surfactant	Surfactant
Small particles	Larger particles	Largest particles
Usually clear	Usually cloudy	Usually a solid color
Stable mixture	Unstable mixture	Limited stability
Solution of hydrogen peroxide	Calamine lotion	Shampoos and conditioners

Table 8–2 Solutions, Suspensions, and Emulsions

Soaps

Soaps are compounds made by mixing plant oils or animal fats with strong alkaline substances. Glycerin is also formed in the process. Potassium hydroxide produces a soft soap, whereas sodium hydroxide forms a hard soap. A mixture of the two alkalis will yield a soap of intermediate consistency. A good soap does not contain excess free alkali and is made from pure oils and fats. Soaps used in the industry may be categorized as deodorant soaps, beauty soaps, medicated soaps, and shaving soaps.

Deodorant soaps include a bactericide that remains on the body to kill the bacteria responsible for odors. One of the most common antiseptic and antibacterial agents used in these soaps is triclocarban. Triclocarban, often listed in the ingredients as TCC, is prepared from aniline. Aniline additives have been known to increase the skin's sensitivity to the sun.

Beauty soaps are intended for the more delicate tissues of the face. They have a more acid pH and are less drying to the skin, yet are able to remove dirt and oil from the skin's surface. Many beauty soaps are transparent and contain large quantities of glycerin. Other beauty soaps contain larger amounts of oils that leave an emollient film on the skin.

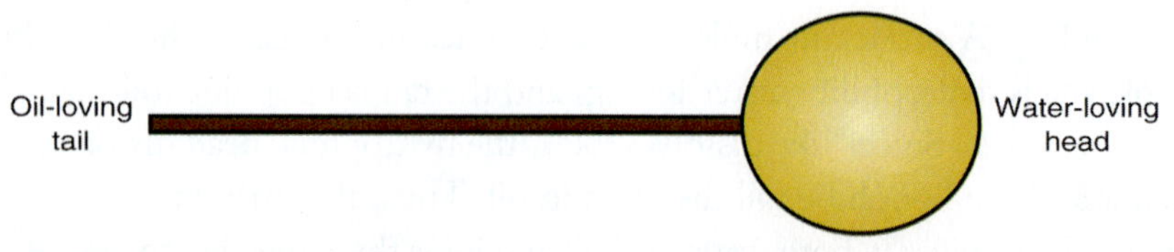

Figure 8–12 Surfactant molecules.

Medicated soaps are designed to treat skin problems such as rashes, pimples, and acne. Many contain small percentages of cresol, phenol, or other antiseptics. Resorcinol is often used as a drying agent in medicated products designed to treat oily conditions. The strongest medicated soaps can be obtained only with a doctor's prescription.

Shaving soaps can be purchased in various forms and shapes. Hard shaving soaps include those sold in cake, stick, or powdered form, and are similar in composition to toilet soaps. They are also available as soft soaps, as in shaving cream in a tube, jar, or press-button container. Liquid soaps are another option that barbers and stylists can utilize. Whatever form of shaving soap is used, it usually contains animal and/or vegetable oils, alkaline substances, and water. The presence of coconut and other plant oils tends to improve the lathering qualities of shaving soap.

Ointments

Ointments are semisolid mixtures of organic substances such as lard, petrolatum, or wax, and a medicinal agent. No water is present. For the ointment to soften, its melting point should be below body temperature (98.6 degrees Fahrenheit). Ointments are prepared by melting an organic substance followed by mixing it with a medicinal agent.

Other Cosmetic Preparations

Astringents may have an alcohol content of up to 35 percent. Astringents cause contraction of tissues and may be used to remove oil accumulation on the skin or to "close the pores" after a facial or shave. Due to the high alcohol content of astringent lotions, some skin types may be sensitive and react with a slight swelling or redness of the skin. Additional astringent ingredients may include one or more of the following: alum, boric acid, sorbitol, water, camphor, and perfumes.

Cake or pancake makeup is generally composed of kaolin, zinc, talc, titanium oxide, mineral oil, fragrances, precipitated calcium carbonate, finely ground pigments, and inorganic pigments such as iron oxides. Cake makeup is used to cover scars and pigmentation defects.

Cleansing creams are used during facials and shaves in the barbershop. The action of a cleansing cream is caused in part by the oil content of the cream, which has the ability to dissolve other greasy substances. Older formulas, such as cold cream, contain relatively few ingredients that may include vegetable or mineral oil, beeswax, water, preservatives, and emulsifiers. The newer cleansing formulations are more skin condition specific and may contain additional degreasers such as lemon juice, synthetic surfactants, emollients, and humectants.

Cleansing lotions serve the same purposes as cleansing creams but are of a lighter consistency and are usually water-based emulsions. They are available in dry-, normal-, and oily-skin formulations. Some ingredients common to cleansing lotions are cetyl alcohol, cetyl palmitate, and sorbitol; perfumes and colorings are added to enhance lotions' marketing value.

Depilatories are preparations used for the temporary removal of superfluous hair by dissolving it at the skin line. Depilatories contain detergents to strip the sebum from the hair and adhesives to hold the chemicals to the hair shaft for the 5 to 10 minutes necessary to remove the hair. During the short processing time, swelling accelerating agents such as urea or melamine expand the hair, helping to break the hair bonds. Finally, chemicals such as sodium hydroxide, potassium hydroxide, thioglycolic acid, or calcium thioglycolate destroy the disulfide bonds. These chemicals turn the hair into a soft, jellylike mass of hydrolyzed protein that can be scraped from the skin. Although depilatories are not commonly used in barbershops, familiarity with them is necessary because many of your customers may use them at home.

Epilators remove hair by pulling it out of the follicle. Two types of wax are currently used for professional epilation: cold and hot. Both products are made primarily of resins and beeswax. Beeswax has a relatively high incidence of allergic reaction; therefore, it is advisable to do a small patch test of the product to be used. Recently, an electrical apparatus made for the home hair-removal market has become available.

Eye lotions or toners are generally formulas of boric acid, bicarbonate of soda, zinc sulfate, glycerin, and herbs. They are designed to soothe and brighten the eyes.

Fresheners, also known as skin freshening lotions, have the lowest alcohol content (0 to 4 percent) of the tonic lotions. They are designed for dry, mature, and sensitive skin types. The formulation of a freshener typically includes some or all of the following: witch hazel, alcohol and camphorated alcohol, citric acid, boric acid, lactic acid, phosphoric acid, aluminum salts, menthol, chamomile, and floral scents.

Greasepaint is a mixture of fats, petrolatum, and a coloring agent that is used for theatrical purposes.

Hair spray is used to hold the finished style. Many new formulations for hair spray contain a variety of polymers, such as acrylic/acrylate copolymer, vinyl acetate, crotonic acid copolymer, PVM/MA copolymer, and polyvinylpyrrolidone (PVP), and plasticizers such as acetyl triethyl citrate, benzyl alcohol, and silicones as stiffening agents. Additional ingredients might include silicone, shellac, perfume, lanolin or its derivatives, vegetable gums, alcohol, sorbitol, and water.

Hairdressings, such as pomades, give shine and manageability to dry or curly hair. They may be applied to either wet or dry hair. Such dressings typically consist of lanolin or its derivatives, petrolatum, oil emulsions, fatty acids, waxes, mild alkalis, and water.

Masks and *packs* are available to serve many purposes and skin conditions including deep cleansing, pore reduction, tightening, firming, moisturizing, and wrinkle reduction. Clay masks typically contain varying combinations of kaolin (china clay), bentonite, purified siliceous (fuller's) earth or colloidal clay, petrolatum, glycerin, proteins, SD alcohol, and water. The primary ingredients typically found in peel-off masks are SD alcohol 40, polysorbate-20, and polymers such as polyvinyl alcohol or vinyl acetate.

Massage creams are used to help the hands to glide over the skin. They contain formulations of cold cream, lanolin or its derivatives, and sometimes casein (a protein found in cheese).

Medicated lotions are available by prescription for skin problems such as acne, rashes, or other eruptions.

Moisturizing creams are designed to treat dryness. They contain humectants, which create a barrier that allows the natural water and oil of the skin to accumulate in the tissues. This barrier also works to protect the skin from air pollution, dirt, and debris. Moisturizers contain a variety of emollients ranging from simple ingredients such as peanut, coconut, or a variety of other oils, to more complex chemical compounds such as cetyl alcohol, cholesterol, dimethicone, or glycerin derivatives.

Pastes are soft, moist cosmetics with a thick consistency. They are bound together with the aid of gum, starch, and water. If oils and fats are present, water is absent. The colloidal mill assists in the removal of grittiness from the paste.

Scalp lotions and ointments usually contain medicinal agents for active correction of a scalp condition such as itching or flakiness. An astringent lotion may be applied to the scalp before shampooing to control oiliness as well as the itching and flakiness of dry scalp conditions. Medicated lotions and ointments for severe scalp conditions must be prescribed by a physician.

Sticks are similar to ointments. They are a mixture of organic substances (oils, waxes, petrolatum) that are poured into a mold to solidify. Sticks are firmer than ointments because they do not contain water. A styptic stick and an eyebrow pencil are examples of stick cosmetics.

Styling aids, such as gels and mousses, typically consist of polymer and resin formulations that are designed to give the hair body and texture. Many incorporate the same ingredients found in hair sprays (see above) but add moisturizers and humectants, such as cetyl alcohol, panthenol, hydrolyzed protein, quats, or a variety of oils to the ingredient list.

Suntan lotions are designed to protect the skin from the harmful ultraviolet rays of the sun. They are rated with a sun protection factor (SPF) that enables sunbathers to calculate the time they can remain in the sun before the skin begins to burn. Suntan lotions are emulsions that might contain para-aminobenzoic acid (PABA), a variety of oils, petrolatum, sorbitan stearate, alcohol, ultraviolet inhibitors, acid derivatives, preservatives, and perfumes.

Toners usually have an alcohol content of 4 to 15 percent and are designed for use on normal and combination skin types.

Wrinkle treatment creams are designed to conceal lines on aging skin either via a crease-filling capacity or through a "plumping up" of the tissues.

Among the many possible ingredients in these treatments are hormones and collagen. Some are made of herbs and other natural ingredients while others are entirely synthetic.

UNITED STATES PHARMACOPEIA (U.S.P.)

The *United States Pharmacopeia* is a book that defines and standardizes drugs used by the public. Some of the most common chemical ingredients used in the formulation of hair and skin products are as follows:

Alcohol is a colorless liquid obtained from the fermentation of starch, sugar, and other carbohydrates. Isopropyl (rubbing) and ethyl (beverage or grain) alcohol are both volatile (readily evaporated) alcohols. These alcohols function as solvents and can be found in shampoos, conditioners, hair colorants, hair sprays, tonics, and styling aids. Fatty alcohols, such as cetyl and cetearyl alcohol, are nonvolatile oils that are used as conditioners. The alcohols most often used in the barbershop are ethyl alcohol and isopropyl alcohol. Seventy percent ethyl alcohol is used to sanitize implements with a fine cutting edge. Fifty to sixty percent isopropyl alcohol is an effective antiseptic that can be applied to the skin.

Alkanolamines (al-kan-all-AM-eenz) are substances used to neutralize acids or raise the pH of hair products. They are often used in place of ammonia because there is less odor associated with their use. Alkanolamines are used as alkalizing agents in hair lighteners and permanent wave solutions.

Alum is an aluminum potassium or ammonium sulphate supplied in the form of crystals or powder; it has a strong astringent action. For this reason, alum can be found in skin tonics and lotions and, in powder or liquid form, as *styptic* that can be used to stop the bleeding of small nicks and cuts.

Ammonia, a colorless gas composed of hydrogen and nitrogen, has a pungent odor. Ammonia is used to raise the pH in permanent waving, haircoloring, and lightening substances. Ammonium hydroxide and ammonium thioglycolate are examples of ammonia compounds that are used to raise solution pH levels for better penetration into the hair.

Ammonia water, as commercially used, is a colorless liquid with a pungent, penetrating odor. It is a by-product of the manufacture of coal gas. As it readily dissolves grease, it is used as a cleansing agent and is also used with hydrogen peroxide in hair lighteners. A 28 percent solution of ammonia gas dissolved in water is available commercially.

Boric acid is used for its bactericidal and fungicidal properties in baby powders, eye creams, mouthwashes, soaps, and skin fresheners. It is a mild healing and antiseptic agent, although the American Medical Association warns of possible toxicity. Severe irritation and poisonings have occurred after application to open skin wounds.

Ethyl methacrylate (ETH-il-meth-u-KRYE-layt) is an ester (compound) of ethyl alcohol and methacrylic acid used in the chemical formulation of many sculptured nails. Inhalation of the fumes is not recommended.

Formaldehyde is a colorless gas manufactured by an oxidation process of methyl alcohol. It is used as a disinfectant, fungicide, germicide, and preservative as well as an embalming solution. In the cosmetics industry, small amounts of formaldehyde are used in soap, cosmetics, and nail hardeners and polishes. Formaldehyde and its derivatives, such as *formalin,* should be used with caution because National Cancer Institute studies indicate that it is toxic, can lead to DNA damage, and is known to react with other chemicals to become a carcinogen.

Glycerin is a sweet, colorless, odorless, oily substance formed by the decomposition of oils, fats, or fatty acids. It is used as a solvent and as a skin moisturizer in cuticle oils and facial creams.

Hydrogen peroxide is a compound of hydrogen and oxygen. It is a colorless liquid with a characteristic odor and a slightly acidic taste. Organic matter, such as silk, hair, feathers, and nails, is bleached by hydrogen peroxide because of its oxidizing power. A hydrogen peroxide solution is used as a bleaching agent for the hair in solutions of 20 to 40 volumes. A 3 to 5 percent solution of hydrogen peroxide possesses antiseptic qualities.

Petrolatum, commonly known as Vaseline, petroleum jelly, or paraffin jelly, is a yellowish to white, semisolid, greasy mass that is almost insoluble in water. It is used in wax epilators, eyebrow pencils, lipsticks, protective creams, cold creams, and many other cosmetics for its ability to soften and smooth the skin.

Phenol, or carbolic acid, is not actually an acid but rather a slightly acidic coal tar derivative. A 5 percent solution is used to sanitize metallic implements.

Phenylenediamine, derived from coal tar, has a succession of derivatives known to penetrate the skin. It is believed to cause cancer.

Potassium hydroxide (caustic potash) is prepared by electrolysis of potassium chloride. It may be used for its emulsifying abilities in formulas for hand lotions, liquid soaps, protective creams, and cuticle softeners.

Quaternary ammonium compounds (quats) are found in many antiseptics, surfactants, preservatives, sanitizers, and germicides. Quats are synthetic derivatives of ammonium chloride. Although quats can be toxic, they are considered safe in the proportions used in the industry.

Silicones are a special type of oil used in hair conditioners and as a water-resistant lubricant for the skin. Silicones are less greasy than plain oils and have the ability to form a "breathable" film that does not cause comedones.

Sodium bicarbonate (baking soda) is a precipitate made by passing carbon dioxide gas through a solution of sodium carbonate. The resulting white powder is used as a neutralizing agent and, when mixed in shampoo, to remove hair spray buildup.

Sodium carbonate (soda ash or washing soda) is found naturally in ores and lake brines or seawater. It is used in shampoos and permanent wave solutions. Sodium carbonate absorbs water from the air.

Witch hazel is a solution of alcohol, water, and powder ground from the leaves and twigs of *Hamamelis virginiana*. It works as an astringent and skin freshener. Because of the alcohol content, it should not be applied directly to an open wound or to the delicate membranes of the eye.

Zinc oxide is a heavy white powder that is insoluble in water. It is used cosmetically in face powder, foundation cream, and sunscreen products for its ability to impart opacity.

chapter glossary

acids	solutions that have a pH below 7.0
alkalis	solutions that have a pH above 7.0
atoms	smallest particles of an element that still retain the properties of that element
bases	also known as alkalis
chemical change	change in the chemical composition of a substance in which new substances are formed
chemical properties	characteristics that can only be determined with a chemical reaction
chemistry	the science that deals with the composition, structures, and properties of matter
compounds	two or more atoms of different elements united chemically with fixed chemical composition, definite proportions, and distinct properties
compound molecules	chemical combinations of two or more atoms of different elements
element	the simplest form of matter
elemental molecules	molecules containing two or more atoms of the same element that are united chemically
emulsions	mixtures of two or more immiscible substances united with the aid of a binder or emulsifier
inorganic chemistry	chemistry dealing with compounds lacking carbon
ion	an atom or molecule that carries an electrical charge
ionization	the separating of a substance into ions
matter	any substance that occupies space, has physical and chemical properties, and exists in the form of a solid, liquid, or gas
molecules	two or more atoms joined chemically
organic chemistry	study of substances that contain carbon
oxidation	chemical reaction that combines an element or compound with oxygen to produce an oxide
oxides	compounds of any element combined with oxygen
pH (potential hydrogen)	relative degree of acidity or alkalinity of a substance
pH scale	a measure of the concentration of hydrogen ions in acidic and alkaline solutions
physical change	change in the form of a substance without the formation of a new substance
physical mixture	combination of two or more substances united physically
physical properties	characteristics of matter that can be determined without a chemical reaction
pure substance	matter that has a fixed chemical composition, definite proportions, and district properties
redox	contraction for reduction—oxidation

reduction	the subtraction of oxygen from, or the addition of hydrogen to, a substance
salts	compounds that are formed by the reaction of acids and bases
suspensions	formulations in which solid particles are distributed throughout a liquid medium

8

chapter review questions

1. Define organic and inorganic chemistry.
2. List the four states of matter.
3. Define elements, compounds, and mixtures.
4. Describe the differences between solutions, suspensions, and emulsions.
5. Define pH and draw a pH scale.
6. Explain oxidation and reduction reactions. Give an example of each.

Learning Objectives

After completing this chapter, you should be able to:

1. Identify and define common electrical terms.
2. Discuss and recognize electrical safety devices.
3. Identify different electrical modalities and their uses.
4. Identify visible and invisible light rays.
5. Explain the effects of ultraviolet and infrared rays.

Key Terms

alternating current
pg. 192

amp
pg. 192

anaphoresis
pg. 198

anode
pg. 196

cataphoresis
pg. 198

cathode
pg. 196

circuit breaker
pg. 193

complete circuit
pg. 191

conductor
pg. 191

converter
pg. 192

disincrustation
pg. 197

direct current
pg. 192

electric current
pg. 191

electrode
pg. 196

electrotherapy
pg. 196

faradic current
pg. 198

fuse
pg. 193

galvanic current
pg. 197

ground fault circuit interrupter
pg. 193

infrared rays
pg. 202

insulator
pg. 191

iontophoresis
pg. 198

modalities
pg. 196

ohm
pg. 193

polarity
pg. 196

rectifier
pg. 192

rheostat
pg. 191

sinusoidal current
pg. 198

Tesla high-frequency current
pg. 198

ultraviolet rays
pg. 199

visible light
pg. 199

volt
pg. 192

watt
pg. 193

wavelength
pg. 199

In today's barbershop, haircutting and other services would not be possible without electricity. It is probably safe to say that most barbers would not like to return to the days of the hand clipper! In this chapter, you will learn some important safety precautions regarding the use of electricity in the barbershop. You will also be introduced to different electrical currents that can be used for scalp and facial electrotherapy treatments.

Light therapy treatments are another service that barbers can offer their clients. Different light rays have different effects on the skin. It is for this reason that barbers need to know when it is appropriate to apply the thermal and chemical properties associated with light therapy to the skin.

ELECTRICITY

Electricity is a valuable tool for the barber, provided it is used carefully and intelligently. Electricity is a form of energy that produces magnetic, chemical, or thermal effects while in motion. It is a flow of electrons, which are negatively charged subatomic particles.

Electrical Terms

An **electric current** is the flow of electricity along a conductor. All substances can be classified as conductors *or* insulators, depending on the ease with which an electric current can be transmitted through them.

A **conductor** is any substance, material, or medium that conducts electricity. Most metals, carbon, the human body, and watery solutions of acids and salts are good conductors of electricity.

An **insulator**, or *nonconductor*, is a substance that does not easily transmit electricity. Rubber, silk, dry wood, glass, and cement are good insulators.

An *electric wire* is composed of fine, twisted metal threads that act as a conductor and a covering of silk or rubber that is the insulator.

A **complete circuit** is the path of electric current from the generating source through conductors and back to its original source (Figure 9–1).

A **rheostat** is an adjustable resistor, such as a light dimmer, that is used for controlling the current in a circuit.

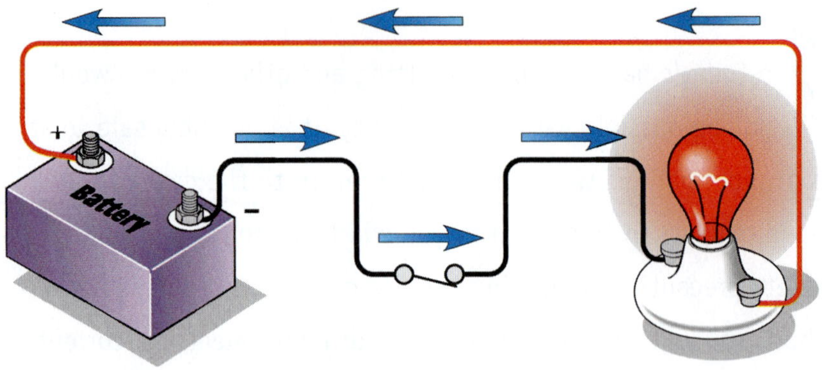

Figure 9–1 A complete electrical circuit.

Types of Electric Current

There are two kinds of electric current: direct current and alternating current.

1. **Direct current** (DC) is a constant, even-flowing current that travels in one direction only and produces a chemical reaction. Battery-operated instruments such as flashlights, cellular phones, and cordless electric clippers use direct current. A **converter** is an apparatus that changes direct current to alternating current. Some cars have converters that allow the use of appliances that would normally be plugged into an electrical wall outlet to be powered by the car's battery.
2. **Alternating current** (AC) is a rapid and interrupted current, flowing first in one direction and then in the opposite direction, that produces a mechanical action. A wall socket utilizes alternating current. Electric clippers, hair-dryers, and other tools that plug into a wall outlet use alternating current. A **rectifier** is an apparatus that changes alternating current to direct current. Cordless electric clippers and battery chargers use a rectifier to convert the AC current from an electrical wall outlet to the DC current needed to recharge the batteries.

Electrical Measurements

In the flow of electric current, individual electrons flow through a wire in the same way that individual water molecules flow through a garden hose.

A **volt** (V), or voltage, is the unit that measures the pressure that pushes the flow of electrons forward through a conductor, much like water pressure pushes water molecules through a hose. A higher voltage indicates more pressure, more force, and more power. If the voltage is lower, the current is weaker (Figure 9–2).

An **amp** (A), or ampere, is the unit that measures the strength of an

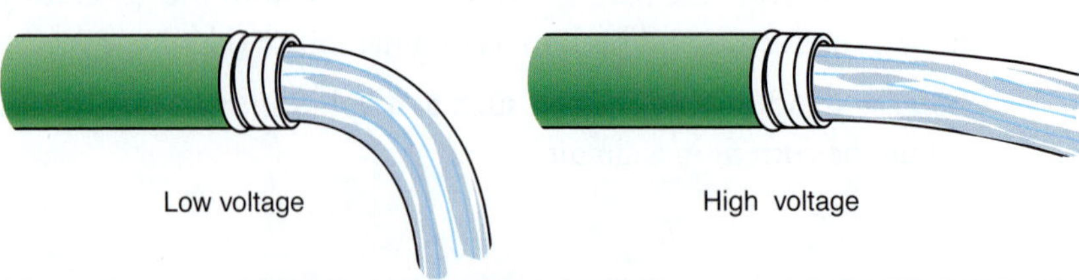

Figure 9–2 Volts measure the pressure or force that pushes on electrons.

electric current. Just as a water hose must be able to expand as the amount of water flowing through it increases, so a wire must expand with an increase in the amount of electrons (amps). A cord must be heavy-duty enough to handle the amps put out by the appliance. For example, a hairdryer rated at 10 amps requires a cord that is twice as thick as one rated at 5 amps. If the current, or number of amps, is too strong, the cord can overheat and cause a fire. If the current is not strong enough, the appliance will not operate correctly.

A *milliampere* is one-thousandth of an ampere. The current for facial and scalp treatments is measured in milliamperes as an ampere current would be much too strong.

An **ohm** (O) is a unit that measures the resistance of an electrical current. Unless the force (volts) is stronger than the resistance (ohms), the current will not flow through the wire.

A **watt** (W) measures how much electric energy is being used in one second. A 40-watt bulb uses 40 watts of energy per second. A *kilowatt* (kW) is 1,000 watts. The electricity in a house is measured in kilowatt- hours (kWh). 1

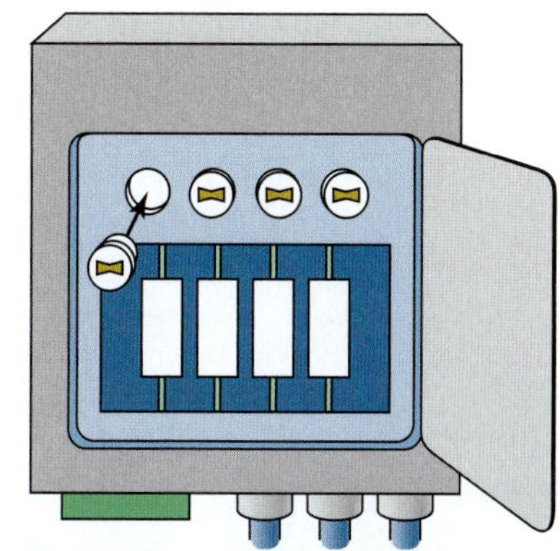

Figure 9-3 Fuse box.

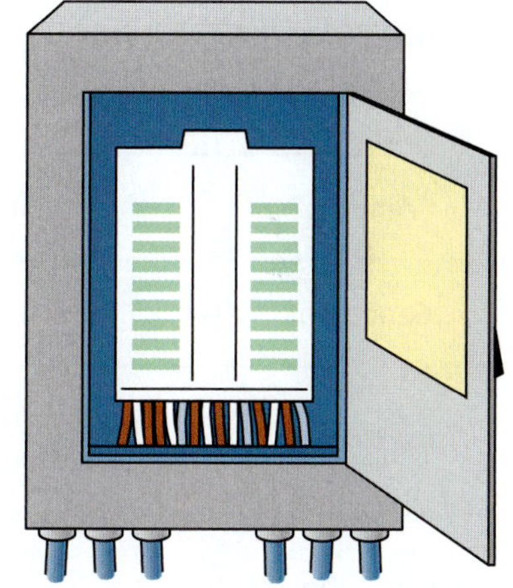

Figure 9-4 Circuit breakers.

Safety Devices

A **fuse** is a safety device that prevents the overheating of electrical wires by preventing excessive current from passing through a circuit. It blows or melts when the wire becomes too hot from overloading the circuit with too much current from too many appliances, for example, or if faulty equipment is used. To re-establish the circuit, the appliance must be unplugged or disconnected and a new fuse inserted in the fuse box (Figure 9–3).

A **circuit breaker** is a switch that automatically interrupts or shuts off an electric circuit at the first indication of an overload (Figure 9–4). In modern electric circuits, circuit breakers have replaced fuses. Circuit breakers supply the same safety control as fuses against overloaded lines and faulty electrical apparatus, but they do not require replacement. They can also be reset. When wires become too hot because of overloading or a faulty piece of equipment, the breaker will click off or disengage, thus breaking the circuit. If an electric appliance malfunctions while in operation, disconnect the appliance from the wall socket immediately and check all connections and insulations before resetting.

A **ground fault circuit interrupter** (GFCI) is a life-saving device that senses imbalances within an electric circuit (Figure 9–5). When it "pops" open, it means that it has sensed a ground fault or current leaking to ground. These devices must be installed properly to operate as intended; otherwise, although the outlet may work, the protection function of their design will be lost.

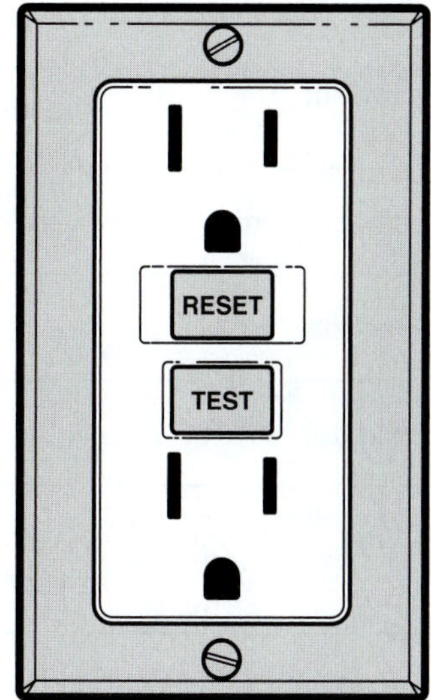

Figure 9-5 Ground fault circuit interrupter (GFCI).

The principle of *grounding* is another important way of promoting electrical safety. All electrical appliances must have at least two electrical connections. The "live" connection supplies current to the circuit. The ground connection completes the circuit and carries the current safely away to the ground.

The different sizes of the prongs on modern electrical plugs guarantee that the plugs can only be inserted one way. This feature provides protection from electrical shock in the event of a short circuit. Some appliance cords have a third, circular prong that provides an additional ground. This extra ground is designed to guarantee a safe path for electricity if the first ground fails or is improperly connected.

2

See Table 9–1 for a summary of electrical terms.

Term	Description
Alternating current	Current that moves in an alternating direction; A to B and B back to A. There is no polarity in alternating current. The current that comes out of a wall socket is an example of alternating current.
Ampere	A unit used to measure the rate of flow of an electrical current.
Conductor	A material that electric current flows through without resistance.
Direct current	A current where electrons flow in the same direction. Direct current has polarity. Iontophoresis is an example.
Electric charge	A basic feature of certain particles of matter that causes them to attract or repel other charged particles.
Electric circuit	The path that an electric current follows.
Electric field	The influence a charged body has on the space around it that causes other charged bodies in that space to experience electric forces
Electrode	A piece of metal, glass, or other conductor through which current enters or leaves an electrical device.
Electromagnetism	A basic force in the universe that involves both electricity and magnetism.
Electron	A subatomic particle with a negative electric charge.
Insulator	A material that opposes the flow of an electric current.
Ion	An atom or group of atoms that has either gained or lost electrons and so has an electric charge.
Kilowatt-hour	The amount of electric energy a 1,000-watt device uses per hour.

Table 9-1 Basics of Electricity

Term	Description
Milliampere meter	An instrument for measuring the rate of flow of an electric current.
Neutron	A subatomic particle in the nucleus that has no electric charge.
Ohm	The unit used to measure a material's resistance to the flow of electric current.
Plug	A two- or three-prong connector at the end of an electrical cord that connects an apparatus into an electrical outlet.
Polarity changer	A switch that reverses with the direction of the current from positive to negative and vice versa.
Proton	A subatomic particle with a positive electric charge, located in the nucleus.
Resistance	A material's opposition to the flow of electric current.
Rheostat	A specific control regulating the strength of the current used; a variable resistor.
Static electricity	An electric charge that is not moving.
Voltage	A type of pressure that drives electric charges through a circuit.
Watt	A unit used to measure the ratio of energy consumption, including electric energy.

Table 9-1 (continued)

Electrical Equipment Safety

The protection and safety of the client should be the primary concern of barbers and stylists. All electrical equipment should be inspected regularly to determine whether or not it is in safe working condition. Careful attention to electrical safety helps to eliminate accidental shock, fire, and burns. A review of the following reminders will help ensure the safe use of electricity in the barbershop.

- All electrical appliances should be UL-certified (Figure 9–6).
- Study the instructions before using any electrical equipment.
- Disconnect appliances when not in use.
- Keep all wires, plugs, and equipment in good repair and inspect all electrical equipment frequently.
- Do not overload outlets (Figure 9–7).
- Avoid getting electrical cords wet.
- When using electrical equipment, protect the client at all times.

UL
®
Underwriters Laboratories (UL) certifies the safety of electrical appliances. Curling irons, hair-dryers, and electric clippers that are UL-approved are certified to be safe when used according to the manufacturers' directions. Always look for the UL symbol on electrical appliances and take the time to read and follow the manufacturers' directions.

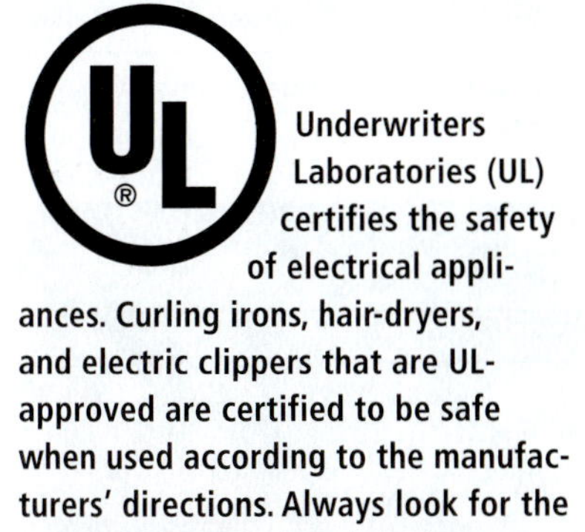

Figure 9-6 A UL symbol as it appears on electrical devices.

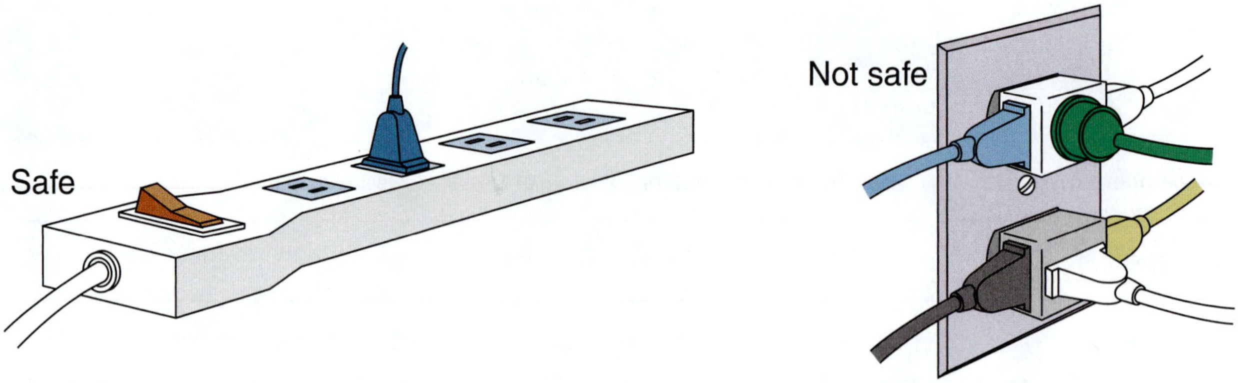

Figure 9-7 One plug per outlet.

- Do not touch any metal while using an electrical appliance.
- Do not handle electrical equipment with wet hands.
- Do not allow the client to touch any metal surfaces while being treated with electrical equipment.
- Do not leave the room while a client is connected to an electrical device.
- Do not attempt to clean around an electric outlet while equipment is plugged in.
- Do not touch two metallic objects at the same time if either is connected to an electric current.
- Do not step on, or set objects on, electrical cords.
- Do not allow electrical cords to become twisted or bent; the fine wires inside the cord will break and the insulation will wear away from the wires.
- Disconnect an appliance by pulling on the plug, not on the cord.
- Do not repair electrical appliances unless you are qualified to do so.

Electrotherapy

Electronic facial and scalp treatments are commonly referred to as **electrotherapy**. Different types of electric currents are used for facial and scalp treatments. These different types of currents are called **modalities** and each one produces a different effect on the skin.

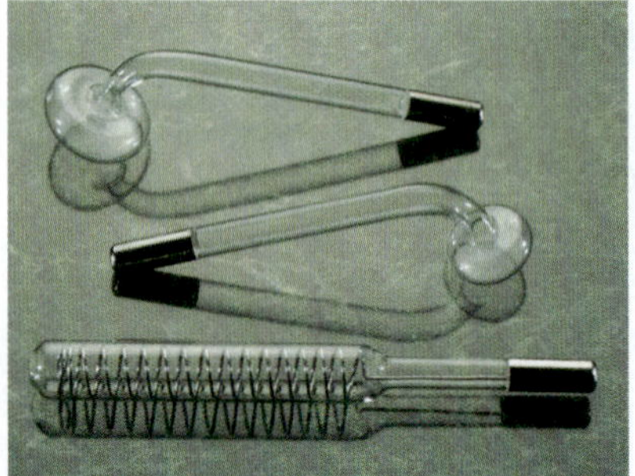

Figure 9-8 Electrodes come in a variety of shapes.

An **electrode** is an applicator used to direct the electric current from the machine to the client's skin. Electrodes are available in many shapes and are usually made of carbon, glass, or metal (Figure 9–8).

Polarities

Polarity indicates the negative or positive pole of an electric current. The positive pole is called an **anode**, is usually red, and may be marked with a "P" or a plus (+) sign (Figure 9–9). The negative electrode is called a **cathode**. It is usually black and marked with an "N" or a minus (–) sign (Figure 9–9).

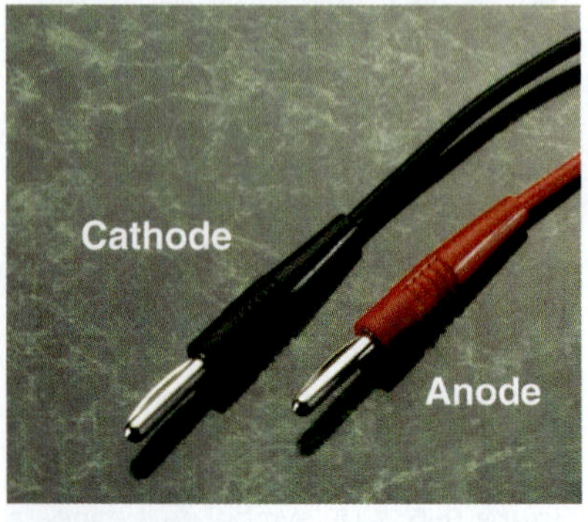

Figure 9-9 Anode and cathode.

If the electrodes are not marked, either of the following tests will help to determine the anode from the cathode electrode.

1. Separate the tips of two conducting cords from each other and immerse them in a glass of salt water. Turn the selector switch of the appliance to galvanic current, and then turn up the intensity. As the water is decomposed, more active bubbles will accumulate at the negative pole than at the positive pole.
2. Place the tips of two conducting cords on two separate pieces of blue moistened litmus paper. The paper under the positive pole will turn red, while the paper under the negative pole will stay blue. If you use red litmus instead of blue, the positive pole will keep the red litmus the same and the negative pole will turn the red litmus blue.

CAUTION

Polarity tests can be dangerous and should not be performed without an instructor's supervision. Do not allow the tips of the conduction cords to touch, which can cause a short circuit.

Modalities

Modalities are the currents used in electronic facial and scalp treatments. The four main modalities used in barbering are the galvanic, sinusoidal, faradic, and Tesla high-frequency currents.

Galvanic Current

The most commonly used modality is the **galvanic current**. It is a constant and direct current (DC), having a negative and positive pole, that is reduced to a safe, low-voltage level. Galvanic current produces chemical changes when passed through body tissues and fluids, and is used to create chemical and ionic reactions in the skin. These reactions depend on the negative or positive polarity that is used (Table 9–2).

Disincrustation is used to facilitate deep pore cleansing. During this process galvanic current is used to create a chemical reaction that acts to

Positive Pole (Anode)	Negative Pole (Cathode)
Produces acidic reactions	Produces alkaline reactions
Closes the pores	Opens the pores
Soothes nerves	Stimulates and irritates the nerves
Decreases blood supply	Increases blood supply
Contracts blood vessels	Expands blood vessels
Hardens and firms tissues	Softens tissues

Note that the effects produced by the positive pole are the exact opposite of those produced by the negative pole.

Table 9-2 Effects of Galvanic Current

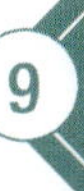

emulsify the sebum and waste in the pores. An electropositive solution is applied to the skin and the negative pole is used to make direct contact with the substance while the client holds the positive pole (see Chapter 13).

Iontophoresis means the introduction of ions. It is a process in which galvanic current is used to introduce water-soluble products into the deeper layers of the skin. Both the positive and negative poles are used in the process. Ionic penetration takes place in two ways: **cataphoresis**, which forces acidic substances into the tissues from the positive toward the negative pole, and **anaphoresis**, which forces liquids into the tissues from the negative toward the positive pole (see Chapter 13).

Faradic Current

Faradic current is an alternating and interrupted current capable of producing a mechanical reaction without a chemical effect. Two electrodes are required to complete the faradic circuit. Faradic current causes muscular contractions and may be used in scalp and facial treatments (see Chapter 13). Some of the benefits of using faradic current include:

- improved muscle tone.
- increased blood circulation.
- increased metabolism.
- removal of waste products.
- stimulation of hair growth.
- invigoration of the area being treated.
- increased glandular activity.
- relief of blood congestion.

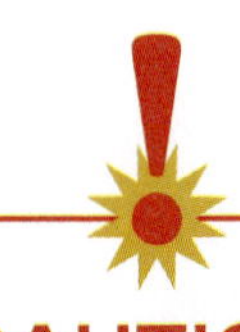

CAUTION

Do not use a sinusoidal current if the face is flushed or if the client has broken capillaries in the skin, high blood pressure, or skin condition with pustules.

Sinusoidal Current

Sinusoidal current, which is similar to faradic current, may be used during scalp and facial manipulations. It is an alternating current that produces mechanical contractions in the muscles and also requires the use of two electrodes (see Chapter 13). Some advantages of using sinusoidal current include:

- supplies greater stimulation, deeper penetration, and is less irritating than faradic current.
- soothes the nerves and penetrates into deeper muscle tissue.

High-Frequency Current

Tesla high-frequency current is characterized by a high rate of oscillation that produces heat. It is commonly called the violet ray and is used for both scalp and facial treatments. Due to its rapid oscillation, Tesla current does not cause muscular contractions. Instead, the physiological effects are either stimulating or soothing, depending on the method of application.

The electrodes are made of glass or metal and only one electrode is used to perform a service. The shapes of the electrodes vary depending on the service: the facial electrode is flat and the scalp electrode is rake-shaped. As the current passes through the glass electrode, tiny violet sparks are emitted. All treatments given with high-frequency current should be started with mild current and gradually increased to the required strength. Approximately five minutes should be allowed for a general facial or scalp treatment, depending upon the condition being treated (see Chapters 12 and 13). As with all other tools and implements, follow manufacturer's directions. The potential benefits of using Tesla high-frequency current are:

- stimulated blood circulation.
- improved glandular activity.
- increased metabolism.
- increased absorption of nutrients and elimination of wastes.
- improved germicidal action.
- relief of congestion.

LIGHT THERAPY

Light therapy refers to the use of light rays to effect treatments. Therapeutic lamps are used to produce artificial light rays for use in the barbershop. Different light rays will produce heat, chemical reactions, or germicidal effects.

Visible light is electromagnetic radiation that we can see. Electromagnetic radiation is also called *radiant energy* because it radiates energy through space on waves. The distance between two successive peaks is called the **wavelength**. Long wavelengths have low frequency, meaning the number of waves is less frequent within a given length. Short wavelengths have a higher rate of frequency because the number of waves is more frequent within a given length (Figure 9–10).

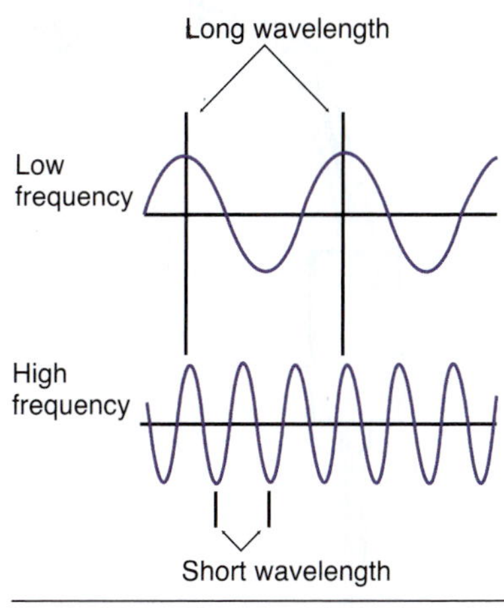

Figure 9–10 Long and short wavelengths.

The entire range of electromagnetic radiation wavelengths is called the *electromagnetic spectrum.* Visible light is the part of the spectrum that we can see and makes up 35 percent of natural sunlight.

Ultraviolet rays and infrared rays are also forms of electromagnetic radiation, but they are invisible to the human eye. Invisible rays make up 65 percent of natural sunlight at the earth's surface.

4

When light passes through a glass prism it produces the seven colors of the rainbow, arrayed in the following manner: red, orange, yellow, green, blue, indigo, and violet (Figure 9–11). Within the visible spectrum of light, violet has the shortest wavelength and red has the longest. In the field of barbering, we are concerned with the rays that produce heat (infrared rays) and those that produce chemical and germicidal reactions (ultraviolet rays).

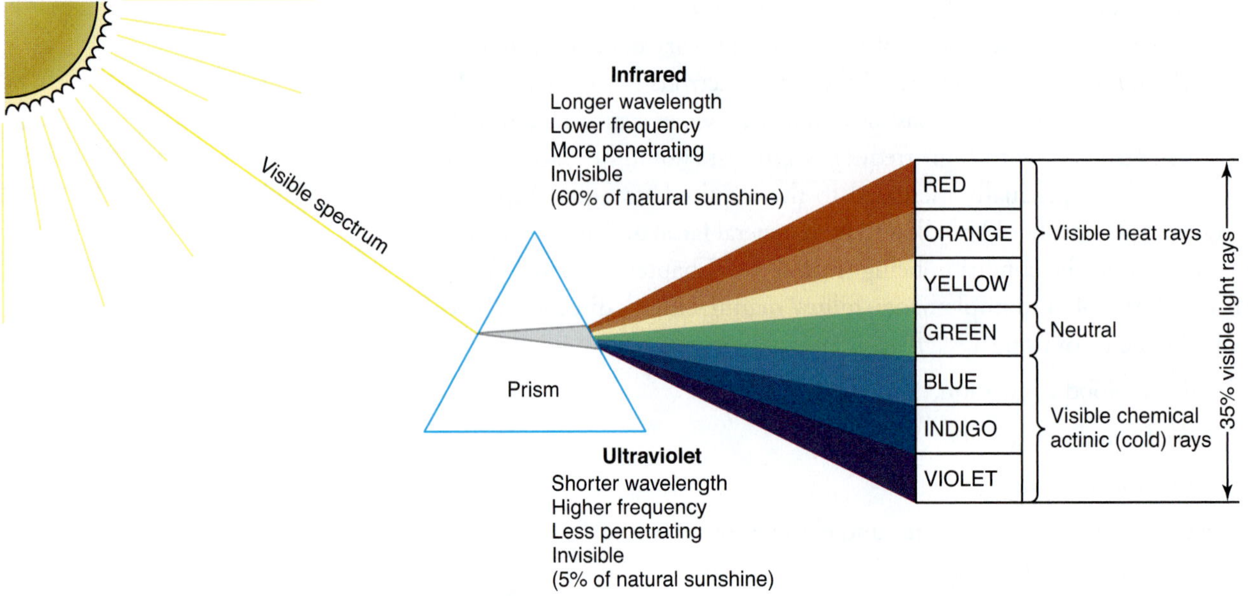

Figure 9–11 The visible spectrum.

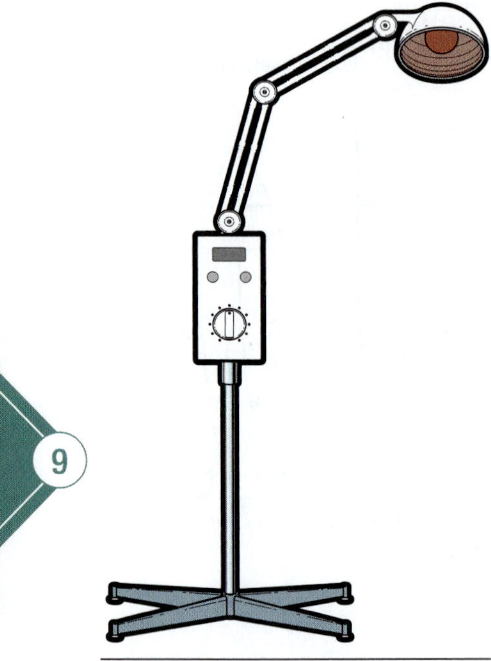

Figure 9–12 Therapeutic lamp.

In the barbershop, artificial light rays are produced through the use of therapeutic lamps. The bulbs in these lamps are capable of producing the same rays that are originated by the sun. Therapeutic lamps that produce infrared and ultraviolet rays are available in either separate or combination units. They are also available in several different styles, which include tabletop and floor models (Figure 9–12).

Visible Light Rays

Visible light rays are the primary light sources used for scalp and facial treatments. The bulbs used for therapeutic visible light therapy are white, red, and blue. *White light* is referred to as a *combination light* because it consists of all the visible rays of the spectrum. *Red light* produces the most heat and penetrates the deepest. It is used on dry skin in combination with oils and creams. *Blue light* contains few heat rays, is the least penetrating, and provides germicidal and chemical benefits. Blue light should be used only on bare, oily skin.

The lamp used to reproduce visible lights is usually a dome-shaped reflector mounted on a pedestal with a flexible neck. The dome is finished with a highly polished metal lining capable of reflecting heat rays. The bulbs used with this lamp come in various colors for different purposes. As with all other lamps, the client's eyes must be protected from the glare and heat of the light. For proper eye protection, the client's eyes are covered with cotton pads saturated with dilute boric acid or witch hazel solution.

- *White light* relieves pain, especially in congested areas, and more particularly around the nerve centers, such as the back of the neck and across the shoulders.

- *Blue light* has a tonic effect on bare skin and a soothing effect on the nerves. It is deficient in heat rays. Blue light should be used only over clear skin, without any cream, oil, or powder present on the skin.
- *Red light* has strong heat rays, creates a stimulating effect, can be used over creams and ointments to soften and relax body tissue, and penetrates the skin more deeply than does blue light. Heat rays aid the penetration of lanolin creams into the skin and are recommended for dry, scaly, and shriveled skin.

INVISIBLE LIGHT RAYS

Ultraviolet Rays

Ultraviolet (UV) rays, also known as cold rays or actinic rays, make up 5 percent of natural sunlight. UV rays have short wavelengths, produce chemical effects, kill germs, and are the least penetrating rays. There are three general types of ultraviolet lamps: the glass bulb, the hot quartz, and the cold quartz.

- The glass bulb lamp is used mainly for cosmetic or tanning purposes.
- The hot quartz lamp is a general, all-purpose lamp suitable for tanning, tonic, cosmetic, or germicidal purposes.
- The cold quartz lamp produces mostly short ultraviolet rays. It is used primarily in hospitals.

UV rays are divided into three categories: UVA, UVB, and UVC. The farther away from the visible light spectrum, the shorter and less penetrating the ultraviolet rays.

- *UVA rays* are the tonic UV rays. UVA rays are closest to the visible spectrum and are the longest of all the UV rays. These rays are used in tanning booths and penetrate deeply into skin tissue. Overexposure can destroy the elasticity of the skin, causing premature aging and wrinkling.
- *UVB rays* are the therapeutic rays in the middle of the UV range, which produce some effects from both ends of ultraviolet rays. Long exposure to UVB rays will burn the skin.
- *UVC rays* are the most germicidal and chemical of the ultraviolet rays, as well as being the farthest away from the visible spectrum. These rays don't penetrate far into the skin but can burn the surface. UVC rays are destructive to bacteria, as well as to skin tissue if the skin is exposed to them for too long a period of time.

Ultraviolet rays are used to treat acne, tinea, and seborrhea, and to combat dandruff. They also promote healing and can stimulate the growth of hair, as well as produce a tan by increasing skin pigment if the skin is exposed in short doses over a long period of time. Table 9-3 summarizes the pros and cons of UV ray treatments

Ultraviolet rays are applied with a lamp at a distance of 30 to 36 inches from the skin. Average exposure can produce skin redness and overdoses will cause blistering. It is best to start with a short exposure of two to three minutes and gradually increase the exposure over a period of days to seven to eight minutes. To receive full benefit from ultraviolet rays, the area to be treated should be clean, with no cream or lotion applied to the skin.

CAUTION

The client's eyes should always be protected when ultraviolet rays are used. Goggles or eye pads saturated with dilute boric acid or witch hazel should be provided for clients, and protective eyewear or sunglasses for the barber.

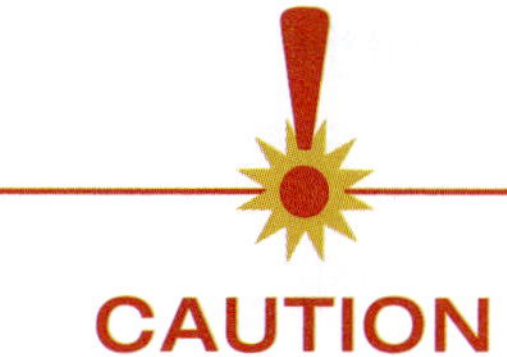

CAUTION

Never leave the client unattended during light therapy treatments.

Benefits of Ultraviolet Ray Treatments	Disadvantages of Ultraviolet Rays
Increases resistance to disease by promoting the production of vitamin D in the skin and increasing the number of red and white cells in the blood.	May destroy hair pigment.
Increases the elimination of waste products and restores nutrition where needed.	Continued exposure to UV rays causes premature aging of the skin.
Stimulates the circulation by improving the flow of blood and lymph.	Continued exposure to UV rays causes painful sunburn.
Increases the fixation of calcium in the blood.	Continued exposure to UV rays causes a higher risk of skin cancer, especially for fair- or light-skinned individuals.

Table 9-3 Benefits and Disadvantages of Ultraviolet Rays

CAUTION

When performing infrared treatments, the length of exposure should not exceed five minutes. It is important to break the path of the rays every few seconds to prevent overexposure. This can be accomplished by the barber moving his hand back and forth across the ray's path between the lamp and the client's skin.

9

Infrared Rays

Beyond the red rays of the spectrum are the **infrared rays**. These are pure heat rays, comprising about 60 percent of sunshine. Infrared rays are long, penetrate more than two inches into the body, and can produce the most heat. Infrared rays produce no light whatsoever, only a rosy glow when active. Special glass bulbs, which can be red or white, are used to produce infrared rays. Most moisturizing skin creams may be used, but check the ingredients for possible contraindications. The lamp should be operated at an average distance of 30 inches and the client's comfort checked frequently.

Infrared ray treatments will heat and relax the skin without increasing the temperature of the body as a whole. These rays will dilate blood vessels in the skin, thereby increasing blood circulation, and increase metabolism and chemical changes within skin tissues. Infrared rays will also soothe nerves, relieve muscular pain, and increase the production of perspiration and oil on the skin.

Electrotherapy and light therapy treatments are special client services that new and established barbers should consider offering. When the services discussed in this chapter are performed professionally and marketed effectively, the barbershop will benefit from increased revenue, client retention, and new-client referrals that can elevate the shop's reputation "a cut above" the rest. 5

chapter glossary

alternating current	rapid and interrupted current, flowing first in one direction then the opposite direction
amp	a unit measures the strength of an electric current
anaphoresis	toward the positive pole
anode	positive electrode
cataphoresis	process of forcing acidic substances into tissues using galvanic current from the positive toward the negative pole
cathode	negative electrode
circuit breaker	switch that automatically interrupts or shuts off an electric circuit at the first sign of overload
complete circuit	the path of an electric current from the generating source through the conductor and back to its original source
conductor	any substance, medium, or material that conducts electricity
converter	an apparatus that changes direct current to alternating current
disincrustation	process used to soften and emulsify oil and blackheads in the hair follicles
direct current	constant current that travels in one direction only and produces a chemical reaction
electric current	the flow of electricity along a conductor
electrode	an applicator used to direct electric current from a machine to the skin
electrotherapy	electronic scalp and facial treatments
faradic current	alternating current that produces a mechanical reaction without chemical effect
fuse	device that prevents excessive current from passing through a circuit
galvanic current	constant and direct current, having a positive and negative pole, that produces chemical changes in tissues and body fluids
ground fault circuit interrupter	a device that senses imbalances in an electric current
infrared rays	invisible rays with long wavelengths and deep penetration; they produce the most heat
insulator	substance that does not easily transfer electricity
iontophoresis	process of introducing water-soluble products into the skin through the use of electric current
modalities	currents used in electric facial and scalp treatments
ohm	the unit that measures the resistance of an electrical current
polarity	negative or positive pole of an electric current
rectifier	apparatus that changes alternating current to direct current

rheostat	an adjustable resistor used for controlling current in a circuit
sinusoidal current	alternating current used in scalp and facial manipulations that produces mechanical contractions
Tesla high-frequency current	thermal or heat-producing current with a high oscillation rate; also known as the violet ray
ultraviolet rays	invisible rays, with short wavelengths and minimal skin penetrating, that produce chemical effects and kill germs; also called actinic or cold rays
visible light	electromagnetic radiation that can be seen by the human eye
volt	unit that measures the pressure or force of electricity
watt	measurement of how much electric energy is used in one second
wavelength	distance between two successive peaks of electromagnetic waves

chapter review questions

1. Describe two types of electrical current.
2. Explain the differences between a fuse, circuit breaker, and GFCI.
3. List and define four electrical modalities used in scalp and facial treatments.
4. Discuss the effects of visible and invisible light rays.
5. Explain the differences between ultraviolet and infrared rays.
6. Explain the effects of ultraviolet and infrared rays.

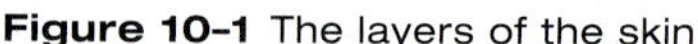

Figure 10–1 The layers of the skin.

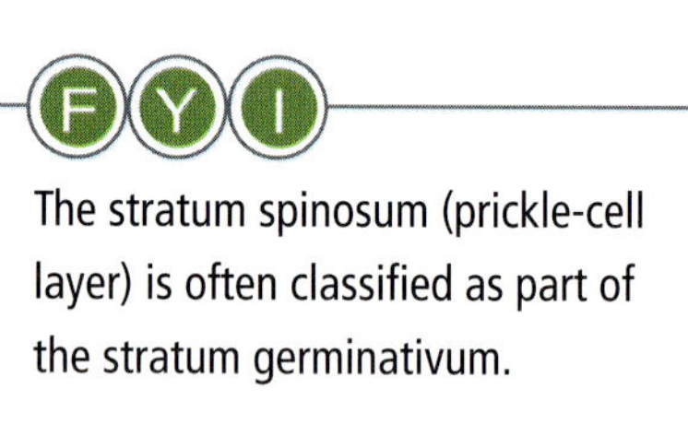

FYI

The stratum spinosum (prickle-cell layer) is often classified as part of the stratum germinativum.

- The **stratum granulosum** (gran-yoo-LOH-sum), or *granular layer*, consists of cells that look like distinct granules. These cells are almost dead and are pushed to the surface to replace cells that are shed from the stratum corneum.
- The **stratum germinativum** (jer-mih-nah-TIV-um), also known as the *stratum mucosum, Malpighian*, or *basal layer*, is the deepest layer of the epidermis. This layer is responsible for the growth of the epidermis and contains a dark pigment called *melanin*, which protects the sensitive cells below from the destructive effects of excessive exposure to ultraviolet rays.

Dermis

The **dermis** (DUR-mis) is the underlying, or inner layer of the skin. It is also called the **derma**, **corium**, **cutis**, or **true skin**. The dermis is about 25 times thicker than the epidermis and consists of a highly sensitive vascular layer of

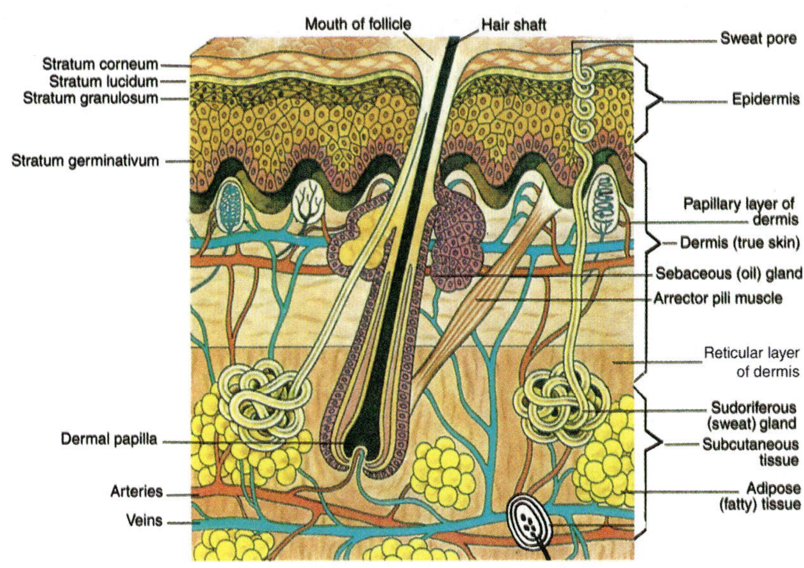

Figure 10–2 Structures of the skin.

connective tissue. Within its structure are numerous blood vessels, nerves, lymph and oil glands, hair follicles, arrector pili muscles, and papillae. The dermis consists of two layers: the papillary, or superficial layer; and the reticular, or deeper layer (Figure 10–2).

- The **papillary** (PAP-uh-lair-ee) **layer** lies directly beneath the epidermis. It contains small, cone-shaped projections of elastic tissue called papillae (puh-PIL-eye) that point upward into the epidermis. Some of these papillae contain looped capillaries or small blood vessels. Others contain small structures called tactile corpuscles with nerve fiber endings that are sensitive to touch and pressure. This layer also contains some melanin (skin pigment).
- The **reticular** (ruh-TIK-yuh-lur) **layer** is the deeper layer of the dermis, which supplies the skin with oxygen and nutrients. It contains the following structures within its network:
    - fat cells
    - sweat glands
    - blood vessels
    - hair follicles
    - lymph glands
    - arrector pili muscles
    - oil glands

Subcutaneous (sub-kyoo-TAY-nee-us) **tissue**, also known as **adipose tissue**, is a layer of fatty tissue found below the dermis that some specialists regard as a continuation of the dermis. Subcutaneous tissue varies in thickness according to age, gender, and general health. It gives smoothness and contour to the body, contains fats for use as energy, and also acts as a protective cushion for the outer skin. 1

10

How the Skin Is Nourished

Blood and lymph supply nourishment to the skin. From one-half to two-thirds of the body's blood supply is distributed to the skin. As the blood and lymph circulate through the skin, they contribute essential materials for growth, nourishment, and repair of the skin, hair, and nails. Networks of arteries and lymphatics in the subcutaneous tissue send their smaller branches to hair papillae, hair follicles, and skin glands.

Nerves of the Skin

The skin contains the surface endings of many nerve fibers, which are classified as follows:

- **Motor nerve fibers**, which are distributed to the arrector pili muscles attached to the hair follicles. These muscles trigger goose bumps when a person is frightened or cold.
- **Sensory nerve fibers**, which react to heat, cold, touch, pressure, and pain (Figure 10–3). These receptors send messages to the brain.
- **Secretory nerve fibers**, which are distributed to the sweat and oil glands of the skin. Secretory nerves regulate the excretion of perspiration from the sweat glands and the flow of *sebum* from the oil glands.

Sense of Touch

The papillary layer of the dermis houses the nerve endings that provide the body with the sense of touch. These nerve endings register basic sensations such as touch, pain, heat, cold, pressure, or deep touch. Nerve endings are most abundant in the fingertips. Complex sensations, such as vibrations, seem to depend on the sensitivity of a combination of these nerve endings.

Skin Elasticity

10

The skin gets its strength, form, and flexibility from protein fibers within the dermis called collagen and elastin. **Collagen** fibers make up a large

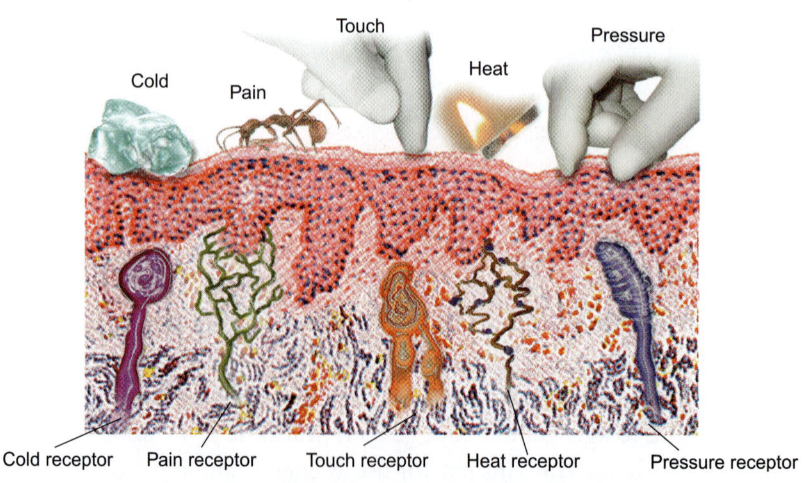

Figure 10-3 Sensory nerve endings in the skin.

portion of the dermis and help to give structural support to the many structures found in this layer. When collagen fibers become weakened, wrinkles and sagging of the skin can occur. **Elastin** gives the skin its elasticity and flexibility and the ability to regain its shape after stretching. When healthy skin expands, it regains its former shape almost immediately. Conversely, one of the most prominent characteristics of aged skin is its loss of elasticity.

Skin Color

The color of the skin, whether fair or dark, depends on two factors: blood supply and melanin. Of the two, blood supply to the skin is least influential to skin color. **Melanin**, however, is the primary source of skin color because the grains of pigment are deposited in the stratum germinativum of the epidermis and the papillary layer of the dermis.

Special cells called *melanocytes* produce the pigment granules that are scattered throughout the germinativum and papillary layers. These granules are called *melanosomes* and they produce the complex protein called melanin, a brown-black pigment that serves as the skin's protective screen from the sun's rays. The color of pigment is a hereditary trait that varies among races and nationalities and from person to person. Dark skin contains more melanin than light skin.

The Glands of the Skin

The skin contains two types of duct glands, the **sudoriferous** (sood-uh-RIF-uh-rus) **glands** or *sweat glands*, and the **sebaceous** (sih-BAY-shus) **glands** or *oil glands* (Figure 10–4), which extract material from the blood to form new substances.

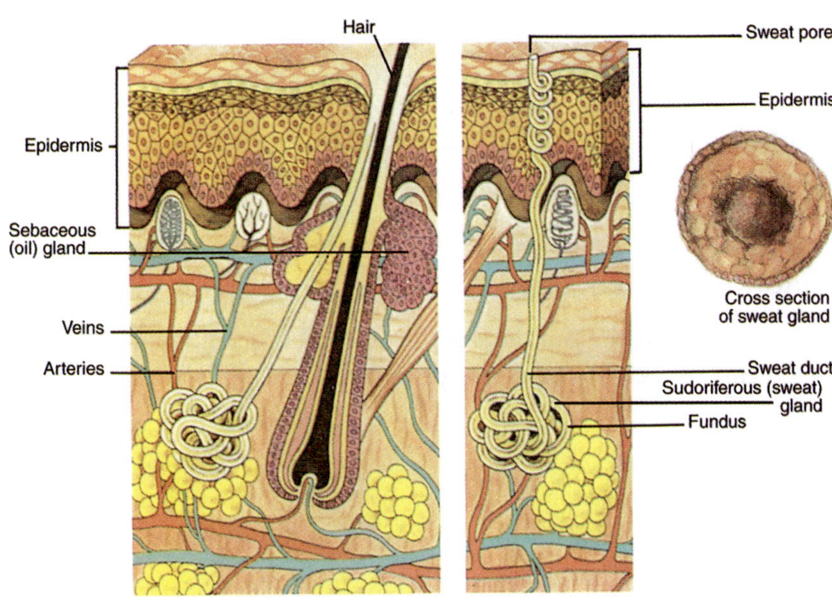

Figure 10-4 Sweat gland and oil gland.

Sudoriferous (Sweat) Glands

The sudoriferous or sweat glands consist of a coiled base (*fundus*) and a tubelike duct that terminates at the skin surface to form the sweat pore. Practically all parts of the body are supplied with sweat glands, although they are more numerous on the palms, soles, forehead, and armpits.

The sweat glands regulate body temperature and help to eliminate waste products from the body. Because the excretion of sweat is under the control of the nervous system, sweat gland activity is greatly increased by heat, exercise, emotion, and certain drugs.

Normally, one or two pints of liquid containing salts are eliminated daily through the sweat pores in the skin.

Sebaceous (Oil) Glands

The sebaceous or oil glands of the skin are connected to the hair follicle. These glands consist of little sacs with ducts that open into the hair follicle where they secrete **sebum**, which lubricates the skin and preserves the softness of the hair. With the exception of the palms and soles, these glands are found in all parts of the body, particularly the face.

Sebum is a semifluid, oily substance produced by the oil glands. Ordinarily it flows through the oil ducts leading to the mouths of the hair follicles. However, when the sebum becomes hardened and the duct becomes blocked, a blackhead is formed. The primary function of sebum is to act as a shield that prevents moisture from evaporating from the skin surface.

Absorption Level of the Skin

Although the skin is an intact outer layer of the body, it is, in fact, indented by hair follicles with their sebaceous glands and by the pores of the sudoriferous glands. These pockets, although normally resistant to bacterial attack (except in certain cases where they show as pimples, boils, blackheads, or acne), will allow the entry of special drugs and chemicals into the body. Chemical preparations such as antiseptic creams and ointments may be absorbed to combat skin infections, or products such as vitamin and hormone creams may be used as skin conditioners to help overcome dry or damaged skin.

Functions of the Skin

The principal functions of the skin are protection, sensation, heat regulation, excretion, secretion, and absorption.

- *Protection.* The skin protects the body from injury and bacterial invasion. The outermost layer of the epidermis is covered with a thin layer of sebum, which renders it waterproof. The skin is resistant to ranges of temperature, minor injuries, chemical substances, and many forms of bacteria.
- *Sensation.* The skin responds to heat, cold, touch, pressure, pain, and location through its sensory nerve endings. Stimulation of a sensory nerve

ending sends a message to the brain, which then stimulates a response. When you scratch an itch or pull away from a hot object, you are responding to the stimulation of sensory nerve endings and the message they conveyed to the brain. Sensory endings responsive to touch and pressure lie in close relation to hair follicles.

- *Heat regulation.* Heat regulation is a function of the skin that protects the body from the environment. A healthy body maintains a constant internal temperature of about 98.6 degrees Fahrenheit. As changes occur in the outside temperature, the blood and sweat glands of the skin make necessary adjustments to facilitate the cooling of the body through the evaporation of sweat.
- *Excretion.* Perspiration is excreted from the skin. Water lost by perspiration carries salt and other chemicals with it.
- *Secretion.* Sebum is secreted by the sebaceous glands and lubricates the skin, keeping it soft and pliable. Sebum also lubricates the hair. Emotional stress may increase the flow of sebum.
- *Absorption.* Absorption is limited, but does occur. Some female hormone creams can enter the body through the skin and influence it to some degree. Fatty materials, such as lanolin creams, are absorbed largely through the hair follicles and sebaceous gland openings. 2

DISORDERS OF THE SKIN

Although barbers are not licensed to perform treatments for medical conditions, the performance of facials and shaves are traditional services well within the barber's scope of expertise. This includes addressing certain skin conditions, such as oily or dry skin, or alleviating minor acne conditions. During the shaving process, barbers need to be able to recognize *hypertrophies* such as moles and warts, or skin conditions that may be aggravated by the shaving procedure. The following section has been compiled to familiarize barbers and barber-stylists with common skin disorders so that they may perform barbering services in a knowledgeable and skillful manner.

Symptoms are signs or indications of disease. Symptoms of skin disorders are generally divided into two groups: *subjective symptoms*, such as itching, burning, or pain that can be felt by the individual; and *objective symptoms*, such as pimples or boils, which can be observed. *Lesions*, in the form of scales, pimples, or pustules, are symptoms that may characterize the skin conditions that barbers see in the performance of their work. Since these symptoms may be similar in appearance to certain contagious disorders, it is important to be able to differentiate between common or noncontagious skin conditions and more serious or communicable ones. This knowledge helps the barber to know which services may or may not be performed in the barbershop.

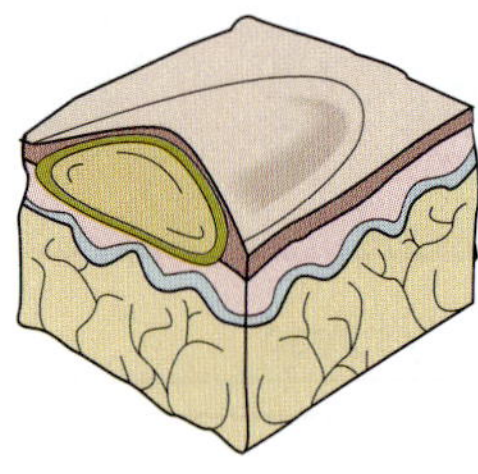

Bulla:
Same as a vesicle only greater than 0.5 cm
Example:
Contact dermatitis, large second-degree burns, bulbous impetigo, pemphigus

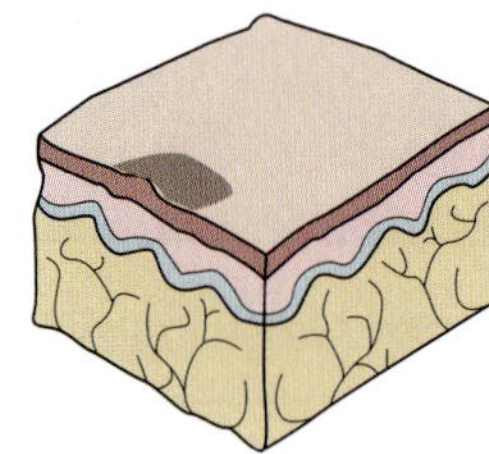

Macule:
Localized changes in skin color of less than 1 cm in diameter
Example:
Freckle

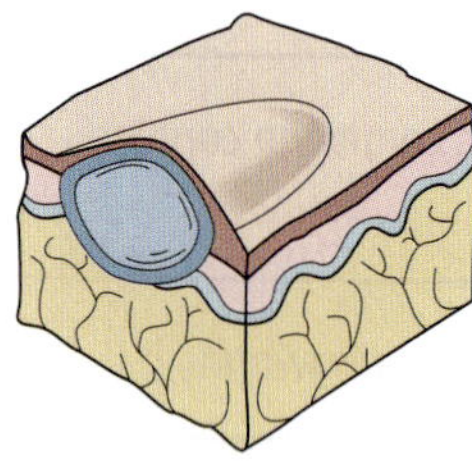

Tubercle:
Solid and elevated; however, it extends deeper than papules into the dermis or subcutaneous tissues, 0.5–2 cm
Example:
Lipoma, erythema, nodosum, cyst

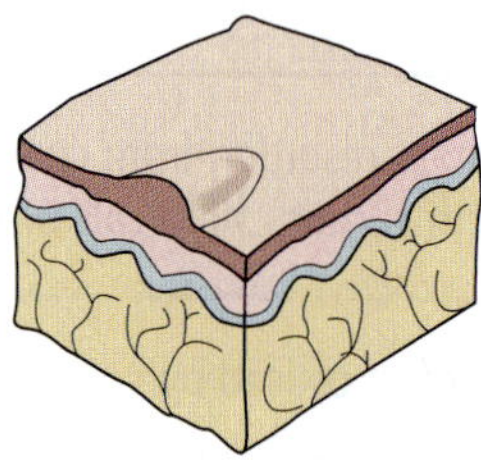

Papule:
Solid, elevated lesion less than 0.5 cm in diameter
Example:
Warts, elevated nevi

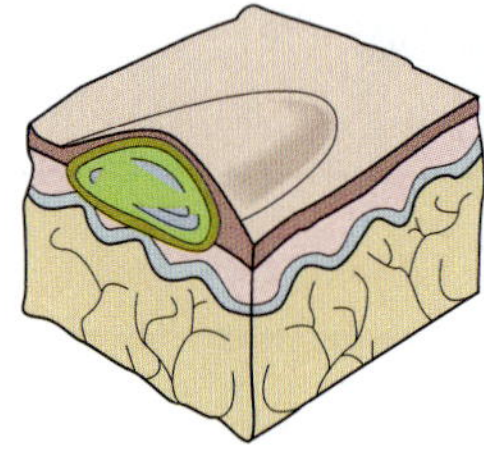

Pustule:
Vesicles or bullae that become filled with pus, usually described as less than 0.5 cm in diameter
Example:
Acne, impetigo, furuncles, carbuncles, folliculitis

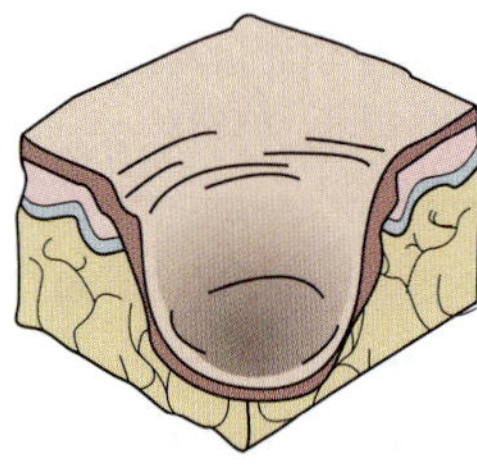

Ulcer:
A depressed lesion of the epidermis and upper papillary layer of the dermis
Example:
Stage 2 pressure ulcer

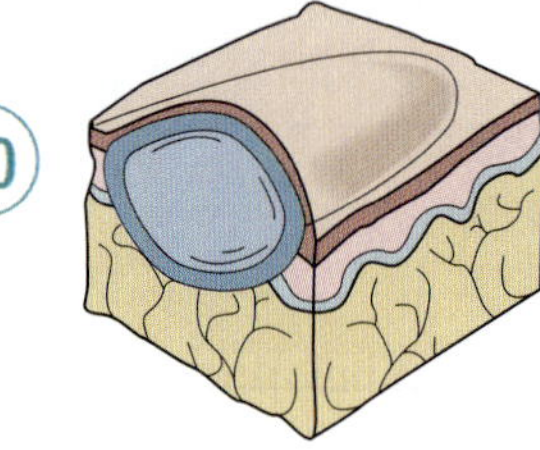

Tumor:
The same as a nodule—a small, knobby growth or calcification—only greater than 2 cm
Example:
Carcinoma (such as advanced breast carcinoma); **not** basal cell or squamous cell of the skin

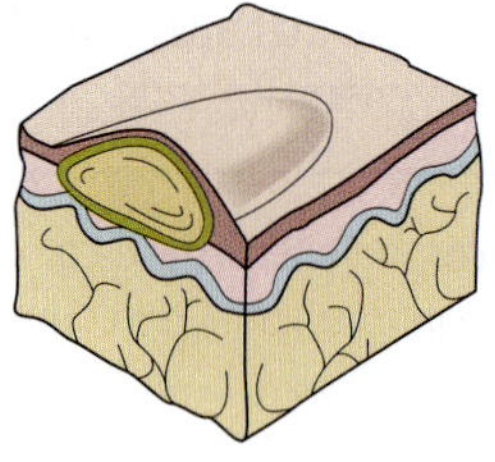

Vesicle:
Accumulation of fluid between the upper layers of the skin; elevated mass containing serous fluid; less than 0.5 cm
Example:
Herpes simplex, herpes zoster, chicken pox

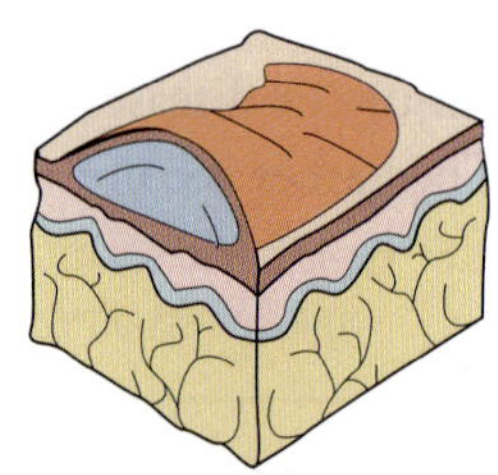

Wheal:
Localized edema in the epidermis causing irregular elevation that may be red or pale
Example:
Insect bite or a hive

Figure 10-5 Primary skin lesions.

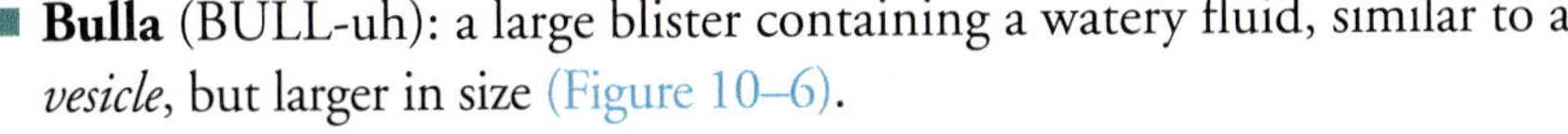

- **Bulla** (BULL-uh): a large blister containing a watery fluid, similar to a *vesicle*, but larger in size (Figure 10–6).
- **Cyst** (SIST): a closed, abnormally developed sac containing fluid, semi-fluid, or morbid matter, above or below the skin.
- **Macule** (MAK-yool): a small, discolored spot or patch on the surface of the skin. Macules are neither raised nor sunken.
- **Papule** (PAP-yool): a small, elevated pimple that contains no fluid, but that may develop pus (Figure 10–7).
- **Pustule** (PUS-chool): an inflamed pimple containing pus (Figure 10–7).
- **Tubercle** (TOO-bur-kul): an abnormal, rounded solid lump larger than a papule that projects above the surface or lies within or under the skin.
- **Tumor** (TOO-mur): an abnormal cell mass varying in size, shape, and color that results from the excessive multiplication of cells. *Nodules* are also referred to as tumors, but they are smaller.
- **Ulcer** (UL-sur): a depressed lesion.
- **Vesicle** (VES-ih-kel): a small blister or sac containing clear fluid lying within or just beneath the epidermis. Poison ivy and poison oak produce small vesicles (Figure 10–8).
- **Wheal** (WHEEL): an itchy, swollen lesion that lasts only a few hours. Hives and insect bites are examples of wheals.

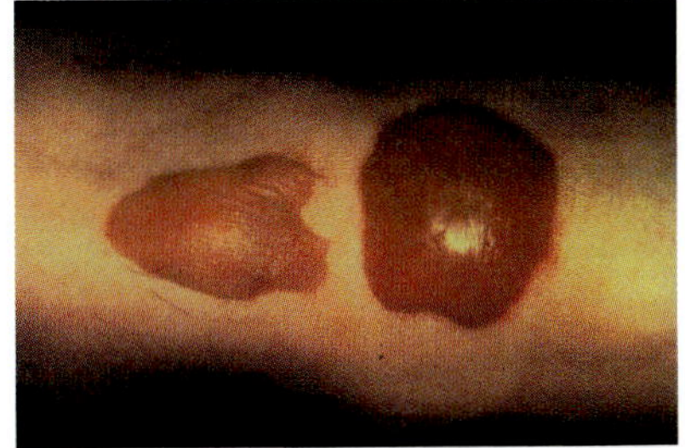

Figure 10-6 Bullae.

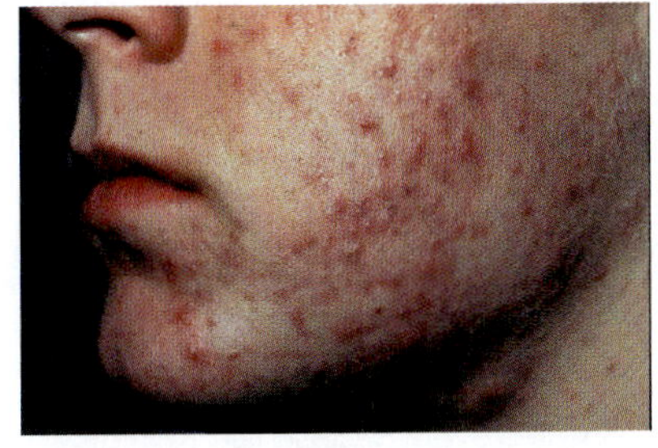

Figure 10-7 Papules and pustules.

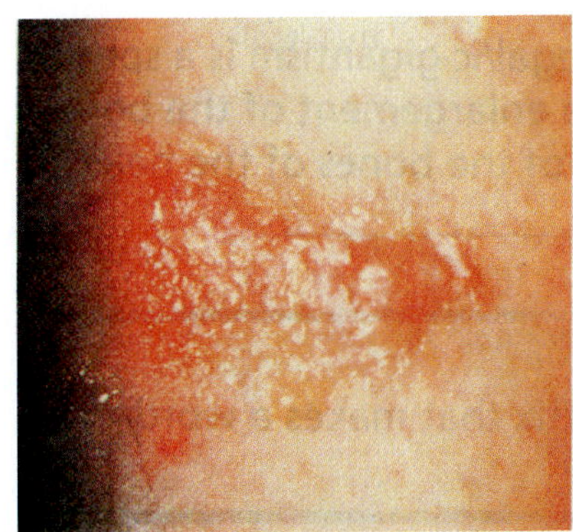

Figure 10-8 Poison oak vesicles.

Secondary Lesions

Secondary lesions are characterized by a collection of material on the skin, such as a scale, crust, or keloid; or by a loss of skin surface as with an ulcer or fissure (Figure 10–9).

- **Crust** or scab: an accumulation of dead cells that forms over a wound or blemish while it is healing; an accumulation of sebum and pus, sometimes mixed with epidermal material.

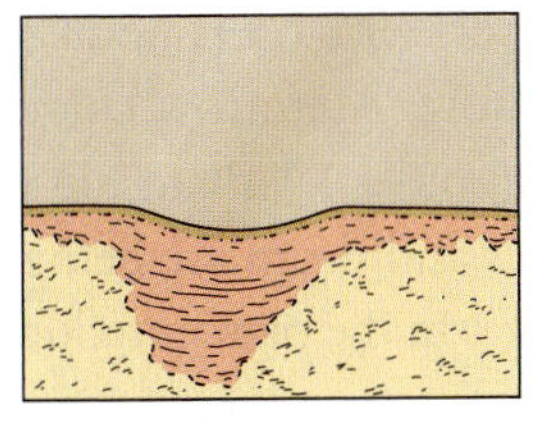

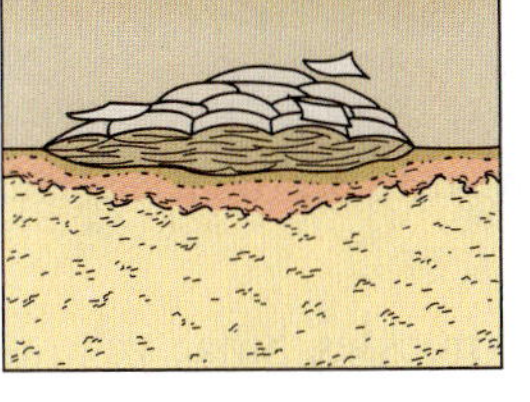

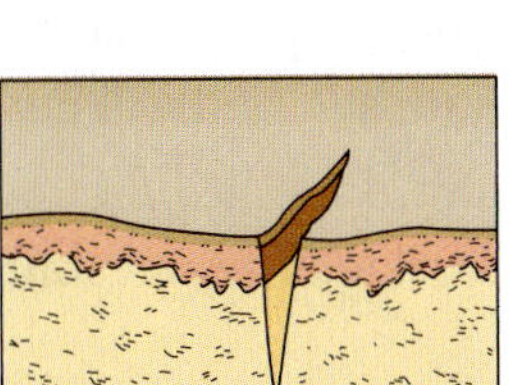

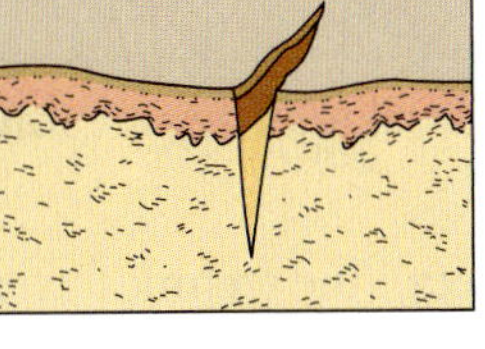

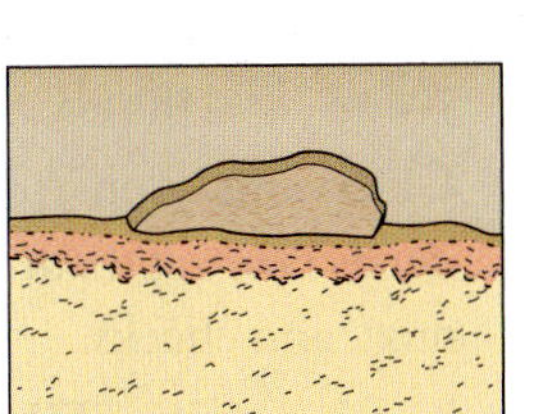

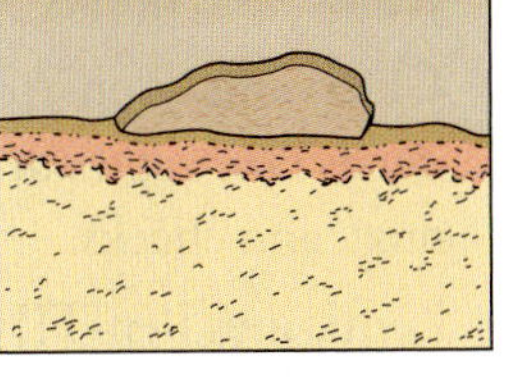

Figure 10-9 Secondary skin lesions.

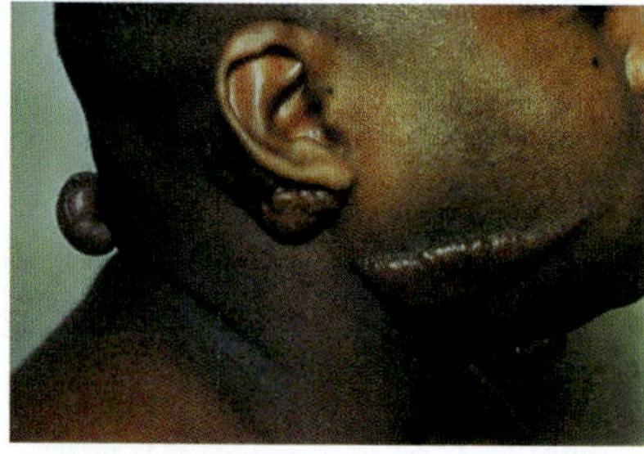

Figure 10–10 Keloids.

- **Excoriation** (ek-skor-ee-AY-shun): a skin sore produced by scratching or scraping. The skin's surface becomes raw due to the loss of superficial skin after an injury.
- **Fissure** (FISH-ur): a crack in the skin that penetrates into the dermis, such as with chapped hands or lips.
- **Keloid** (KEE-loyd): a thick scar resulting from excessive growth of fibrous tissue (Figure 10–10).
- **Scale**: any accumulation of dry or greasy flakes, such as abnormal or excessive dandruff.
- *Scar* or **cicatrix** (SIK-uh-triks): a light-colored, slightly raised mark that is formed after an injury or skin lesion has healed.

Hypertrophies of the Skin

A **hypertrophy** (hy-PUR-truh-fee) of the skin is an abnormal growth of skin tissue that is usually benign or harmless.

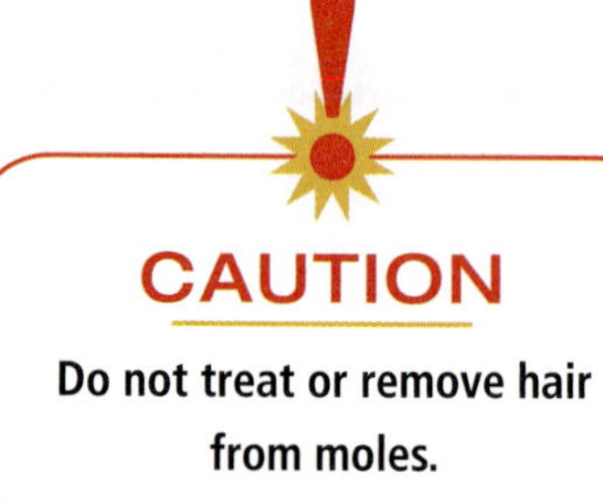

- **Keratoma** (kair-uh-TOH-muh): an acquired, superficial, thickened patch of skin commonly known as a *callus* that is caused by continued pressure or friction; frequently occurring in regions subject to friction, such as the hands and feet.
- **Mole**: a small, brownish spot or blemish on the skin ranging in color from pale tan to brown to bluish black. Some moles are small and flat, resembling freckles, while others are more deeply seated and darker in color. Large, dark hairs often grow in moles. If a mole grows in size, gets darker, or becomes sore or scaly, medical attention is needed.
- **Verruca** (vuh-ROO-kuh): the technical term for wart and a hypertrophy of the papillae and epidermis. Caused by a virus, it is infectious to the person who has one and can spread from one location to another, particularly along a scratch in the skin.

10

Pigmentations of the Skin

Pigment may be affected by internal factors within the body or by external conditions such as prolonged sun exposure. Abnormal colors are seen in every skin disease and in many systemic disorders. A change in pigmentation can be observed when certain substances and drugs are being taken internally. The following terms relate to changes in the pigmentation of the skin.

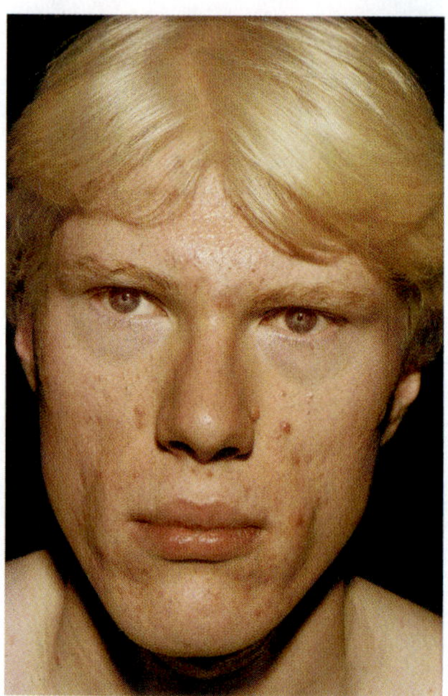

Figure 10–11 Albinism.

- **Albinism** (AL-bi-niz-em): a congenital leukoderma or absence of melanin pigments in the body, including the skin, hair, and eyes. This condition may be partial or complete. The hair is silky and white or pale yellow. The skin is pinkish-white, and will not tan (Figure 10–11).
- **Chloasma** (kloh-AZ-mah): also called *liver spots*, are caused by increased deposits of pigment in the skin. They are found mainly on the forehead, nose, and cheeks.
- **Lentigines** (len-TIJ-e-neez): the technical term for freckles. Small yellow-to-brown colored spots appearing on the skin when exposed to sunlight and air.

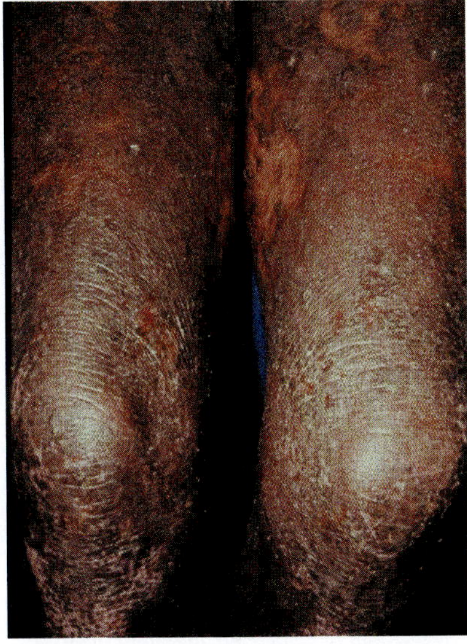

Figure 10–12 Vitiligo.

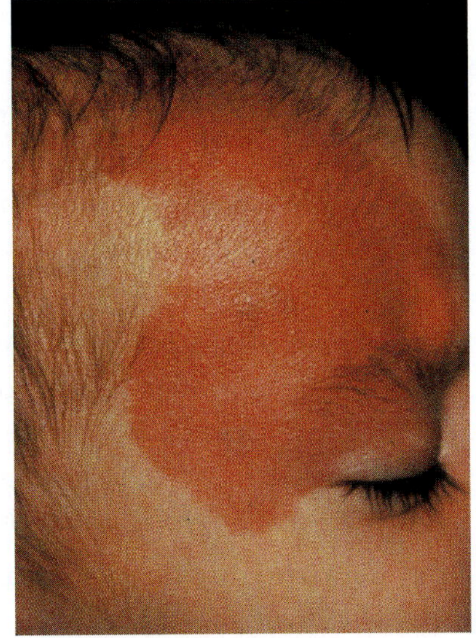

Figure 10–13 Port wine stain.

- **Leukoderma** (loo-koh-DUR-muh): a skin disorder characterized by abnormal white patches; caused by a burn or congenital pigmentation defects. It is classified as albinism and **vitiligo** (Figure 10–12).
- **Nevus** (NEE-vus): a small or large malformation of the skin due to abnormal pigmentation or dilated capillaries; commonly known as a birthmark.
- **Stain**: an abnormal brown or wine-colored skin discoloration with a generally circular and irregular shape. Its permanent color is due to the presence of darker pigment. Stains occur during aging, after certain diseases, and after the disappearance of moles, freckles, and liver spots. The cause is unknown (Figure 10–13).
- **Tan**: a change in the pigmentation of the skin caused by exposure to ultraviolet rays from the sun or from tanning lamps.

Inflammations of the Skin

- **Anthrax** (AN-thraks): an inflammatory skin disease characterized by the presence of a small, red papule, followed by the formation of a pustule, vesicle, and hard swelling. It is accompanied by itching and burning at the point of infection and is contagious. It can be spread in the barbershop through the use of an infected shaving brush.
- **Dermatitis** (dur-muh-TY-tis): the general term for an inflammatory condition of the skin. The lesions may appear in various forms, such as vesicles or papules.
- **Dermatitis venenata** (VEN-uh-nah-tuh): an eruptive skin infection that is characteristic of the abnormal conditions resulting from occasional or frequent contact with chemicals or tints. Individuals may develop allergies to certain ingredients in cosmetics, antiseptics, disinfectants, and aniline derivative tints used in the barbering profession. This occupational

Figure 10-14 Eczema.

disorder or disease may be minimized by using rubber gloves or protective creams whenever possible.

- **Eczema** (EG-zuh-muh): an inflammatory skin disease that may be acute or chronic in nature and present in many forms of dry or moist lesions. Eczema is frequently accompanied by itching or burning and all cases should be referred to a physician for treatment. Its cause is unknown (Figure 10–14).
- **Herpes simplex** (HER-peez SIM-plex): a recurring viral infection that produces fever blisters or cold sores characterized by a single vesicle or group of vesicles with red, swollen bases. The blisters usually appear on the lips, nostrils, or other part of the face, and rarely last more than a week. Herpes simplex is contagious (Figure 10–15).
- **Ivy dermatitis**: a skin inflammation caused by exposure to poison ivy, poison oak, or poison sumac leaves. Blisters and itching develop soon after contact occurs. The condition can be spread to other parts of the body by contact with contaminated hands, clothing, objects, and anything that was exposed to the plant itself. If the irritating plant oil remains on the skin, it also can be spread from one person to another by direct contact. Serious cases should be referred to a physician.
- **Psoriasis** (suh-RY-us-sis): a chronic, inflammatory skin disease characterized by dry red patches covered with coarse, silvery scales. Psoriasis usually occurs on the scalp, elbows, knees, chest, or lower back, but rarely on the face. If irritated, bleeding points occur. It is not contagious and the cause is unknown (Figure 10–16).

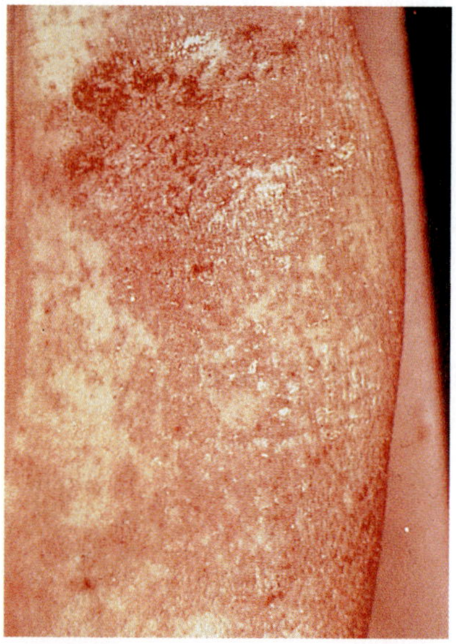

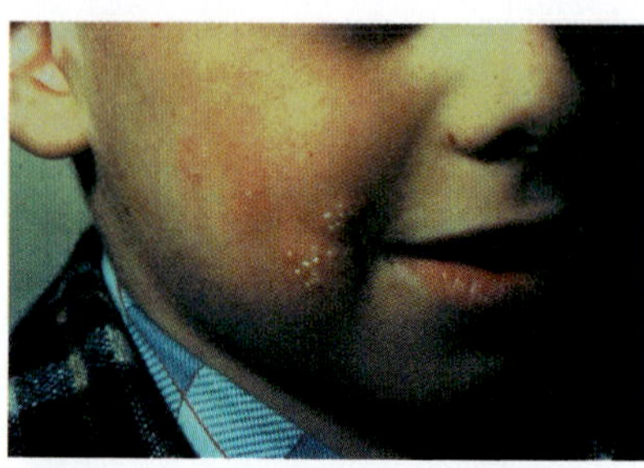

Figure 10-15 Herpes simplex.

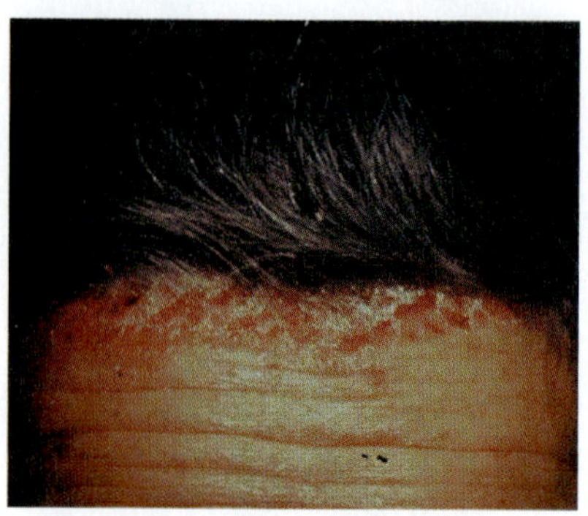

Figure 10-16 Psoriasis.

Disorders of the Sebaceous (Oil) Glands

There are several common disorders of the sebaceous glands that barbers and stylists should be able to identify and understand.

- **Acne** (AK-nee): a skin disorder characterized by chronic inflammation of the sebaceous glands from retained secretions. It occurs most frequently on the face, back, and chest. Although the cause of acne is generally held to be microbic in nature, factors such as adolescence and disturbances of the digestive tract can trigger inflammations. The two basic types of acne are acne simplex, or common pimples, and acne vulgaris, which is a more serious and deep-seated skin condition. It is always advisable to seek diagnosis and treatment by a competent physician before any facial service is given in the barbershop (Figure 10–17).
- **Asteatosis** (as-tee-ah-TOH-sis): a condition of dry, scaly skin, characterized by the absolute or partial deficiency of sebum. It can be the result of old age, exposure to cold or alkalies, or bodily disorders.
- *Comedone* (KAHM-uh-dohn) or blackhead: a mass of hardened sebum in a hair follicle, appearing most frequently on the face, forehead, and nose. The hardened sebum creates a blockage at the mouth of the follicle and should be removed only by using proper extraction procedures (Figure 10–18).

- **Milia** (MIL-ee-uh), also known as whiteheads: small, whitish masses in the epidermis, due to the retention of sebum. Milia can occur on any part of the face and neck, and occasionally on the chest and shoulders and they are often associated with dry skin types (Figure 10–19).
- **Rosacea** (roh-ZAY-shee-uh), formerly called *acne rosacea*: a chronic, inflammatory congestion of the cheeks and nose. It is characterized by redness, dilation of the blood vessels, and the formation of papules and pustules. The cause of rosacea is unknown, but certain factors are known to aggravate the condition in some individuals. These include consumption of hot liquids, spicy foods, or alcohol; being exposed to extremes of heat and cold; exposure to sunlight; and stress (Figure 10–20).
- **Seborrhea** (seb-oh-REE-ah): a skin condition due to overactivity and excessive secretion of the sebaceous glands. An itching or burning sensation may accompany it. An oily or shiny nose, forehead, or scalp indicates the presence of seborrhea. On the scalp, it is readily detected by the presence of an unusual amount of oil on the hair (Figure 10–21).
- **Steatoma** (stee-ah-TOH-muh): a sebaceous cyst or fatty tumor that is filled with sebum. It is a subcutaneous tumor of the sebaceous glands that can range in size from a pea to an orange. A steatoma usually occurs on the scalp, neck, or back and is sometimes called a *wen* (Figure 10–22).

Disorders of the Sudoriferous (Sweat) Glands

- **Anhidrosis** (an-hih-DROH-sis): lack of perspiration, often a result of fever or certain skin diseases. It requires medical attention.

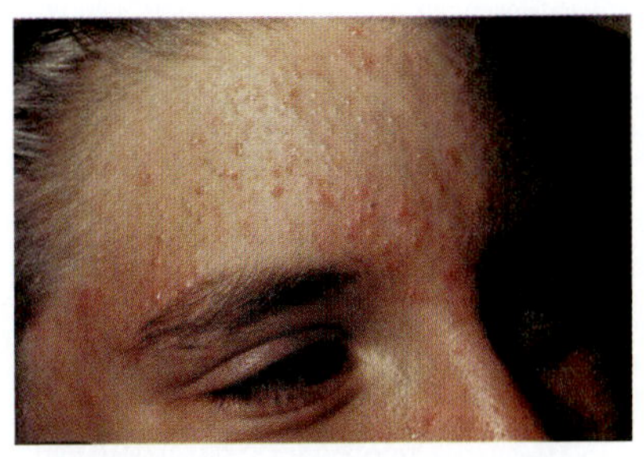

Figure 10-17 Acne.

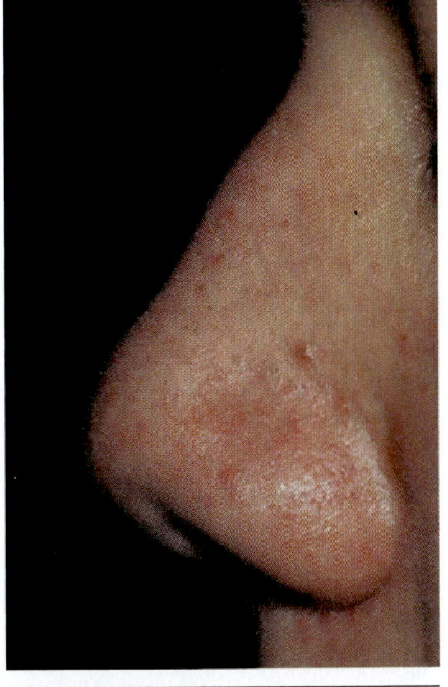

Figure 10-18 Comedones.

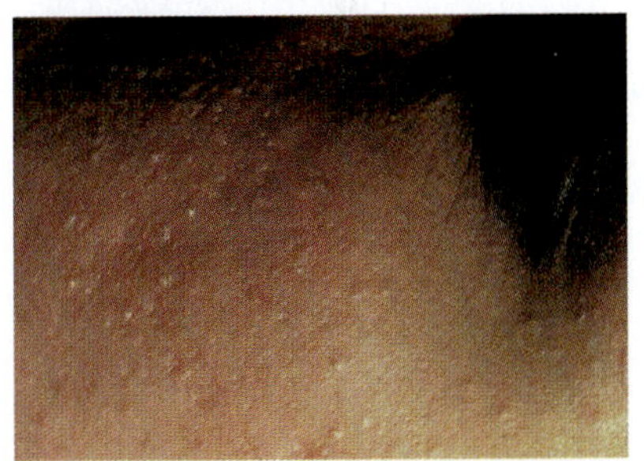

Figure 10-19 Milia.

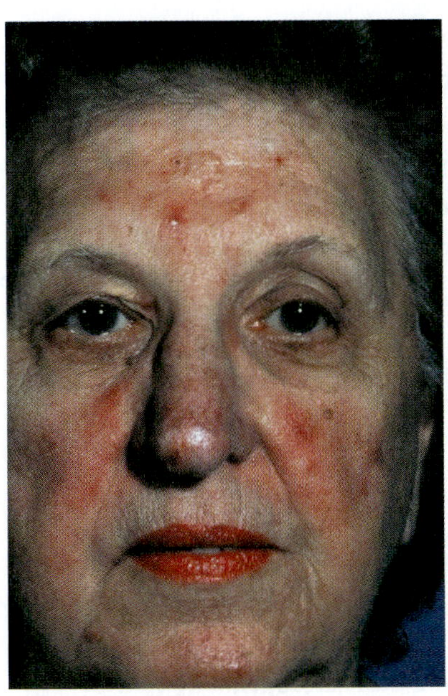

Figure 10-20 Rosacea.

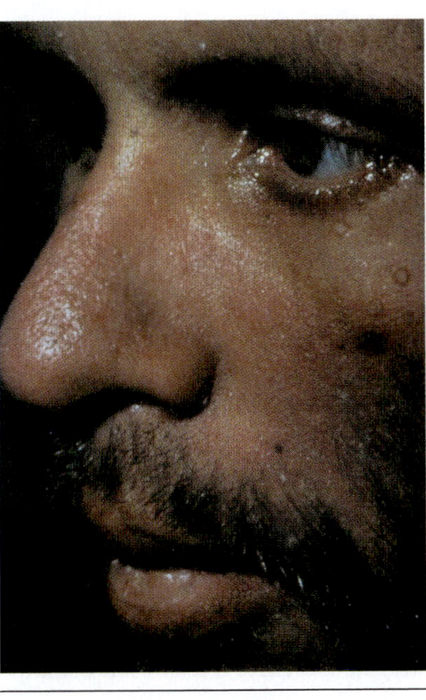

Figure 10-21 Seborrhea.

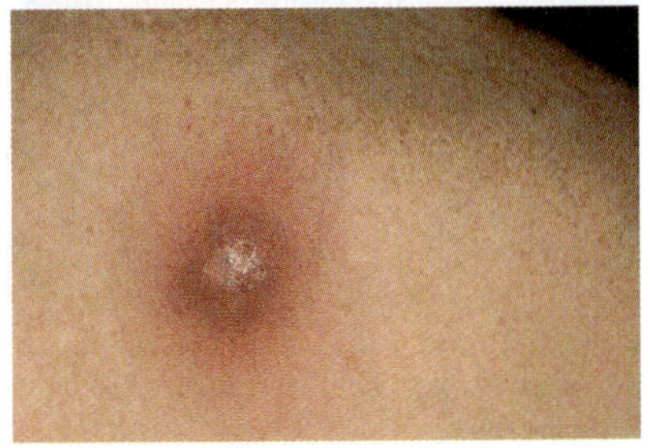

Figure 10-22 Steatoma.

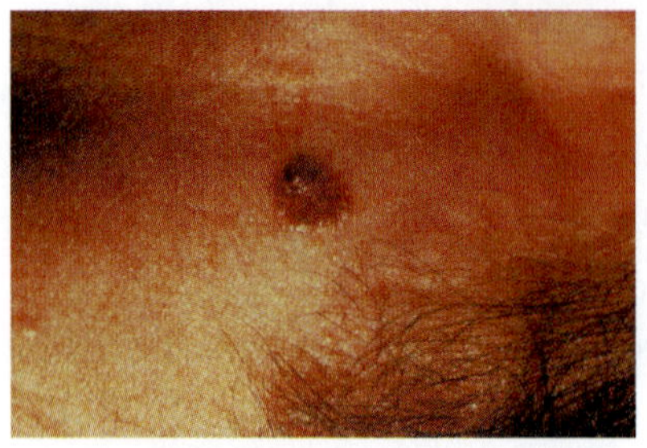

Figure 10–23 Basal cell carcinoma.

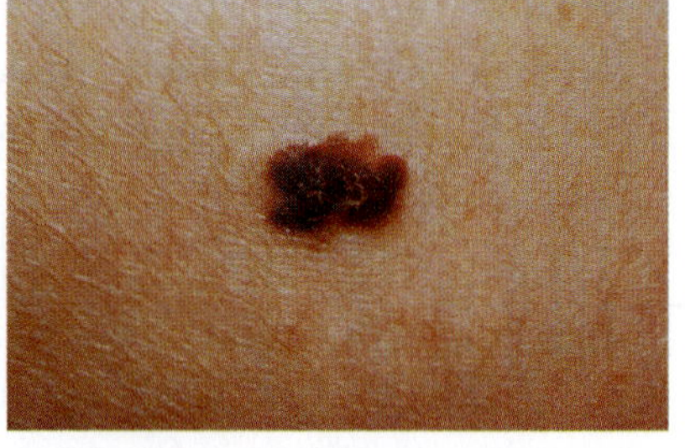

Figure 10–24 Malignant melanoma.

- **Bromhidrosis** (broh-mih-DROH-sis): refers to foul-smelling perspiration, usually noticeable in the armpits or on the feet.
- **Hyperhidrosis** (hy-per-hi-DROH-sis): excessive perspiration caused by excessive heat or general body weakness. The parts of the body most commonly affected are the armpits, joints, and feet. It requires medical treatment.
- **Miliaria rubra** (mil-ee-AIR-ee-ah ROOB rah): *prickly heat*, an acute inflammatory disorder of the sweat glands characterized by the eruption of small, red vesicles, accompanied by burning and itching of the skin. It is caused by exposure to excessive heat.

Skin Cancer

Skin cancer from overexposure to the sun comes in three distinct forms that vary in severity. Each is named for the type of body cells that it affects.

- **Basal cell carcinoma**: the most common type and the least severe skin cancer. It is often characterized by light or pearly nodules (Figure 10–23).
- **Malignant melanoma**: the most serious form of skin cancer, often characterized by dark brown or black patches on the skin. The patches may appear jagged, raised, or uneven in texture. Malignant melanomas often appear on individuals who do not receive regular sun exposure and is sometimes termed the "city person's cancer." Although the least common, malignant melanoma is the most dangerous type of skin cancer (Figure 10–24).
- **Squamous cell carcinoma**: a skin cancer that is more serious than basal cell carcinoma and is often characterized by scaly red papules or nodules (Figure 10–25).

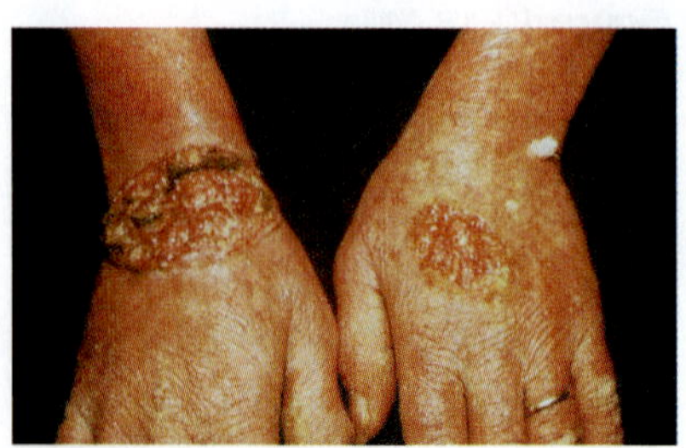

Figure 10–25 Squamous cell carcinoma.

If detected early, most cases of skin cancer respond to medical treatment. It is important for the barber or stylist to be able to recognize the appearance of serious skin disorders in order to better serve clients. Although barbers should not attempt to diagnose skin disorders, they should be aware of changes in their clients' skin so that they can sensitively suggest that the client seek the advice of a dermatologist. 3

Maintaining the Health of the Skin

Diet is the major factor involved in maintaining the skin's overall health and appearance. Proper and beneficial dietary choices help to regulate hydration, oil production, and the function of cells.

- *Foods:* Eating a well-balanced diet of the three basic food groups of fats, carbohydrates, and proteins is the best way to support the health of the skin.
- *Vitamins and supplements:* Various nutrients aid in healing, softening, and fighting diseases of the skin. Vitamin A supports the overall health of the skin, vitamin C is important to skin and tissue repair, vitamin D promotes healthy and rapid healing of the skin, and vitamin E helps to fight against the harmful effects of the sun's rays.
- *Water:* Ingesting plenty of fluids sustains the health of the cells, aids in the elimination of toxins and waste, helps to regulate the body's temperature, and aids in proper digestion.

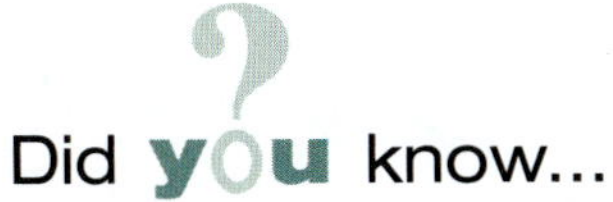

It is estimated that 75 percent of Americans are chronically dehydrated. Research suggests that the benefits of water on human health and functioning are many.

- Even mild dehydration will slow metabolism by as much as 3 percent.
- Drinking lots of water can help stop hunger pangs for many dieters.
- Lack of water is the number-one cause of daytime fatigue.
- A 2 percent drop in body water can trigger fuzzy short-term memory and trouble with basic math, and can cause difficulty focusing on a computer screen or printed page.

chapter glossary

acne	skin disorder characterized by chronic inflammation of the sebaceous glands from retained secretions
adipose tissue	also know as subcutaneous tissue; lies beneath the dermis
albinism	congenital leukoderma or absence of melanin pigment of the body
anhidrosis	deficiency or lack of perspiration
anthrax	inflammatory skin disease characterized by the presence of a small, red papule, followed by the formation of a pustule, vesicle, and hard swelling
asteatosis	condition of dry, scaly skin due to lack of sebum
basal cell carcinoma	most common and least severe type of skin cancer
bromhidrosis	foul-smelling perspiration
bulla	large blister containing a watery fluid
chloasma	nonelevated spots due to increased pigmentation in the skin
cicatrix	technical term for scar
collagen	fibrous protein that gives the skin form and strength
corium	another name for the dermis
crust	dead cells that have accumulated over a wound
cuticle	another name for the epidermis
cutis	another name for the dermis
cyst	closed, abnormally developed sac containing fluid or morbid matter, above or below the skin
derma	technical name for skin; also another name for the dermis
dermatitis	an inflammatory condition of the skin
dermatitis venenata	an eruptive skin condition due to contact with irritating substances such as tints or chemicals
dermatology	medical science that deals with the study of the skin
dermis	second or inner layer of the skin; also known as the derma, corium, cutis, or true skin
eczema	inflammatory skin condition characterized by painful itching; dry or moist lesion forms
elastin	protein base similar to collagen that forms elastic tissue
epidermis	outermost layer of the skin; also called the cuticle or scarf skin
excoriation	skin sore or abrasion caused by scratching or scraping
fissure	a crack in the skin that penetrates to the dermis

herpes simplex	fever blister or cold sore; recurring viral infection
hyperhidrosis	excessive perspiration or sweating
hypertrophy	abnormal skin growth
ivy dermatitis	a skin inflammation caused by exposure to poison ivy, poison oak, or poison sumac
keloid	thick scar resulting from excessive tissue growth
keratoma	technical name for callus, caused by pressure or friction
lentigines	technical name for freckles
lesion	a structural change in the tissues caused by injury or disease
leukoderma	skin disorder characterized by abnormal white patches
macule	spot or discoloration of the skin such as a freckle
malignant melanoma	most severe form of skin cancer
melanin	coloring matter or pigment of the skin; found in the stratum germinativum of the epidermis and in the papillary layers of the dermis
milia	technical name for a whitehead
miliaria rubra	technical name for prickly heat
mole	small brownish spot on the skin
motor nerve fibers	nerve fibers distributed to the arrector pili muscles, which are attached to the hair follicles
nevus	technical name for a birthmark
papillary layer	outer layer of the dermis, directly beneath the epidermis
papule	pimple
psoriasis	skin disease characterized by red patches and silvery-white scales
pustule	inflamed pimple, containing pus
reticular layer	deeper layer of the dermis
rosacea	chronic congestion of the skin characterized by redness, blood vessel dilation, papules, and pustules
scale	an accumulation of dry or greasy flakes on the skin
scarf skin	another name for the epidermis
sebaceous glands	oil glands of the skin connected to hair follicles
seborrhea	skin condition caused by excessive sebum secretion

sebum	an oily substance secreted by the sebaceous glands
secretory nerve fibers	regulate the excretion of perspiration from the sweat glands and the flow of sebum from the oil glands
sensory nerve fibers	react to heat, cold, touch, pressure, and pain, and send messages to the brain
squamous cell carcinoma	type of skin cancer more serious than basal cell carcinoma, but not as serious as malignant melanoma
stain	abnormal brown or wine-colored skin discoloration
steatoma	sebaceous cyst or fatty tumor
strata	plural of stratum; layers
stratum corneum	outermost layer of the epidermis; the horny layer
stratum germinativum	innermost layer of the epidermis, also known as the basal or Malpighian layer
stratum granulosum	granular layer of the epidermis beneath the stratum lucidum; grainy layer
stratum lucidum	clear layer of the epidermis, directly beneath the stratum corneum
subcutaneous tissue	fatty tissue layer that lies beneath the dermis; also called adipose tissue
sudoriferous glands	sweat glands of the skin
symptoms	signs of disease that can be felt (subjective) or seen (objective)
tan	darkening of the skin due to exposure to ultraviolet rays
true skin	another name for the dermis
tubercule	abnormal solid lump, above, within, or below the skin
tumor	abnormal cell mass resulting from excessive multiplication of cells
ulcer	open skin lesion accompanied by pus and loss of skin depth
verruca	technical name for wart
vesicle	small blister or sac containing clear fluid
vitiligo	an acquired leukoderma of the skin characterized by milky-white spots
wheal	itchy, swollen lesion caused by insect bites or plant irritations, such as nettle

chapter review questions

1. Briefly describe healthy skin.
2. Name two main divisions of the skin and describe the layers within each division.
3. Identify the appendages of the skin.
4. How is the skin nourished?
5. Name three types of nerve fibers found in the skin.
6. What determines the color of the skin?
7. Identify two types of glands found in the skin and describe their functions.
8. List the six important functions of the skin.
9. Define lesion.
10. List the primary lesions of the skin.
11. List the secondary lesions of the skin.
12. List the characteristics of the following: eczema, herpes simplex, psoriasis, and dermatitis venenata.
13. List and describe the disorders of the sebaceous glands.
14. List and describe the disorders of the sudoriferous glands.
15. Explain three ways to maintain healthy skin.

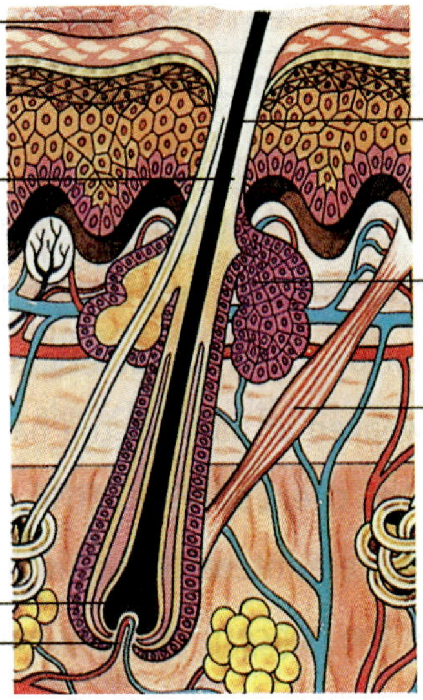

Epidermis or outer layer of the skin
Hair root
Hair follicle
Sebaceous or oil gland
Arrector pili
Hair bulb
Dermal papilla

Figure 11-1 Structures of the hair.

hair follicles are favorite breeding places for germs and the accumulation of sebum and dirt.

The follicle does not run straight down into the skin or scalp. It is set at an angle so that the hair above the surface has a natural flow to one side. This natural flow is sometimes called the *hair stream* since the hair emerges from the scalp and slants naturally in a particular direction.

The **hair bulb** is a thickened, club-shaped structure that forms the lower part of the hair root. The lower part of the hair bulb is hollow and fits over and covers the dermal papilla.

The **dermal papilla** (puh-PIL-uh) is a small, cone-shaped elevation at the base of the hair follicle that fits into the hair bulb. It consists of many tiny capillaries that are responsible for supplying oxygen and nutrients to the epidermal tissue that lines the hair follicle. Eventually, the epidermal tissue completely surrounds the papilla and forms the hair bulb. This rich blood and nerve supply is vital to the growth and regeneration of the hair, since it is through the papilla that nourishment reaches the hair bulb. As long as the papilla is healthy and well nourished, new hair will grow.

The *sebaceous glands* consist of small, saclike structures with ducts that are attached to each hair follicle. They secrete an oily substance called sebum that gives the hair luster and pliability. The overproduction of sebum can bring on a common form of oily dandruff, which, in turn, may become a contributing factor to hair loss or baldness.

Some of the factors that influence sebum production are subject to personal control. These factors are diet, blood circulation, emotional disturbance, stimulation of the endocrine glands, and certain drugs.

- *Diet* influences the general health of the hair. Overindulgence in sweet, starchy, and fatty foods may cause the sebaceous glands to become overactive and to secrete too much sebum.

- *Blood circulation* is a factor because the hair derives its nourishment from the blood supply, which in turn depends upon the foods eaten for certain elements. In the absence of necessary food elements, the health of the hair declines.
- *Emotional disturbances* are linked with the health of the hair through the nervous system. The hair's condition is affected by stress. Healthy hair is an indication of a healthy body.
- *Endocrine glands* are ductless glands. Their secretions go directly into the bloodstream, which in turn influences the welfare of the entire body. The condition of the endocrine glands influences their secretion. During adolescence, endocrine glands are very active; after middle age, their activity usually decreases. Endocrine gland disturbances influence the hair as well as other aspects of health.
- *Drugs*, such as the hormones and certain medications, may adversely affect the hair.

The **arrector pili** (ah-REK-tor PY-ly) is a minute, involuntary muscle fiber in the skin attached to the underside and base of the hair follicle. Fear or cold causes it to contract, which makes the hair stand up straight, resulting in "goose bumps." Eyelash and eyebrow hairs lack arrector pili muscles. 1

Structures of the Hair Shaft

The three main layers of the hair shaft are the cuticle, cortex, and medulla (Figure 11–2).

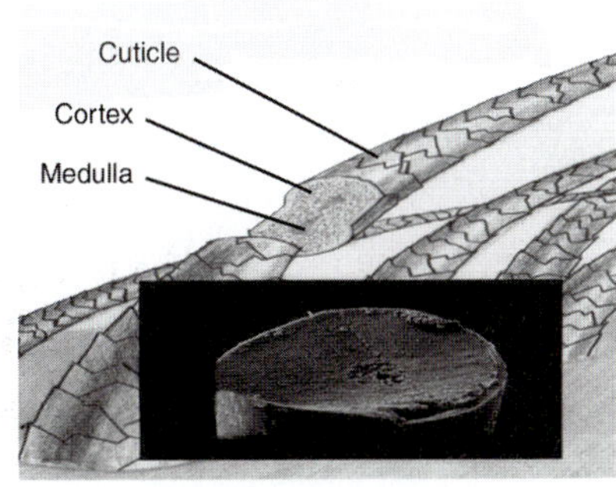

Figure 11-2 Cross section of hair.

The term **cuticle** is also used to identify the outermost layer of hair and should not be confused with the cuticle of the skin. The cuticle of the hair consists of a single overlapping layer of transparent, scalelike cells that point away from the scalp toward the hair ends. A healthy, compact cuticle layer is the hair's primary defense against damage. Conversely, certain chemical solutions soften and raise these scales to allow for absorption into the cortex.

A lengthwise cross section of hair shows that although the cuticle scales overlap, each individual cuticle scale is attached to the cortex (Figure 11–3). However, it is important to note that the hair has only one cuticle layer. Swelling the hair raises the cuticle layer and opens the spaces between the scales, which allows liquids to penetrate. If there were more than one cuticle layer stacked upon each other, solutions would not be able to penetrate the hair. Oxidation tints, permanent waving solutions, and chemical hair relaxers must have an alkaline pH in order to penetrate the cuticle layer to reach the chemical structure within the cortex.

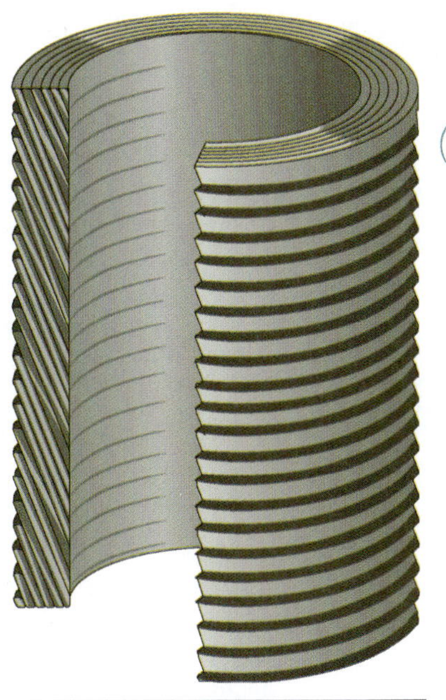
Figure 11-3 The cuticle layer.

The **cortex** is the middle layer of the hair. It is a fibrous protein core formed by elongated cells that contain melanin pigment. About 90 percent of the total weight of the hair comes from the cortex. Its unique protein structure provides strength, elasticity, and natural color to the hair. The changes that take place in the hair during chemical services occur within the cortex.

The **medulla** is the innermost layer and is sometimes referred to as the *pith* or *marrow* of the hair. It is composed of round cells. Although mature male beard hair contains a medulla, this layer of the hair may be absent in very fine and naturally blond hair. 2

The Chemical Composition of Hair

Hair is composed of protein that grows from cells that originate within the hair follicle. This is where the hair shaft begins. When these living cells form they begin a journey upward through the follicle, where they mature through a process called keratinization. As the newly formed cells mature, they fill up with a fibrous protein called **keratin**, move upward, lose their nucleus, and die. By the time the hair shaft emerges from the scalp, the cells are completely keratinized and no longer living. The hair shaft that we see is a nonliving fiber composed of keratinized protein.

Hair is approximately 91 percent protein. The protein is made up of long chains of amino acids, which are made up of elements. The elements found in human hair are carbon, oxygen, hydrogen, nitrogen, and sulfur. These five elements, often referred to as the COHNS elements because of their scientific abbreviations, are also found in skin and nails. As illustrated in Table 11–1, the chemical composition of average hair is 51 percent carbon, 21 percent oxygen, 6 percent hydrogen, 17 percent nitrogen, and 5 percent sulfur. The chemical composition varies with color. Light hair contains less carbon and hydrogen and more oxygen and sulfur. Conversely, dark hair has more carbon and less oxygen and sulfur.

The Nature of Hair Protein

Hair is a complex structure that varies greatly from one person to another. The diameter, elasticity, and configuration of the bonds of each strand all help to determine what the keratinized protein we call hair will look and

Element	Percentage in Normal Hair
Carbon	51%
Oxygen	21%
Hydrogen	6%
Nitrogen	17%
Sulfur	5%

Table 11–1 The COHNS Elements

feel like. Although there are many variations, all hair types have certain common factors that include proteins, amino acids, polypeptide chains, and bonds.

Proteins are essential organic compounds necessary for life, and hair is approximately 91 percent protein. Proteins are made of long chains of chemical units known as **amino acids**. Each amino acid is joined end-to-end in a definite order by chemical bonds known as **peptide bonds** or **end bonds** (Figure 11–4).

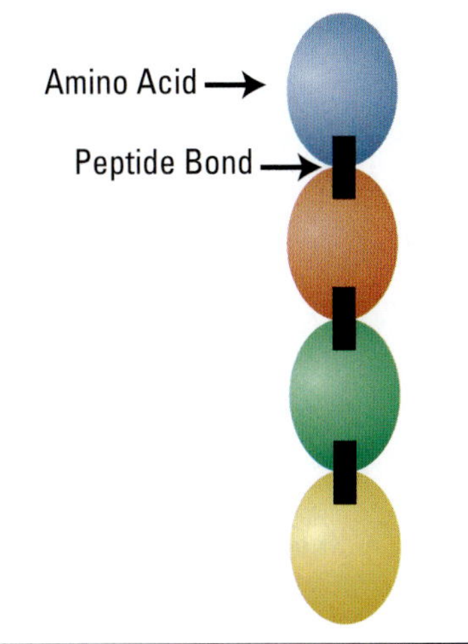

Figure 11-4 Amino acids joined by peptide bonds.

The peptide bonds are the strongest chemical bonds in the cortex as they join each amino acid to form the polypeptide chain. Most of the strength and elasticity of the hair is attributed to these chemical bonds. When even a few bonds are broken through overstretching or the use of strong acidic or alkaline solutions, the hair can become weakened or damaged to the point of breakage. Once the end bonds are broken, there is no way of re-forming them. This is just one reason why barbers need to be aware of the potential damage that rough treatment or chemical overprocessing can have on the structure of the hair.

A long chain of amino acids joined by peptide bonds is called a *polypeptide* or **polypeptide chain**. The polypeptide chains intertwine around each other to create a coil or spiral of protein called a *helix* (Figure 11–5).

Cross Bonds of the Hair Cortex

Within the hair cortex, a more complex structure is formed when millions of polypeptide chains are cross-linked by three types of *side* or **cross bonds** to form a ladderlike structure (Figure 11–6). The cross bonds consist of hydrogen, salt, and disulfide bonds, which account for the strength and elasticity of human hair. They are also essential to blow-drying and wet sets, thermal styling, and chemical processes. Table 11–2 summarizes the properties of the three types of side bonds as well as the peptide bond.

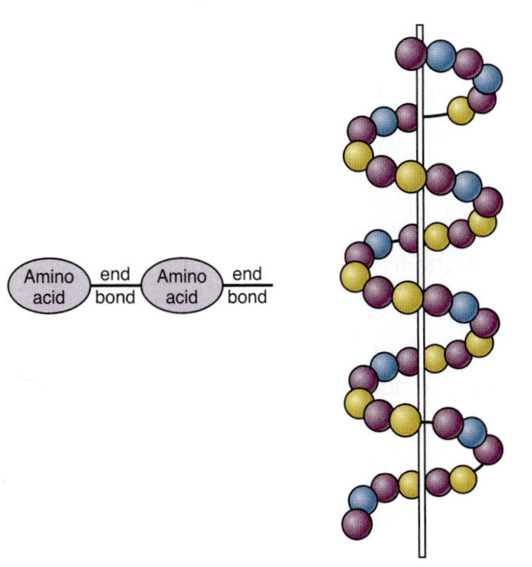

Figure 11-5 A polypeptide chain.

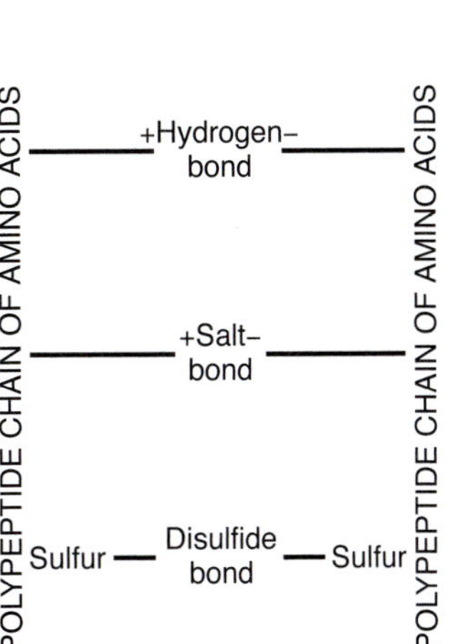

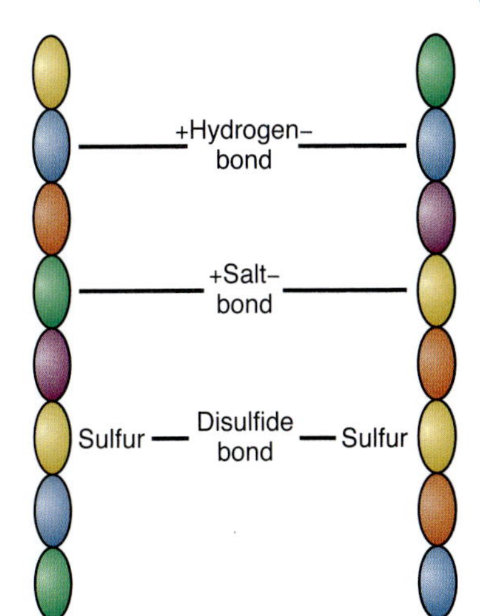

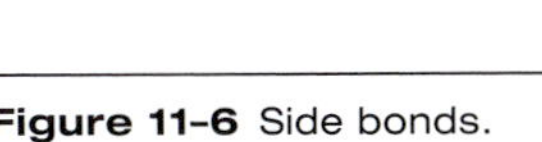

Figure 11-6 Side bonds.

Bond	Type	Strength	Broken By	Re-formed By
hydrogen	side bond	weak physical	water or heat	drying or cooling
salt	side bond	weak physical	changes in pH	normalizing pH
disulfide	side bond	strong chemical	1. thio perms and thio relaxers 2. hydroxide relaxers	1. oxidation with neutralizer 2. converted to lanthionine bonds
peptide	end bond	strong chemical	chemical depilatories	not re-formed; hair dissolves

Table 11-2 Bonds of the Hair

A **hydrogen bond** is a special type of ionic cross bond that is easily broken by water or heat. Although individual hydrogen bonds are weak, they are so numerous in the hair that they account for about one-third of the hair's overall strength.

Hydrogen bonds add body to the hair and also help to keep the parallel chains of polypeptides together. The physical breaking of the hydrogen bonds when shampooing and rinsing causes the cuticle to swell. When the hair is set on rollers, the cortex shrinks into a new position as it dries around the rollers. This is also true of blow-drying techniques when the barber works with a comb or brush to style the hair into place while drying. Since hydrogen bonds reflect physical change in the hair fiber, they are also referred to as physical bonds or H-bonds. Water, dilute alkali, neutral, and acid solutions will break hydrogen bonds. Drying and dilute acids will reform them.

A **salt bond** is also a physical cross bond, but it reacts to changes in pH. Salt bonds depend on pH and account for another one-third of the hair's total strength. These bonds are easily broken by strong acidic or alkaline solutions.

A **disulfide** (dy-SUL-fyd) **bond**, also known as a *sulfur bond*, is a covalent bond, which is different from the ionic bonding found with hydrogen or salt bonds. Disulfide bonds join the sulfur atoms of two neighboring cysteine amino acids to create cystine. Although there are fewer disulfide bonds in the hair, they are stronger than hydrogen or salt bonds and account for a third of the hair's total strength.

Unlike hydrogen and salt bonds, disulfide bonds are not broken by heat or water. Because the disulfide bonds create chemical cross bonds between the polypeptide chains, chemical solutions are required to change or restructure them. Ammonium thioglycolate permanent waves break disulfide bonds, which are then re-formed with neutralizers. Sodium hydroxide chemical hair relaxers also break disulfide bonds, which are converted to lanthionine bonds when the relaxer is rinsed from the hair. Disulfide bonds broken by hydroxide relaxers are permanently broken and cannot be re-formed. The more disulfide bonds in the hair, the more resistant it will be to chemical processes. Disulfide or sulfur bonds are also known as S-bonds and may be referred to as cystine bonds.

Hair Pigment

Natural hair color is the result of the *melanin* pigment found within the cortex. There are two different types of melanin: eumelanin and pheomelanin.

Eumelanin (yoo-MEL-uh-nin) provides brown and black color to hair. **Pheomelanin** (fee-oh-MEL-uh-nin) provides natural hair colors that range from red and ginger to yellow and light blond tones. All natural color is dependent on the ratio of eumelanin to pheomelanin, along with the total number and size of the pigment granules.

The number of hairs on the head varies with the color of the hair. The approximate amounts for different hair colors are: blond, 140,000; brown, 110,000; black, 108,000; and red, 90,000.

Wave Pattern

The **wave pattern** of the hair refers to the amount of movement in the hair strand and is described as straight, wavy, curly, and coiled (Figure 11–7). Although an individual's particular wave pattern is the result of genetics and racial background, the four wave patterns can be found in each racial or ethnic group.

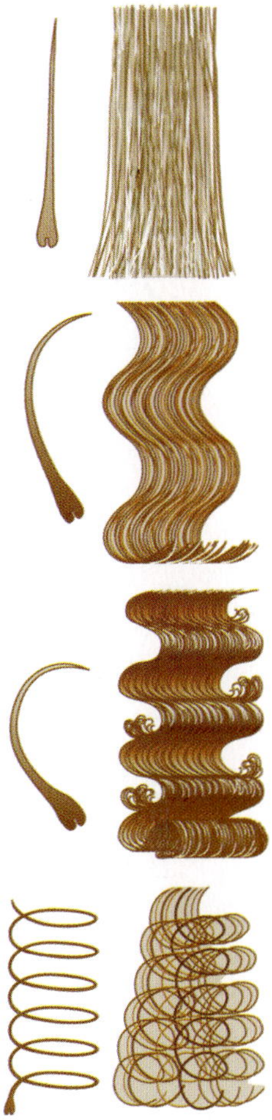

Figure 11–7 Straight, wavy, curly, and coiled strands.

Generally speaking, hair has one of three shapes. As hair grows out it may assume the shape, size, and direction of the follicle, although there is no strict rule regarding cross-sectional shapes of hair. Wavy, straight, or curly hair has been found in all shapes. A cross-sectional view of hair under the microscope reveals that straight hair is usually round, wavy hair is usually oval, and extremely curly hair is usually almost flat.

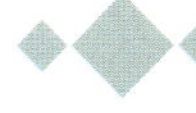

HAIR GROWTH

Hair is found all over the body except on the palms, soles, lips, and eyelids. There are three main types of hair on the body: vellus or lanugo hairs, primary terminal hair (Figure 11–8), and secondary terminal hair.

1. **Vellus** or **lanugo** hair is the short, fine, and soft downy hair found on cheeks, forehead, and nearly all areas of the body. It helps in the efficient evaporation of perspiration.
2. **Primary terminal hair** is the short, thick hairs that grow on the eyebrows and eyelashes. Eyebrows divert sweat from the eyes and eyelashes help protect the eyes from foreign bodies and light.

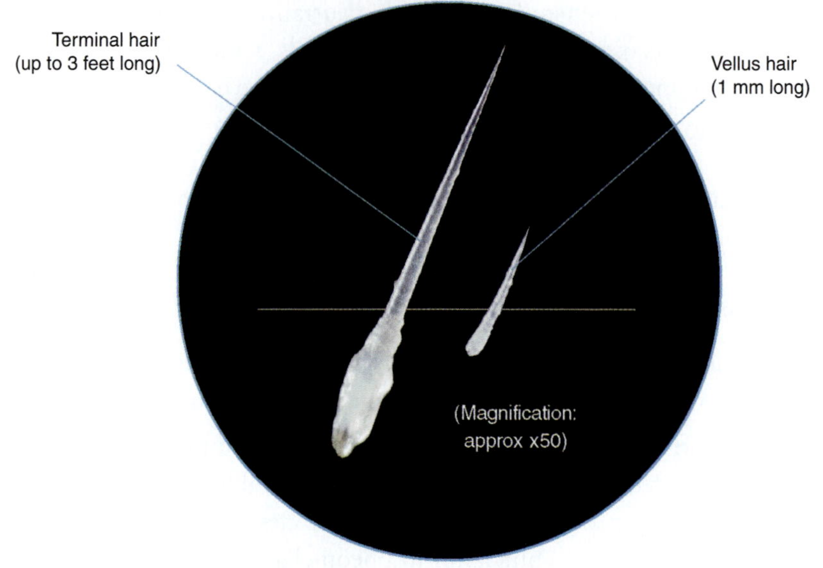

Figure 11-8 Terminal and vellus hair.

3. **Secondary terminal hair** is the long hair found on the scalp, beard, chest, back, and legs.

The average growth of healthy hair on the scalp is about one-half inch per month. The rate of growth will differ on specific parts of the body, between sexes, among races, and with age. The growth of scalp hair occurs more rapidly between the ages of 15 and 30, and declines sharply between 50 and 60. Hair growth is also influenced by such factors as the seasons of the year, nutrition, and hormonal changes within the body. Temporary climatic conditions will also affect the hair: moisture in the air will deepen the natural wave, cold air causes the hair cuticle to contract, and heat will cause the hair to swell or expand, and absorb moisture.

Hair growth is not increased by shaving, trimming, cutting, or singeing, or by the application of ointments or oils. Oils act as lubricants to the hair shaft, but do not feed the hair.

Normal Hair Shedding

It is normal to lose an average of 75 to 100 hairs per day. This shedding process makes room for new hair that is in the process of growing. Hair loss beyond this estimated average indicates some problem. Eyebrow hairs and eyelashes are replaced every four to five months.

Growth Patterns

It is important when cutting and styling hair to consider the hair's natural growth patterns. Doing so will produce a more natural-looking haircut and a style that the client will have less trouble duplicating for everyday wear. Growth patterns result in hair streams, whorls, and cowlicks.

- A **hair stream** is hair that flows in the same direction. It is the result of follicles being arranged and sloping in a uniform manner. When two such streams slope in opposite directions, they form a natural part in the hair.

- A **whorl** is hair that forms in a circular or swirl pattern. Whorls are most often seen at the crown.
- A **cowlick** is a tuft of hair that stands straight up. Cowlicks are usually more noticeable at the front hairline, but they may be located anywhere on the scalp. Styles should be chosen to minimize their upright effects.

The Growth Cycles of Hair

In normal and healthy hair, each individual strand goes through a cycle of events: growth, fall, and replacement. These three phases are known as the anagen, catagen, and telogen phases (Figure 11–9).

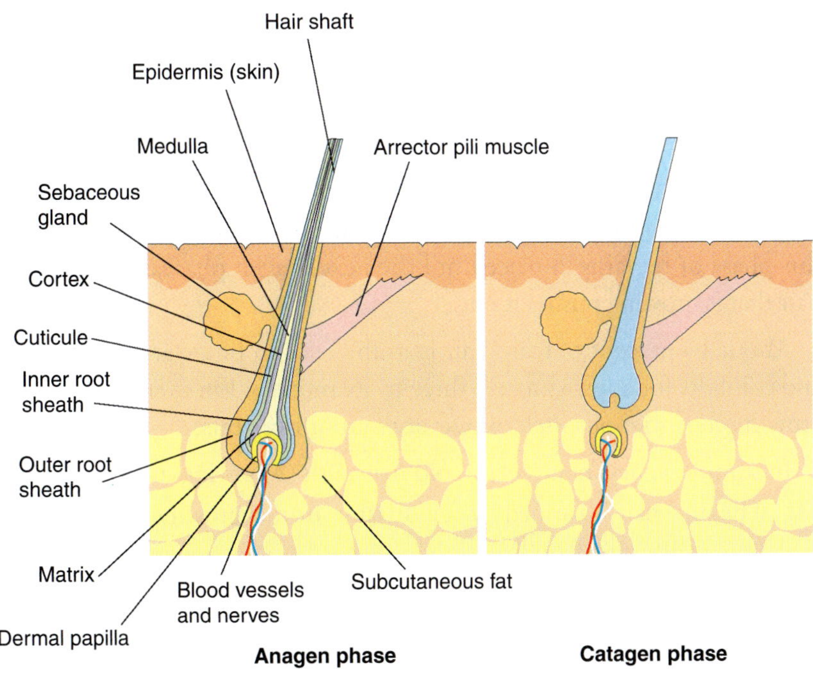

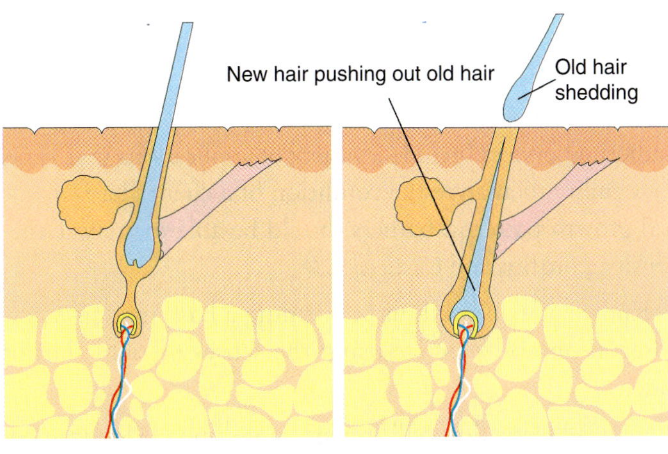

Figure 11-9 Cycles of hair growth.

Anagen: The Growth Phase

During the **anagen** (AN-uh-jen) or growth **phase**, new hair is produced. The stem cells actively manufacture new keratinized cells in the hair follicle. About 90 percent of scalp hair is growing in the anagen phase at any one time and this generally lasts from three to five years.

Catagen: The Transition Phase

The **catagen** (KAT-uh-jen) **phase** is a transition period between the growth and resting phases of a hair strand. During this phase the follicle shrinks, the hair bulb disappears, and the shrunken root end forms a rounded club. Also during the catagen phase, the follicle is preparing for new growth by making germ cells. They surround the club and await the signal to renew the anagen phase. Lasting from one to three weeks, less than 1 percent of the hair is in the catagen phase at any one time.

Telogen: The Resting Phase

The **telogen** (TEL-uh-jen) or resting **phase** is the final phase of the hair cycle, lasting until the fully grown hair is shed. The hair is either shed during this phase or remains in place until the next anagen phase, when the new hair that is growing pushes it out.

About 10 percent of scalp hair is in the telogen phase at any one time, and this lasts for approximately three to six months. On average, the entire growth process repeats itself once every four or five years.

In summary, new hair replaces old hair in the following ways:

1. The new hair is formed by cell division from a growing point at the root around the papilla.
2. The bulb loosens and separates from the papilla.
3. The bulb moves upward in the follicle.
4. The hair moves slowly to the surface, where it is shed.

HAIR ANALYSIS

Barbering services include a variety of applications that benefit from a barber's ability to analyze the condition of a client's hair. In addition to wave and growth patterns, barbers should be able to analyze the hair's texture, density, porosity, and elasticity.

Knowledge and skill in performing a hair analysis can be acquired by observation and practice using the senses of sight, hearing, smell, and touch.

- *Sight.* Observation will impart some knowledge immediately, such as whether the hair looks dry or oily. Sight alone, however, will not provide an accurate judgment of hair's quality. The sense of sight comprises approximately 15 percent of the process of hair analysis.

- *Hearing.* Some clients will volunteer information about their hair, health problems, or experiences with products and medications. Since all of these factors are important when deciding how to treat the hair, it is advisable to listen carefully.
- *Smell.* Certain scalp disorders will create an odor. If the client is in general good health and the scalp is clean, the hair should be odor-free.
- *Touch.* The sense of touch is key to analyzing hair condition and texture. Without developing this sense to its fullest capacity, the barber cannot provide truly professional services.

Hair Texture

Hair texture refers to the degree of coarseness or fineness of individual hair strands, which may vary on different parts of the head. Hair texture is measured by the diameter of the hair strand and is classified as coarse, medium, or fine.

Coarse hair has the largest diameter and tends to be stronger than fine hair. It also has a stronger structure that may require more processing or stronger products than medium or fine hair during chemical services. Generally, it is more difficult for hair lighteners, haircolors, waving solutions, and relaxing creams to penetrate coarse hair.

Medium hair texture is the most common and is the standard to which other hair is compared. Medium hair is considered normal and does not usually pose any special problems or concerns.

Fine hair has the smallest diameter and is generally more fragile, easier to process, and more susceptible to damage from chemical services than is coarse or medium hair. Some fine or very fine hair does not possess a medulla, which helps to account for a smaller diameter of the strand.

Wiry hair, whether coarse, medium, or fine, has a hard, glassy finish because the cuticle scales lie flat against the hair shaft. It usually takes longer to give this type of hair a chemical service.

Hair texture can be determined by feeling a single strand of dry hair between the fingers. Hold the strand securely with one hand while rolling it between the thumb and forefinger of the other hand. With practice, you will be able to feel the difference between coarse, medium, and fine hair textures.

Hair Density

Hair density measures the amount of individual hair strands per square inch of scalp area. It can be classified as thick, average, or thin; or, high, medium, and low density. Hair density is different from hair texture in that individuals with the same hair texture can have different densities or different amounts of hair per square inch.

The average hair density is approximately 2,200 per square inch, with the average head of hair containing about 100,000 individual strands. The number of hairs on the head varies with the color of the hair—blonds usually have the highest density and redheads the least density per square inch.

Hair Porosity

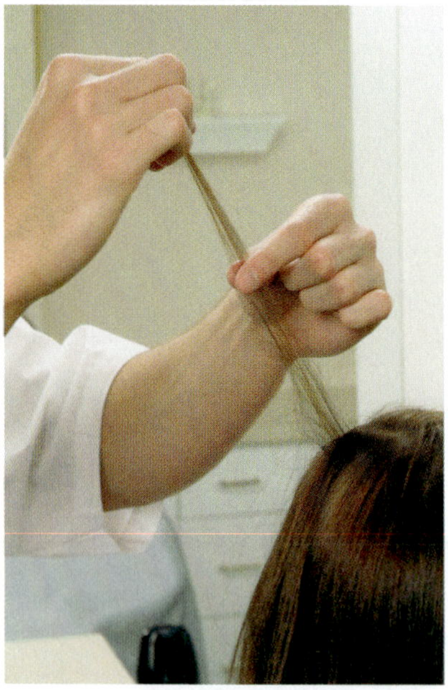

Hair porosity is the ability of the hair to absorb moisture. The degree of porosity is directly related to the condition of the cuticle layer of the hair. A compact cuticle layer is naturally more resistant to penetration, whereas porous hair has a raised cuticle layer that easily absorbs water. The porosity level of hair can be classified as moderate, poor, and porous; or, average, low, and high porosity.

Hair that has moderate or average porosity is considered normal. This hair type presents no special problems and chemical applications usually process as expected.

Hair with a high porosity level is considered overly porous and is usually the result of previous overprocessing. Hair in this condition absorbs liquids quickly and requires special care.

Hair that is classified as having poor or low porosity is considered resistant. This hair type absorbs the least amount of moisture and may require a more alkaline solution than other hair types.

Figure 11-10 Testing for hair porosity.

The porosity of the hair can be checked by holding multiple strands of dry hair between the fingers while sliding the thumb and forefinger of the other hand down toward the scalp (Figure 11–10). If the hair feels smooth and the cuticle is compact, it is considered resistant. If you can feel a slight roughness or the imbrications of the cuticle scales, the hair is porous. Should the hair break or feel very rough, the hair is probably overporous.

Hair Elasticity

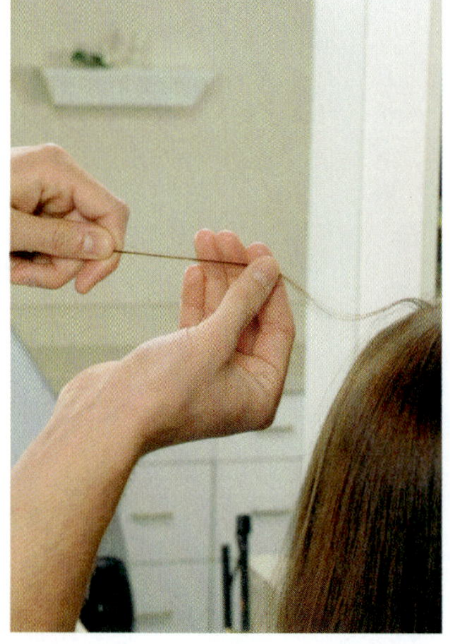

Figure 11-11 Testing for hair elasticity.

Hair elasticity is the ability of the hair to stretch and return to its original length without breaking. Hair with normal elasticity is springy and has a live and lustrous appearance. Wet hair with normal elasticity, especially curly or wavy hair, will stretch up to 50 percent of its original length and return to that length without breaking. Test for hair elasticity by gently tugging a few strands of hair as shown in Figure 11–11.

Hair elasticity is an indication of the strength of the cross bonds in the hair. Hair with normal elasticity tends to hold the curl from sets and permanent waves without excessive relaxing of the curl. Hair with low or poor elasticity is brittle and breaks easily. Hair in this condition may have been overprocessed during previous chemical applications or may be the result of poor nutrition or internal disorders.

HAIR LOSS

As previously discussed, we all lose some hair every day as a result of the normal shedding that takes place during the hair's natural growth and replacement cycle. Over 63 million people in the United States suffer from **alopecia** (al-oh-PEE-shah), the technical term for any abnormal hair loss.

Although the medical community does not recognize hair loss as a medical condition, many individuals who have a hair loss condition feel an anguish that is all too real and often overlooked. A study that investigated the perceptions of bald and balding men, compared to men who had hair, revealed that bald men were perceived as:

- less physically attractive (by both sexes).
- less assertive.
- less successful.
- less personally likeable.
- older.

The perceptions that bald men had of themselves, as compared to those with moderate hair loss, revealed that they:

- experience more negative and emotional effects.
- are more preoccupied with their baldness.
- make some effort to conceal or compensate for their hair loss.

For women, abnormal hair loss is particularly devastating. Studies indicate that women usually have a greater *emotional* investment in their appearance than men; therefore conditions of alopecia can be very traumatic. Most women with abnormal hair loss felt anxious, helpless, and less attractive.

Types of Abnormal Hair Loss

Alopecia may appear in different forms as a result of a variety of abnormal conditions. These forms include androgenic alopecia, alopecia areata, alopecia senilis, and alopecia syphilitica.

Androgenic Alopecia

11

Androgenic (an-druh-JEN-ik) **alopecia** is hair loss that occurs as a result of genetics, age, and hormonal changes that cause the miniaturization of terminal hair, converting it to vellus hair (Figure 11–12). Androgenic alopecia can begin as early as the teens (**alopecia prematura**) and is frequently seen by the age of 40. Almost 40 percent of men and women show some degree of hair loss by age 35.

In men, androgenic alopecia is known as male pattern baldness, which usually progresses to the familiar horseshoe-shaped pattern or fringe of hair (Figure 11–13). In women, it shows up as a generalized thinning in the crown area.

Alopecia Areata

Alopecia areata (air-ee-AH-tah) is characterized by the sudden falling out of hair in round patches that create bald spots. It is a highly unpredictable

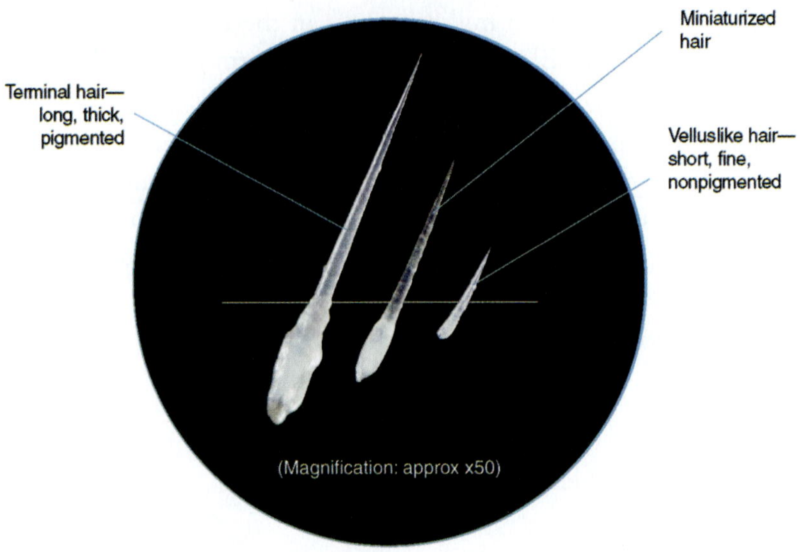

Terminal hair—
long, thick,
pigmented
Miniaturized
hair
Velluslike hair—
short, fine,
nonpigmented
(Magnification: approx x50)

Figure 11-12 Miniaturization of the hair follicle.

GRADUAL LOSS OF HAIR
1
2
3
4
5
6
7
8

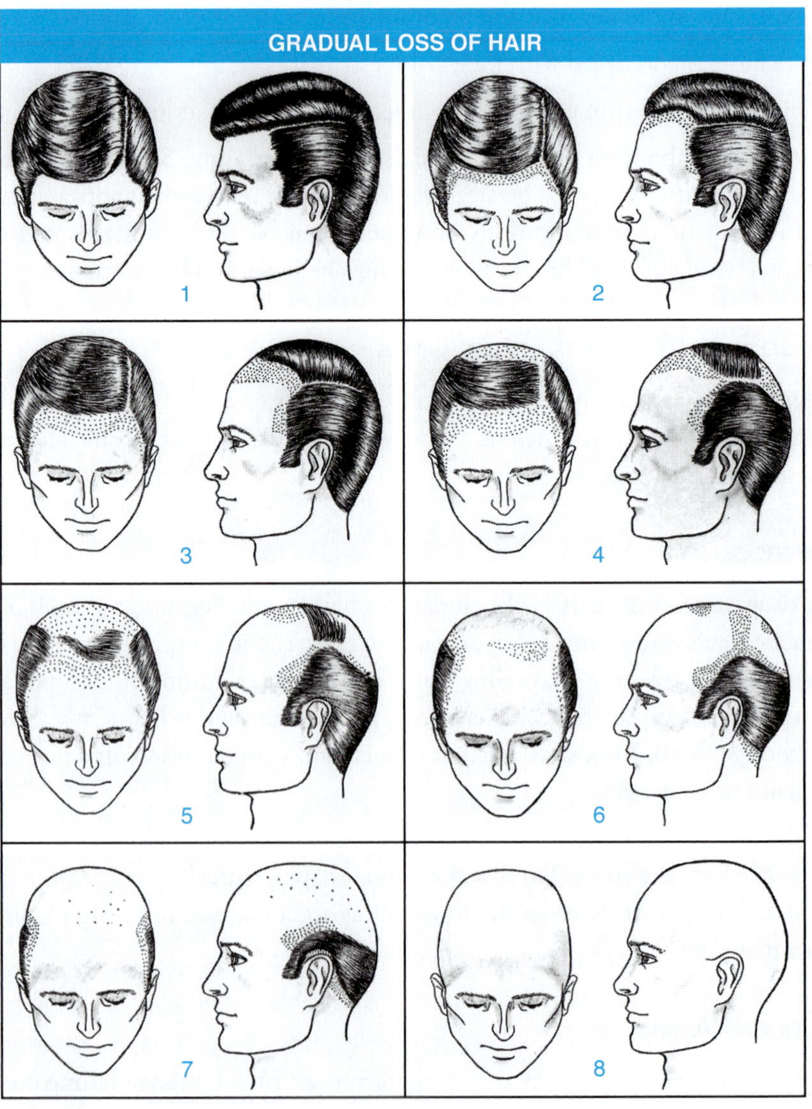

Figure 11-13 Gradual balding process.

skin disease that may occur on the scalp and elsewhere on the body (Figure 11–14).

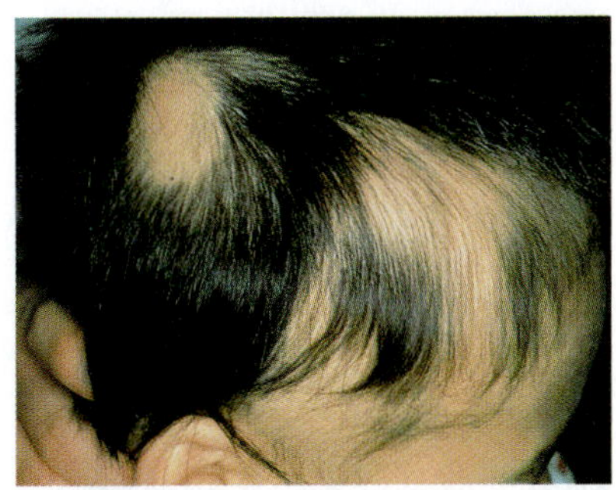

Figure 11-14 Alopecia areata.

Due to certain similarities with other autoimmune disorders, it is suggested that alopecia areata is an autoimmune disease. Alopecia areata causes the affected hair follicles to be attacked by the person's own immune system, as white blood cells stop hair growth during the anagen phase. The hair loss usually begins with one or more small, round, smooth bald patches on the scalp that can progress to total scalp hair loss (alopecia totalis) or complete body hair loss (alopecia universalis). Although hair regrowth may occur within a year, the new growth may or may not be permanent.

There have been cases where a form of temporary alopecia areata has occurred as a result of anemia, scarlet fever, typhoid fever, nervous conditions, or malnutrition. Clients who exhibit symptoms of alopecia areata should be referred to a physician.

Alopecia Senilis

Alopecia senilis is the normal loss of scalp hair occurring in old age. The loss of hair is permanent.

Alopecia Syphilitica

Alopecia syphilitica is caused by syphilis. The non-inflamed bald areas look molted or moth-eaten and may also affect the beard and eyebrow areas. The hair usually grows back. 6

Hair Loss Treatments

The only two hair loss treatments that have been proven to stimulate hair growth and that are approved by the FDA are minoxidil and finasteride.

Minoxidil is a topical treatment that is applied to the scalp twice a day. It is sold over the counter as a nonprescription drug and is available for both men and women. It is available in two different strengths, 2 percent regular and 5 percent extra strength, and is not known to have any negative side effects.

Finasteride is an oral prescription medication for men only. Although it is considered more effective and convenient than minoxidil, its possible side effects include weight gain and loss of sexual function.

In addition to the medicinal treatments described above, there are also several surgical options available. Transplants, or hair plugs, are probably the most common permanent hair replacement technique. The process consists of removing small sections of hair that include the follicle, papilla, and bulb from areas of thick hair growth, and transplanting them into the bald area. Only licensed surgeons may perform this procedure and several surgeries are usually necessary to achieve the desired results. The cost of each surgery ranges from about $8,000 to over $20,000.

Barbers and stylists can offer other nonmedical or nonsurgical options to their clients. These include wigs, toupees, hair weaving, and hair extensions (see Chapter 16).

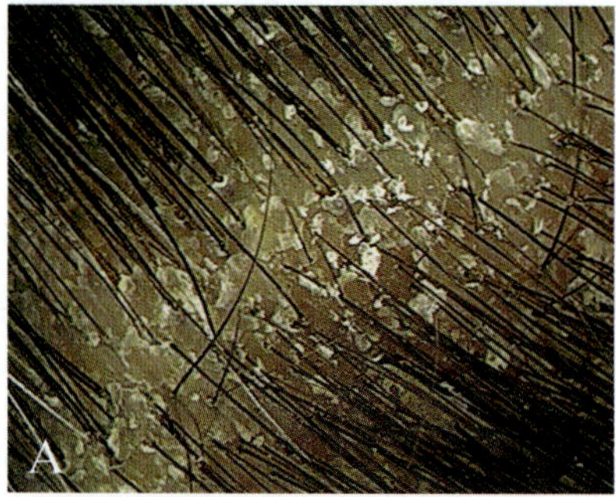

Figure 11-15a Pityriasis capitis simplex. Photo courtesy of P & G. Beauty.

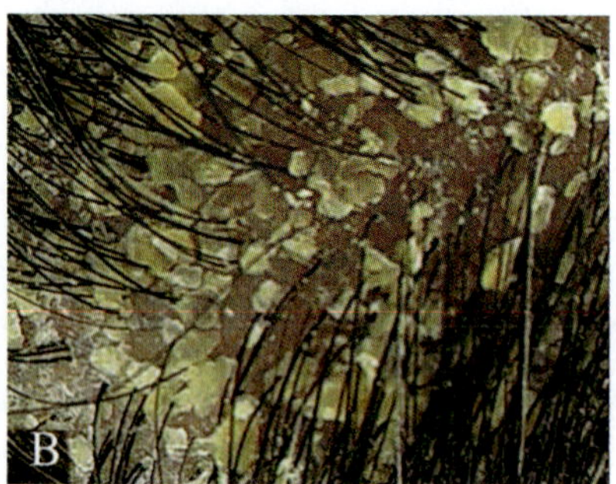

Figure 11-15b Pityriasis steatoides. Photo courtesy of P & G. Beauty.

DISORDERS OF THE SCALP

The common disorders of the scalp include dandruff, vegetable parasitic infections (tinea), animal parasitic infections, and staphylococci infections.

Dandruff

Dandruff is the presence of small, white scales that usually appear on the scalp and hair. The medical term for dandruff is pityriasis (pit-ih-RY-uh-sus). Just as the skin on other parts of the body is continually being shed and replaced, the uppermost layer of the scalp goes through the same process. Skin cells in the outer layer of the scalp flake off and are replaced by new cells from below. Ordinarily, these scales loosen and fall off freely so the natural shedding of the scalp's dead scales should not be mistaken for dandruff.

Dandruff is characterized by the excessive production, shedding, and accumulation of surface cells. Instead of growing to the surface and falling off, these horny scales accumulate on the scalp. A sluggish scalp due to poor circulation, infection, injury, improper diet or poor personal hygiene can contribute to this accumulation, as does the use of strong shampoos and/or insufficient rinsing of the hair.

The two principal types of dandruff are pityriasis capitis simplex and pityriasis steatoides.

- **Pityriasis capitis simplex** is the technical term for classic dandruff characterized by scalp irritation, large flakes, and an itchy scalp (Figure 11–15a). The scales may be attached to the scalp in masses or scattered loosely throughout the hair. Treatments include the use of mild or medicated shampoos, scalp massage and treatments, and antiseptic or medicated scalp ointments.
- **Pityriasis steatoides** (stee-uh-TOY-deez) is a more severe form of dandruff that is characterized by an accumulation of greasy or waxy scales mixed with sebum (Figure 11–15b). This excessive shedding of the scales mixed with sebum causes the dandruff to stick to the scalp in patches, where it causes itching and irritation. If the greasy scales are torn off, bleeding or oozing of sebum may follow. Medical treatment is advisable for clients with this condition.

At one time, dandruff was thought to be contagious; however, the latest research has determined that it is not. Regardless of whether or not dandruff is contagious, the common use of tools and implements from one client to another is prohibited. Barbers must always practice approved sanitation and disinfection procedures in the barbershop before and after each client service.

11

Did you know...

Current research confirms that dandruff is the result of a fungus called **malassezia** (pityrosporum ovale) that is present on all human skin. This fungus develops symptoms of dandruff when it grows out of control and can worsen when aggravated by factors such as stress, age, hormones, or poor hygiene. Long neglected, severe forms of dandruff may cause injury to hair follicles, which in turn can lead to hair loss.

Vegetable Parasitic Infections (Tinea)

Tinea (TIN-ee-uh) is the medical term for ringworm. Ringworm is caused by vegetable parasites such as fungi and is characterized by itching, scales, and, sometimes, painful circular lesions. A case usually starts with a small, reddened patch of little blisters that spread outward and then heal in the middle, with a scalelike appearance. If the ringworm has spread, several patches may be present at one time.

All forms of tinea are contagious and can be easily transmitted from one person to another. Infected skin scales or hair containing the fungi are known to spread the disease; public showers, swimming pools, and unsanitary articles are also sources of transmission. Sanitation and proper disinfection procedures must be used to help prevent the spread of ringworm. All cases of tinea should be referred to a physician.

- **Tinea capitis** is commonly known as *ringworm of the scalp* (Figure 11–16). It is characterized by red papules, or spots, at the openings of the hair follicles. The patches spread; the hair becomes brittle and lifeless, and breaks off leaving a stump, or falls from the enlarged, open follicles.
- **Tinea sycosis** (SIGH-koh-sis), or *barber's itch*, is a fungal infection occurring chiefly over the bearded area of the face. Beginning as small, round, slightly scaly, inflamed patches, the areas enlarge, clearing up somewhat at the center with elevation at the borders. As the parasites invade the hairs and follicles, hard, lumpy swellings develop. In severe cases, pustules form around the hair follicles and rupture, forming crusts. In the later stage, the hairs become dry, break off, and fall out, or are readily extracted. Tinea sycosis is highly contagious and medical treatment is required.
- **Tinea favosa** (fah-VOH-suh) is also known as tinea favus (FAY-vus) or honeycomb ringworm. It is characterized by dry, sulfur-yellow, cuplike crusts on the scalp, having a peculiar, musty odor. Scars from favus are bald patches, pink or white, and shiny. It is very contagious and should be referred to a physician.

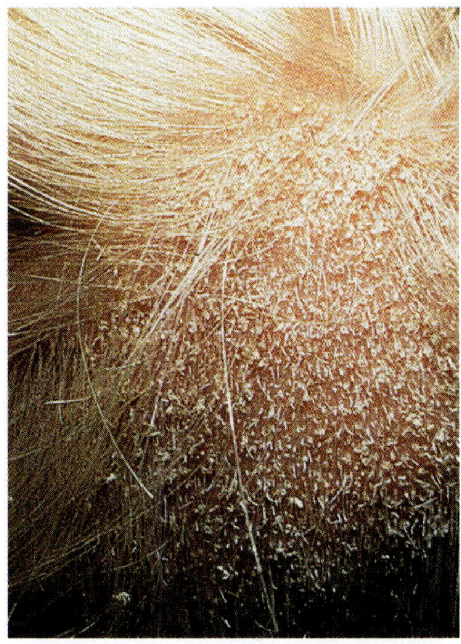

Figure 11–16 Tinea capitis.

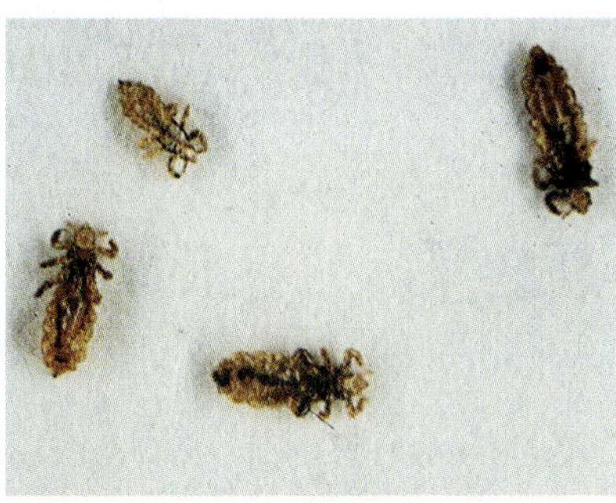

Figure 11–17 Head lice.

11

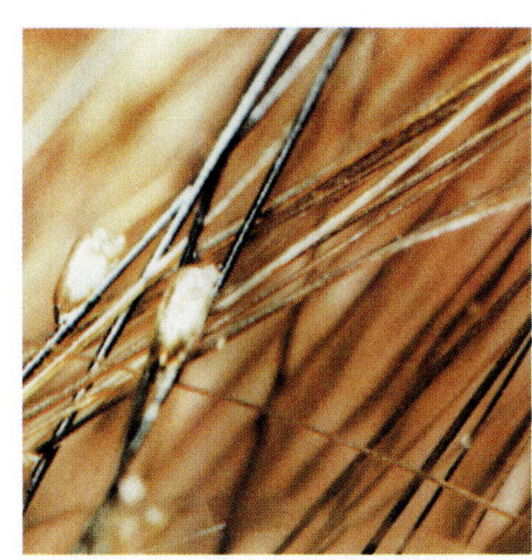

Figure 11–18 Nits (lice eggs).

Animal Parasitic Infections

The two most common animal parasitic infections that barbers may see in the barbershop are pediculosis capitis and scabies.

- **Pediculosis** (puh-dik-yuh-LOH-sis) **capitis** is the infestation of the hair and scalp with head lice (Figures 11–17 and 11–18). The parasites feed on the scalp and cause severe itching. The head louse is transmitted from one person to another by contact with infested hats, combs, brushes, and other personal items.

  There are several commercially prepared products sold over the counter for the treatment of head lice. Head lice are tenacious creatures

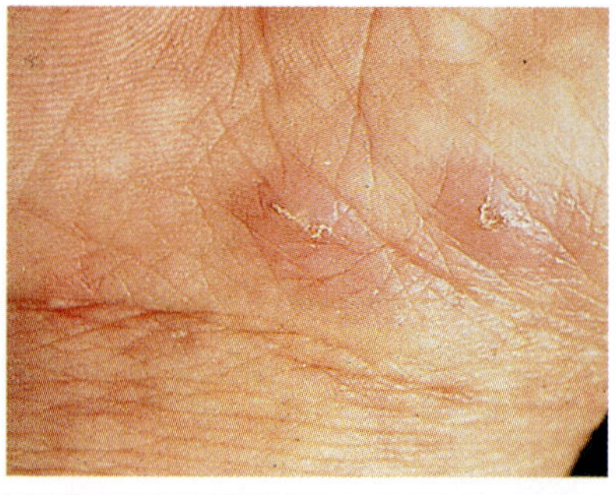

Figure 11–19 Scabies.

that can live off of the human body for up to 48 hours, so it is important to disinfect all household and personal items to avoid reinfestation. Cases of head lice should not be treated in the barbershop—the client should be referred to a physician.

NOTE: Remember to thoroughly disinfect the barber chair, capes, tools, workstation, and the reception area when a case of pediculosis capitis has been recognized in the barbershop.

- *Scabies* is a highly contagious skin disease caused by the itch mite. Vesicles and pustules usually form from the irritation caused by the parasites, or from scratching the affected areas (Figure 11–19). A client with this condition should be referred to a physician for medical treatment. As with all disorders and diseases, the practice of approved sanitation and disinfection procedures will help to limit the spread of scabies.

Staphylococci Infections

There are three bacterial staphylococci infections that barbers may encounter in the barbershop. They are sycosis vulgaris, furuncles, and carbuncles.

- **Sycosis vulgaris** is a chronic bacterial infection involving the follicles of the beard and mustache areas. It is transmitted by the use of unsanitary towels or implements, and it can be worsened by irritation, such as from shaving or a continual nasal discharge. The main lesions are papules and pustules pierced by hairs. The surrounding skin is tender, reddened, swollen, and itchy. Medical treatment is required and a client with this condition should be referred to a physician.

  NOTE This infection must not be confused with tinea sycosis, which is due to ringworm fungus.

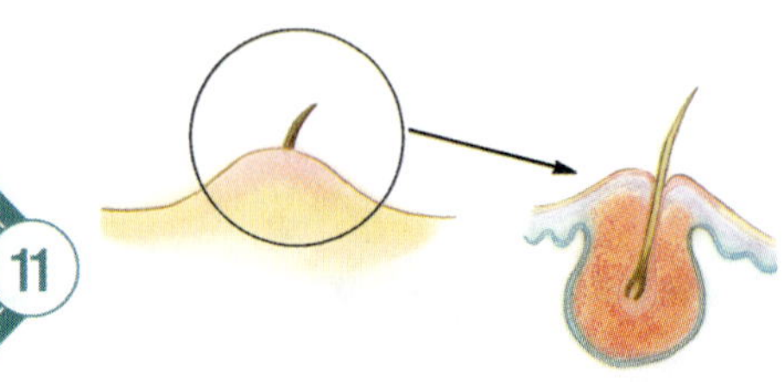

Figure 11–20 Furuncle (boil).

- A **furuncle** (FYOO-rung-kul), or boil, is an acute bacterial infection of a hair follicle, producing constant pain. A furuncle is the result of an active inflammatory process limited to a definite area that subsequently produces a pustule perforated by a hair (Figure 11–20). A client with this condition should be referred to a physician.
- A **carbuncle** (KAHR-bung-kul) is the result of an acute, deep-seated bacterial infection in the subcutaneous tissue. It is similar to a furuncle, or boil, but is larger. A client with this condition should be referred to a physician.

Folliculitis and **pseudofolliculitis** barbae are inflammations of the follicle caused by bacteria or irritation. Staphylococcus aureus and yeast are common bacterial causes of folliculitis. Irritants that cause folliculitis include work-related chemical exposure and mechanical irritation caused by improper shaving, hair breakage, or ingrown hairs.

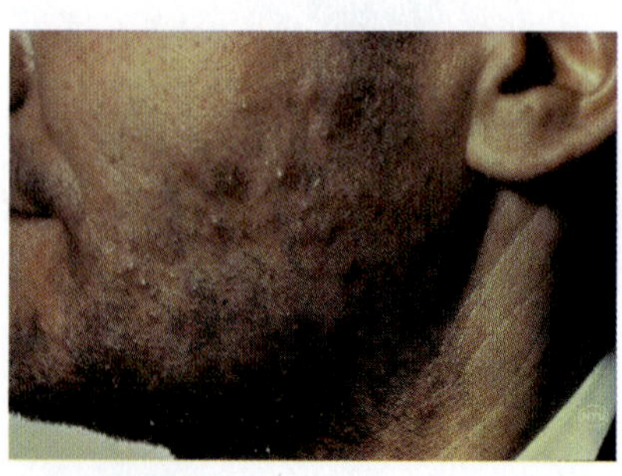

Figure 11–21 Regular facial treatments incorporating masks can help rid clients of folliculitis.

Folliculitis is often accompanied by inflammation and pus as a result of the hair growing slightly under the skin, rather than up and out onto the skin surface. Treatment for this condition should include the drying up and disinfection of the pustules and the desensitizing of the area. Clear gel masks that soothe and heal have also proven to be beneficial (Figure 11–21).

Pseudofolliculitis barbae, also referred to as "razor bumps," resembles folliculitis without the pus. This condition can be caused by improper shaving or by broken hair below the skin surface that grows into the side of the follicle, causing irritation and swelling that cuts off oxygen to the bottom of the follicle. Bacteria then have a perfect environment for growth that can lead to the development of pus and folliculitis. Pseudofolliculitis barbae is prevented by shaving in the direction of the hair growth and by avoiding close shaving. Electric razors can help and special razors are available that cut hair above the skin.

With an understanding of the causes of folliculitis and pseudofolliculitis, the barber can help the client to determine if the condition is caused by chemical or mechanical means. Preparations that contain salicylic acid to break up impactions and kill bacteria are available for the prevention of ingrown hairs. Physicians may prescribe topical and oral antibiotics for more serious conditions. When mechanical causes, such as improper shaving, are the source of the condition, the barber can offer the client some instruction in proper shaving techniques. 7

DISORDERS OF THE HAIR

Hair disorders are usually noncontagious conditions, which include canities, hypertrichosis, trichoptilosis, trichorrhexis nodosa, monilethrix, and fragilitas crinium.

- **Canities** (kah-NISH-ee-eez) is the technical term for gray hair. Canities is due mainly to the loss of the hair's natural melanin pigment in the cortical layer. Other than the absence of pigment, gray hair is the same as pigmented hair. Gray hair is really mottled hair; spots of white or whitish-yellow are scattered about in the hair shafts. Normally, gray hair grows out in this condition from the hair bulb; therefore, graying does not take place after the hair has grown. The two main types of canities are congenital and acquired; a third form is known as ringed hair.

  Congenital canities exists at or before birth. It occurs in albinos and occasionally in persons with perfectly normal hair. The patchy type of congenital canities may develop slowly or rapidly, depending on the cause of the condition.

  Acquired canities may be due to the natural aging process and genetics, or it may be premature. Other causes of acquired grayness are worry, anxiety, nervous strain, prolonged illness, and heredity.

  Ringed hair is a third form of canities that is characterized by alternating bands of gray and pigmented hair throughout the length of the hair strand.

- **Hypertrichosis** (hi-pur-trih-KOH-sis) or hirsuties (hur-SOO-shee-eez) is a condition of abnormal hair growth. It is characterized by the development and growth of terminal hair in those areas of the body that would normally grow only vellus hair. A mustache or light beard on a woman is

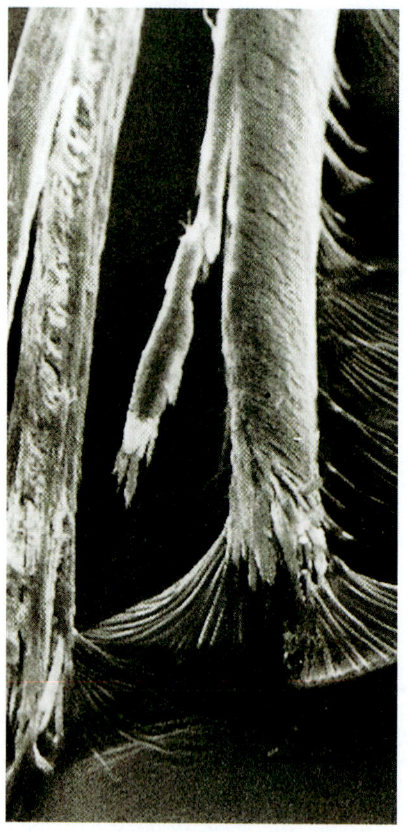

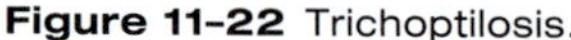

Figure 11-22 Trichoptilosis.

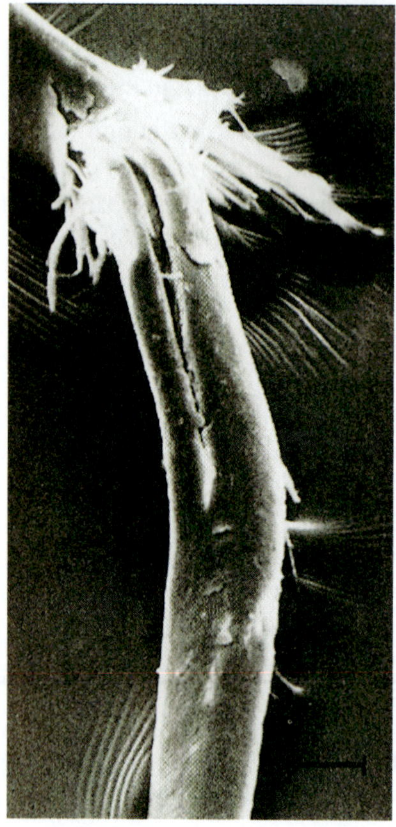

Figure 11-23 Trichorrhexis nodosa.

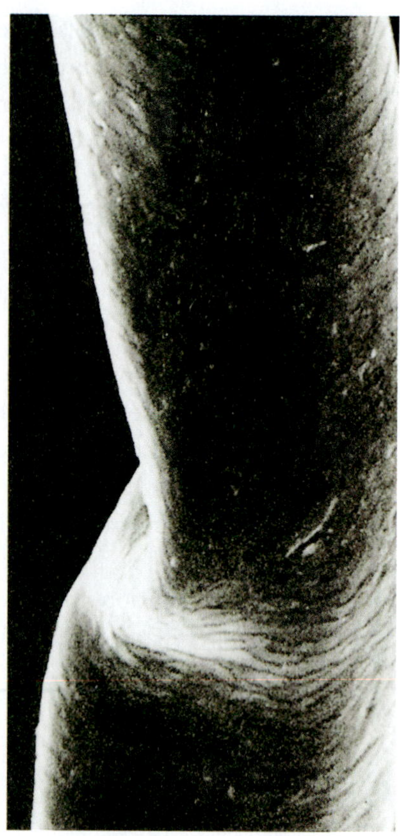

Figure 11-24 Monilethrix.

an example of hypertrichosis. Treatments include tweezing, depilatories, waxing, shaving, mechanical epilators, and electrolysis.

- *Trichoptilosis* (trih-kahp-tih-LOH-sus) is the technical term for split ends (Figure 11–22). The split ends may be removed by cutting, or conditioning treatments may be used to soften and lubricate dry ends.
- *Trichorrhexis nodosa* (trik-uh-REK-sis nuh-DOH-suh) is the technical term for knotted hair (Figure 11–23). It is characterized by brittleness and the formation of nodular swellings along the hair shaft. Treatments include softening the hair with conditioners and moisturizers.
- *Monilethrix* (mah-NIL-ee-thrixs) is the technical term for beaded hair (Figure 11–24). The hair breaks easily between the nodes; treatments include hair and scalp conditioning.
- *Fragilitas crinium* (fruh-JIL-ih-tus KRI-nee-um) is the technical term for brittle hair. The hairs may split along any part of their length. Treatments include hair and scalp conditioning. 8

chapter glossary

alopecia	the technical name for hair loss
alopecia areata	the sudden falling out of hair in patches or spots
alopecia prematura	hair loss that occurs before middle age
alopecia senilis	hair loss occurring in old age
alopecia syphilitica	hair loss as a result of syphilis
amino acids	the building blocks or units of structure in protein
anagen phase	growth phase in the hair cycle
androgenic alopecia	hair loss that occurs as a result of genetics, age, and hormonal changes; male pattern baldness
arrector pili	involuntary muscle fiber attached to the follicle
canities	technical term for gray hair
carbuncle	the result of an acute, deep-seated bacterial infection in the subcutaneous tissue
catagen phase	transition phase of the hair growth cycle
cortex	middle layer of the hair shaft
cowlick	tuft of hair that stands straight up
cross bonds	also known as side bonds; hydrogen, salt, and sulfur bonds in the hair cortex
cuticle	outermost layer of the hair shaft
dermal papilla	small, cone-shaped elevation located at the base of the hair follicle that fits into the hair bulb
disulfide bond	also known as a sulfur bond; a type of chemical cross bond found in the hair cortex
end bonds	also known as peptide bonds; chemical bonds that join amino acids end to end
eumelanin	melanin that gives brown and black color to hair
follicle	tubelike depression in the skin that contains the hair root
folliculitis	skin condition in which the hair grows slightly under the skin, causing a bacterial infection with pus
furuncle	an acute bacterial infection of a hair follicle, producing constant pain; also known as a boil
hair bulb	club-shaped structure that forms the lower part of the hair root
hair density	the amount of hair per square inch of scalp
hair elasticity	the ability of the hair to stretch and return to its original length
hair porosity	the ability of the hair to absorb moisture
hair root	the part of the hair that is encased in the hair follicle

hair shaft	the part of the hair that extends beyond the skin
hair stream	hair that flows in the same direction
hair texture	measures the diameter of a hair strand; coarse, medium, fine
hydrogen bond	a physical cross bond in the hair cortex
hypertrichosis	a condition of abnormal hair growth
keratin	the protein of which hair is formed
lanugo	vellus hair
medulla	innermost or center layer of the hair shaft
pediculosis capitis	the infection of the hair and scalp with head lice
peptide bonds	end bonds; chemical bonds that join amino acids end to end
pheomelanin	melanin that gives red to blond color to hair
pityriasis capitis simplex	dry dandruff type
pityriasis steatoides	waxy or greasy dandruff type
polypeptide chain	long chain of amino acids linked by peptide bonds
primary terminal hair	short, thick hairs that grow on the eyebrows and lashes
pseudofolliculitis	a form of folliculitis without pus known as "razor bumps"
salt bond	a physical cross bond within the hair cortex
secondary terminal hair	long hair found on the scalp, beard, chest, back, and legs
sycosis vulgaris	bacterial infection of the bearded areas of the face
telogen phase	resting phase of the hair growth cycle
tinea	technical name for ringworm
tinea capitis	ringworm of the scalp
tinea favosa	ringworm characterized by dry, sulfur-yellow crusts on the scalp
tinea sycosis	ringworm of the bearded areas on the face; barber's itch
trichology	the science dealing with the hair, its diseases, and care
vellus	soft, downy hair that appears on the body
wave pattern	amount of movement in the hair strand; straight, wavy, curly, and coiled
whorl	hair that grows in a circular pattern

chapter review questions

1. Why is the study of hair important to the barber?
2. Identify the technical term for the study of hair.
3. Describe the differences between the hair root and hair shaft.
4. List the structures of the hair root.
5. Identify the layers of the hair shaft.
6. What are amino acids?
7. What are peptide bonds?
8. List the cross bonds in the hair.
9. Identify ways in which peptide bonds and cross bonds can be broken.
10. What is melanin?
11. Define wave pattern.
12. Define hair stream, whorl, and cowlick.
13. Define and explain the anagen, catagen, and telogen phases of hair growth.
14. List and define the characteristics of hair used in hair analysis.
15. List and describe different types of hair loss.
16. List and describe common disorders of the scalp.
17. List and describe disorders of the hair.
18. Identify the causes and characteristics of folliculitis and pseudofolliculitis.

part 3

PROFESSIONAL BARBERING

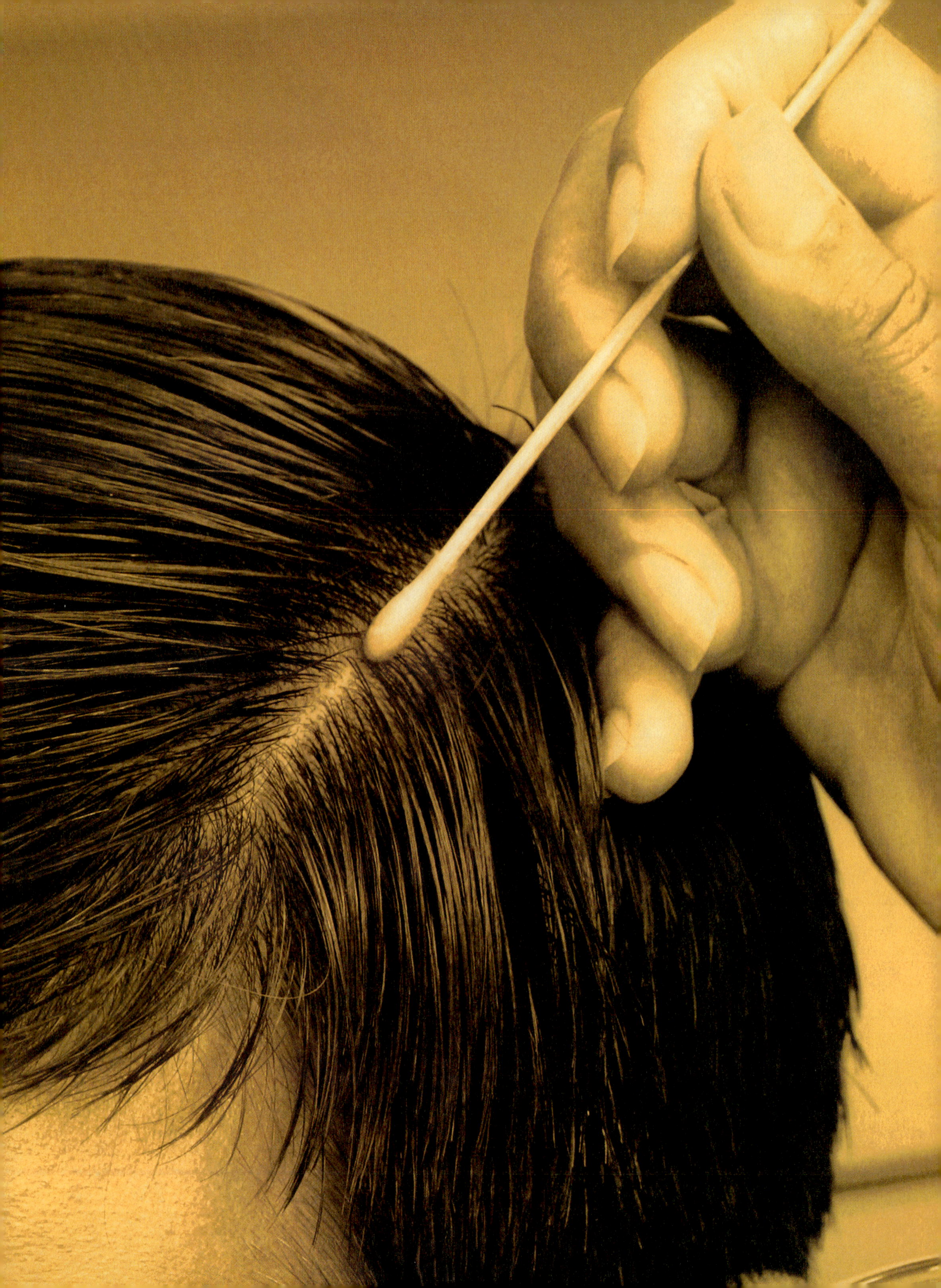

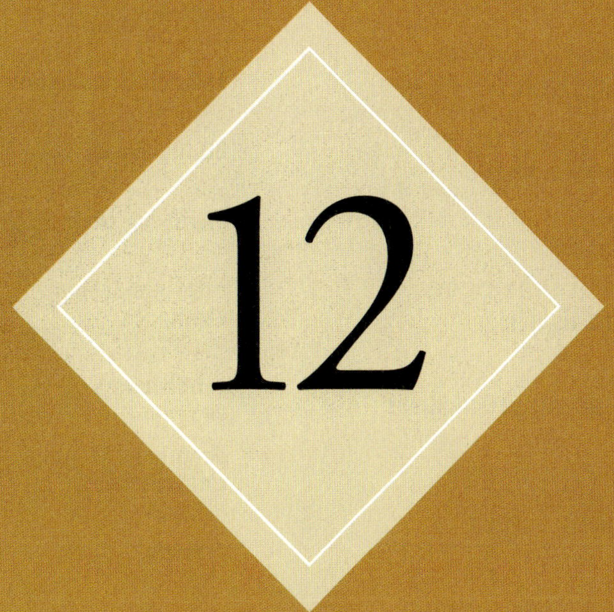

TREATMENT OF THE HAIR AND SCALP

Chapter Outline

Shampoos and Conditioners • Draping • The Shampoo Service

The Shampoo Procedure • Scalp Treatments

Learning Objectives

After completing this chapter, you should be able to:

1. Identify services associated with the treatment of the hair and scalp.
2. Discuss pH factor as it relates to hair care products.
3. Identify different types of shampoos, conditioners, rinses, and tonics.
4. Demonstrate proper draping procedures for hair services.
5. Demonstrate the shampoo service.
6. Demonstrate scalp massage techniques and treatments.

Key Terms

The treatment of the hair and scalp includes regular shampoo and scalp massage services as well as special treatments for hair and scalp conditions. These services provide additional opportunities for barbers to perform relaxing and effective procedures that help to ensure the health of the client's hair and scalp from one shop visit to another.

The shampoo service can be one of the most relaxing and enjoyable services that a client receives in the barbershop (Figure 12–1). Professionally delivered scalp massage during the shampoo offers hygienic and circulatory benefits to the client and prepares the hair for the haircutting service. Shampoo services ensure that the barber is working with clean hair that is free from oils and hair products that can interfere with cutting tools and final haircut results. Follow-up hair conditioning treatments after the shampoo help to keep the hair in a healthy and manageable condition for the client and the barber.

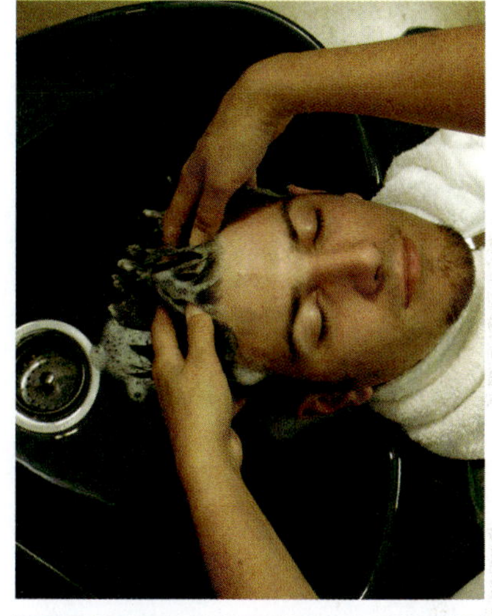

Figure 12–1 The shampoo service.

Special services, such as deep-penetrating conditioners or electrotherapy and light therapy treatments for scalp conditions, help to maintain the health of the scalp and hair. These services can also help to promote hair growth and may reduce the occurrence of hair loss.

Many of today's barbershop owners are aware of the positive impact and results that these services can provide for their patrons from both physiological and psychological standpoints. In addition, the performance of professional hair and scalp treatments can increase client retention and referral, while promoting a positive reputation for the barber and the barbershop. 1

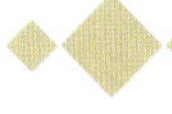

SHAMPOOS AND CONDITIONERS

The purpose of a shampoo product and service is to cleanse the scalp and hair. This may seem an obvious fact, but many barbers still encounter clients who use bar soap or other detergent products that can leave the hair dry or coated with soap residues. Conversely, **shampoos** are specially formulated solutions for the hair and scalp; they do not contain the harsh alkalis found in soaps and detergents and therefore tend to leave the hair in a more manageable condition.

Conditioners refer to either hair conditioners or scalp conditioners. Generally, hair conditioners moisturize the hair and help to restore some of the natural oils and proteins; scalp conditioners are available for overall scalp maintenance or to treat conditions requiring a medicinal product.

Shampoos

There are many types of shampoo products on the market. As a professional barber, you will need to become skilled at selecting shampoo products that best serve the condition of the client's hair and scalp. Make it a standard operating procedure to read manufacturer's labels so that an informed choice can be made. In addition, display and use the barbershop's retail products at the workstation or shampoo sink back bar. Doing so not only promotes product sales, but also demonstrates to clients that the barber endorses the product and its effectiveness inside and outside the barbershop.

To be effective, a shampoo must remove all dirt, oil, perspiration, and skin debris, without adversely affecting either the scalp or the hair. The hair collects dust particles, natural oils from the sebaceous glands, perspiration, and dead skin cells that can accumulate on the scalp. This accumulation creates a breeding ground for disease-producing bacteria, which can lead to scalp disorders. The hair and scalp should be thoroughly shampooed as frequently as is necessary to keep them clean, healthy, and free from bacteria.

Four requirements of an effective shampoo product are as follows:

- It should cleanse the hair of oils, debris, and dirt.
- It should work efficiently in hard as well as soft water.
- It should not irritate the eyes or skin.
- It should leave the hair and scalp in their natural condition.

The barber should select a shampoo product according to the condition of the client's hair and scalp. Hair is usually characterized as being dry, normal, oily, or chemically treated. The scalp is usually described as being dry, normal, oily, or requiring treatments for certain disorders, such as dandruff conditions. For example, a client may have an oily scalp due to overactive sebaceous glands, but a dry hair condition due to overprocessing of chemical services. An accurate analysis of the hair and scalp as discussed in Chapter 11 will assist in the selection of shampoo products for clients.

Shampoo Chemistry

Chapter 8 provided an overview of important chemistry basics such as pH and surfactants. Now this information will be used as it relates to shampoo products and the barber's selection of different formulations for different hair types and conditions.

Shampoos and pH

As it applies to barbering services and products, the pH of a solution is the value used to indicate the acidity or alkalinity of water-based solutions. The acidity or alkalinity of cosmetic products, such as a shampoo, is important because it influences how that product will affect various layers of the hair and skin. Acidic solutions (below pH 7.0) will shrink, constrict, and harden the cuticle scales of the hair shaft. An alkaline solution (above pH 7.0) will soften, swell, and expand the hair shaft cuticle scales. Remember, the lower the pH, the greater the degree of acidity of a solution; and the higher the pH, the greater the degree of alkalinity of a solution (Figure 12–2).

Shampoos are emulsions that usually range between 4.5 and 7.5 on the pH scale. Since the normal pH range for hair and skin is 4.5 to 5.5, mild or more acidic shampoos are found closer to this range. Conversely, stronger or more alkaline shampoos are found beyond 6.0 on the pH scale. 2

Shampoo Molecules

Shampoos consist of two main ingredients: water and surfactants. Shampoo molecules are the result of combining water with a **surfactant**, or base detergent, which creates a surfactant molecule. These molecules are composed of a head and tail, each with its own special function.

The tail of the shampoo (surfactant) molecule attracts dirt, grease, debris, and oil, but repels water. The head of the shampoo molecule attracts water, but repels dirt. Working together both parts of the molecule effectively cleanse the hair (Figures 12–3 through 12–6).

Additional ingredients in the forms of moisturizers, preservatives, foam enhancers, perfumes, and others are added to base surfactants to create a variety of shampoo formulations. Along with water and the base surfactant,

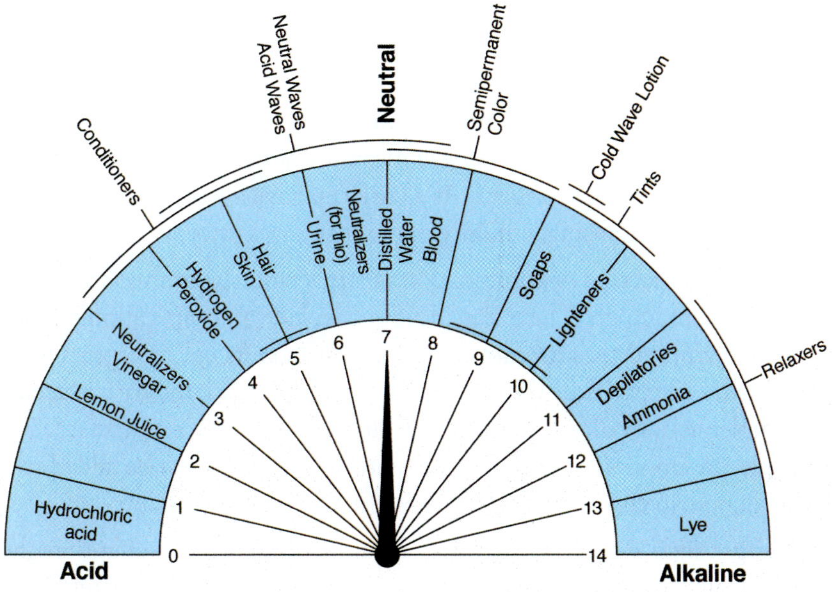

Figure 12-2 The pH scale.

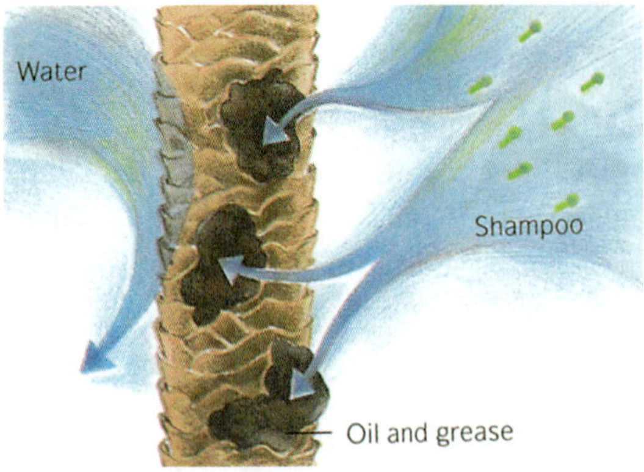

Figure 12-3 The tail of the shampoo molecule is attracted to oil and dirt.

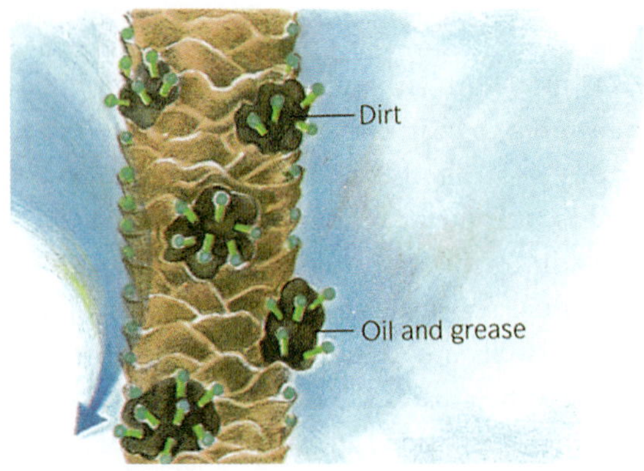

Figure 12-4 Shampoo causes oils to run up into small globules.

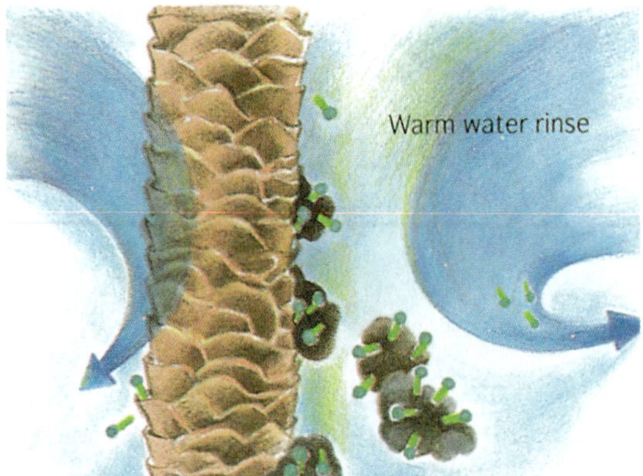

Figure 12-5 During rinsing, the heads of the shampoo molecules attach to water molecules and cause debris to roll off.

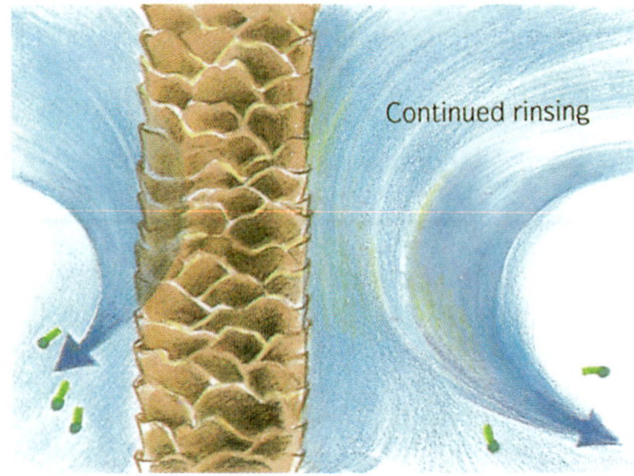

Figure 12-6 Thorough rinsing washes away debris and excess shampoo.

these ingredients are listed on product labels in descending order according to the percentage of each ingredient in the shampoo.

Surfactants

Next to water, surfactants are the second most common ingredient found in shampoos. *Surfactant* and *detergent* mean the same thing and refer to the cleansing or *surface-active* agent. As a surface-active agent, surfactants can take the form of cleansing, emulsifying, or foaming agents.

The base surfactant or combination of surfactants determines the classification of a shampoo. These classifications include anionic, cationic, nonionic, and ampholytic surfactants. Most manufacturers use detergents from more than one classification. It is customary to use a secondary surfactant to complement, or offset, the negative qualities of the base surfactant. For example, an amphoteric that is nonirritating to the eyes can be added to a harsh anionic to create a product that is more comfortable to use.

- *Anionics*, such as sodium lauryl sulfate and sodium laureth sulfate, are the most commonly used detergents. Sodium lauryl sulfate is a relatively harsh cleanser that produces a rich foam. It is suitable for use in hard or soft water because it rinses easily from the hair. Sodium laureth sulfate is also a strong, rich, foaming detergent but, because it is less alkaline than the lauryl sulfates, it is often used in shampoos that are designed to be milder or less drying to the hair shaft.

- *Cationics* are made up almost entirely of quaternary ammonium compounds or quats. Practically all quaternary compounds have some antibacterial action so they are sometimes included in the chemical composition of dandruff shampoos.
- *Nonionics* are valued as surfactants for their versatility, stability, and ability to resist shrinkage, particularly in cold temperatures. They have a mild cleansing action and low incidence of irritation to human tissues. Cocamide (DEA, MEA) is one of the most widely used nonionics in the industry, not only in shampoos but also in lipsticks and permanent waving lotions.
- *Ampholytes* can behave as an anionic or a cationic substance, depending on the pH of the solution. Ampholytic surfactants have a slight tendency to cling to hair and skin, which aids in hair manageability. They also possess germicidal properties that vary between derivatives. Amphoteric surfactants are used in several baby shampoos because they do not sting the eyes. Many amphoterics are identified on the ingredient list as Amphoteric I-20.

A familiarity with these four classifications of detergents or surfactants and their use in shampoo products should assist the barber in making professional decisions when selecting the appropriate product for use on a client's hair and scalp.

Water

For efficiency in shampooing, it is important for barbers to know what type of water is available in the barbershop and whether the water is hard or soft.

Soft water is rain water or water that has been chemically softened, containing very small amounts of minerals. It therefore lathers freely. For this reason, it is preferred for shampooing.

Hard water contains certain minerals, and as a result shampoo does not readily lather in it. Depending on the kind of hard water available in the community, it can usually be softened by chemical processes and made suitable for shampooing.

Types of Shampoos

Shampoo products account for the highest dollar expenditure in hair care products and are available in liquid, liquid-dry, and dry or powder formulations. Until a few decades ago, shampoo (and conditioner) choices were limited to a few types and brands. The standard shampoos then included the plain, liquid cream, castile, egg, and green soap shampoos.

Today, barbers have a wide variety of products that are suitable for most hair and scalp conditions. There are shampoos for dry, oily, normal, fine, coarse, limp, or chemically treated hair. There are shampoos that add a slight amount of color to hair and those that cleanse the hair of mineral deposits and product buildup. Many manufacturers have become more "hair condition conscious" so that even medicated shampoos are less drying to the hair and scalp.

A visit to your local barber supply will introduce you to a wide variety of products for use in the barbershop. The following provides basic information that may be needed to make an informed choice concerning the *categories* of shampoos.

Liquid shampoos are available in cream or clear (plain) forms. *Liquid cream* shampoos are usually fairly thick white liquids that contain either soap or soap jelly. Magnesium stearate is also used as a whitening agent. These shampoos often contain oily compounds to make the hair feel silky and softer. Use this type of shampoo as directed by your instructor or the manufacturer. *Plain shampoos* are usually clear and may be an amber shade or a greenish yellow. They may contain a plain liquid soap or a detergent-based product. These shampoos seldom have lanolin or other special agents used to leave a gloss on the hair. A plain shampoo may be used on hair that is in good condition, but not on color-treated hair because it may strip or fade the color.

Liquid-dry shampoos are cosmetic products used for cleansing the scalp and hair when the client is prevented by illness from having a regular shampoo. Some have an astringent quality that allows the product to evaporate quickly.

Dry or powder shampoos can be used when the client's health will not permit a wet shampoo or the service is too uncomfortable. Powder or dry shampoos may contain orris root powder and cleanse the hair without the use of water. The shampoo is sprinkled into the hair where it picks up dirt and oils as it is brushed through the hair. Always follow manufacturer's directions and never give a dry shampoo prior to a chemical service.

Most of today's shampoos can be classified as belonging to one of the following shampoo types.

Acid-balanced shampoos are balanced to the pH level of hair and skin and usually contain citric, lactic, or phosphoric acid. These shampoos are mild and are formulated to prevent the stripping of hair color from the hair. They have a low alkaline content, which makes them a good choice for normal, chemically treated, and fragile hair. Follow the manufacturer's directions, but most acid-balanced shampoos can be used daily.

Moisturizing or conditioning shampoos are usually mild, cream shampoos that contain moisturizing agents (*humectants*) designed either to "lock in" the moisturizing properties of the product or to draw moisture into the hair. They are formulated to make the hair smooth and shiny and to avoid damaging chemically treated hair. Protein and biotin are conditioning agents that help restore moisture and elasticity, strengthen the hair shaft, and add volume. Like acid-balanced shampoos, moisturizing shampoos will not remove artificial color from the hair.

Clarifying shampoos contain an acidic ingredient such as cider vinegar to cut through product buildup that can coat and flatten hair. They provide thorough cleansing and should be used only when buildup is evident. Once- or twice-weekly applications should suffice, depending on how much styling product the client uses. These shampoos are also helpful in preparing the hair for chemical services or to remove medication or hard-water mineral buildup from the hair.

Balancing shampoos are designed for oily hair and scalp. These shampoos wash away excess oiliness while keeping the hair from drying out.

Medicated shampoos contain a medicinal or antiseptic agent such as sulfur, tar, cresol, or phenol. They are usually effective in reducing dandruff or relieving scalp conditions. Although sold without a prescription, they are generally quite strong and can affect the color of tinted or lightened hair. *Therapeutic medicated shampoos* contain special chemicals or drugs that are very effective in reducing excessive dandruff. They must be used only by prescription and instructions should be followed carefully.

Organic shampoos are some of the most recent to be available on the market, yet their origins are centuries old. True organic formulations will contain natural, organic substances such as herbs, flowering or other plants, and/or minerals. Aloe vera, nettles, chamomile, or jojoba are just some of the ingredients that may be formulated into these shampoos, which are usually pH balanced.

Color-enhancing shampoos are created by combining the surfactant with basic colors. They are attracted to porous hair and provide only slight color changes, which are removed with plain shampooing. Color shampoos are used to brighten the hair, add slight color, and eliminate unwanted color tones.

Conditioners

Much like shampoos in past decades the availability of commercial conditioners was limited. Products such as olive oil preparations, cholesterol, and cream rinses represented the usual choice range.

Conditioners are special chemical agents that are applied to hair to deposit protein or moisture, restore hair strength and body, or protect against possible damage. Conditioners range from 3.0 to 5.5 on the pH scale. They are temporary remedies for hair that feels dry or is damaged. Conditioners do not heal damaged hair, nor can they permanently improve the quality of new hair growth.

Excessive use of conditioners, or using the wrong type of conditioner, can lead to a buildup of product on the hair that makes it heavy and oily. For this reason, the barber needs to know when to choose between a cream rinse for detangling and a reconstructor for damaged hair.

Conditioners are available in three basic types: instant, treatment or repair, and leave-in. The barber must decide the type to use based on the texture and condition of the hair and the desired results.

Instant conditioners are applied to the hair following a shampoo and are rinsed out after one to five minutes. They usually have a lower pH than the hair, which helps to close the cuticle scales. The typical instant conditioner does not penetrate into the hair shaft but may add oils, moisture, and sometimes protein to the cuticle scales of the hair. Finishing, detangling, and cream rinses are examples of instant conditioners.

Moisturizing conditioners contain chemical compounds called humectants that absorb and promote the retention of moisture in the hair. They can also seal moisture inside damp hair by coating the cuticle. Moisturizing conditioners are usually heavier than instant conditioners and have a longer application time of 10 to 20 minutes. They often contain the same ingredients as instant conditioners, but are formulated to be more penetrating. Some require the use of heat for deeper penetration and longer lasting results. Quaternary ammonium compounds are included in the formulation of moisturizers for their ability to attach to hair fibers. Natural moisturizing ingredients may include oils, essential fatty acids, sodium PCA, and sometimes herbs. Coating moisturizers usually contain wax or glycerin in addition to other ingredients.

Protein conditioners are available in a cream form with moisturizers and oils and in a concentrated liquid-protein form. Both utilize hydrolized protein for its ability to pass through the cuticle to penetrate the cortex, where the keratin has been lost from the hair. These conditioners improve texture, equalize porosity, and help to increase elasticity in the hair. The hair should be well rinsed prior to cutting, setting, or drying, as excess conditioner may coat or weigh down the hair.

Deep-conditioning treatments are chemical mixtures of concentrated protein in the heavy cream base of a moisturizer. They penetrate several layers of the cuticle and are the preferred therapy when an equal degree of moisturizing and protein treatment is desired. As with the previously discussed conditioners, deep-conditioning treatments require thorough rinsing prior to other services.

Synthetic polymer conditioners are special formulations for use on badly damaged hair. A polymer is a compound consisting of many repeating units that form a chain. Hair is a natural polymer and when it is so severely damaged that normal protein conditioners cannot recondition it, a synthetic polymer may be necessary to prevent breakage and correct excessive porosity.

Leave-in conditioners, such as spray-on thermal protectors (blow-drying sprays), are products that should not be rinsed out of the hair. Some are designed for use with thermal tools, while others are included with some chemical service products to equalize the porosity of the hair shaft.

Scalp conditioners are available in a variety of formulations and for different purposes. Cream-based products with moisturizers and emollients are usually used to soften and improve the health of the scalp. *Medicated scalp lotions* are conditioners that promote the healing of the scalp. *Astringent scalp tonics* help to remove oil accumulation on the scalp and are used after a scalp treatment.

Rinses

Although the application of a conditioning agent is usually the second step in a shampoo service, the application of color or bluing rinses is a profitable service that can be easily learned and applied at the shampoo bowl.

A hair **rinse** is an agent that is used to cleanse or condition the hair and scalp, bring out the luster of the hair, or add highlights.

Water rinses are obviously used to wet and rinse the hair during the shampoo service. Warm water should be used to thoroughly rinse and remove any shampoo residue on the hair.

Medicated rinses are formulated to control minor dandruff and scalp conditions. A dandruff rinse is a commercial product that is applied following a shampoo to remove and control dandruff. Some rinses are used in a prepared form while others are diluted with water. Always follow the manufacturer's directions.

Bluing rinses are preparations that contain a blue base color. The bluing counteracts yellowish or dull gray tones in the hair, neutralizing them to silvery gray or white tones. These rinses are available in cream shampoo form or as a temporary hair color rinse in liquid form. Both are applied at the shampoo bowl. The cream shampoo type is rinsed from the hair, however, while the temporary color rinse is not.

> *NOTE:* The porosity of the hair must be taken into consideration to avoid a two-toned effect on the porous ends or shaft of the hair. Follow the manufacturer's directions when mixing to achieve the desired silver or slate tone.

It is the barber's responsibility to be knowledgeable about the products used in the shop or salon. Basic product knowledge can be easily obtained from product labels, distributors, trade show demonstrations, and manufacturer representatives. Table 12–1 lists products suitable for different hair types.

12

Tonics

The term hair **tonic** indicates almost any type of cosmetic solution that stimulates the scalp, helps to correct a scalp condition, or is used as a grooming aid. There are numerous hair tonics on the market so it is important to understand the ingredients, specific actions, and use of each type. The barber should also be prepared to advise clients concerning the use of tonics and the specific purpose of each.

Hair tonics are used to groom the hair, stimulate the scalp, maintain a healthy scalp, and to correct dandruff and itchy-scalp conditions. They are available in nonalcoholic, alcoholic, emulsion, and oil mixture formulations.

- *Nonalcoholic tonics* usually contain an antiseptic solution, with hair-grooming ingredients added.

Hair Type	Fine	Medium	Coarse
Straight	Volumizing shampoo Detangler, if necessary Protein treatments	Acid-balanced shampoo Finishing rinse Protein treatments	Moisturizing shampoo Leave-in conditioner Moisturizing treatments
Wavy, Curly, Extremely Curly	Fine-hair shampoo Light leave-in conditioner Protein treatments Spray-on thermal protectors	Acid-balanced shampoo Leave-in conditioner Moisturizing treatment	Moisturizing shampoo Leave-in conditioner Protein and moisturizing treatments
Dry & Damaged (Perms, Color, Relaxers, Blow-drying, Sun, Hot Irons)	Gentle cleansing shampoo Light leave-in conditioner Protein and moisturizing repair treatments Spray-on thermal protection	Shampoo for chemically treated hair Moisturizing conditioner Protein and moisturizing repair treatments	Deep-moisturizing shampoo for damaged hair Leave-in conditioner Deep-conditioning treatments and hair masks

Table 12–1 Matching Products to Hair Types

- *Alcoholic tonics* consist of an antiseptic and alcohol combination that acts as a mild astringent.
- *Cream tonics* are emulsions containing lanolin and mineral oils.
- *Oil mixture tonics* contain considerable amounts of alcohol with a small portion of oil floating on the top. These tonics are used as a grooming agent.

  NOTE: For maximum benefit, a scalp massage should be used in conjunction with tonic applications.

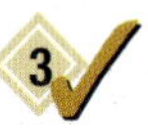

12

DRAPING

The comfort and protection of the client must always be considered during barbering services. **Draping** protects the client's skin and clothing and assures clients that the barber is conscientious about their comfort and safety.

There are two main types of drapes used to perform barbering services: waterproof or plastic capes, also known as shampoo capes; and haircutting capes, also known as chair cloths.

- Waterproof capes are used to protect the client's skin and clothing from water or other liquids and from chemical processes.
- The preferred haircutting capes are made of nylon or synthetic materials. These draping fabrics are usually more comfortable for the client because they do not hold in as much body heat in as plastic capes are prone to do. From the barber's standpoint, these fabrics are more effective in shedding

fective in shedding wet and dry hair. Wet hair has a tendency to stick to plastic capes, making it more difficult to shake loose hairs off the drape.

Draping Methods

The method of draping to be used depends on the service to be performed. Several draping methods are presented in this text, although those taught by your instructor are also appropriate. Regardless of the draping method or the service to be provided, several important steps apply to all draping procedures, as consideration for the client should always be one of your highest priorities.

The purpose of the towel or neck strip in draping procedures is to prevent the cape from having direct contact with the client's skin and to maintain sanitation standards. The application of this barrier between the client's skin and the drape is a requirement of every state's barber law, rules, and regulations.

Important steps for draping a client for any type of service are as follows:

1. Prepare materials and supplies for the service.
2. Sanitize your hands.
3. Ask the client to remove all neck and hair jewelry, and store it in a safe place.
4. Remove objects, if any, from the client's hair.
5. Turn the client's collar to the inside.
6. Proceed with the appropriate draping method.

Draping for Wet and Chemical Services

Wet hair services include shampooing, hair and scalp treatments, and all chemical applications.

1. Fold a towel in a lengthwise and diagonal manner. Place the towel lengthwise across the client's shoulders, crossing the ends beneath the chin (Figure 12–7).
2. Drape the plastic or waterproof cape over the towel and fasten it at the back so that the cape does not touch the client's skin. Position and flatten the top edge of the towel down over the neckline of the cape (Figure 12–8).
3. Place another towel over the cape and secure it in front with a chair cloth clip (Figure 12–9).

12

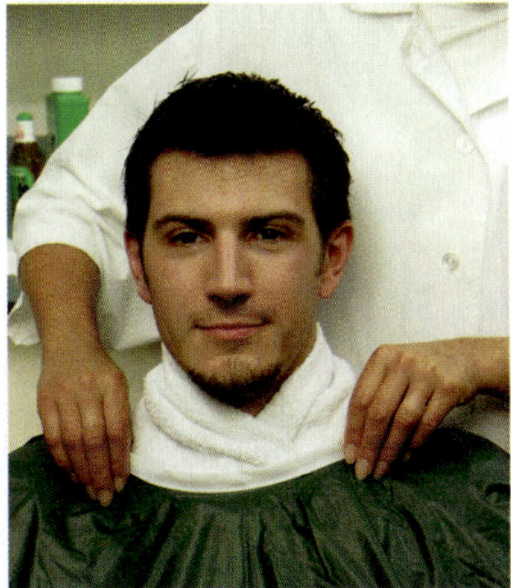

Figure 12-7 Cross the towel ends beneath the client's chin.

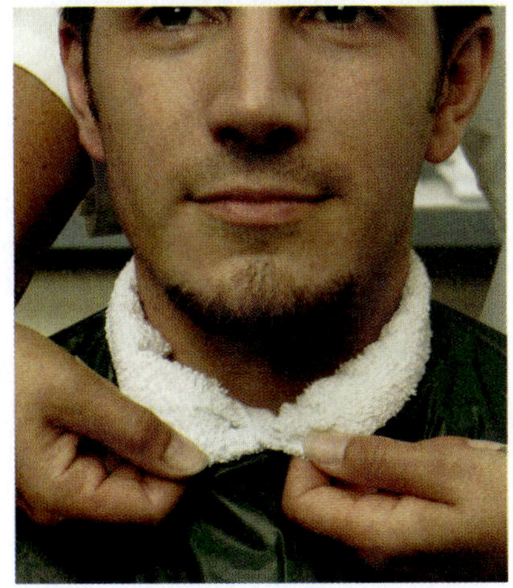

Figure 12-8 Position and flatten top edge of towel over cape neckline.

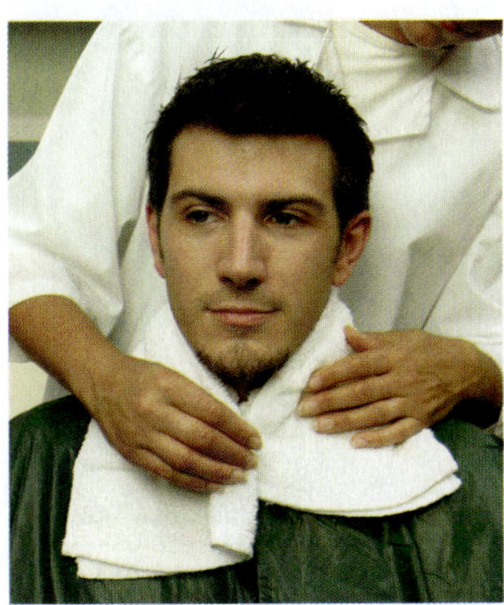

Figure 12-9 Place second towel over cape and secure with clip.

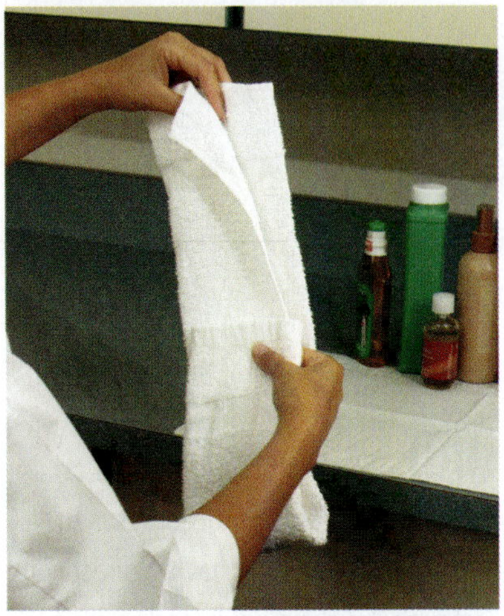

Figure 12-10 Fold towel in thirds.

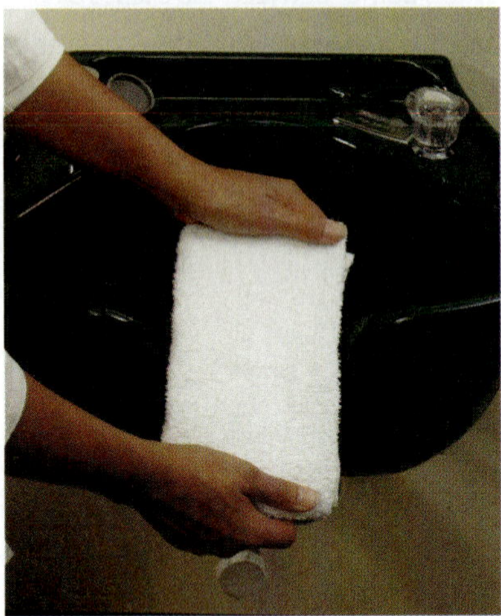

Figure 12-11 Create a barrier in the neck rest of the shampoo bowl.

NOTE: Step 3 above is optional for the *shampoo* service. If two towels are too bulky at the shampoo bowl, fold the second towel in thirds and place it in the neck rest of the shampoo bowl to create a barrier between the client and the sink (Figures 12–10 and 12–11).

Use a third towel for blotting purposes after the shampoo.

NOTE: Two towels, one under the cape and one over the cape as in Figure 12–9, should always be used for *chemical* services. A third towel from a clean, closed cabinet is used at the shampoo bowl for blotting purposes after rinsing chemical products from the hair.

Draping for Haircutting Services

Haircut draping requires a towel or neck strip and a nylon or cotton chair cloth. If a shampoo service precedes the haircut, remove the waterproof cape and towel. Replace the towel with a neck strip as this allows the hair to fall more naturally without obstruction. Replace the plastic cape with a nylon or cotton chair cloth. Follow the steps below as illustrated in Figures 12–12 through 12–14.

1. Drape the chair cloth loosely across the client's chest and shoulders. Place neck strip around the client's neck from front to back. Hold one end of the neck strip against the client's skin at the back or side of the neck while wrapping the rest of the strip. Secure the second neck strip end by tucking it neatly into the rest of the neck strip (Figure 12–12).
2. Lift the chair cloth from across the client's shoulders, slide into place around the neck, and fasten at the back of the neck (Figure 12–13).
3. Fold and flatten the top edge of the neck strip over the neckline of the chair cloth to prevent the client's skin from touching the drape (Figure 12–14). 4

12

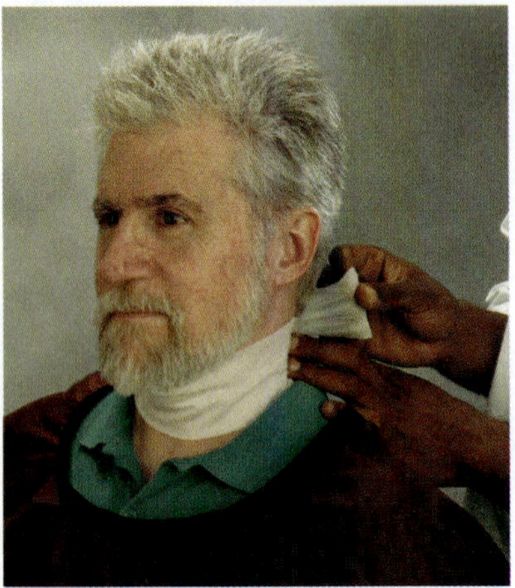

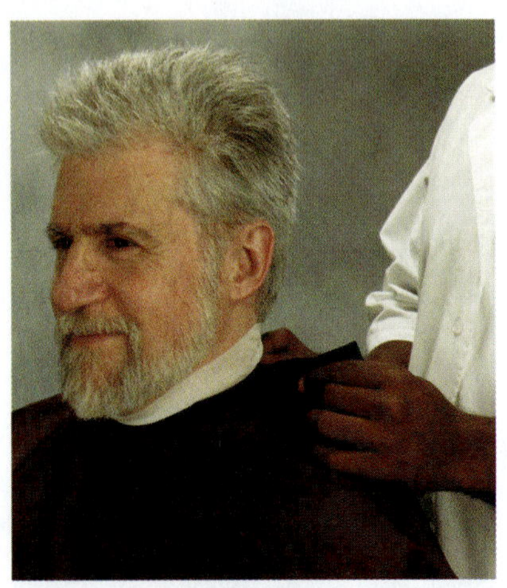

Figure 12-12 Drape chair cloth loosely and position neck strip around the neck.

Figure 12-13 Fasten drape.

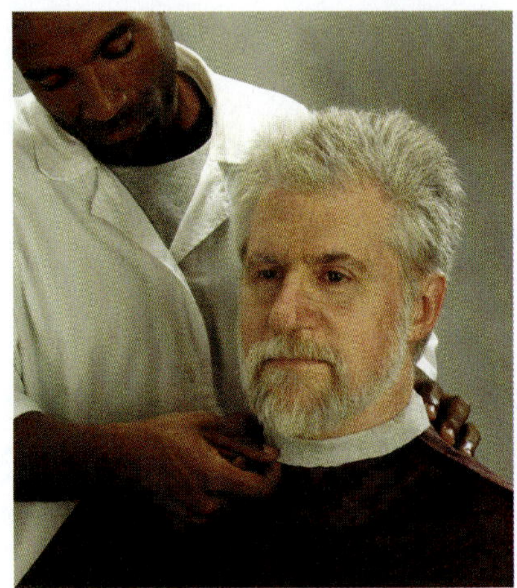

Figure 12-14 Fold and smooth neck strip.

THE SHAMPOO SERVICE

The shampoo service requires proper draping and positioning of the client, scalp manipulations to facilitate the shampoo procedure, and proper body positioning of the barber. Most barbershops are equipped with shampoo bowls either within a working booth area or in a separate section of the shop. Typically, the barber stands beside the client and shampoo bowl while performing the shampoo. Some shops have been equipped, however, with the European-style shampoo bowl, which is a free-standing unit that allows the barber to stand in back of the client's head.

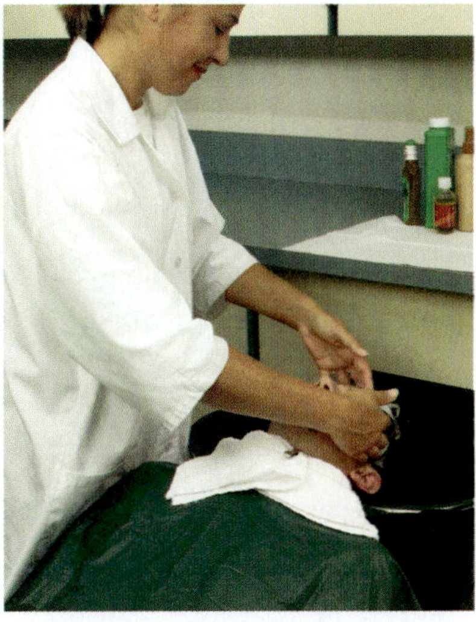

Figure 12–15 Reclined method.

Methods of Shampooing and Rinsing

Two methods are used for shampooing and rinsing: reclined and inclined.

- The *reclined method* of shampooing is the most commonly used. The hydraulic or shampoo chair is reclined with the client's head positioned in the neck rest of the shampoo bowl (Figure 12–15). This method is favored because it is more comfortable for the client and permits greater speed and efficiency for the barber.
- The *inclined method* can be used when a standard shampoo bowl is not available or when the client cannot use the reclined method. This method requires the client to bend his head forward over the shampoo bowl or sink (Figure 12–16). The client may sit on a stool or chair positioned close to the sink.

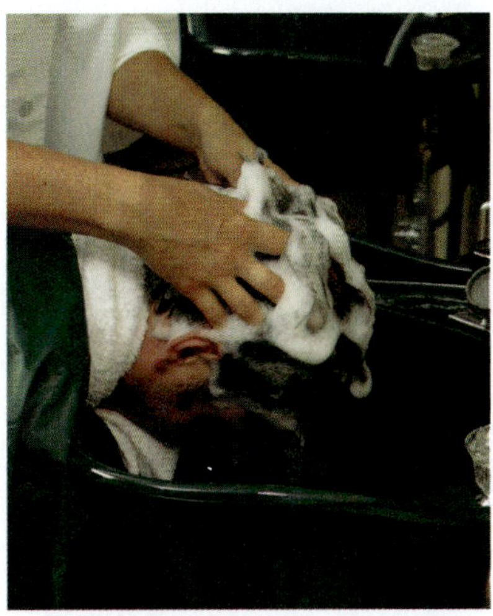

Figure 12–16 Inclined method.

Physical Presentation

To prevent muscle aches, back strain, and fatigue it is important to maintain good posture at the shampoo bowl. Review the following suggestions to maintain a good posture while shampooing.

1. Stand as close as possible to the back of the client's head.
2. Flex the knees slightly and position your body directly over your feet to maintain good balance.
3. Try to keep your chin parallel to the floor to avoid neck strain. The head should be raised, with the chest up, abdomen flat, and the shoulders relaxed.
4. Do not bend or twist sideways from the waist or lean too far forward.

Superior Shampoo Service

Excellence in performing the shampoo service requires barbers and stylists to give individual attention to each client's needs. In addition to selecting the shampoo best suited to the condition of the scalp and hair, the effectiveness of the shampoo will depend on the manner in which the shampoo is applied, the quality of the scalp massage, and the manner in which the shampoo is rinsed from the hair.

A client may find fault with the shampoo service for any of the following reasons:

- Improper shampoo selection
- Insufficient scalp massage
- Extreme water temperatures, either too hot or too cold
- Shampoo or water that runs onto client's face, ears, or eyes
- Wetting or soiling the client's clothing
- Scraping or scratching the client's scalp with fingernails
- Improper hair blotting
- Insufficient cleansing and rinsing

In addition to learning what a superior shampoo service is all about, you will also need to become familiar with such aspects of the shampoo service as the set-up, selection of products, water temperature, application of shampoo, and shampoo massage manipulations.

Set-Up and Preparation

Adequate preparation is the first step in performing a good shampoo. Before starting, the barber should assemble all necessary supplies or have them stored in an area convenient to the shampoo bowl. Shampoo service supplies include cleansing and conditioning products, waterproof drapes, and terry cloth towels.

Product Selection

It is essential that the barber is knowledgeable about the products used in the shop. Always read product labels and follow the manufacturer's directions. To determine which product to use, the barber *must* perform a hair and scalp analysis. Six characteristics of the hair and scalp should be considered before choosing products:

1. Condition of the scalp: dry, oily, normal, abrasions or disorders present
2. Condition of the hair: dry, brittle, fragile, oily, normal, or chemically treated
3. Hair density: thin, medium, thick
4. Hair texture: fine, average, coarse
5. Hair porosity: average porosity, porous, nonporous
6. Hair elasticity: poor, average, very good

With practice and experience, barbering students learn the effects of certain products on the hair and scalp. For example, moisturizing shampoos are not alkaline enough to cleanse an oily scalp and hair condition. Also, heavy, cuticle-coating conditioners can "weigh down" fine hair, leaving it flat or oily, while coarse hair may require a humectant-rich, moisturizing conditioner to increase manageability (refer to Table 12–1).

Water Temperature

The water should be comfortably warm for the client. Cold water, in addition to causing discomfort, tends to reduce lathering. Hot water can cause the scalp to flake or become dry. Warm water is not only comfortable and relaxing for the client, it also reacts favorably during the foaming process.

Application of Shampoo

Following a warm-water rinse to dampen the hair, the shampoo product should be dispensed into the barber's hand and then dispersed over both palms to facilitate spreading it throughout the client's hair. Spread sections of the hair apart with the thumbs and fingers to apply the shampoo directly onto the scalp. Make sure that the entire scalp is covered. The shampoo should be massaged completely into the scalp and hair. Warm water is added gradually to work up a rich, creamy lather. As the lather is created and the scalp manipulated, be careful to avoid getting shampoo lather on the client's face.

All shampoo movements must be executed with the cushion tips of the fingers. The scalp manipulations are repeated several times, until the lather is completely worked into the hair and scalp. The excess lather is then removed by a sweep of the palm from the front to the back of the head and rinsed from the barber's hand. The hair is then rinsed thoroughly with a strong spray.

Shampoo Massage Manipulations

The proper way to massage the scalp during a shampoo is as follows:

1. Stand behind or to the side of the client at the shampoo bowl as the style of sink allows.
2. Wet the hair, protecting the client's face, ears, and neck (Figures 12–17 through 12–19).
3. Lather the hair, starting at the front hairline and working along the sides toward the back and nape areas (Figure 12–20).
4. Use rotary movements over the entire head area (Figures 12–21 through 12–23).
5. Repeat these movements for each section several times.

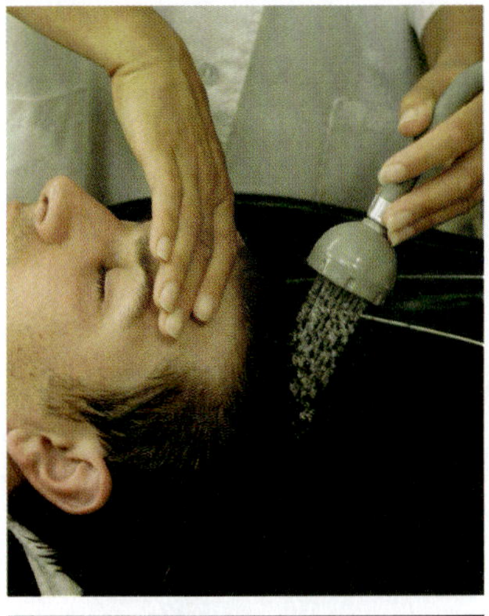

Figure 12-17 Protecting the face.

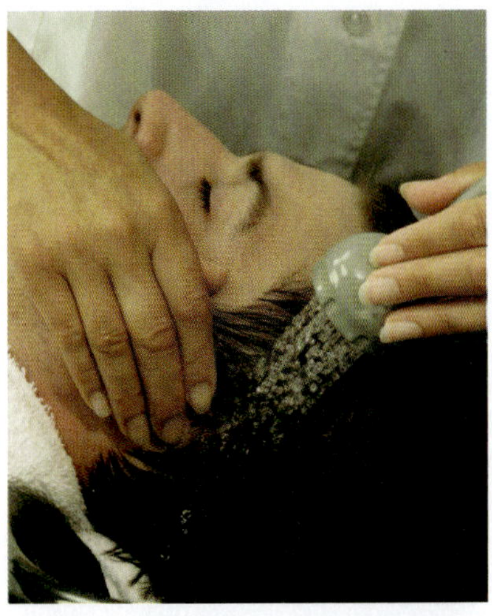

Figure 12-18 Protecting the ears.

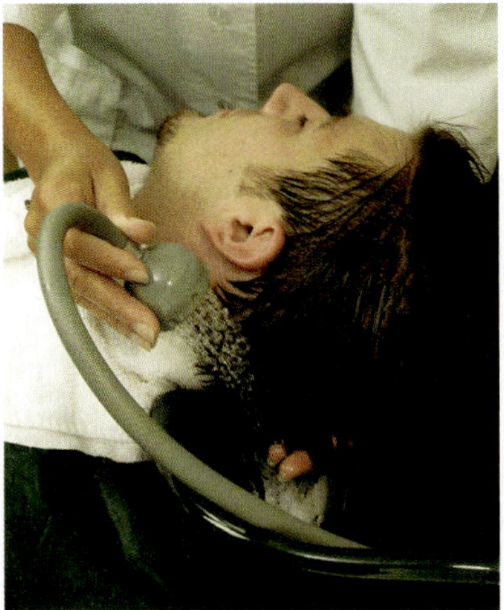

Figure 12-19 Supporting and protecting the neck.

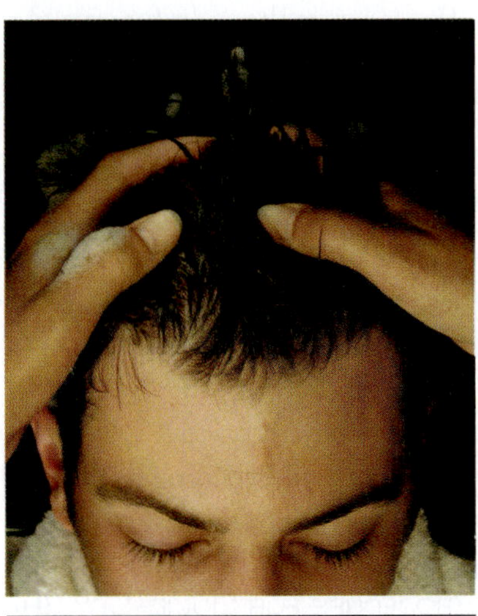

Figure 12-20 Lathering the hair.

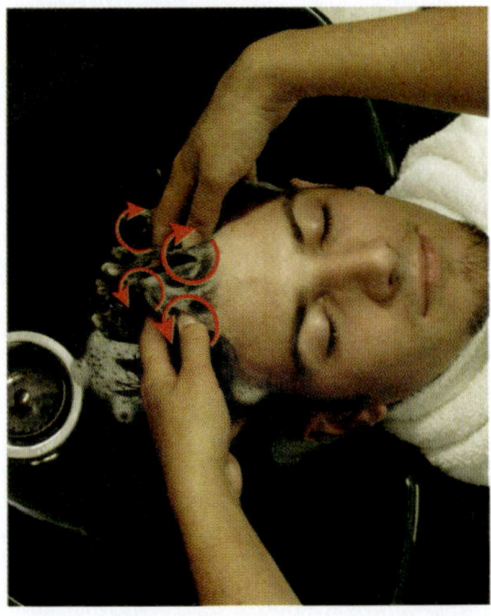

Figure 12-21 Rotary movements on top of head.

12

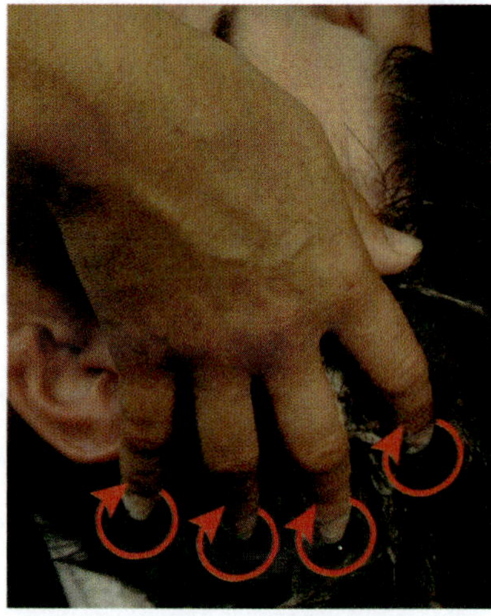

Figure 12-22 Rotary movements at sides of head.

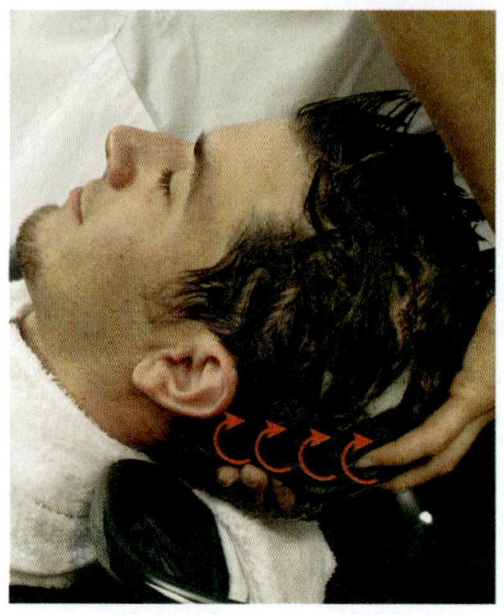

Figure 12-23 Rotary movements at back of head.

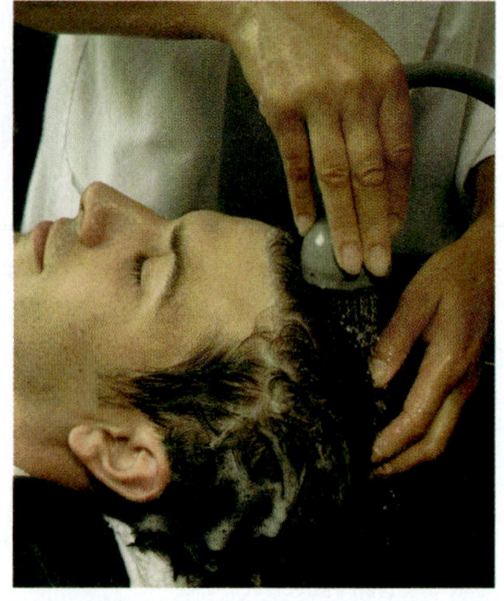

Figure 12-24 Rinse the hair thoroughly with warm water.

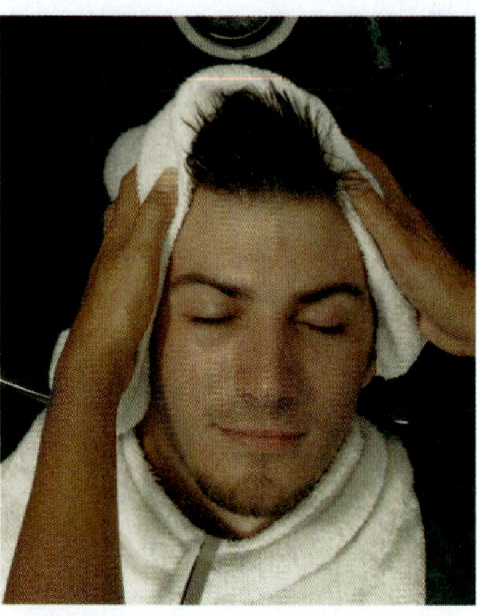

Figure 12-25 Blot the hair.

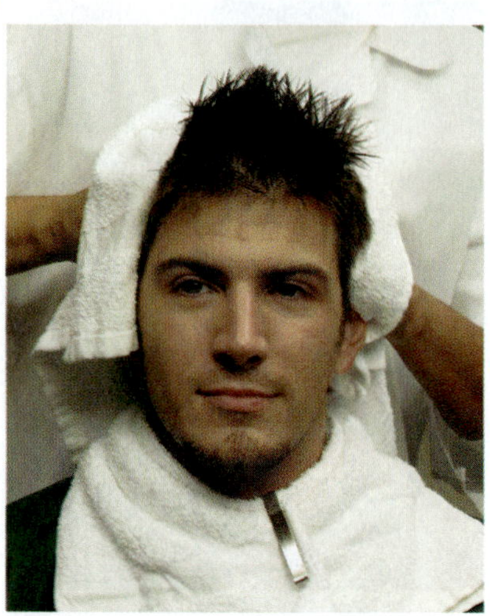

Figure 12-26 Lightly towel dry the hair.

THE SHAMPOO PROCEDURE

1. Seat the client in a comfortable and relaxed position.
2. Drape the client according to textbook or instructor's procedures.
3. Consult with the client about products, hair and scalp problems, or any questions they have about their hair or scalp.
4. Examine the condition of the client's hair and scalp. Briefly massage the scalp to loosen epidermal scales, debris, and scalp tissues.
5. Decide on the type of products to be used.
6. Position the client for the shampoo service. Drape back of cape over the chair back.
7. Wet the hair with warm water.
8. Apply shampoo to all parts of the scalp.
9. Massage the scalp for several minutes as described in the preceding section.
10. Rinse the hair thoroughly with warm water and repeat the lathering if necessary. (Suggest a hair rinse or conditioner at this time.)
11. Rinse the hair thoroughly with warm water (Figure 12–24).
12. Blot the hair (Figure 12–25).
13. Raise client to a sitting position and lightly towel dry the hair; wipe face and ears if necessary (Figure 12–26).
14. Comb hair into position for cutting (Figure 12–27).

   Note: With practice, you will develop a set-up routine for the shampoo service and become comfortable with asking clients questions that relate to the service. 5

Procedure for Liquid-Dry Shampoo

1. Brush the hair thoroughly and comb it lightly.
2. Part the hair into small sections.

3. Saturate a piece of cotton with the liquid-dry shampoo, squeeze it out lightly, and apply to the scalp along each part line. Follow by swiftly rubbing the scalp with a towel along the same area. Repeat this procedure over the entire head.
4. Saturate more cotton with the product and apply down the length of the hair strands.
5. Rub the hair strands with a towel to remove the soil.
6. Remoisten the hair lightly with liquid, and comb it into the desired style.

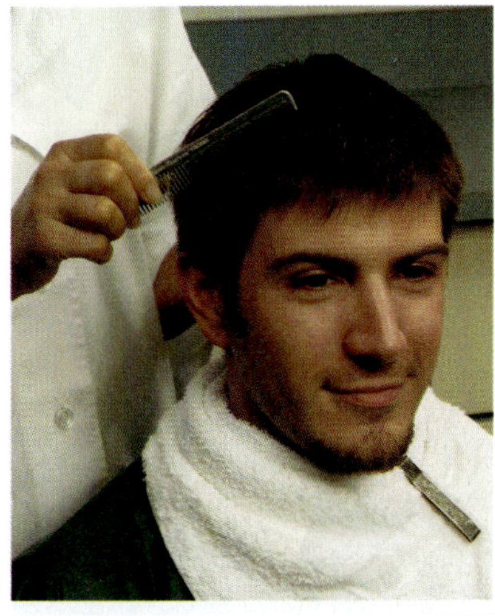

Figure 12-27 Comb the hair.

Procedure for Dry or Powder Shampoo

A dry or powder shampoo is usually given when the client's health will not permit a wet shampoo. Sprinkle the product into the hair and work it in one section at a time. Next, brush the hair to remove the powder.

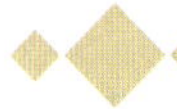

SCALP TREATMENTS

The purpose of scalp and hair treatments is to preserve the health and appearance of the hair and scalp. These treatments also help to prevent and combat scalp disorders such as dandruff, dryness, oiliness, or hair loss.

Cleanliness and stimulation are the essential basic requirements for healthy hair and scalp. Because the scalp and hair are so interrelated, many scalp disorders need correction in order to maintain the health of the hair. A healthy scalp will help to maintain a healthy head of hair.

Scalp treatments may be given separately or combined with hair treatments. In many cases, a product that is good for the scalp is also good for the hair. In other cases, separate products may need to be used. Conditions caused by neglect, such as a tight scalp, overactive or underactive oil glands, and tense nerves may be corrected by proper scalp treatments. Depending on the client's needs, the scalp treatment may include:

1. Cleansing with a suitable shampoo.
2. Massage with the hands or electrical appliance.
3. Use of electrical appliances, such as an electric steamer, infrared lamp, ultraviolet lamp, high-frequency current, or dermal lamp.
4. The application of cosmetic preparations, such as hair tonics, astringents, antiseptics, or ointments.

CAUTION

Do not suggest a scalp treatment if abrasions or lesions are present. Advise clients with serious or contagious scalp disorders to consult a physician.

Scalp Steam

The **scalp steam** is effective in preparing the scalp for scalp massage manipulations and treatments. Steam relaxes the pores, softens the scalp and hair, and increases blood circulation. A scalp steamer assures a constant and controlled source of steam; however, steam towels can also be used effectively. To use a scalp steamer, fill the container with water, fit the hood over the client's head, and turn on the current. Many hoods have openings on the side so the barber's hands can be inserted to perform a scalp massage during the scalp steam.

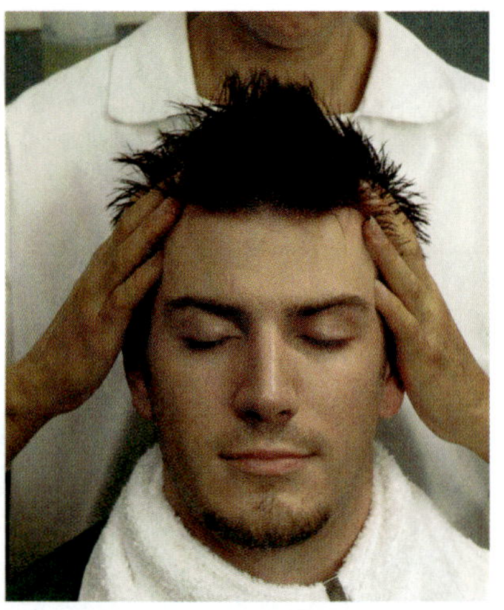

Figure 12-36 Ear-to-crown movement.

Refer to Table 12–2 to review the muscles, nerves, and arteries affected by scalp massage.

Scalp Treatment with an Electric Massager

An electric massager, sometimes called a vibrator or hand massager, is an electrical tool that is used to perform a stimulating scalp massage. Before using, adjust the vibrator on the back of the hand, leaving the thumb and fingers free. Then turn on the current. The vibrations are transmitted through the cushions of the fingertips. The same movements are followed as for a regular hand scalp massage. When using the vibrator on the scalp, be careful to regulate the intensity and duration of the vibrations, as well as the pressure applied (Figure 12–37).

Scalp massage is most effective when given in a series of treatments and may be advised for general scalp maintenance, to promote hair growth, or to correct a scalp condition.

Scalp Treatment for Normal Scalp and Hair

The purpose of a general scalp treatment is to keep the scalp and hair clean and healthy. Regular scalp treatments can also help to prevent baldness.

1. Drape the client.
2. Brush the hair for a few minutes to loosen dead skin cells.
3. Part the hair and apply a scalp conditioner or ointment directly to the scalp with a cotton pledget or cotton swab (Figure 12–38).

Massage and Its Influence on the Scalp

Massage Movements	Muscles	Nerves	Arteries
Sliding Movement (Fig. 12–31)	Auricularis superior	Posterior auricular	Frontal & Parietal
Neck-to-Crown Movement (Fig. 12–32)	Auricularis posterior	Greater occipital	Occipital
Forehead-to-Crown Movement (Fig. 12–33)	Frontalis	Supra-orbital	Frontal
Front Hairline Movement (Fig. 12–34)	Frontalis	Supra-orbital	Frontal & Parietal
Rotary Movement (Fig. 12–35)	Auricularis posterior	Greater occipital	Posterior auricular & Parietal
Ear-to-Crown Movement (Fig. 12–36)	Auricularis anterior & superior	Temporal auricular	Frontal & Parietal

Table 12-2 Massage and Its Influence on the Scalp

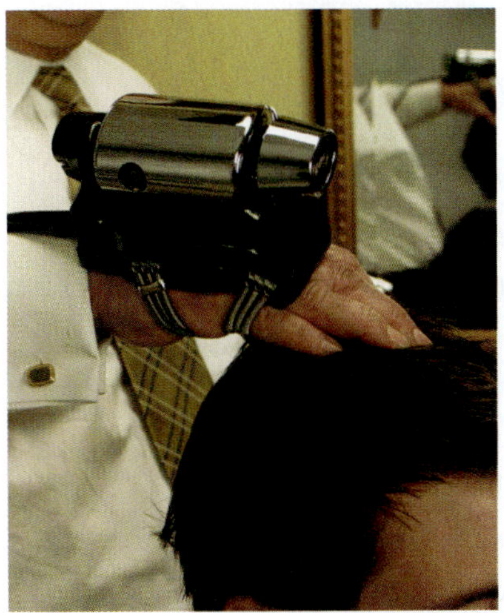

Figure 12-37 Hand-held electric massager.

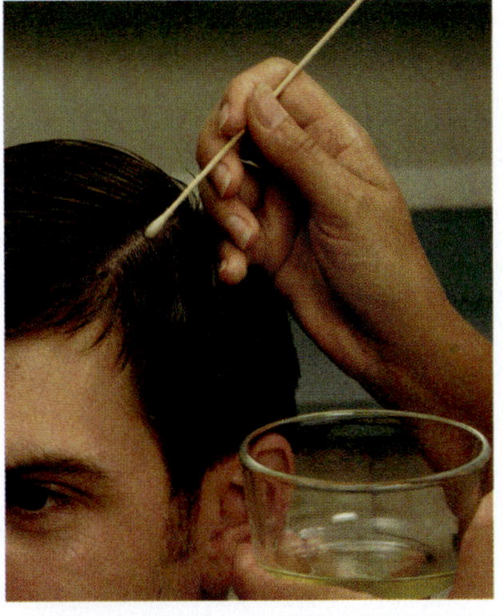

Figure 12-38 Apply scalp conditioner.

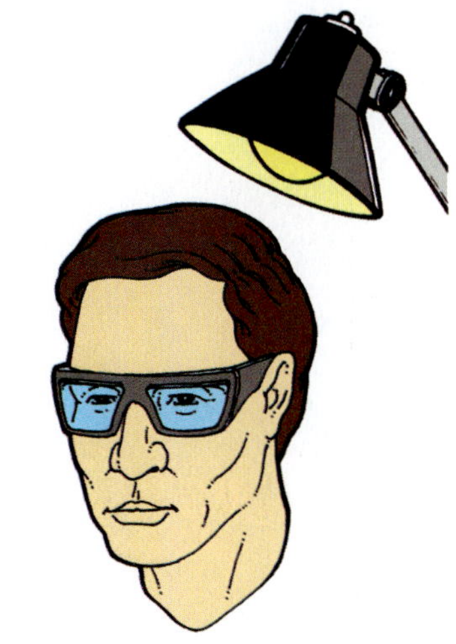

Figure 12-39 Apply infrared lamp.

4. Apply infrared lamp for three to five minutes (Figure 12–39).
5. Massage the scalp for 10 minutes.
6. Shampoo the hair and towel dry.
7. Optional step: Stimulate the scalp with high-frequency current for two to three minutes.
8. Apply a suitable scalp lotion or tonic and work it well into the scalp.
9. Comb and style the hair.

CAUTION

Never use a scalp or hair treatment product that contains alcohol *before* applying high-frequency current. Such products can be safely applied only *after* the high-frequency treatment.

Dry-Scalp and -Hair Treatment

Inactivity of the oil glands, or the excessive removal of natural oil, produces dry hair and scalp conditions. Other causes contributing to dry hair and scalp are an indoor lifestyle, frequent washing with strong soaps or shampoos, and the continued use of drying tonics or lotions. Select scalp preparations that contain moisturizing and emollient agents. Avoid the use of strong soaps, preparations containing a mineral or sulfonated oil base, greasy preparations, and lotions with a high alcohol content.

1. Drape the client.
2. Brush the client's hair.
3. Massage and stimulate the scalp for three to five minutes.
4. Apply a scalp preparation for this condition.
5. Steam the scalp with hot towels or scalp steamer for 7 to 10 minutes.
6. Shampoo the hair using a mild shampoo suitable for dry scalp and hair.
7. Towel dry the hair, making sure the scalp is thoroughly dried.
8. Apply scalp cream sparingly with a rotary, frictional motion.
9. Apply an infrared lamp over the scalp for three to five minutes.
10. Stimulate the scalp with direct high-frequency current, using a glass rake electrode, for about five minutes (Figure 12–40).

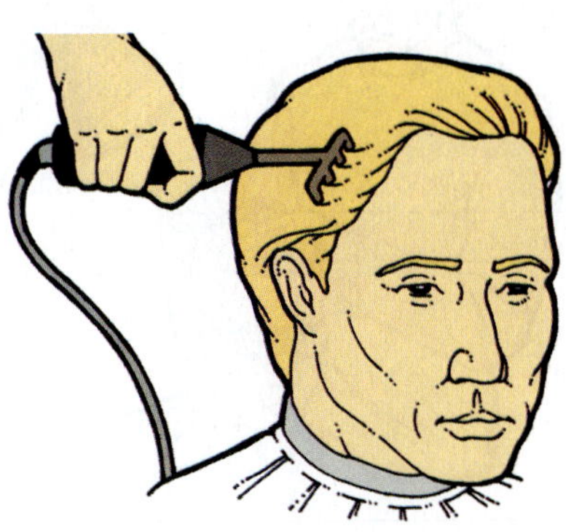

Figure 12-40 Applying high-frequency current.

11. Rinse the hair thoroughly.
12. Comb the hair into the desired style.

Oily-Scalp and -Hair Treatment

The main cause of an oily scalp is overactive sebaceous glands. Manipulating the scalp will increase circulation and help to release hardened sebum from the follicles.

1. Drape the client.
2. Brush the hair.
3. Apply a medicated scalp lotion to the scalp only.
4. Apply infrared lamp or scalp steamer for three to five minutes.
5. Massage the scalp. (Option: Faradic or sinusoidal current may be used.)
6. Shampoo with a product suitable for oily scalp and hair.
7. Towel dry the hair.
8. Apply direct high-frequency current for three to five minutes.
9. Apply a medicated lotion or astringent to the scalp only.
10. Comb the hair into the desired style.

Dandruff Scalp Treatment

The principal signs of dandruff are the appearance of white scales on the hair and scalp accompanied by itching. Dandruff may be associated with either a dry (pityriasis capitis simplex) or a more severe oily condition (pityriasis steatoides). Other contributing causes of dandruff are poor blood circulation to the scalp, improper diet, and lack of hygienic practices.

1. Drape the client.
2. Shampoo with an antidandruff shampoo, according to the type of dandruff.
3. Towel dry the hair.
4. Apply antidandruff conditioner or antiseptic lotion to the scalp.
5. Apply steam towels or scalp steamer for three to five minutes.
6. Massage the scalp.
7. Shampoo again with an antidandruff shampoo.
8. Both the barber and the client should put on tinted safety goggles.
9. Expose the scalp to ultraviolet rays (for its germicidal effects) for five to eight minutes, parting the hair every half inch (Figure 12–41).
10. Apply antidandruff conditioner or lotion to the scalp.
11. Expose the scalp to an infrared lamp for five minutes to help penetration of the lotion.
12. Comb hair into desired style.

Alternate Step: In place of Step 11, high-frequency current may be applied for three to five minutes. Be sure, however, that the antidandruff conditioner or lotion used in Step 10 does not contain alcohol.

12

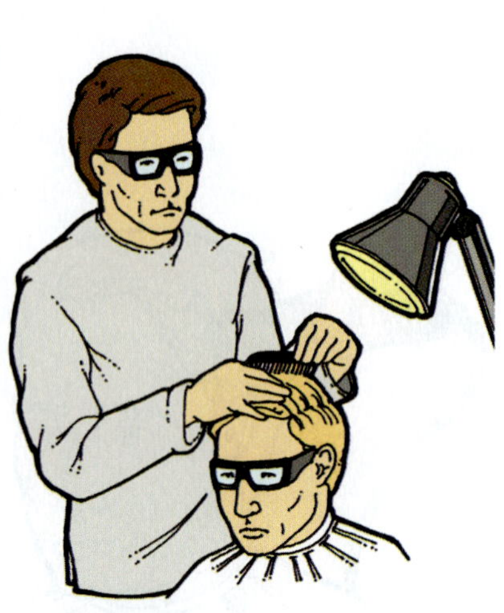

Figure 12–41 Applying ultraviolet rays.

Scalp Treatment for Alopecia

Alopecia is the term used to describe hair loss. The chief causes of alopecia are heredity, poor circulation, lack of proper stimulation, improper nourishment, certain infectious skin diseases such as ringworm, or constitutional disorders. Conditions of alopecia may benefit from stimulation of the blood supply to the germinal papilla through scalp treatments.

1. Apply regular scalp manipulations.
2. Shampoo the hair and scalp as required (dry or oily).
3. Dry the scalp thoroughly.
4. Protect the client's and barber's eyes with goggles.
5. Expose the scalp to ultraviolet rays for about five minutes.
6. Apply a medicated scalp ointment as directed by a physician.
7. Apply indirect high-frequency current (with the client holding the wire glass electrode between both hands) for about five minutes.
8. Comb the hair into the desired style.

Corrective Hair Treatment

A corrective hair treatment deals with the hair shaft, rather than the scalp. Dry and damaged hair can be greatly improved by reconditioning (corrective) treatments that make the hair soft and pliable. Dry hair may be softened quickly with a reconditioning preparation applied directly on the outside of the hair shaft. The product used for this purpose is usually an emulsion containing cholesterol and related compounds.

1. Drape the client.
2. Massage and stimulate the scalp for three to five minutes.
3. Apply a mild shampoo and rinse thoroughly.
4. Blot the hair with a towel.
5. Apply a deep-conditioning agent according to the manufacturer's directions.
6. Rinse conditioner thoroughly.
7. Comb the hair into the desired style.

Hair Tonic Treatments

Scalp steamers, steam towels, vibrators, and scalp manipulations may all be used with hair tonics. During scalp steams, apply the tonic after the scalp has been steamed and before combing the hair into the desired style.

For a hair tonic treatment, massage the scalp, apply scalp steam, massage again with hands or a vibrator, and comb the hair into the desired style. 6

chapter glossary

acid-balanced shampoos	shampoo that is balanced to the pH of hair and skin (4.5–5.5)
balancing shampoos	designed for hair and scalp conditions
bluing rinses	temporary colors or shampoo products with a blue base used to offset yellow and gray tones in hair
clarifying shampoos	shampoos containing an acidic ingredient that cuts through product buildup
color-enhancing shampoos	created by combining surfactant bases with basic dyes
conditioners	chemical agents used to deposit protein or moisturizers in the hair
deep-conditioning treatments	chemical mixtures of concentrated protein and moisturizers
draping	covering the client's clothing with a cape or chair cloth
dry or powder shampoos	shampoos that cleanse the hair without water
instant conditioners	conditioners that typically remain on the hair from one to five minutes and are rinsed out
leave-in conditioners	conditioners and thermal protectors that can be left in the hair without rinsing
liquid shampoos	available in cream or clear forms and contain soap or soap jelly
liquid-dry shampoos	liquid shampoos that evaporate quickly and do not require rinsing
medicated rinses	rinses formulated to control minor dandruff and scalp conditions
medicated shampoos	shampoos containing medicinal agents for control of dandruff and other scalp conditions
moisturizing or conditioning shampoo	products formulated to add moisture to dry hair
moisturizing shampoo	mild cream shampoos containing humectants
organic shampoos	formulated from natural organic ingredients
powder or dry shampoos	may contain orris root powder and cleanse the hair without water; powder is brushed out of the hair.
protein conditioners	products designed to slightly increase hair diameter with a coating action and to replace lost proteins in hair
rinse	an agent used to cleanse or condition the hair and scalp
scalp conditioners	cream-based products and ointments used to soften and improve the health of the scalp
scalp steam	process of using steam towels or steaming unit to open scalp pores
shampoos	hair cleansers
surfactant	a base detergent
synthetic polymer conditioners	formulations designed to repair extremely damaged hair
tonic	product used to groom the hair or to maintain the health of the scalp

chapter review questions

1. Identify the parts and functions of the shampoo molecule.
2. Describe the chemical composition of shampoo.
3. List the three basic types of shampoo.
4. Explain the characteristics of anionic, cationic, nonionic, and amphoteric surfactants.
5. Why is the acidity or alkalinity of products important to the barber?
6. Explain the effect of acidic solutions on hair and skin; of alkaline solutions.
7. List seven types of conditioners.
8. Identify the hair type that may require a synthetic polymer.
9. List the different types of hair tonics.
10. Explain the purpose of draping a client.
11. Explain the purpose of the towel or neck strip in draping.
12. Describe the type of cape that should be used for wet and chemical services. Why?
13. Describe the type of cape that is preferred for haircutting services. Why?
14. Outline the important steps in giving a shampoo.
15. Outline the massage manipulations applied to the scalp during a shampoo.
16. Compare the massage manipulations used in a shampoo service to the manipulations used in a scalp massage.
17. List the scalp treatments that use ultraviolet rays; infrared rays.
18. Identify three important CAUTIONS associated with scalp treatments.

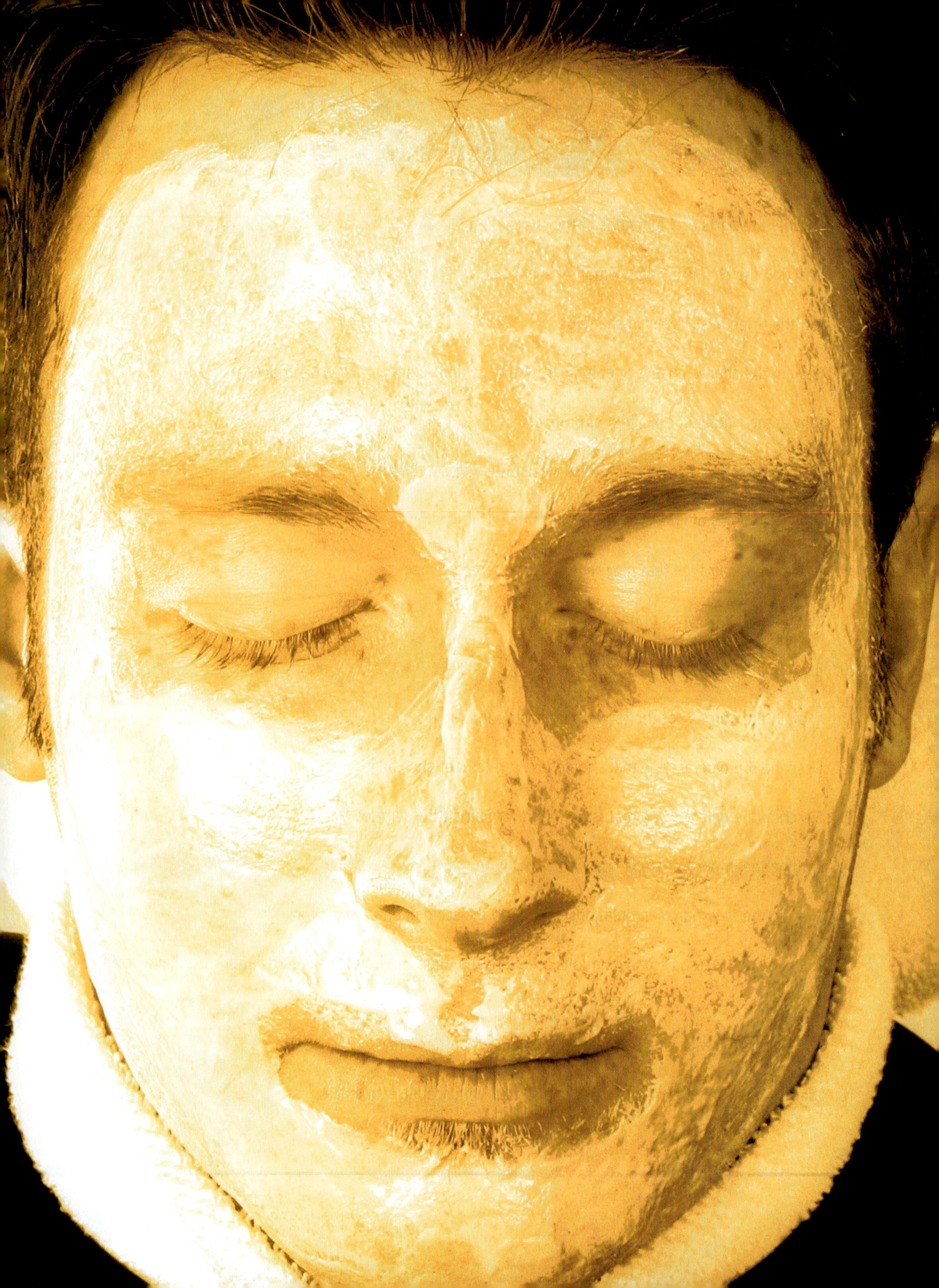

MEN'S FACIAL MASSAGE AND TREATMENTS

Chapter Outline

Arteries Affected by Facial Massage

An artery is a tubular, thick-walled, elastic vessel that, like capillaries and veins, is part of the circulatory system that transports blood from the heart to all parts of the body. Blood returns to the heart through the veins. The primary arteries that are affected by facial massage are presented in Table 13–4.

Artery	Arterial Branches and Blood Supply Areas	
Common carotids Main sources of blood supply to the head, face, and neck; located at the sides of the neck	Internal division: supplies the brain, eye sockets, eyelids, and forehead External division: supplies superficial parts of the head, face, and neck	
External maxillary (facial artery) supplies the lower region of the face, mouth, and nose	Submental: supplies chin and lower lip Inferior labial: supplies lower lip Angular: supplies side of the nose Superior labial: supplies upper lip, septum, and the wings of the nose	
Superficial temporal	Continuation of External Carotid	Supplies muscles, skin, and scalp on the front, side, and top of the head
	Frontal	Supplies the forehead
	Parietal	Supplies the crown and sides of the head
	Transverse facial	Supplies the masseter
	Middle temporal	Supplies the temples and eyelids
	Anterior auricular	Supplies the anterior part of the ear
Occipital	Supplies the scalp and back of the head up to the crown	
	Sternocleidomastoideus	Supplies the sternocleidomastoideus muscle
Posterior auricular	Supplies the scalp, behind and above the ear	
	Auricular	Supplies the skin in back of the ear

Table 13–4 Arteries Affected by Facial Massage

Veins Affected by Facial Massage

The deoxygenated blood returning to the heart from the head, face, and neck flows on each side of the neck in two principal veins: the internal jugular and the external jugular. The most important veins are parallel to the arteries and take the same names as the arteries. Both the internal and external jugular veins serve the areas of head, face, neck, and chest.

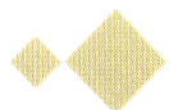

THEORY OF MASSAGE

Most clients enjoy a properly administered facial treatment for its stimulating and relaxing effects. Facial massage involves the external manipulation of the face and requires a skillful touch. This is accomplished with the hands, or with the aid of electrical appliances such as electric massagers or vibrators. Each massage movement is executed in such a way as to obtain a specific result.

The benefits of massage depend upon the type, intensity, and extent of the manipulations used. Massage must be performed systematically and never in a casual or irregular manner. The condition of the skin and the general physical condition of the client should always be considered. Normal skin may receive soothing, mildly stimulating, or strongly stimulating massage treatments. Sensitive, inflamed skin could be further damaged, however, by massage. If massage is desired, the manipulations must be gentle and soothing to damaged or sensitive skin. Massage should be used with judgment and moderation.

Massage should never be recommended or employed when the following conditions are present:

- Inflammation of the skin
- Severe skin lesions
- Pus-containing pimples
- High blood pressure
- Skin infection

Massage Manipulations

When massaging any part of the head, face, or neck, any pressure should be applied in an upward direction. This rule should be followed in all massage manipulations, whether they are intended to stimulate, relax, or soothe the skin. When applying rotary manipulations, the same rule applies because the pressure should be applied on the upward swing of the movement.

An understanding of the motor points of the face is important in the performance of an effective facial massage. A motor point is a point on the skin over a muscle where pressure or stimulation will cause contraction of that muscle. A review of the motor points as illustrated in Figure 13–1 will assist in the manipulation of the facial muscles during a treatment.

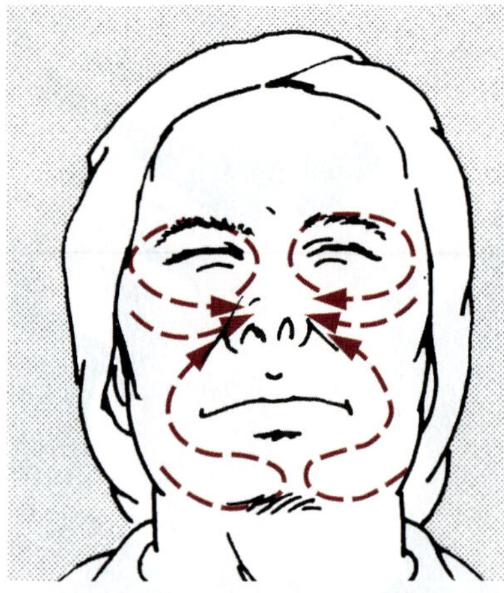
Figure 13-8 Applying cleansing cream.

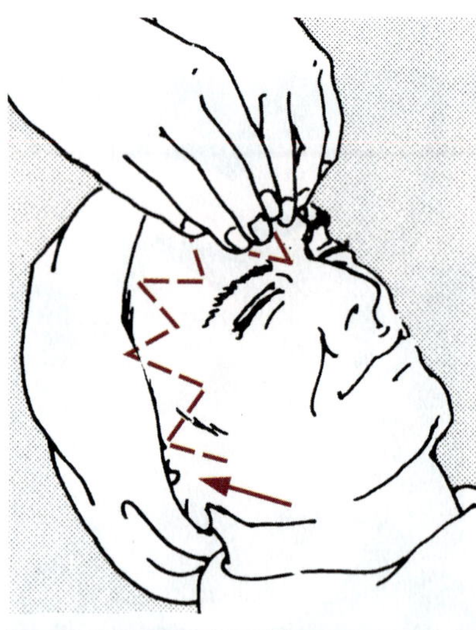
Figure 13-9 Using up-and-down movements across forehead.

- The activity of the skin and scalp glands is stimulated.
- The skin is rendered soft and pliable.
- The nerves are soothed and rested.
- Pain is sometimes relieved.

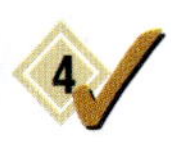

Facial Massage Manipulations

When performing facial massage manipulations, remember that an even tempo or rhythm induces relaxation. Once the manipulations have begun, one or both of the hands should remain on the skin at all times. When it becomes necessary to remove the hands, avoid abrupt motions and gently feather-off the hands from the skin.

Remember that massage movements are directed from the insertion toward the origin of a muscle to avoid damage to muscular tissues. Refer to Figure 13–1 and apply minimal pressure on the motor points of the face when performing the massage manipulations listed below.

Figures 13–8 through 13–16 show different massage movements that may be used on the various parts of the face and neck. Your instructor may employ a massage manipulation procedure that is equally correct. The following massage techniques correlate to the illustrations pictured in Figures 13–8 through 13–16.

1. Apply cleansing cream lightly over the face with stroking, spreading, and circulatory movements (Figure 13–8).
2. Stroke fingers across forehead with up-and-down movements (Figure 13–9).
3. Manipulate fingers across the forehead with a circular movement (Figure 13–10).
4. Stroke fingers upward along sides of nose (Figure 13–11).
5. Apply a circular movement over sides of nose and use a light, stroking movement around the eyes (Figure 13–12).

13

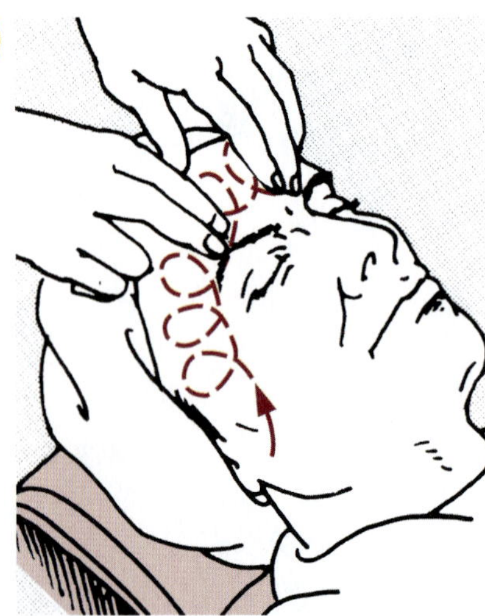
Figure 13-10 Circular movement across the forehead.

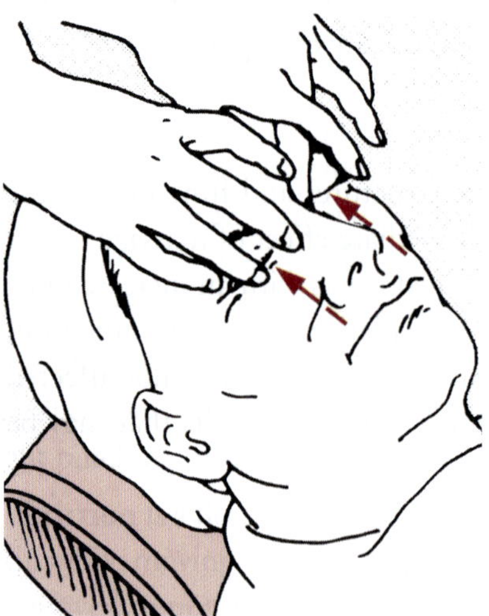
Figure 13-11 Stroking movement along side of nose.

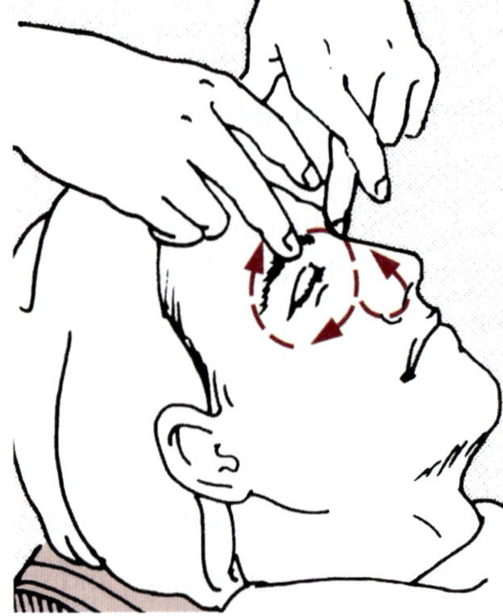
Figure 13-12 A combination of circular and stroking movements.

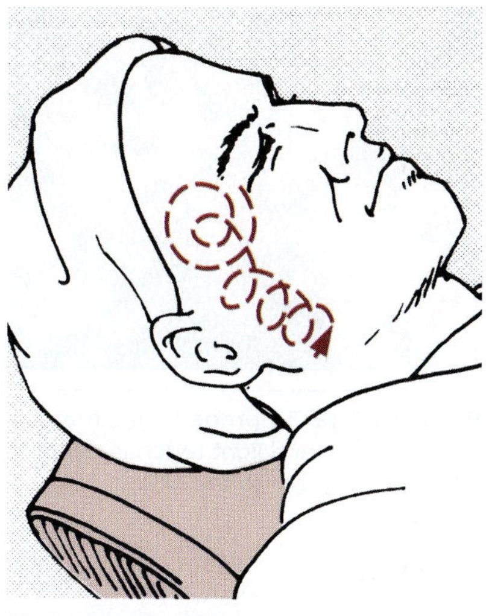

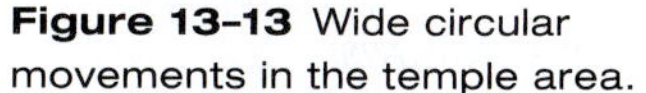

Figure 13–13 Wide circular movements in the temple area.

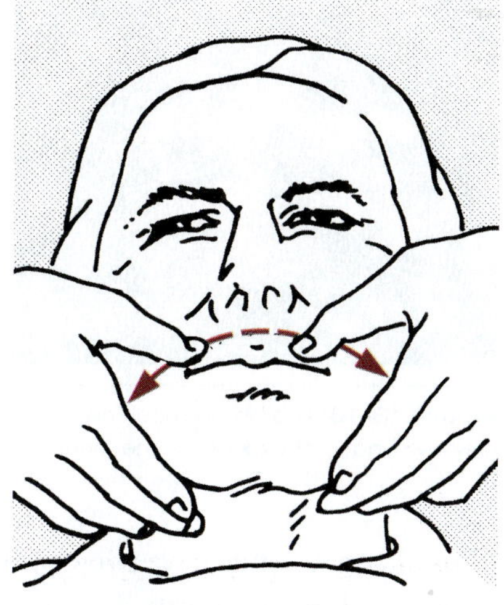

Figure 13–14 Stroking movement across upper lip.

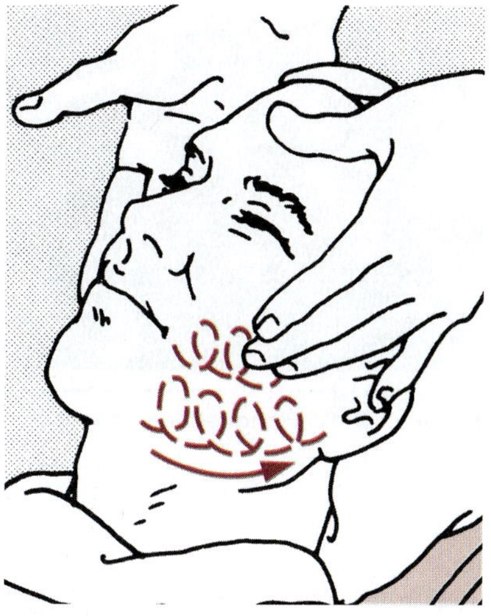

Figure 13–15 Rotary circular movements on the lower face.

6. Manipulate the temples, and then the front and back of the ears, with a wide circular movement (Figure 13–13).
7. Gently stroke both thumbs across upper lip (Figure 13–14).
8. Manipulate fingers from the corners of the mouth to the cheeks and temples with a rotary (circular) movement. Manipulate fingers along the lower jaw from the tip of the chin to the ear using the same technique (Figure 13–15).
9. Stroke fingers above and below lower jawbone from the chin to the ear. Manipulate fingers from under the chin and neck to the back of the ears and up to the temples (Figure 13–16). 5

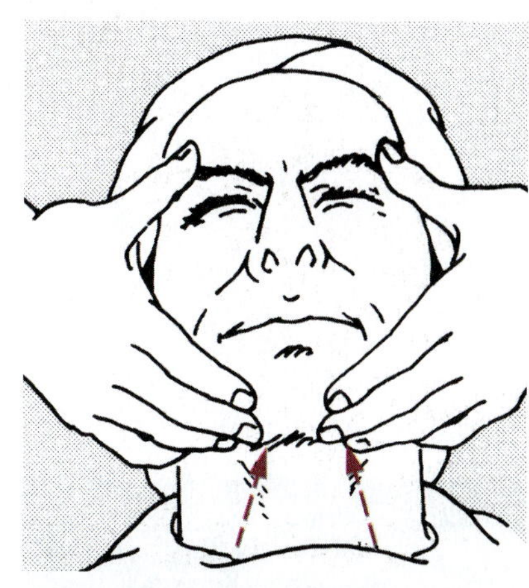

Figure 13–16 Manipulating fingers from under chin to back of ears to temples.

EQUIPMENT FOR MASSAGE TREATMENTS

In addition to massage techniques performed with the hands, appliances such as massagers or vibrators, brush machines, electrical modalities, and light rays can be used to enhance the facial treatment service.

The **electric massager** most often used in barbershops is a handheld unit that transmits vibrations through the barber's hand to the client's skin and muscles (Figure 13–17). This type of massaging technique is used over heavy muscle tissue such as the scalp and shoulders to produce a succession of stimulating impulses. It has an invigorating effect on muscle tissue, increases the blood supply to the parts treated, is soothing to the nerves, increases glandular activity, and stimulates the skin and scalp. When used correctly, electric massagers can be used to perform vibratory facials. CAUTION: Some hand massager appliances are heavy and cumbersome for smaller hands. Always "try one on for size" before purchasing.

The *brush machine* helps to stimulate, cleanse, and lightly exfoliate the skin. Many different models are available by a variety of manufacturers.

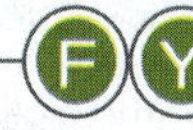

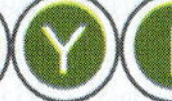

FYI

Massage manipulations on the face are usually performed with upward movements; however, the presence of facial hair may require a different approach. Direct massage movements in the direction of beard growth. Massage manipulations that go against or across the grain may cause discomfort to the client.

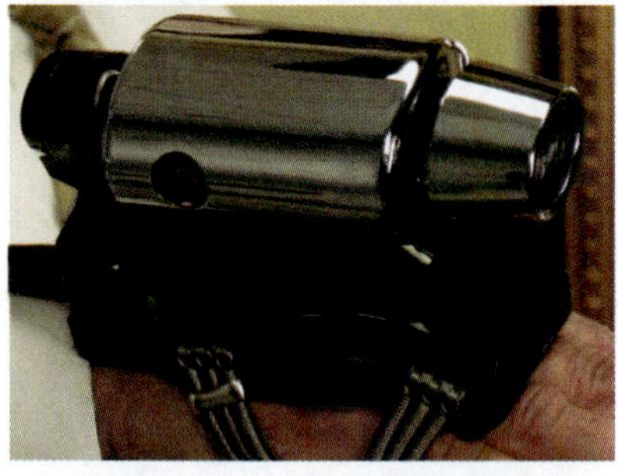

Figure 13-17 Handheld massager.

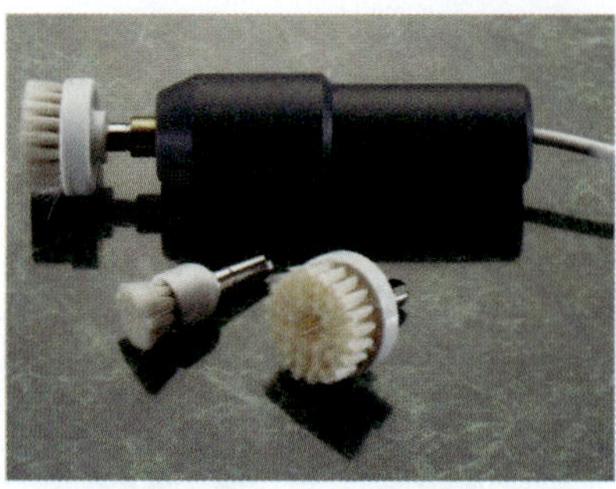

Figure 13-18 The brush machine helps cleanse and lightly exfoliate the skin.

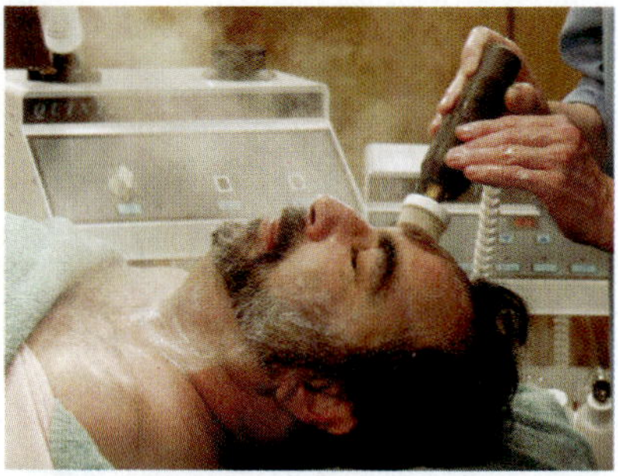

Figure 13-19 To properly use the brush machine, a light touch is used, with no pressure on the skin.

Typically these units have two or three small brush attachments that can be rotated at different speeds (Figure 13–18).

The procedure for using a rotary brush machine is as follows:

1. Perform a light cleansing on the skin.
2. Insert the appropriate size brush for the face into the handheld device.
3. Apply more cleanser to the skin.
4. Dip the brush into water and begin the pattern of movement at the forehead.
5. Continue the rotation down the cheeks, nose, upper lip, chin, jaw, and neck areas. No pressure should be applied with the bristles of the brush remaining straight (Figure 13–19).
6. Remoisten the brush as needed during the process. Dryer skin types require a slow, steady rotation. Thicker, oily skin types can tolerate a faster speed. CAUTION: The rotary brush *is not* recommended for use on inflamed or acne-prone skin.

Steamers are electrical devices that produce and project moist, uniform steam that can be positioned over sections of the head or face for softening and cleansing purposes. The steam warms the skin, inducing the flow of both oil and sweat, and has an antiseptic effect for problematic skin.

Steamers may be used in place of hot towels for scalp and hair reconditioning treatments. When positioned over the scalp, the steam softens the skin, increases perspiration, and promotes the effectiveness of applied scalp tonics and lotions.

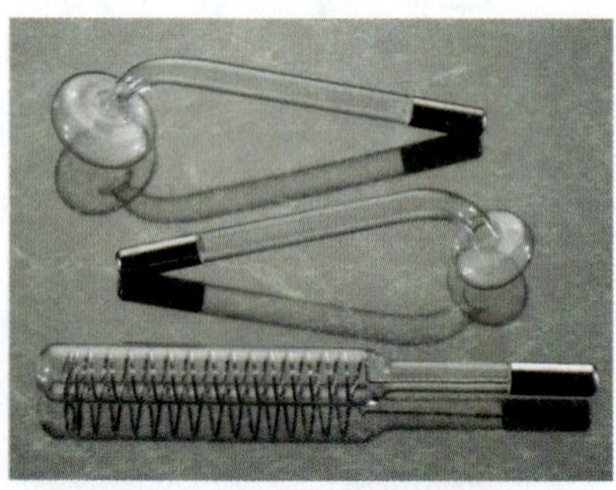

Figure 13-20 Electrodes for the high-frequency machine.

13

Facial treatments performed with *electric facial machines* are a form of electrotherapy. As you learned in Chapter 9 there are several electrical currents, or modalities, used in electrotherapy: high-frequency, galvanic, faradic, and sinusoidal currents. Some electric facial machines can generate all four currents and others may produce only one or two.

Electrical modality machines require an *electrode* to apply and direct the current to the client's skin. Except for the high-frequency modality (Figure 13–20), each of the currents requires two electrodes, one positive and one negative, to conduct the flow of electricity through the body. A positive electrode (anode) is red and a negative electrode (cathode) is black, with plus- and minus-sign markings respectively (Figure 13–21).

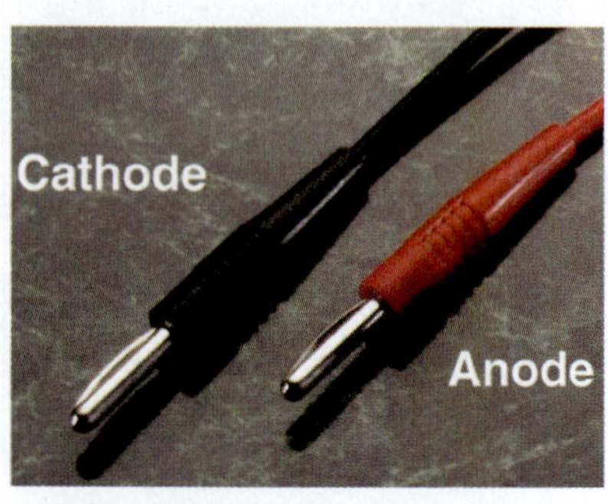

Figure 13-21 Anode and cathode.

Type of Light	Beneficial Effects
Ultraviolet	Increases the elimination of waste products Improves the flow of blood and lymph Has a germicidal and antibacterial effect Produces vitamin D in the skin Can be used to treat rickets, psoriasis, and acne Produces a tan
Infrared	Heats and relaxes the skin Dilates blood vessels and increases circulation Produces chemical changes Increases metabolism Increases production of perspiration and oil Deep penetration relieves pain in sore muscles Soothes nerves
White Light	Relieves pain in the back of the neck and shoulders Produces some chemical and germicidial effects Relaxes muscles
Blue Light	Soothes nerves Improves skin tone Provides some chemical and germicidal effects Used for mild cases of skin eruptions Produces little heat
Red Light	Improves dry, scaly wrinkled skin Relaxes muscles Penetrates the deepest Produces the most heat

Table 13-5 Effects of Light Therapy

Light rays are used to impart light therapy treatments on the skin. Infrared, ultraviolet, white, blue, and red rays are used to produce different effects through the use of therapeutic lamps. Single-function and combination units are available in floor and tabletop models as discussed in Chapter 9. Table 13–5 provides a summary of the types of light used in treatments and their beneficial effects.

High-Frequency Machine

High-frequency or Tesla current is characterized by a high rate of oscillation that is used for both scalp and facial treatments. Although it is sometimes called the violet ray because of its color, there are no ultraviolet rays in high-frequency current.

The primary actions of high-frequency current are thermal and antiseptic. Its rapid vibrations do not produce muscular contractions or chemical changes so the physiological effects are either stimulating or soothing, depending on the method of application.

CAUTION

When performing electrotherapy treatments, the barber and the client must avoid contact with metals or water.

The electrodes for high-frequency machines are made of glass or metal. Their shapes vary from the flat facial electrode to the rake-shaped scalp electrode. As the current passes through the glass electrode, tiny violet sparks are emitted. All high-frequency treatments should be started with a mild current, which is gradually increased to the required strength. The length of the treatment depends upon the condition to be treated. For general facial or scalp treatments, no more than five minutes should be allowed.

The high-frequency machine is a versatile tool that can benefit the client's skin in the following ways:

1. Stimulates blood circulation
2. Helps to oxygenate the skin
3. Increases glandular activity
4. Aids in elimination and absorption
5. Increases cell metabolism
6. Promotes antiseptic and germicidal action
7. Generates a warm feeling that has a relaxing effect on the skin

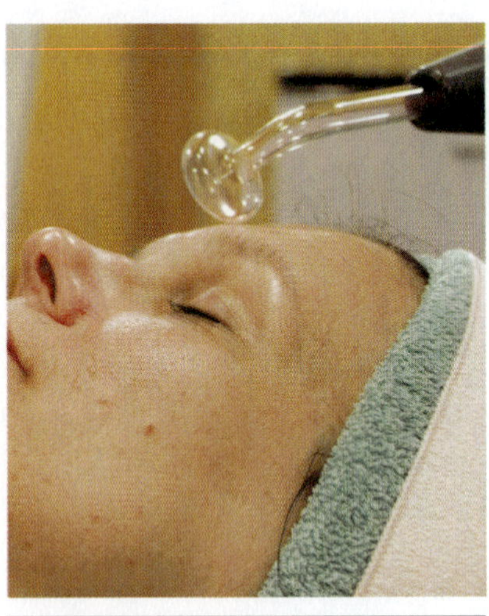

Figure 13-22 Direct application method using high frequency.

Application of High-Frequency Current

For proper use, follow the instructions provided by the manufacturer. There are three methods of using Tesla high-frequency current: direct surface application, indirect application, and general electrification.

Direct surface application is performed with the mushroom or rake-shaped electrodes for its calming and germicidal effect on the skin (Figure 13–22). The heat that is generated has a sedative effect, and oily and acne-prone skin benefit from its germicidal action. The germicidal benefits of high-frequency current are produced only with the direct application method. This method can be used on clean, dry skin, over facial creams, and over gauze for a sparking effect.

When applying high-frequency current to the face using the facial electrodes, movements are started on the neck and worked upward to the jaw, cheeks, chin, nose, and forehead. The procedure for direct surface application during a facial treatment is as follows:

1. Place the mushroom-shaped electrode into the handheld device.
2. Adjust the rheostat to the proper setting. If in doubt, start at a low setting and increase as needed.
3. Place an index finger on the glass electrode.
4. Apply the electrode directly onto the client's skin beginning on the neck.
5. Glide the electrode over the skin in circular, upward movements on the neck toward the jaw, then cheeks, chin, nose, and forehead areas.

   NOTE: If the electrode tends to drag, place gauze between the skin and the electrode.
6. To remove from the skin, place an index finger over the glass and remove it. Turn the power switch off.

Indirect application is performed with the client holding the wire glass electrode between both hands (Figure 13–23). To prevent shock, the power is turned on after the client is holding the electrode firmly and turned off before the electrode is removed from the client's hand. At no time is the electrode held by the barber or stylist. Indirect application of the current produces both a toning and stimulating effect on the skin that is ideal for aging and sallow skin.

The procedure for indirect application during a facial treatment is as follows:

1. Apply cream to client's face.
2. Instruct the client to hold the wire glass electrode with both hands.
3. The barber places the fingers of one hand on the client's forehead.
4. With the opposite hand, the barber turns the high-frequency machine on to a low setting.
5. Using both hands, the barber performs tapping (tapotement) motions in a systematic manner over the client's face.
6. To discontinue the high-frequency service, the barber removes one hand from the skin and turns the power off. CAUTION: Do not lose contact with the client's skin during this procedure while the current is on.

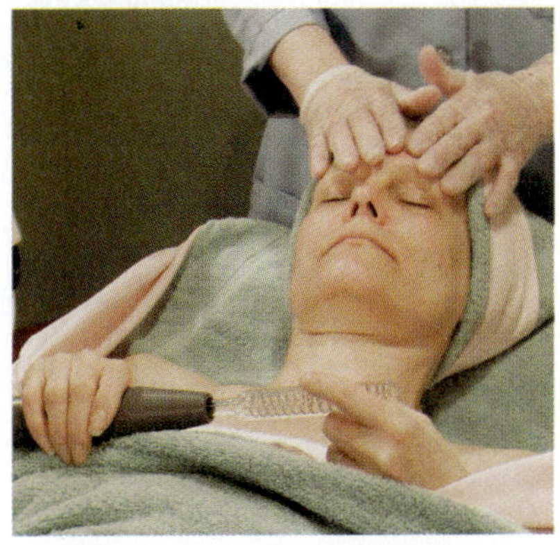

Figure 13-23 Indirect application method using high frequency.

General electrification is performed with the client holding a metal electrode. This method charges the client's body with electricity without being touched by the barber. Calm, sedative, or soothing effects are produced with the general electrification method of application.

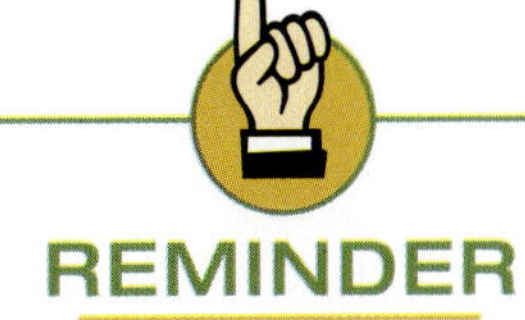

REMINDER

When using high-frequency current, never use a skin or scalp lotion that contains alcohol prior to the electrical treatment.

Disinfection and Maintenance

After each use, clean the glass electrode by wiping it with a soap and water solution. Do not immerse the electrode directly in water. Next, place the end only of the electrode into a disinfectant solution for 20 minutes. Rinse with cool water, but do not get the metal parts wet. Dry with a clean towel and store in a covered container. CAUTION: Do not place electrodes in an ultraviolet-ray cabinet sanitizer or autoclave.

13

Galvanic Machine

The galvanic machine converts the oscillating current received from an outlet into a direct current (Figure 13–24). The electrons then flow continuously in the same direction. This produces a relaxation response that can be regulated to target specific nerve endings in the epidermis. Galvanic current is used to produce chemical (disincrustation) and ionic (iontophoresis) reactions in the skin. This treatment is beneficial for oily or acne skin problems.

The galvanic machine has two poles, a negative (−) and a positive (+). Both are used for different effects. Several types of electrodes are available for the galvanic machine. The most popular are the disincrustator and the ionizing roller. To make proper contact, each electrode must be covered with cotton and the client must hold the opposite pole electrode.

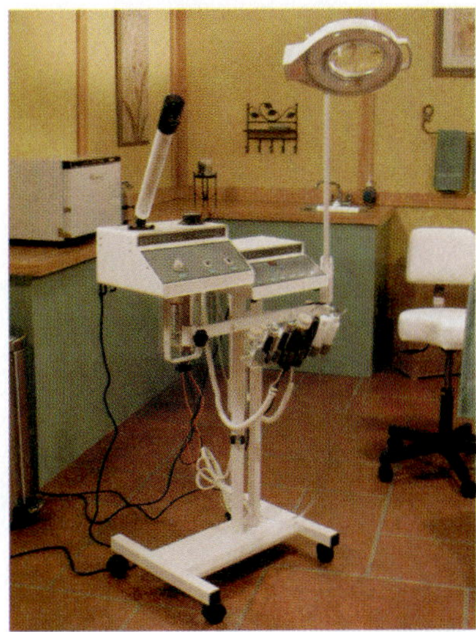

Figure 13-24 "Five-in-one" machine, including galvanic electrodes.

Applications of Galvanic Current

Disincrustation is used to facilitate deep pore cleansing. During this process, the galvanic current is used to create a chemical reaction that helps to emulsify or liquefy sebum and waste. To perform disincrustation, an acid-based solution is placed onto the skin's surface. When this current passes through certain solutions containing acids and salts, or passes through the tissues and fluids of the body, it produces chemical changes.

The procedure for the disincrustation services is as follows:

1. Gently cleanse the skin prior to treatment.
2. Instruct the client to remove any jewelry from the hand that will be used to hold the electrode. Cover the electrode held by the client with a moistened sponge or piece of dampened cotton. This electrode is connected to the red wire (positive).
3. Prepare the disincrustator electrode (negative) by placing a dampened sponge or cotton pad into the black ring, then slide the ring back onto the electrode.
4. Dip the electrode into the disincrustation solution and apply the electrode to the client's forehead. Turn the switch to negative and set at 0.05 micro-amps. Gradually turn the rheostat clockwise to increase the intensity of the current. At this point the client will usually experience a metallic taste in the mouth and a slight prickling sensation, which indicate that the current is strong enough. Be sure to explain to the client the sensations he will experience and DO NOT increase the current once these sensations are felt. The alkaline disincrustation solution will be attracted to the positive pole in the client's hand.
5. Gently glide and rotate the electrode over the facial areas that are oily. Before moving the electrode to another section of the face, the current is reduced back to zero and the process is repeated. The time spent doing the disincrustation part of the facial treatment will depend on the condition of the skin. Anywhere from 3 to 10 minutes may be required for normal to oily and acne-prone skin.
6. Upon completion, turn the machine off and remove the electrode. Use cotton pads or sponges to rinse the skin with warm water. Proceed with extractions of blackheads and pustules.

Iontophoresis means the introduction of ions. This process uses galvanic current to apply water-soluble solutions into the deeper layers of the skin. The current flows through conductive solutions by means of positive and negative polarities, or ionization. Once the charge of the solution is determined, the machine is set to the appropriate setting (Table 13–6). The client holds

13

Positive Pole (Anode)	Negative Pole (Cathode)
causes an acid reaction	causes an alkaline reaction
calms or soothes nerve endings	stimulates nerve endings
decreases blood circulation	increases blood circulation; softens and relaxes tissue

Table 13-6 Possible Skin Reactions During Ionization

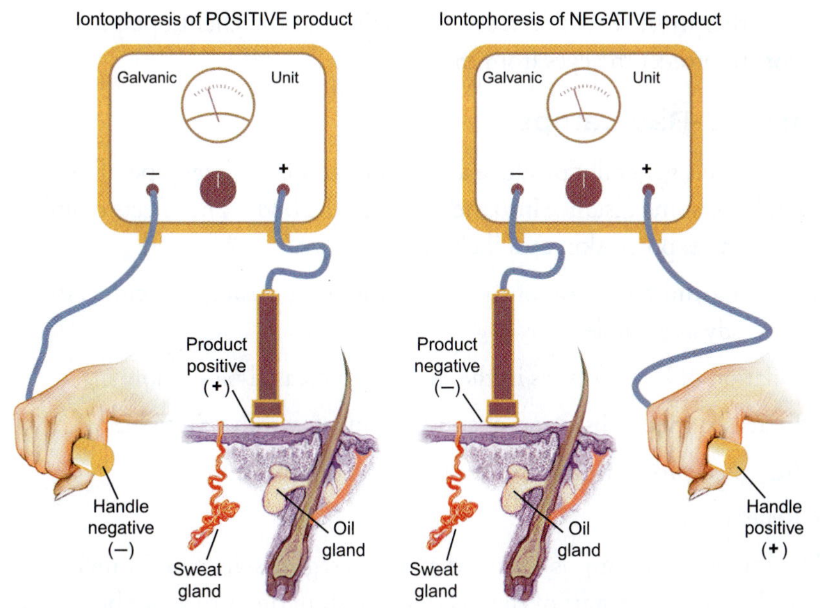

Figure 13-25 Iontophoresis of positive and negative products.

an electrode with the opposite charge (Figure 13–25). Moistened sponges or cotton pads are also used in this process.

Phoresis is the process of forcing chemical solutions into unbroken skin by way of a galvanic current. The process of ionic penetration takes place in two forms: cataphoresis and anaphoresis.

Cataphoresis is the use of the positive pole (anode) to introduce an acid pH product, such as an **astringent** solution, into the skin. Products that have a slightly acid pH are considered positive. The positive pole may also be used to close the follicles or pores after the treatment; decrease redness, as in mild acne; prevent inflammation after comedone and blemish treatment (decrease blood supply); soothe nerves; and harden tissues.

Anaphoresis is the use of the negative pole (cathode) to force an alkaline pH product, such as disincrustation lotion, into the skin. Products with an alkaline pH are considered to be negative. The negative pole may be used to stimulate the circulation of blood to dry skin, stimulate nerves, and soften tissues. The procedure for ionization is the same as that used in the disincrustation process.

Ultraviolet-Ray Lamps

Ultraviolet rays are used to treat acne, tinea, seborrhea, and dandruff. Their germicidal effect helps to promote healing and stimulate hair growth. Ultraviolet-ray lamps deliver these shortest light rays of the spectrum. The benefits of these shorter rays are obtained when the lamp is is placed 30 to 36 inches from the skin.

Average exposure to ultraviolet rays may produce redness of the skin, and overdoses may cause blistering. It is better to start with a two- or three-minute exposure, and gradually increase the time to seven or eight minutes.

The barber must wear tinted safety goggles and the client opaque eye protectors to protect the eyes from the rays.

Infrared-Ray Lamps

Infrared rays generally produce a soothing and beneficial type of heat that extends for some distance into the tissues of the body. The effects of infrared rays on the exposed skin area include:

- Heating and relaxation of the skin without increasing the temperature of the body as a whole
- Dilation of blood vessels in the skin and increased blood flow
- Increased metabolism and chemical changes within skin tissues
- Increased production of perspiration and oil on the skin
- Relief of pain

The infrared-ray lamp is operated at an average distance of 30 inches. It is placed closer at the start of the treatment and, in order to avoid burning the skin, is then moved back gradually as the surface heat becomes more pronounced. Always protect the eyes of the client during exposure. Place pads saturated with dilute boric acid or witch hazel solution over the client's eyelids.

Safety Precautions for Using Electrical Equipment

- Disconnect any appliances when they are not being used.
- Study instructions before using any electrical equipment.
- Keep all wires, plugs, and equipment in a safe condition.
- Inspect all electrical equipment frequently.
- Avoid getting electric cords wet.
- Sanitize all electrodes properly.
- Protect the client at all times.
- Do not touch any metal while using electrical appliances.
- Do not handle electrical equipment with wet hands.
- Do not allow the client to touch metal surfaces when electrical treatments are being performed.
- Do not leave the room when the client is attached to any electrical device.
- Do not attempt to clean around an electric outlet when equipment is plugged in.
- Do not touch two metallic objects at the same time while connected to an electric current.
- Do not use any electrical equipment without first obtaining full instruction in its care and use.

The protection and safety of the client are the primary concern of the barber. All electrical equipment should be inspected regularly to determine whether it is in good working condition. Carelessness may result in shocks or burns. Barbers who practice safety precautions help to eliminate accidents, assuring greater comfort and satisfaction for their clients. 6

With a basic knowledge of the anatomical structure of the head, face, and neck and the primary subdermal systems, and the ability to perform massage manipulations manually or with electrical devices, you are now ready to engage in the analysis and performance of skin care.

FACIAL TREATMENTS

The barber does not treat skin diseases but should be able to recognize various skin disorders so as to differentiate between those that can be serviced in the barbershop and those that should be referred to a physician. Facials performed in the barbershop are considered to be either preservative or corrective treatments.

Preservative treatments are intended to help maintain the health of facial skin. The performance of correct cleansing, massage, and electrical treatments can increase circulation, relax the nerves, activate skin glands, and increase cell metabolism.

Corrective treatments are used to correct skin conditions such as dryness, oiliness, blackheads, aging lines, and minor acne. In general, facial treatments are beneficial because they:

1. cleanse the skin.
2. increase circulation.
3. activate glandular activity.
4. relax tense nerves.
5. maintain muscle tone.
6. strengthen weak muscle tissue.
7. correct certain skin disorders.
8. help prevent the formation of wrinkles and aging lines.
9. improve skin texture and complexion.
10. help to reduce fatty tissues.

To perform the full range of facial treatments presented in this text, the barber will require access to hot and cold water, soft terry cloth towels, therapeutic lamps, and a variety of preparations designed for facial treatments. These preparations include such items as facial creams, tonics, exfoliants, lotions, oils, packs, and masks.

Skin Types

There are four basic skin types that the barber will need to recognize before the appropriate products can be chosen for a facial treatment. Skin type is primarily based on the amount of oil that is produced in the follicles from the sebaceous glands and the amount of lipids found between the cells. Skin types include dry, normal, combination, and oily. Any of these skin types can be *sensitive* to products, irritation, or the environment.

Dry skin does not produce enough oil, which is needed to protect the skin from environmental damage and aging. Dry skin needs extra care because it does not have this protection. The stimulation of oil production and protection of the skin surface is the objective of a facial treatment for dry skin. In some cases, dry skin is also *dehydrated* skin that lacks water. In addition to drinking plenty of water, hydrating the skin with moisturizers and humectants can help minimize the negative effects of dryness and dehydration.

Normal skin has a good water/oil balance. The follicles are a normal size and the skin is free of blemishes. Maintenance and preservative care is the goal for this type of skin.

Combination skin can be both oily and dry at different areas of the face. The T-zone is the section of the face that incorporates the forehead, nose, and chin area. These areas tend to have more sebaceous glands and larger pores. The cheek and outer areas of the face tend to be dry. Water-based products work best for combination skin types.

Oily skin is characterized by excess sebum (oil) production. The follicle size is larger and contains more oil. Oily skin requires more cleansing and exfoliation than other skin types, yet overcleansing can strip and irritate the skin. If the skin is overdried, it is not balanced and the body will try to produce additional oil to compensate for the dryness on the surface. Proper exfoliation and a water-based hydrator will help keep oily skin clean and balanced.

Wrinkles are depressions in the skin that have developed from repetitious muscle action moving in the same direction. Other factors that influence the formation of wrinkles are:

- loosening of the elastic skin fibers due to abnormal tension or relaxation of the facial muscles
- shrinking of the skin tissue as a result of aging
- excessive dryness of the skin
- improper facial care

Skin Analysis

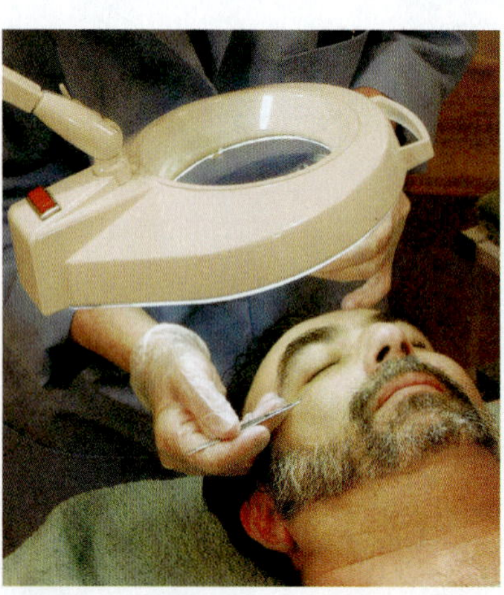

Figure 13-26 Using a magnifying light to analyze the skin.

A knowledge of skin types and conditions is helpful in performing an accurate skin analysis. It is preferable to analyze the skin with a magnifying lamp/light (Figure 13–26), but if one is not available, a close inspection of the skin will suffice. When analyzing the skin it is important to note the client's skin type and conditions and the skin's visible appearance and texture. Be sure to record this information on a client record card for future use (Figures 13–27 and 13–28). Follow guidelines 1–4 when performing a skin analysis:

1. Observe the client's skin type, condition, and appearance; feel the texture.
2. Ask questions of the client relating to the skin's appearance and home care routine.
3. Discuss the facial procedure and/or treatment plans, the products that will be used, and why.
4. Encourage the client to ask questions and then determine a course of action together.

CONSULTATION CARD				
Name ________				Date of Consultation
Address ________				D.O.B.
City ________	State ________	Zip ________		Occupation
Tel. (Home) ________	(Business) ________			Ref. by
				Contraindications
Medical History				
Current Medication				
Previous treatments				
Home Care Products used				
SKIN TYPE	Oily	Normal	Dry	Combination
SKIN CONDITION	Clogged pores	Sensitive	Dehydrated	Mature
Skin Abnormalities				
Remarks				

Figure 13-27 Client consultation card (front).

FACIAL RECORD			
Date	Type of treatment	By	Products purchased
2/14	Cleansing, Peel - Relaxing Massage		Moisturizer with sunscreen
3/16	Cleansing, Peel Modelage Mask		Cleanser, Tonic Lotion
4/5	Cleansing, Peel High Frequency indirect		Moisturizer
4/26 5/13	Cleansing, Peel Massage Cleansing, Peel Iontophoresis Skin is showing marked improvement.	John	Dry skin cream
6/1	Cleansing, Peel Relaxing Massage	Mary	

Figure 13-28 Client consultation card (back).

Skin Care Products

The type of facial treatment will determine the products needed to complete the procedure. Three essential skin care preparations, however, should be used before or after a shave service and during full facial treatments. These essential preparations are cleansers, toners, and moisturizers. Additional products such as exfoliating scrubs, masks, and treatment creams are used in conjunction with the essential preparations during the full facial treatment.

- *Cleansers* should be mild and easy to rinse from the skin. They are available as face washes, lotions, and creams for all types of skin and skin conditions. Face washes are usually water-based products with a neutral or slightly acidic pH effective on oily and combination skin types. Cleansing lotions are water-based emulsions for normal and combination skin that contain emollients or oils to soften the skin. Cleansing creams are oil-based emulsions that are used primarily to dissolve dirt and makeup. Because cleansing creams are heavier than cleansing lotions, performers use these products to remove heavy stage makeup.
- **Toners**, *fresheners,* and *astringents* are used after cleansing and prior to the application of a moisturizer. These tonic lotions vary in strength and alcohol content and therefore vary in pH.

  Fresheners usually have the lowest alcohol content (0 to 4 percent) and are beneficial for dry, mature, and sensitive skin. Toners are designed to tone or tighten the skin and may be used on normal and combination skin types. The alcohol content range of toners is usually 4 to 15 percent. Astringents may contain up to 35 percent alcohol and are used for oily and acne-prone skin. Toners, fresheners, and astringents all help to remove cleanser residue and have a temporary tightening effect on the skin. Some restore the skin's natural pH after cleansing and others can help certain skin conditions.
- *Moisturizers* are the third essential product needed to perform a facial. Moisturizers are formulated to add moisture to the skin and are available for various skin types. They are also available in water-based and oil-based formulations.

  NOTE: The use of cleansers, toners, and moisturizers during the shave service is discussed in Chapter 14.

There are other types of products for specific applications:

- *Exfoliating scrubs* are used to physically rub or remove dead cells from the skin surface. Granular scrubs for normal to dry skin may be used two times per week. Scrubs are available in cream, lotion, and gel forms for a variety of skin types.
- *Masks and packs* draw impurities out of pores, tighten, tone, hydrate, soothe, and nourish the skin, depending on the ingredients. They are available in cream, gel, or clay forms and should be used according to skin type.

Face packs and masks differ in their composition and usage. A mask is usually a setting product, which means that it dries after application, providing complete closure to the environment on top of the skin. Masks are most often applied directly to the skin and are known for their tightening and sebum-absorbing effects. Packs, also referred to as cream or gel masks, are usually applied to the skin over layers of gauze to hold the product in place over the skin. They are beneficial for sensitive skin and have excellent hydrating properties. Applied with a mask brush, they are allowed to set for about 10 minutes.

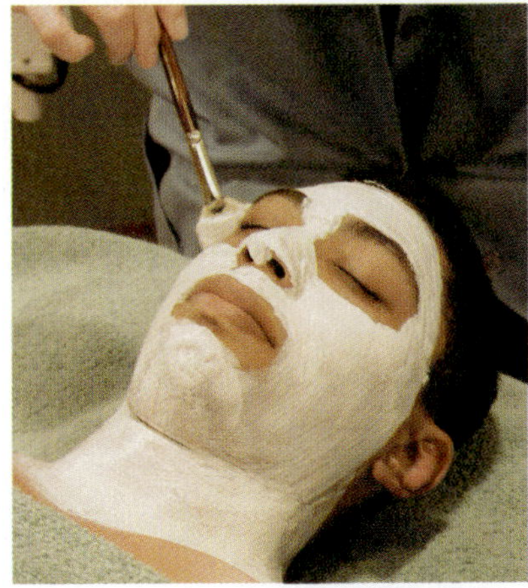

Figure 13-29 Mask application.

High-quality packs and masks should feel comfortable while producing slight tingling and tightening sensations. Always follow the manufacturer's directions for preparation, application, and removal of the product from the skin.

Clay masks are clay preparations used to stimulate circulation and temporarily contract the skin pores. They absorb sebum and are used on oily and combination skin types. Applied with a mask brush, they are allowed to set until dry, usually about 10 minutes (Figure 13–29).

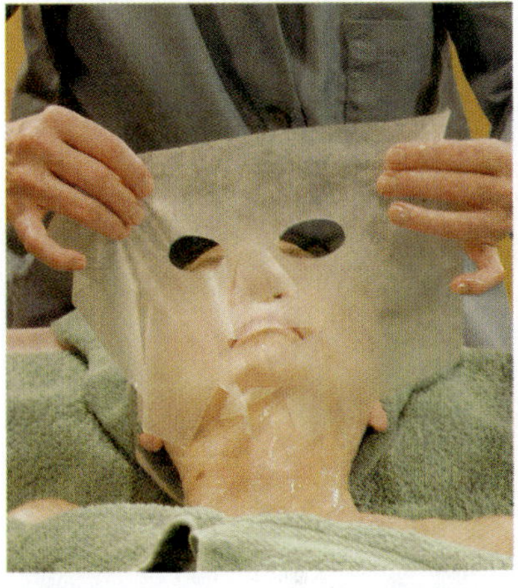

Figure 13-30 Placing gauze on the client's face.

Paraffin wax masks actually employ the pack application method. Specially prepared paraffin is melted at slightly more than body temperature before application. The client's skin is prepared by cleansing, followed by the application of a treatment cream. Eye pads are used and the paraffin is applied over gauze to avoid the facial hair from sticking to the wax (Figures 13–30 and 13–31).

There are various facial masks and packs available for use in the barbershop. Hot-oil masks, milk and honey, egg white, and witch hazel packs have been around for many years. For proper use, the barber should always read the manufacturer's claims and directions. Judge the merits of the mask or pack before recommending it to a client.

- *Massage creams* are creams, lotions, or oils that provide slip during a massage while also nourishing and treating skin conditions.
- **Rolling cream** is a thick, smooth, and usually pink facial cleanser that has been used in barbershops for decades. It is applied in a thin layer over the skin, after which it is rolled off with a firm, stroking motion. As the rolling takes place, loose flaky skin and trapped impurities are lifted from the skin surface. The skin is left soft and smooth with increased circulation to the surface.

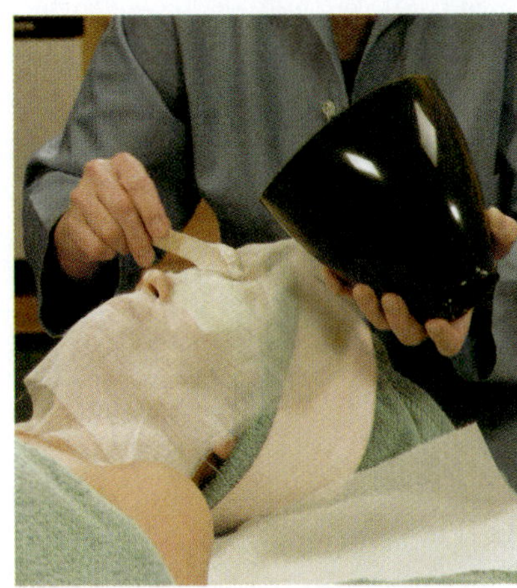

Figure 13-31 Applying a mask over the gauze.

In terms of skin care products and the order in which they will be used during full facial treatments in this text, a general outline is as follows:

1. Cleanser
2. Exfoliant (scrub or rolling cream)
3. Massage cream
4. Cleanser
5. Freshener (low alcohol content)
6. Mask

13

7. Toner
8. Moisturizer

   NOTE: Your instructor's recommended order of product application is equally correct.

Men's Skin Care Products

Several decades ago, men's personal care products consisted of basic items such as cologne, hair tonics or creams, deodorants, shaving creams, and after-shave lotions. The high-end versions of these basic items were often created as spin-off products from clothing designers. Even men's hair sprays were almost nonexistent before the 1960s. Today, however, products that have been developed specifically with the male in mind are abundant on retail shelves and in shops and salons. The male consumer is finally getting the attention he deserves and each year more men are experiencing the benefits of using skin care products on a regular basis.

When choosing men's skin care products for use in the barbershop, it is important to think about the specific characteristics of a product that might appeal to men. For example, men in general do not appreciate highly fragranced or multistep products. Creams should be simple, nonfragranced, and absorbent with a matte finish. Most men do not like the greasy or oily feeling of some products. Men also prefer simpler routines and multipurpose products. For example, a toner that serves as an after-shave will usually be chosen over the purchase and use of two separate products.

Although the quality of the product must be the barber's and the client's first consideration in product choices, packaging characteristics also need to be taken into consideration. Typically, tube packaging is preferred over jars, and size can also be a factor for the client who travels in his profession. One option is to stock barbershop retail shelves with larger containers for the client's home use and smaller, convenient sizes for travel. As a general rule, use the products you retail for services performed within the shop. *Note:* Smaller packaged goods can also be used for promotions and marketing strategies in the barbershop (see Chapter 21). 7

The Basic Facial

The basic facial, sometimes known as the *scientific rest facial,* is beneficial for its cleansing and stimulating action on the skin that also exercises and relaxes the facial muscles. The procedural steps listed below represent one routine that is used to perform a basic facial. It may be changed to conform to your instructor's method or new procedures in the industry.

Procedure

Preparation and performance of a basic facial in the barbershop includes the following steps:

1. Arrange all necessary supplies in a convenient location.
2. Drape the client and engage in client consultation.

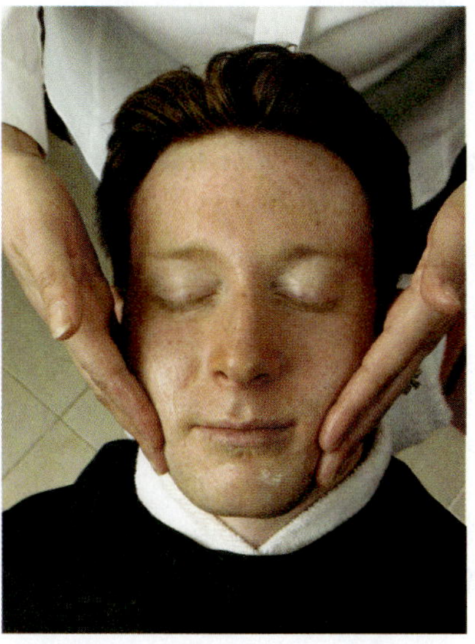

Figure 13-32 Applying cleansing cream.

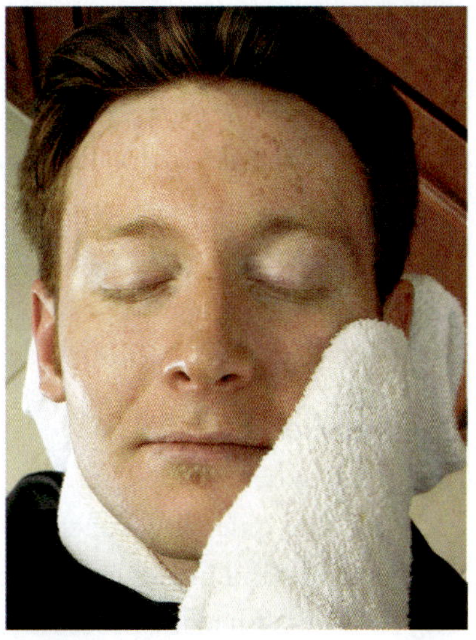

Figure 13-33 Removing cleansing cream.

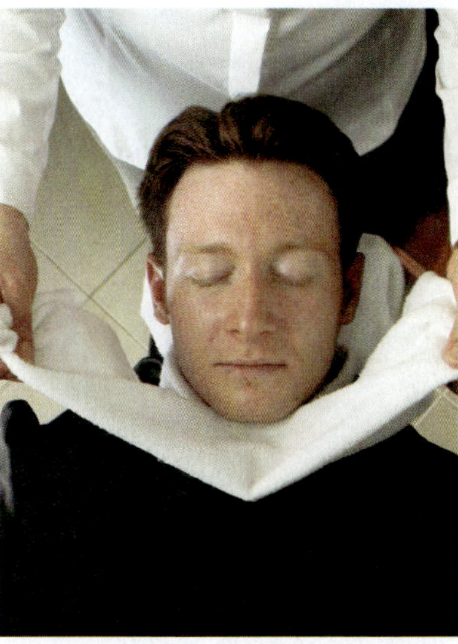

Figure 13-34 Steam towels.

3. Perform skin analysis and make product selection.
4. Place a towel or paper barrier between the client's head and the headrest. Adjust the headrest and recline the hydraulic chair. Make sure the client is comfortable.
5. Protect the client's hair with a towel or cap.
6. Wash your hands.

   NOTE: All products should be removed from their containers with a sanitized spatula. Do not dip the fingers into the containers, which may contaminate the product.
7. Apply cleansing cream over the face, using stroking and rotary movements (Figure 13–32).
8. Remove the cleansing cream with a warm, damp towel (Figure 13–33).
9. Apply two or three steam towels to open pores and loosen imbedded dirt and oils (Figure 13–34).
10. Reapply cleansing cream to the skin with the fingertips.
11. Gently massage the face, using continuous and rhythmic movements (Figures 13–35 and 13–36).

    NOTE: The brush machine may also be used at this time.
12. Wipe off excess cleansing cream with a warm towel.
13. Apply an exfoliating product and lightly massage over the skin.
14. Apply steam towel. Wipe off excess product until the skin is free of exfoliating residue.
15. Gently wipe toner or astringent over the face, then pat dry (Figure 13–37).
16. Apply mask or pack and allow to dry (Figure 13–38).
17. Apply tepid to warm towel to moisten mask/pack. Wipe off product until free of mask/pack.
18. Again, gently wipe toner or astringent over the face and pat dry.

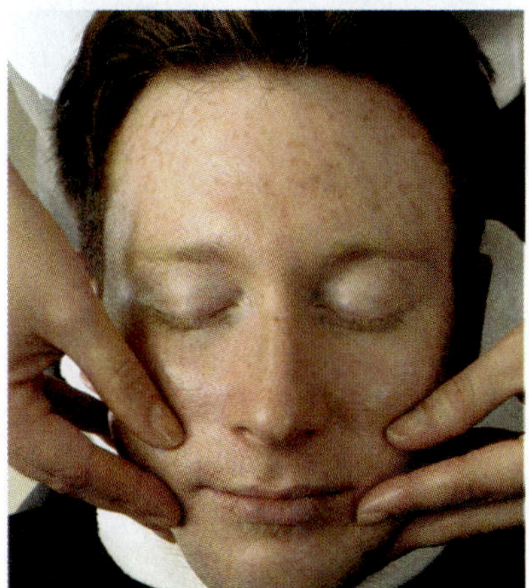

Figure 13-35 Massage the face.

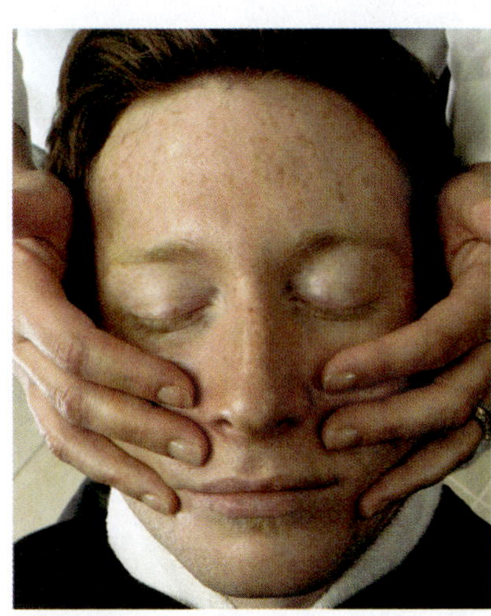

Figure 13-36 Use continuous and rhythmic movements.

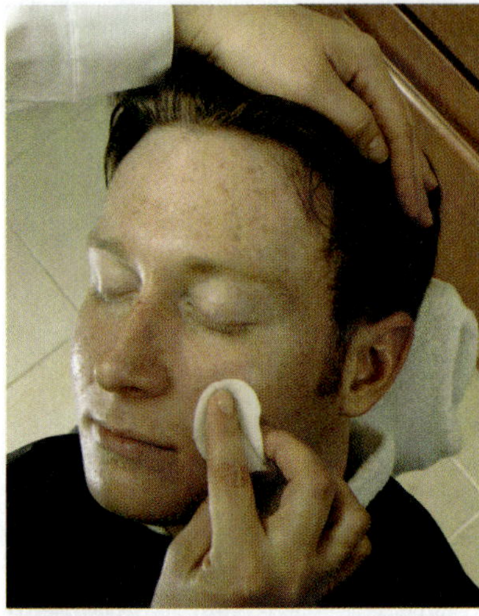

Figure 13-37 Apply toner or astringent.

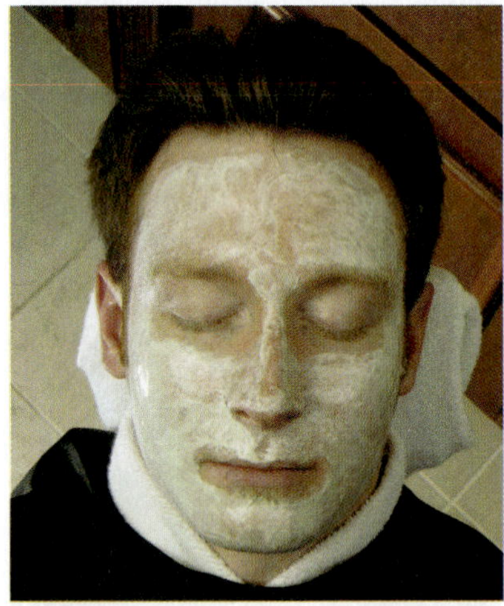

Figure 13-38 Apply mask, allow to dry.

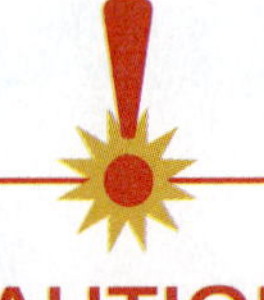

CAUTION

The vibrator should never be used when there is a known weakness of the heart or in cases of fever, abscesses, or skin inflammations.

19. Apply a light coat of moisturizer using the effleurage movement.
20. Apply a light dusting of talc if the client desires it. Remove any excess.
21. Slowly raise the hydraulic chair and assist client to a sitting position.
22. Discard all disposable supplies and materials.
23. Wipe containers and close tightly. Store in appropriate place.
24. Sanitize all nondisposable implements and tools.
25. Wash and sanitize your hands.

Points to Remember

1. Strive to have the client relax.
2. Provide a quiet atmosphere.
3. Organize and maintain supplies in a clean, orderly fashion.
4. Follow a systematic procedure.
5. Perform the facial massage properly.

Actions to Avoid

1. Harming or scratching the skin
2. Excessive or rough massage
3. Product in the client's eyes
4. Using towels that are too hot
5. Breathing into the client's face
6. Not being careful or sanitary
7. Disinterest in the client's skin problems or conversation
8. Leaving excess product on the skin
9. Excessive talking that does not facilitate client relaxation
10. Leaving the chair to obtain materials or supplies
11. Heavy, rough, or cold hands

Vibratory Facial

When using an electric massager on the face, avoid heavy contact with the client's skin. Delicate areas around the nose and upper cheek require a special technique using both of the barber's hands. The right-handed barber will attach the massager to his or her right hand. The left hand is placed on the client's skin. Next, the barber places his or her right hand on top of the left and the vibrations travel through this hand to the client's skin. Direct contact with the barber's right hand can be made to less delicate areas such as the forehead and jaw line, but pressure still needs to be avoided.

Massage Movements

The following steps outline massage movements to use with an electric massager:

1. Adjust the massager on the right hand and place the fingertips of the left hand on the client's left nostril. Place the vibrating right-hand fingers over the left-hand fingers to vibrate through the left hand.

2. Vibrate the skin with a few light up-and-down movements on the left side of the nose.
3. Gently slide the fingers along the upper cheek area and direct them toward the center of the forehead.
4. Place the vibrating right hand onto the skin and perform rotary movements toward the left temple. Pause for a moment.
5. Continue the rotary movements down along the jaw line toward the tip of the chin.
6. Vibrate from the chin back toward the cheek, using wider, firmer movements.
7. Continue with a slow, light stroke at the temple, around the left ear, over the jawbone, toward the center of the neck, and then below the chin.
8. Vibrate rotary movements over the neck, behind the ear, up to the temple, and then toward the center of the forehead.
9. Repeat Steps 2 through 8 on the right side of the face.
10. Repeat Steps 2 through 8 on both sides of the face again and proceed with Step 5 of the vibratory facial procedure that follows.

Procedure

The procedure for a vibratory facial is similar to the basic facial with minor variations. Again we emphasize that the following procedure may be changed to conform with your instructor's routine.

1. Prepare the client as for a basic facial.
2. Apply steam towels.
3. Apply massage cream.
4. Administer the massage using the electric massager as described in the preceding section.
5. Apply cleansing cream with light hand manipulations.
6. Remove cleansing cream with a warm towel.
7. Follow with a mild witch hazel steam.
8. Apply one or two cool towels.
9. Apply a moisturizing face lotion.
10. Dry thoroughly and apply powder if desired.

Rules for Using an Electric Massager

1. Regulate the number of vibrations to avoid overstimulation.
2. Do not use the vibrator for too long in any one spot.
3. Vary the amount of pressure in accordance with the results desired.
4. Do not use a vibrator over the upper lip, as the vibrations may cause discomfort.
5. For soothing and relaxing effects, give very slow, light vibrations for a very short time.
6. For stimulating effects, give light vibrations of moderate speed and time.
7. To reduce fatty tissues, give moderate, fast vibrations with firm pressure.

Rolling Cream Facial

The facial massage most often identified with the barbershop is the rolling cream facial. The rolling cream facial is designed to cleanse and stimulate the skin. Due to the drying qualities of the rolling cream and the application process, this type of facial should be recommended only to clients with normal, oily, or thick skin. It should not be performed on skin that is dry, acne-prone, sensitive, or thin in texture.

Procedure

1. Prepare the client.
2. Moderately steam the face with two or three warm towels.
3. Apply dabs of rolling cream to the chin, cheeks, and forehead. Dampen the fingertips of both hands with water and spread the cream evenly over the face and neck with a smooth, stroking movement.
4. Massage the face and neck with uniform, rotary, stroking and rubbing movements with the cushion tips of the fingers, until most of the cream has rolled off.
5. Apply a small amount of cleansing cream to the face and neck, using lighter manipulations.
6. Remove the cream with a warm towel.
7. Apply a witch hazel steam to the face and neck with one or more hot towels, following with one or two cool towels to close the pores.
8. Apply astringent or toner. Dry and powder the face and neck.
9. Finish as for a basic facial.

Facial for Dry Skin

Dry skin is caused by an insufficient flow of sebum from the sebaceous glands. The objective of a facial for dry skin is to help moisturize it. Dry-skin facials can be performed using infrared rays, galvanic current, or high-frequency current.

Procedure with Infrared Rays

1. Prepare the client as for a basic facial.
2. Apply cleansing cream; remove cream with a warm, moist towel.
3. Sponge the face with a mild tonic lotion.
4. Apply massage cream.
5. Apply lubricating oil, or eye cream, over and under the eyes.
6. Apply lubricating oil over the neck.
7. Cover the client's eyes with cotton pads moistened with witch hazel or a nonalcoholic freshener.
8. Expose the face and neck to infrared rays for not more than five minutes.
9. Perform massage manipulations three to five times.
10. Remove the massage cream and oil with tissues, or with a warm, moist towel.

11. Apply tonic lotion suitable for dry skin. Blot the face dry with tissues or a towel
12. Apply moisturizer.
13. Complete and clean up as for a basic facial.

CAUTION

Do not permit infrared rays to remain on the body tissues for more than a few seconds at a time. Move your hand back and forth across the rays' path to break constant exposure on the client's skin. The total exposure time should not exceed five minutes.

Procedure with Galvanic Current

The procedure for giving a dry-skin facial with galvanic current is similar to the procedure for giving a dry-skin facial with infrared rays, with a few changes:

1. Repeat Steps 1 through 4 of the procedure used with infrared rays.
2. Apply a thick layer of ionized, oil-free gel to the face and neck.
3. Apply negative galvanic current for five to seven minutes, to open the pores.
4. Reapply gel to the face and neck.
5. Apply positive galvanic current for four to six minutes, to close the pores.
6. Repeat Steps 4 through 6 of the procedure used with infrared rays.
7. Repeat Steps 9 through 13 of the procedure used with infrared rays.

Procedure with Indirect High-Frequency Current

1. Follow Steps 1 through 6 of the procedure for a facial with infrared rays.
2. Have client hold electrode in his right hand.
3. Perform manipulations, using the indirect method of applying high-frequency current, for 7 to 10 minutes. Do not use tapping movements and do not lift hands from the client's skin.
4. Apply two or three cool towels to the face and neck.
5. Follow Steps 10 to 13 of the procedure for a facial with infrared rays.

Facial for Oily Skin and Blackheads

Oily skin and/or blackheads (comedones) are caused by hardened masses of sebum formed inside a follicle. The sebaceous material in the follicle darkens when exposed to oxygen thus forming a blackhead.

Procedure

1. Prepare the client as for a basic facial.
2. Apply cleansing lotion and remove it with a warm, moist towel or facial sponges.
3. Place moistened eye pads on the client's eyes, then analyze the skin under a magnifying lamp.
4. Steam the face with three or four moist, warm towels, or a facial steamer to open the pores.
5. Wear gloves and cover your fingertips with cotton and gently press out blackheads. Do not press so hard as to bruise the skin tissue.
6. Sponge the face with astringent or toner.
7. *Optional:* Cover the client's eyes with pads moistened with a mild astringent. Apply ultraviolet light over the skin for three to five minutes.

8. Apply massage cream suitable for the skin condition and perform massage manipulations.
9. Remove cream with a warm, moist towel, cotton pads, or facial sponges.
10. Moisten a cotton pledget with an astringent lotion. Apply it to the face and neck with upward and outward movements to constrict the pores. Blot the excess moisture with tissues. For male clients with beards, use downward and outward movements in the same direction as the hair growth.
11. Apply moisturizer or protective lotion according to skin type.
12. Complete and clean up as for basic facial procedure.

Facial for Acne

Acne is a disorder of the sebaceous glands and serious cases require medical direction. If the client is under medical care, the role of the barber is to perform facial treatments as prescribed by the client's physician. If in doubt, contact the physician directly. With a prescribed treatment plan, treatment of acne conditions by barbers should be limited to the following procedures:

1. Reduction of oily skin by local and topical applications
2. Removal of blackheads using proper procedures
3. Cleansing of the skin
4. Application of medicated and/or prescribed preparations

Procedure

Because acne contains infectious matter, it is advisable to use rubber or latex gloves and disposable materials such as cotton cleansing pads.

1. Prepare the client as for a basic facial.
2. Cleanse the client's face as in a basic facial.
3. Place cotton eye pads over the client's eyes; then analyze the skin under the magnifying lamp.
4. Apply warm, moist towels to the face to open the pores for deep cleansing.
5. Extract comedones as in a facial for oily skin.
6. Cleanse the face with a cotton pad or sponge that has been sprinkled with astringent. CAUTION: If high-frequency current is used as in step 7, use a nonalcoholic toner in place of the astringent.
7. *Optional:* Apply high-frequency current with direct application over the affected area for up to five minutes. Or, cover the client's eyes with goggles and apply ultraviolet light over the skin for three to five minutes for its germicidal effects. Be guided by your instructor.
8. Apply prescribed acne treatment cream if available. *Optional:* Leave the eye pads in place and apply infrared lamp for five to seven minutes to promote penetration of the treatment cream.
9. Leave the eye pads in place and apply a treatment mask that is suitable for the skin condition for 8 to 10 minutes.
10. Remove the mask with moist towels or sponges.

11. Apply astringent to the face with a wet cotton pad or sponge.
12. Apply protective fluid or special acne lotion.
13. Complete cleanup and sanitation procedures as for basic facial procedures.

> **CAUTION**
> Overexposure to ultraviolet rays can destroy skin tissue. Start with a two- or three-minute exposure time and gradually increase to seven or eight minutes.

Hot-Oil Mask

The hot-oil mask can be used for extremely dry, parched, and scaly skin that is prevalent during dry, hot, or windy weather. Although there are many commercially prepared products on the market, some older clients may request this service to soften, smooth, and stimulate skin tissues.

Formula for a Hot-Oil Mask

2 tablespoons of olive oil

1 tablespoon of castor oil (refined grade)

¼ teaspoon of glycerin

Mix the oils in a small container and warm.

Procedure

1. Prepare the client as for a basic facial.
2. Prepare the mask. Saturate cotton pads (4" x 4") or an 18–inch square of gauze with the warm oil mixture.
3. Follow Steps 1 through 11 as in basic facial.
4. After the manipulations do not remove the massage cream. Place eye pads and gauze in position over the face.
5. Use red dermal light or an infrared lamp for 8 to 10 minutes.

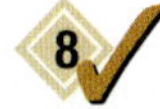

6. Remove the mask and cream.
7. Finish as for a basic facial.

chapter glossary

astringent	tonic lotions with an alcohol content of up to 35 percent; used to remove oil accumulation on oily and acne-prone skin
direct surface application	high-frequency current performed with the mushroom- or rake-shaped electrodes for its calming and germicidal effect on the skin
effleurage	light, continuous stroking movement applied with the fingers (digital) or the palms (palmar) in a slow, rhythmic manner
electric massager	massaging unit that attaches to the barber's hand to impart vibrating massage movements to the skin surface
friction	deep rubbing movement requiring pressure on the skin with the fingers or palm while moving it over an underlying structure
general electrification	high-frequency current application in which the client holds a glass or metal electrode so the body is charged without being touched by the barber
indirect application	high-frequency current performed with the client holding the wire glass electrode between both hands
muscles	system that covers, shapes, and supports the skeleton; contracts and moves various parts of the body
percussion	another name for tapotement
pétrissage	kneading movement performed by lifting, squeezing, and pressing the tissue with a light, firm pressure
phoresis	the process of forcing chemical solutions into unbroken skin by way of a galvanic current
rolling cream	cleansing and exfoliating product used in facials to lift dead skin cells and dirt from the skin surface
tapotement	most stimulating massage movement, consisting of short, quick tapping, slapping, and hacking movements
toners	in relation to massage, toners are tonic lotions with an alcohol content of 4 to 15 percent; used on normal and combination skin types
vibration	in massage, the rapid shaking of the body part while the balls of the fingertips are pressed firmly on the point of application

chapter review questions

1. Identify three characteristics of the skin that may benefit from regularly scheduled facial services.
2. List seven sources capable of stimulating muscular tissue.
3. List and locate the facial muscles associated with facial massage.
4. Explain what stimulation of the nerves achieves.
5. List the ways in which nerves may be stimulated.
6. How many pairs of cranial nerves are there?
7. Identify three cranial nerves that are important to massaging the head, face, and neck.
8. Identify the main arteries that supply blood to the entire head, face, and neck.
9. Identify the principal veins by which the blood from the head, face, and neck is returned to the heart.
10. List and describe five basic massage movements and their effects on the skin.
11. List the benefits of facial treatments.
12. List the electrical equipment that can be used in the performance of facial massage.
13. List and describe the basic skin types.
14. List and describe the use of facial products.
15. List the steps involved in the performance of a basic facial.
16. Read and list the CAUTION and REMINDER boxes presented in this chapter.

principles that will require consideration. For example, the application of hot towels is a standard procedure in preparing the beard for shaving. Nevertheless, some clients may not tolerate a hot towel on their skin. Other individual characteristics such as hair texture, hair growth patterns, and product sensitivity are variables that barbers must consider and make educated judgments about before proceeding with the shave service.

CAUTION

Sideways sawing movements with changeable-blade razors will cause injury to the skin. Instead, employ a gentle scraping motion with this type of razor.

General Sanitation and Safety Precautions of Shaving

Some general rules to be observed when shaving include the following:

1. Always sanitize tools before using.
2. Once the client is in position for the shave, lock the chair.
3. Always use a forward sawing motion with the point of the blade leading when using a conventional straight razor.
4. Always observe the hair growth pattern and shave with it, not against it.
5. Heavy beard growth requires more care in the lathering process and more steam towels than usual to effectively prepare it for the shave.
6. Lather against the grain gently to place the facial hair in a position to be shaved.
7. Lather should be neatly applied to the areas to be shaved and replaced as necessary.
8. The fingers of the hand opposite the hand holding the razor should be kept dry in order to grasp, stretch, and hold the skin firmly during the shave service.
9. Hot towels should not be used on skin that is chapped or blistered from heat or cold, or on skin that is thin and sensitive.
10. When astringents are too harsh for sensitive skin, pH-balanced fresheners or toners should be used.
11. Clients that have an infection in the area to be shaved should not be served because doing so could spread the infection to other parts of the face or to the barber.
12. Curly facial hair requires special care as its growth characteristics may cause problems if the shave isn't performed correctly. Ingrown hairs are often the result of improper hair removal by a razor, tweezers, or trimmer. Curly hair has the tendency to grow in a "looped" direction and as it grows out of the skin, it can bend back into the skin surface. Excessively close shaving, coupled with excessive pressure, with clippers, trimmers, or razors can damage skin to the point that new hair growth is trapped under the injured tissue. This can result in infected bumps on and under the skin surface (folliculitis) or scar tissue, or it may initiate a keloid condition.
13. Take special precautions when shaving beneath the lower lip, lower part of the neck, and around the Adam's apple. These facial areas are usually the most tender and sensitive and easily irritated by very close shaving.
14. When small cuts and nicks occur, pat dry with a sterile cotton pledget and apply **styptic powder**.
15. Keep the skin moist while shaving.

1

Some states may require the use of protective gloves while shaving a client. Be guided by your instructor and state board regulations.

14

CAUTION: Never use a styptic pencil or other astringent that will come into contact with another person's face.

Four Standard Shaving Positions and Strokes

The correct angle of cutting the beard with a straight razor is called the **cutting stroke**. To achieve the best cutting stroke, the razor must glide over the surface at an angle *with the grain of the hair*. It should be drawn in a forward movement with the point of the razor in the lead.

The first step in performing a professional shave is to master the fundamentals of handling the razor. This includes learning how to open and close the razor without injury. To open the razor, grasp the back of the razor's blade between the thumb and index finger of the dominant hand while holding the handle with the opposite thumb and index finger. As the blade and handle separate by way of the pivot (Figure 14–1), reposition the little finger of the dominant hand to rest on the tang as the handle is placed in an upward position (Figure 14–2). When closing the razor, be careful that the cutting edge does not strike the handle (Figure 14–3).

To shave the face with ease and efficiency, the barber employs four standard positions and strokes:

- Freehand position and stroke
- Backhand position and stroke
- Reverse freehand position and stroke
- Reverse backhand position and stroke

Each of the four standard shaving positions and strokes requires consideration and practice of the following:

1. When to use a particular shaving stroke
2. How to hold the razor for each stroke
   a) the position of the right hand in relation to the razor
   b) the position of the left hand in relation to the razor
3. How to stroke the razor

   NOTE: If using a conventional straight razor, review the proper honing and stropping methods before learning each shaving stroke.

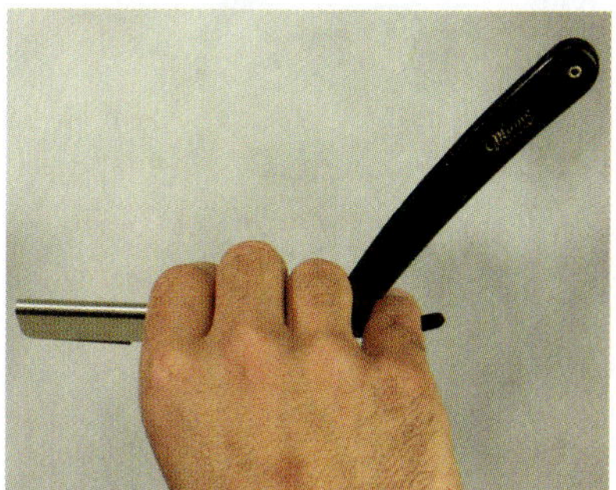

Figure 14–2 Positioning of the little finger.

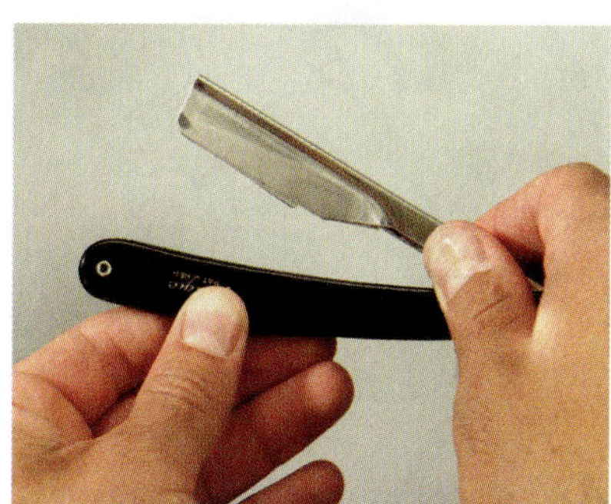

Figure 14–3 Close the razor carefully.

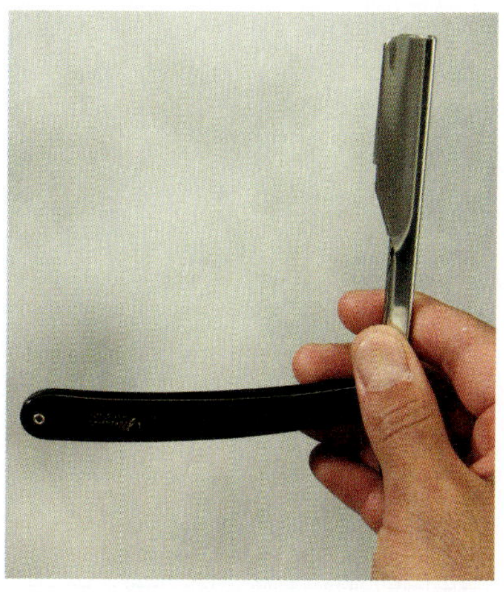

Figure 14–1 Opening the razor.

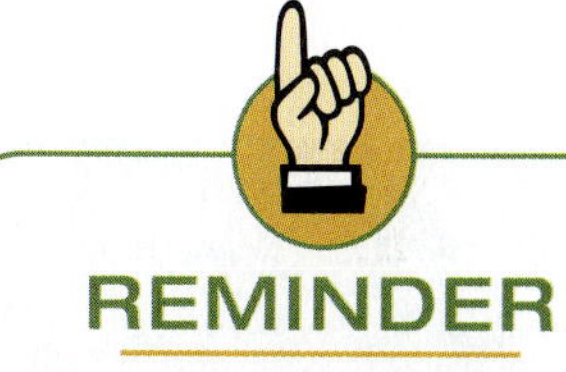

REMINDER

Be careful that the cutting edge does not strike the handle when closing the razor.

Some states prohibit the use of conventional straight razors and allow only changeable-blade razors. Be guided by your state barber board rules and regulations.

14

CAUTION

Always handle razors with extreme care. Warped or loose handles may cause the blade to pass through to the fingers when closing the razor.

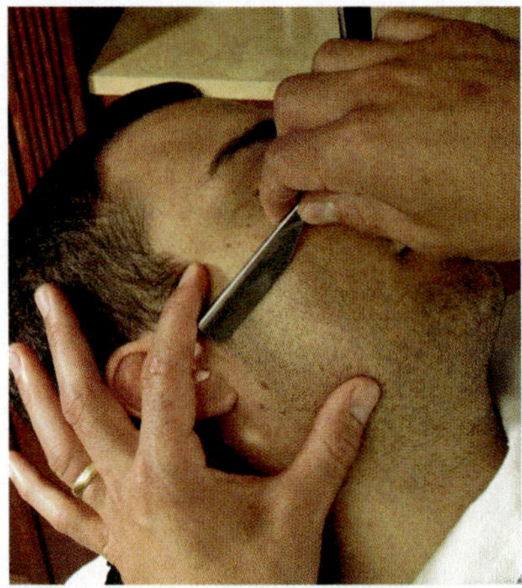

Figure 14-4 Holding position of razor for freehand stroke.

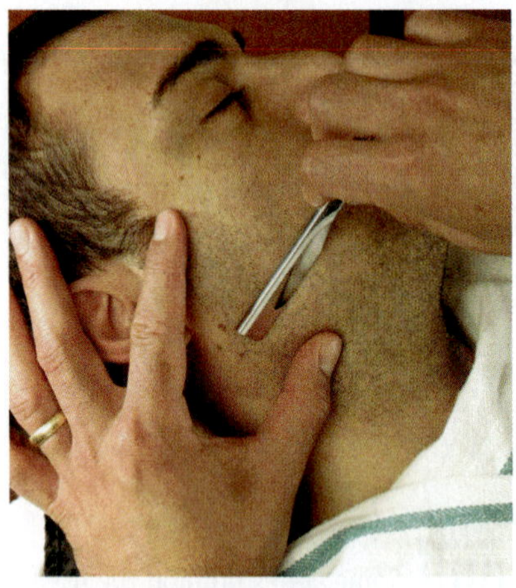

Figure 14-5 Stretch the skin gently with the left hand.

To master the correct hand and finger placement, razor control, and cutting strokes requires practice. Use the following exercises to become comfortable and proficient with a straight razor. The holding positions and strokes that barbers most often employ during the shave service are the freehand, backhand, reverse freehand, and reverse backhand.

Exercise No. 1:

FREEHAND POSITION AND STROKE

1. How to hold the razor.
   The position of the right hand is as follows:
   a) Take the razor in the right hand. Hold the handle of the razor between the third and fourth fingers, with the tip of the small finger resting on the tip of the tang of the razor. The thumb should rest on the side of the shank near the shoulder of the blade. The third finger lies at the pivot of the shank and the handle with the first and second fingers in front of it on the back of the shank (Figure 14–4).
   b) Raise the right elbow to be level with the shoulder. This is the position used in the arm movement.

   The position of the left hand is as follows:
   c) Keep the fingers of the left hand dry in order to prevent them from slipping on the face.
   d) Use the left hand to stretch the skin under the razor (Figure 14–5).
2. How to perform the **freehand stroke** in the freehand position:
   a) Use a gliding stroke, toward you.
   b) Direct the stroke toward the point of the razor in a forward, sawing movement.
3. When to use the freehand stroke.

The freehand position and stroke is used in 6 of the 14 shaving areas. See Nos. 1, 3, 4, 7, 11, and 12 in Figures 14–6 through 14–8.

NOTE: Be guided by your instructor when identifying the numbered shaving areas of 6, 7 and 8 illustrated in Figure 14-6 so that the procedure complies with your state barber board practical exams.

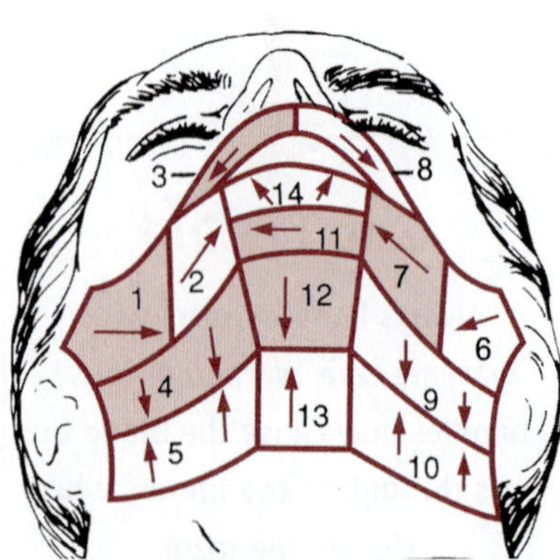

Figure 14-6 Diagram of shaving areas of the face.

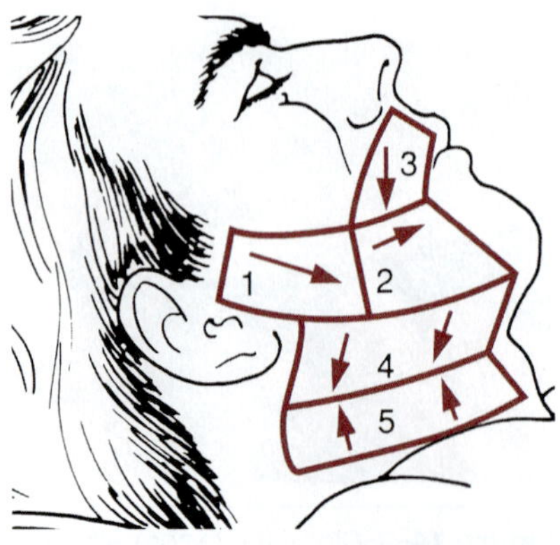

Figure 14-7 Diagram of shaving areas on the right side of the face.

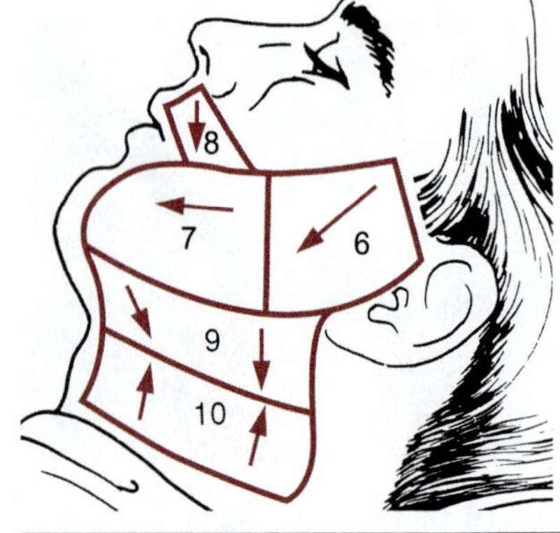

Figure 14-8 Diagram of shaving areas on the left side of the face.

Exercise No. 2:

BACKHAND POSITION AND STROKE

1. How to hold the razor.
   The position of the right hand is as follows:
   a) Hold the shank of the razor firmly with the handle bent slightly back.
   b) Rest the shank of the razor on the first two joints of the first three fingers. Hold the thumb on the underside of the shank. Rest the end of the tang inside the first joint of the third finger as in Figure 14–9. The little finger remains idle. An alternative holding position is shown in Figure 14–10.
   c) Turn the back of the hand away from you and bend the wrist slightly downward. Then raise the elbow so that you can move the arm freely. This is the position used for the backhand stroke with the arm movement. Some practitioners prefer to use a wrist movement, in which case the arm is not held as high.

   The position of the left hand is as follows:
   d) Keep the fingers of the left hand dry in order to prevent them from slipping.
   e) Stretch the skin under the razor.
2. How to perform the **backhand stroke** in the backhand position:
   a) Use a gliding stroke away from you.
   b) Direct the stroke toward the point of the razor in a forward, sawing movement or gentle scraping movement depending on the type of razor used.
3. When to use the backhand stroke.

The backhand stroke is used in 4 of the 14 basic shaving areas and if preferred in area 12. See Nos. 2, 6, 8, and 9 in Figures 14–7 through 14–9.

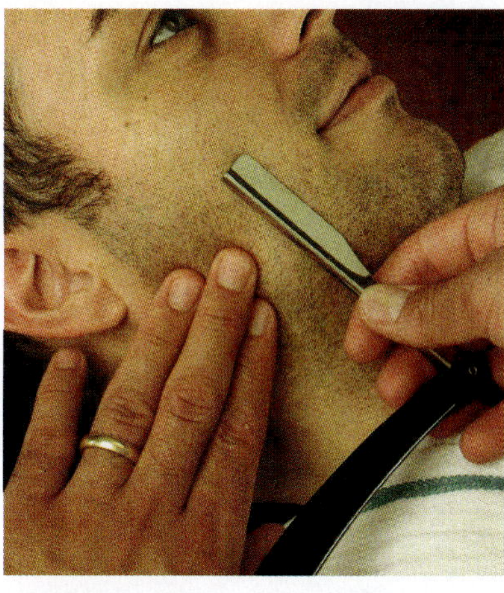

Figure 14-9 Backhand holding position.

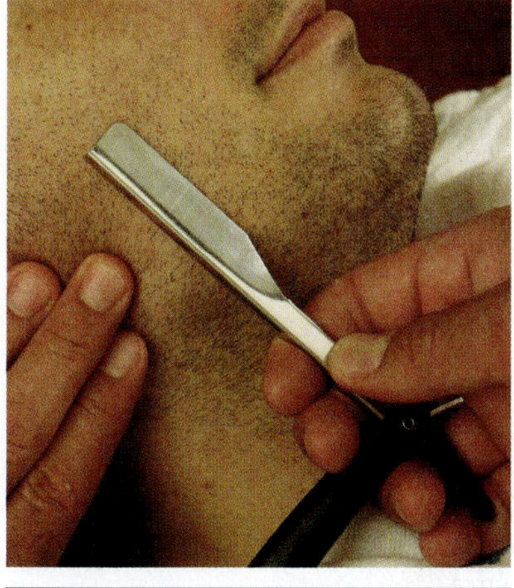

Figure 14-10 Alternative backhand holding position.

Exercise No. 3:

REVERSE FREEHAND POSITION AND STROKE

The **reverse freehand stroke** hand and razor position is similar to the freehand stroke. The stroke movement, however, is performed in an upward rather than a downward direction.

1. How to hold the razor.
   The position of the right hand is as follows:
   a) Hold the razor firmly, as in a freehand position.
   b) Turn the hand slightly toward you so that the razor edge is turned upward (Figure 14–11).

   The position of the left hand is as follows:
   c) Keep the hand dry and use it to pull the skin taut under the razor.
   d) The left hand will be the hand closest to the barber's body in this position.

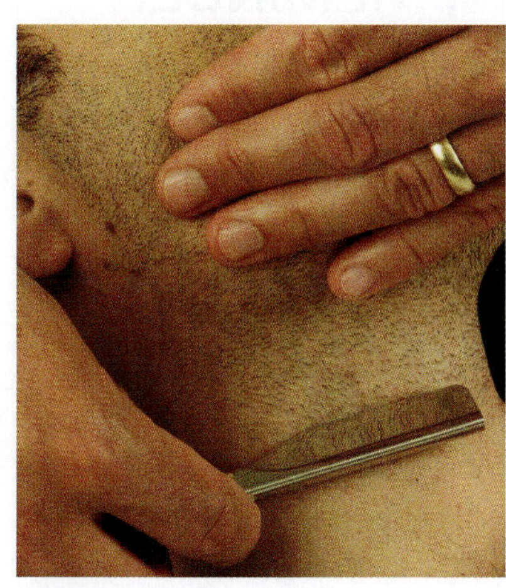

Figure 14-11 Reverse freehand stroke.

14

2. How to perform the reverse freehand stroke in the reverse freehand position:
   a) Use an upward, semi-arc stroke toward you.
   b) The movement is from the elbow to the hand with a slight twist of the wrist.
3. When to use the reverse freehand stroke.

The reverse freehand stroke is used in 4 of the 14 basic shaving areas. See Nos. 5, 10, 13, and 14 on Figures 14–7 through 14–9.

Exercise No. 4:

REVERSE BACKHAND POSITION AND STROKE

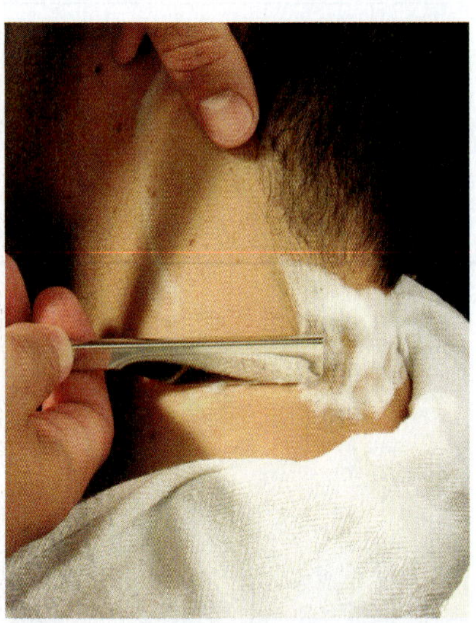

Figure 14-12 Reverse backhand stroke.

The reverse backhand position and stroke require diligent practice to master. The holding position of the razor is the same as that for the backhand stroke except the elbow is positioned downward and the forearm in held upward. When using this stroke, make short cutting strokes in an upward (or downward, depending on shaving area) and slightly outward direction.

1. How to hold the razor.
   The position of the right hand is as follows:
   a) Hold the razor firmly, as in the backhand position.
   b) Turn the palm of the hand to the right so that it faces upward.
   c) Drop the elbow close to the side.
   The position of the left hand is as follows:
   d) Position the left hand so as to be able to draw the skin taut under the razor.
   e) The barber's hand will be positioned above the razor (Figure 14–12).
2. How to perform the **reverse backhand stroke** in the reverse backhand position:
   a) Use a smooth gliding stroke, directed downward toward the point of the razor.
   b) Proceed with short cutting strokes directed downward and slightly outward.
3. When to use the reverse backhand stroke.

The reverse backhand stroke is only used for making the left sideburn outline, and for shaving the left side behind the ear during a neck shave while the client is sitting in an upright position.

The cutting strokes described in the preceding section illustrate the holding and stroking positions that should be employed by the right-handed barber. The left-handed barber will need to reverse the starting position as outlined in Table 14–1. 2

14

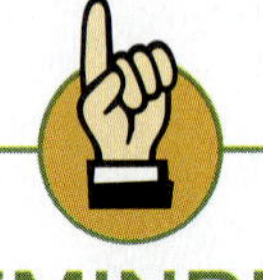

REMINDER

The beard should be shaved at an angle with the grain of the hair; therefore, the barber must determine when the reverse hand positions and strokes are the correct procedure for shaving the client's beard. For example: When the hair in shaving area No. 5 grows downward, the freehand stroke is a better choice than the reverse freehand stroke.

The Professional Shave

A professional shave consists of preparation, shaving, and finishing. The following exercises explain these procedural steps in detail.

Movement	Area of Face for a Left-handed Barber	Position	Direction	Area of Face for a Right-handed Barber
1	Left sideburn	Freehand	Down	Right sideburn
2	Left side of cheek	Backhand	Down	Right side of cheek
3	Left upper lip	Freehand	Down	Right upper lip
4	Left side below jaw	Freehand	Down	Right side below jaw
5	Left side of neck	Reverse freehand	Up	Right side of neck
6	Right upper lip	Backhand	Down	Left sideburn
7	Right sideburn	Freehand	Down	Left side of cheek
8	Right side of cheek	Backhand	Down	Left upper lip
9	Right side below jaw	Backhand	Down	Left side below jaw
10	Right side of neck	Reverse freehand	Up	Left side of neck
11	Across chin R. to L.	Freehand	Across	Across chin L. to R.
12	Below chin	Freehand or backhand	Down	Below chin
13	Middle of neck	Reverse freehand	Up	Middle of neck
14	Lower lip	Reverse freehand	Up	Lower lip

Table 14–1 Shaving Movements for Left-handed and Right-handed Barbers

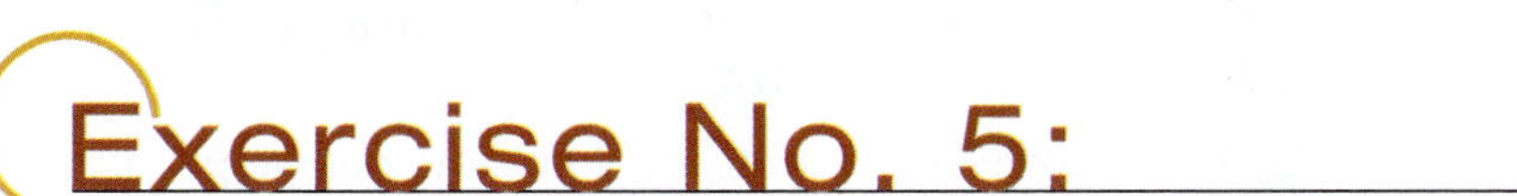

HOW TO PREPARE A CLIENT FOR SHAVING

1. Seat the client comfortably in the chair.
2. Ask the client to loosen his collar. Lay the drape over the client's clothing from the front.
3. Change the headrest cover and adjust it to the proper height.
4. Lower, adjust, and lock the chair to the proper height and level.

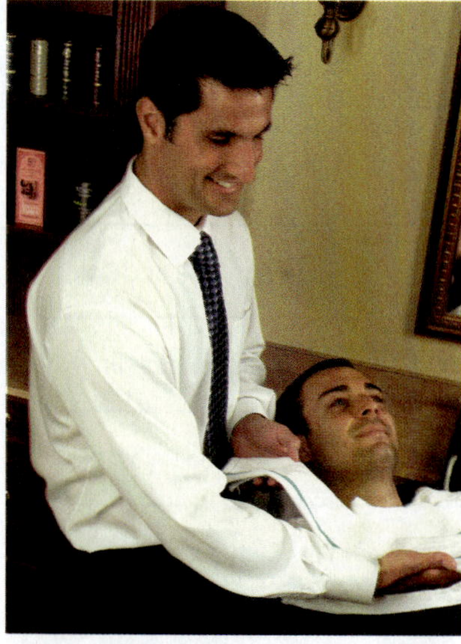

Figure 14–13 Draping second towel across the chest.

5. Wash your hands with soap and warm water, and dry them thoroughly.
6. Unfold a clean towel, and lay it diagonally across the client's chest.
7. Tuck one corner of the towel along the right side of the client's neck, securing the edge tucked inside the neckband with a sliding movement of the forefinger of the left hand. The lower end of the towel is crossed over to the other side of the client's neck and tucked under the neckband, with a similar sliding motion. A second towel or paper strip that is used during the shave to wipe the razor clean of shaving cream and facial hair should be tucked into the neckband and laid across the chest (Figure 14–13).

Exercise No. 6:

HOW TO PREPARE THE FACE FOR SHAVING

CAUTION

Do not use a hot steam towel if the skin is sensitive, irritated, chapped, or blistered.

Lathering and steaming the face are very important steps to preparing the skin for shaving. *Lathering* serves to cleanse the skin, soften the hair, hold the hair in an upright position, and create a smooth, flat surface over which the razor can glide more effectively. *Steaming* the face helps to soften the hair cuticle, provides lubrication by stimulating the action of the oil glands, and relaxes the client. If the client has a mustache, trim and shape it prior to the shave service to prepare it for finish work with the razor.

The face is prepared for shaving as follows:

1. Warm shaving lather is usually prepared in an electric latherizer. Transfer a quantity of lather into the hand and spread it evenly over the bearded areas of the face and neck to be shaved.
2. Use a rotary movement to briskly rub lather into the bearded area with the cushion tips of the fingers. Start at the neck and rub lather up to the right side of the face. Then gently turn the head with the left hand by lightly grasping the top of the head or the back of the head near the crown. Rub lather on the other side of the face and continue lathering until the bearded areas are covered. Rubbing time is from one to two minutes, depending on the stiffness and density of the beard. (Figure 14–14)
3. To prepare a steam towel, fold a clean towel in half lengthwise (Figure 14–15). Then fold it in half again by bringing both ends of the towel together (Figure 14–16).
4. Place the folded towel under a stream of hot water or wrap it around the faucet or hose spray, until it becomes thoroughly saturated and heated (Figure 14–17).
5. Wring out the towel.
6. Standing behind the client, position the steam towel in front of the chin area. Unfold the towel, holding it by the ends. Place the center of the towel over the client's mouth, under the chin, and across the lower part of the neck (Figure 14–18).

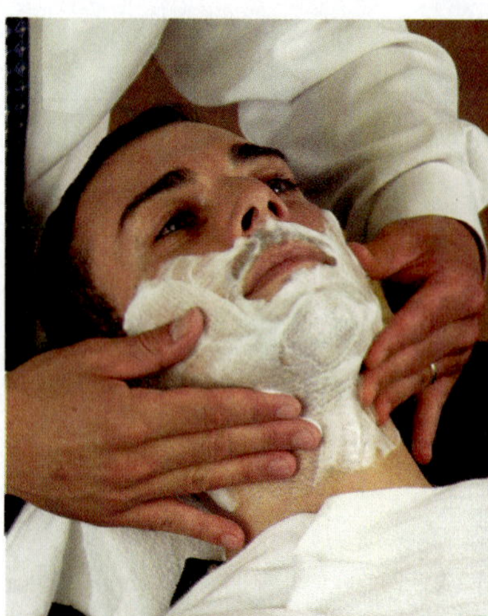

Figure 14–14 Use rotary movements to lather the face.

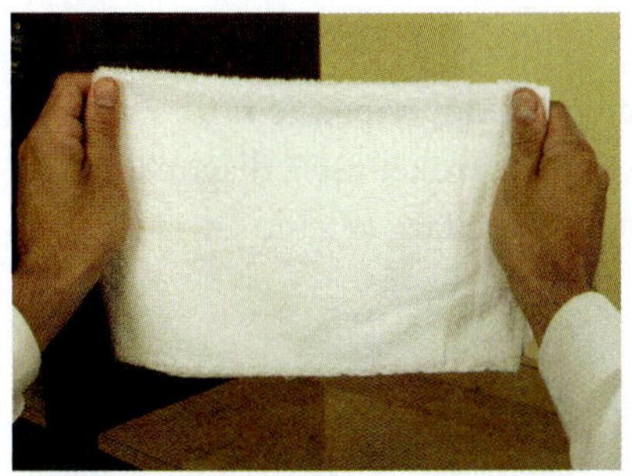

Figure 14–15 Step 1: Fold a clean towel in half, lengthwise.

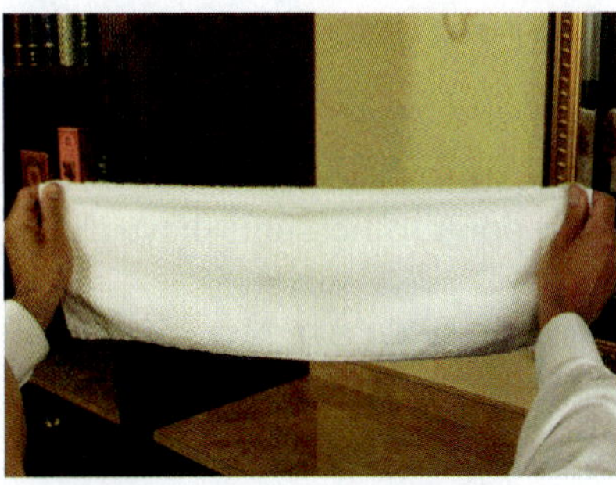

Figure 14–16 Step 2: Fold the towel in half again.

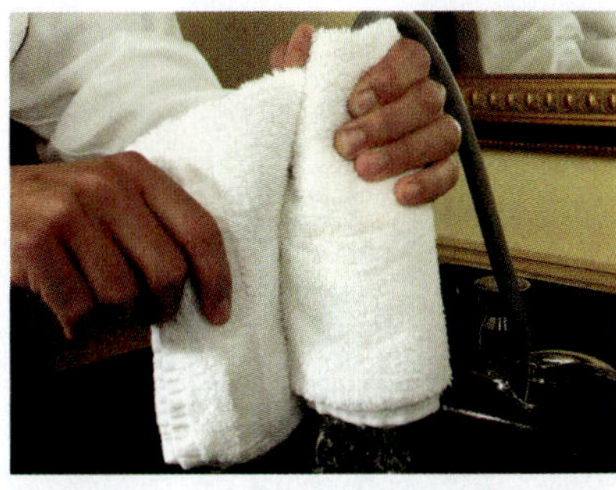

Figure 14–17 Step 3: Wrap the towel around a stream of hot water.

Carefully wrap the towel around the face, leaving the nostrils exposed. Finally, fold the ends over each other on the forehead, covering the eyes (Figure 14–19). Repeat the steaming process if the beard is extremely coarse and/or dense.

7. While the steam towel is on the client's face, strop the razor (if using a conventional straight razor) and immerse it in sanitizing solution.

   NOTE: New blades for changeable-blade razors do not guarantee a sanitized blade. Sanitize this style razor as well. Then wipe the razor dry on a clean towel, and place it in a dry sanitizer or clean, closed container until ready for use.

8. Remove the steam towel and wipe the lather off in one operation.
9. Relather the beard, then wipe the soap from your hands.
10. Standing on the client's right side, begin the shave process.

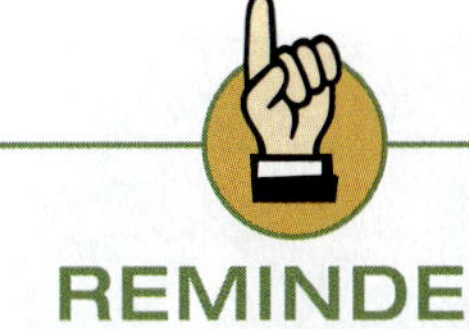

REMINDER

Be sure to sanitize the hose, spray nozzle, and sink *prior* to preparing the steam towel.

Exercise No. 7:

POSITION AND STROKES IN SHAVING

Razor strokes should be correct and systematic. Proper coordination of both hands is necessary. While the right hand holds and strokes the razor, the fingers of the left hand gently stretch the skin area that is being shaved. A taut skin allows the beard hair to be cut more easily.

Loose skin tends to push out in front of the razor and can result in cuts or nicks. Stretching the skin too tightly, however, will cause irritation. The skin must be held firmly, neither too loosely nor too tightly, to create a correct shaving surface for the razor. To prevent slipping, use an alum block to help keep the fingers of the left hand dry at all times.

Shaving Area No. 1

Freehand stroke. Standing at the right side of chair, gently turn the client's face to the left. With the second finger of the left hand, remove the lather from the hairline. Hold the razor as for a freehand stroke. Use long, gliding, diagonal strokes, with the point of the razor leading. Beginning at the hairline on the right side, shave downward toward the jawbone (Figure 14–20).

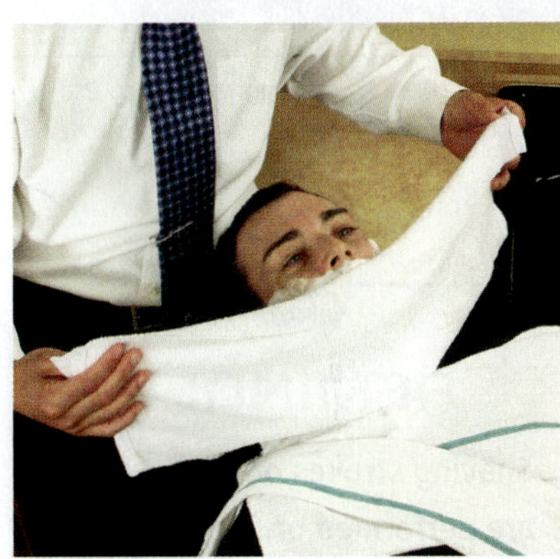

Figure 14–18 Apply the steam towel.

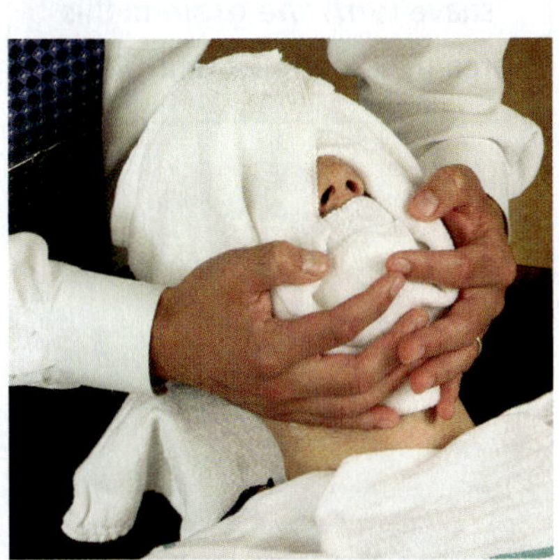

Figure 14–19 Wrap the towel around the face, leaving the nostrils exposed.

Figure 14-20 Shaving area No. 1: freehand stroke.

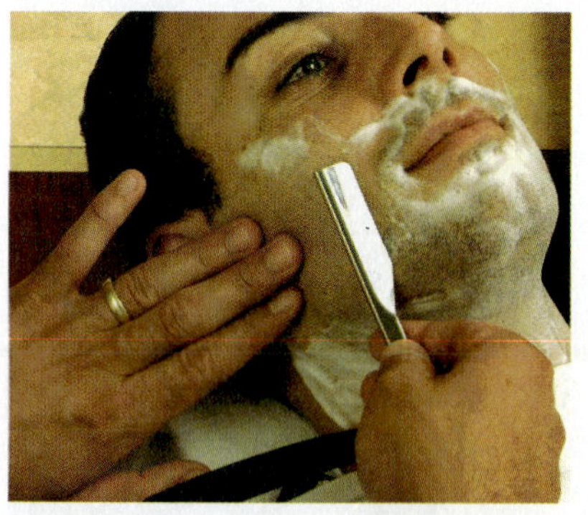

Figure 14-21 Shaving area No. 2: backhand stroke.

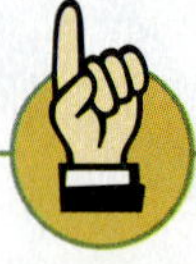

REMINDER

Shaving strokes on the upper lip are performed on a slight diagonal to follow the curves of the face; however, remember to shave *with the grain* in this area (Figures 14-22 and 14-27).

Shaving Area No. 2

Backhand stroke. Remaining in the same position, wipe the razor clean on lather paper. Hold the razor as for a backhand stroke; use a diagonal stroke from point to heel and shave the right side of the face (Figure 14–21).

Shaving Area No. 3

Freehand stroke. Maintaining the same position, wipe the razor clean. Holding it in the same manner as for a freehand stroke, shave underneath the nostrils and over the right side of the upper lip, using the fingers of the left hand to stretch the underlying skin. When shaving underneath the nostril, slightly lift the tip of the nose, taking care not to interfere with breathing. To stretch the upper lip, place the fingers of the left hand against the nose, while holding the thumb below the lower corner of the lip (Figure 14–22). If the client has a mustache, shave the outline with the razor at this time.

Shaving Area No. 4

Freehand stroke. Start at the level of the chin and shave that portion below the jawbone down to the change in the grain of the beard. Be sure to hold the skin taut between the thumb and fingers of left hand (Figure 14–23).

Shaving Area No. 5

Reverse freehand stroke. Move behind the chair. Hold the razor as for a reverse freehand stroke. Shave the remainder of the beard upward with the grain (Figure 14–24). This movement completes shaving of the right side of the face.

Shaving Area No. 6

Backhand stroke. Stand slightly back from the client. Gently turn the face to the right. Relather the left side of the face. Using the thumb, wipe lather from the hairline. Stretch the skin with the fingers of the left hand and shave downward to the lower part of the ear, and slightly forward on the face (Figure 14–25).

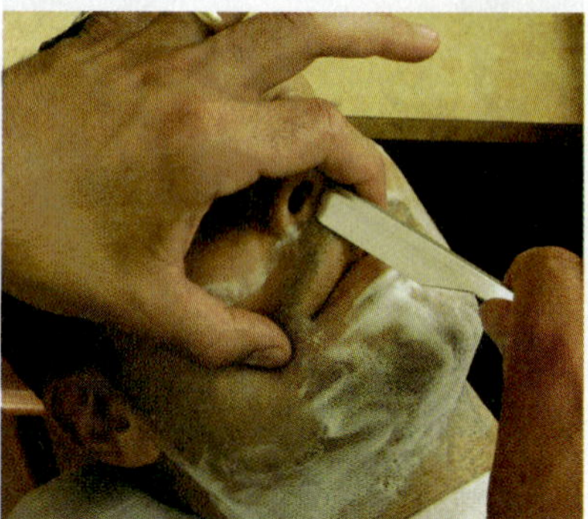

Figure 14-22 Shaving area No. 3: freehand stroke.

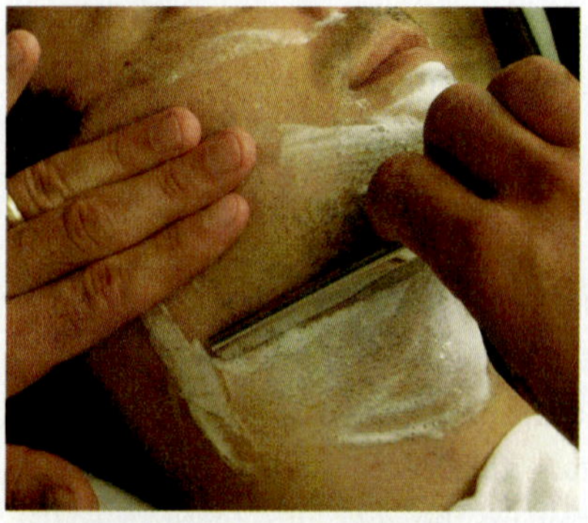

Figure 14-23 Shaving area No. 4: freehand stroke.

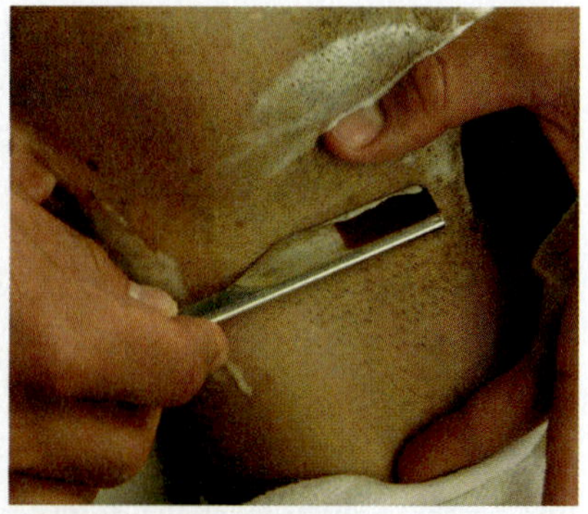

Figure 14-24 Shaving area No. 5: reverse freehand stroke.

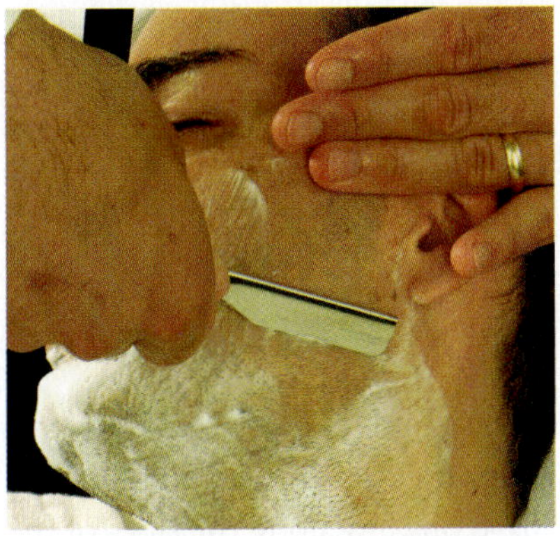

Figure 14-25 Shaving area No. 6: backhand stroke.

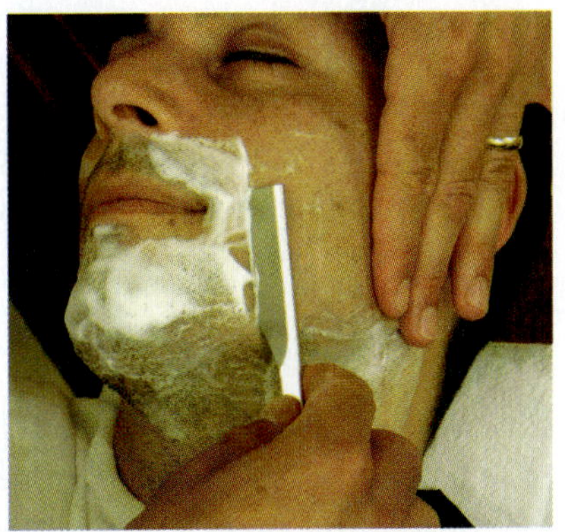

Figure 14-26 Shaving area No. 7: freehand stroke.

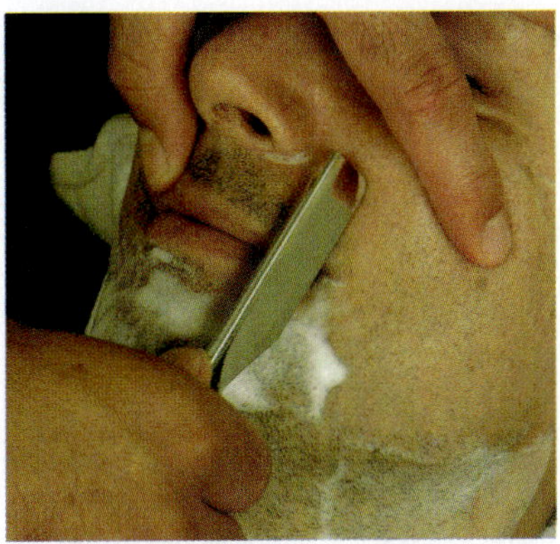

Figure 14-27 Shaving area No. 8: backhand stroke.

NOTE: The skin must be stretched taut to prevent the razor from digging in along the ear.

Shaving Area No. 7

Freehand stroke. Wipe off the razor. Stand to the client's right. Hold the razor as for a freehand stroke. Shave downward on the left side of the face toward the jawbone and point of the chin (Figure 14–26).

Shaving Area No. 8

Backhand stroke. Wipe the razor clean and strop if necessary. Stand to the right side of the client and turn the client's face upward, so that you can shave the left upper lip. Hold the razor as for a backhand stroke. While gently pushing the tip of the nose to the right with the thumb and fingers of the left hand, shave the left side of upper lip (Figure 14–27).

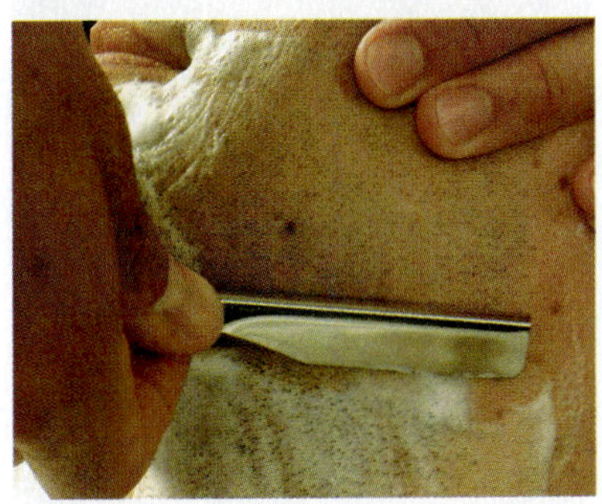

Figure 14-28 Shaving area No. 9: backhand stroke.

Shaving Area No. 9

Backhand stroke. Wipe off the razor. Maintaining the same position, hold the razor as for the backhand stroke. With the fingers of the left hand stretching the skin, shave downward to a point where the grain of the beard changes on the neck (Figure 14–28).

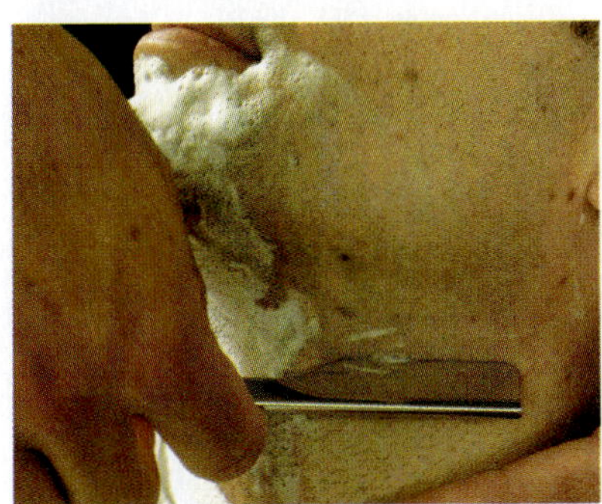

Figure 14-29 Shaving area No. 10: reverse freehand stroke.

Shaving Area No. 10

Reverse freehand stroke. Wipe off the razor. Stand slightly back from the client. Hold the razor as for the reverse freehand stroke. Stretching the skin with the left hand, shave the left side of the neck upward (Figure 14–29).

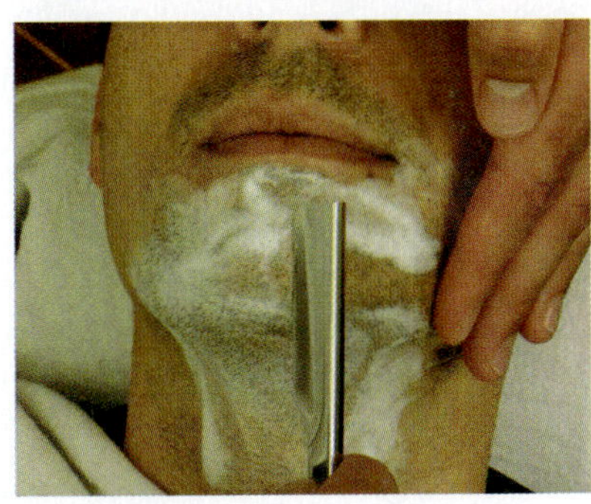

Figure 14-30 Shaving area No. 11: freehand stroke.

Shaving Area No. 11

Freehand stroke. Stand at the client's side and turn the head so the face is pointing up. Holding the razor as for the freehand stroke, shave across the upper part of the chin. Continue shaving across the chin until it has been shaved to a point below the jawbone. The skin is stretched with the left hand (Figure 14–30).

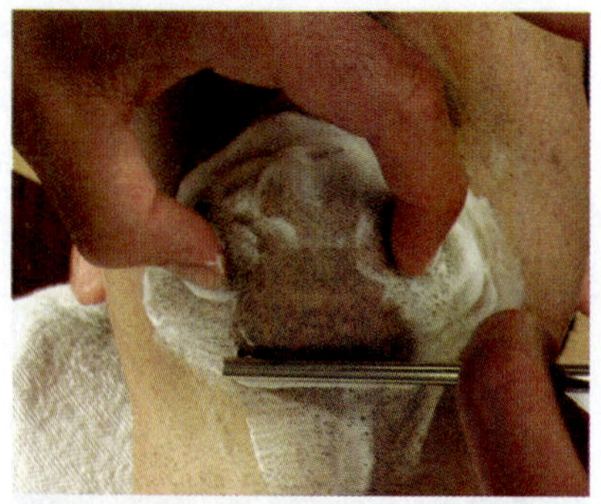

Figure 14-31 Shaving area No. 12: freehand stroke.

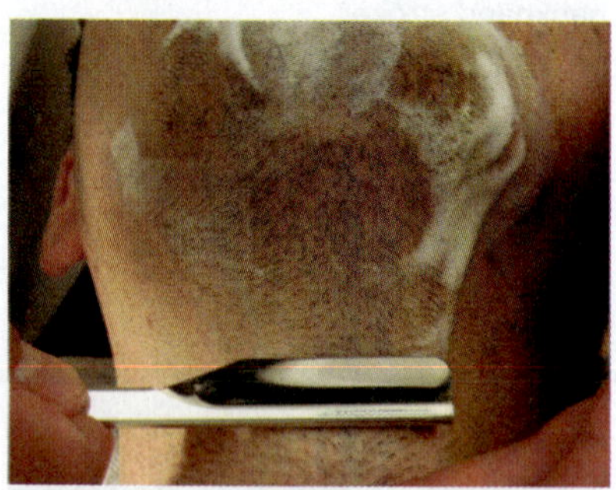

Figure 14-32 Shaving area No. 13: reverse freehand stroke.

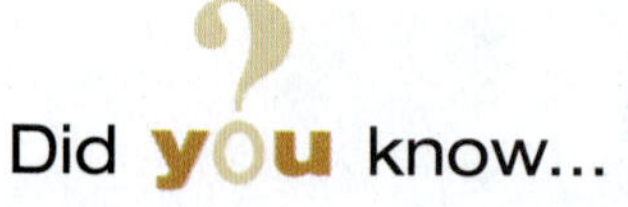

In shaving areas 11 and 14, the client can help to stretch the skin if he rolls his bottom lip slightly over his bottom teeth. This may be known as *balling-the-chin.*

14

Shaving Area No. 12

Freehand stroke. Stretch the skin with the left hand and shave the area just below the chin until the change in the grain of the beard is reached (Figure 14–31). Alternate method: some barbers prefer to use the backhand stroke in shaving area No. 11.

Shaving Area No. 13

Reverse freehand stroke. Move behind the chair. Hold the razor for the reverse freehand stroke. Stretch the skin below the chin and shave upward on the lower part of the neck (Figure 14–32). Shave upward along the sides of the Adam's apple on a slight diagonal to prevent nicks (Figure 14–32).

Shaving Area No. 14

Reverse freehand stroke. Remain behind the chair. Shave upward from the chin toward the lower lip with a few short reverse freehand strokes (Figure 14–33). Wipe off the razor and discard the towel or paper strip.

The Once-Over Shave

The **once-over shave** requires less time for a complete shave service and was once used when men patronized barbershops for their daily shaves. To perform a once-over shave, shave a few more strokes *across the grain* while completing each shaving movement. This will assure a complete and even shave with a single lathering.

The Second-Time-Over Shave

The second-time-over shave follows a regular shave and serves to remove any rough or uneven spots. Using water instead of lather, shave with or across the grain to remove any residual facial hair. This technique may be considered a form of close shaving and care should be taken to avoid irritation or injury to the skin.

The Close Shave

Close shaving is the practice of shaving the beard *against the grain* of the hair during the second-time-over phase of the shave. This practice is undesirable because it may irritate the skin and lead to infection or ingrown hairs. For this reason, barbers and barber-stylists do not traditionally employ close-shaving methods. However, should the client request it, first remove all traces of lather with a steam towel following the first-time-over shave. Turn the towel over and place it on the face. After removing the steam towel remoisten the bearded part of the face and proceed with the second-time-over shave, shaving against the grain. Use free-hand and reverse free-hand strokes as necessary to access the different shaving areas of the face.

When employing the reverse free-hand stroke, stand slightly behind the client. Stroking the grain of the beard sideways will help to facilitate positioning the facial hair to be shaved in this manner. When finished, wipe off the razor on lather paper, a neck strip, or a paper towel. Follow up with the final steps of the shave service, but do not offer to perform a deep cleansing facial at this time as doing so may irritate the skin. Discard all soiled papers in a closed container.

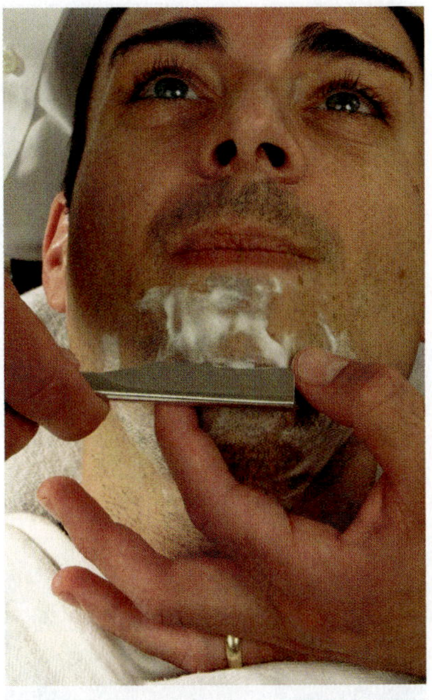

Figure 14-33 Shaving area No. 14: reverse freehand stroke.

Exercise No. 8:

FINAL STEPS OF THE FACIAL SHAVE

The final steps in shaving require attention to a number of important details.

1. Following the shave, apply light facial cream or moisturizing lotion with effleurage massage movements.
2. Prepare a moderately warm towel and apply it over the face. CAUTION: Avoid excessively hot steam towels, as the skin may be sensitive after the shave service.

   NOTE: A complete facial treatment may be performed at this time if the client desires the service.
3. Remove the towel from the face.
4. Apply a toner or other mild astringent using cotton pledgets or a soft tissue. Pat gently; do not wipe or scrape against the skin.
5. Remove the towel from the client's chest and position yourself behind the chair.
6. Spread the towel over the client's face. Pat dry the lower part, then the upper part of the face. Remove the towel and fan the face dry.
7. Move to the right side of the chair and wrap a clean dry towel around your hand, as described in Exercise No. 9.
8. Sprinkle a small amount of talcum powder on the towel and apply evenly to the face.
9. Slowly raise the chair to an upright position.
10. Perform a neck shave if requested, as described in Exercise No. 10.
11. Comb the hair neatly as desired.
12. Wipe off loose hair, lather, or powder from the client's face and clothing. Proceed with mustache trim if not performed before shave service. Remove draping.

4

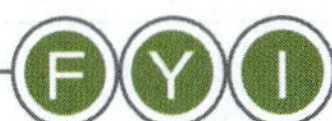

Apply powdered styptic with a cotton swab to nicks or cuts that occur while shaving.

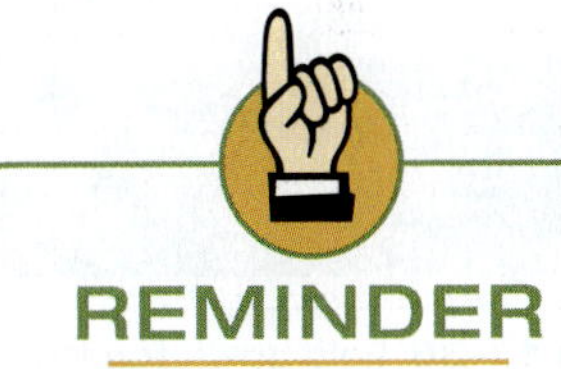

REMINDER

After-shave lotion and witch hazel are astringent preparations commonly used in the barbershop.

14

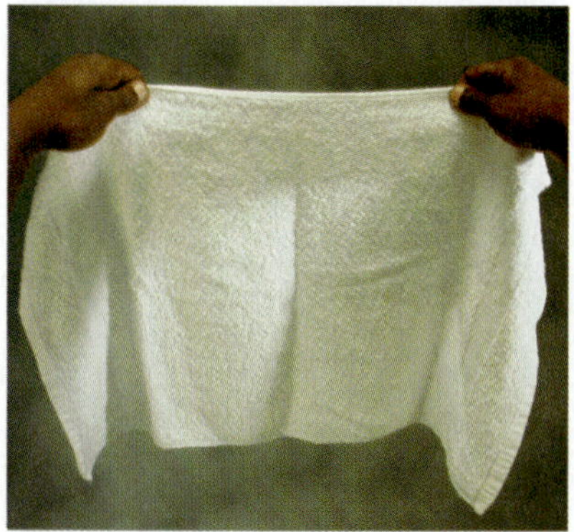
Figure 14-34 Grasp towel lengthwise.

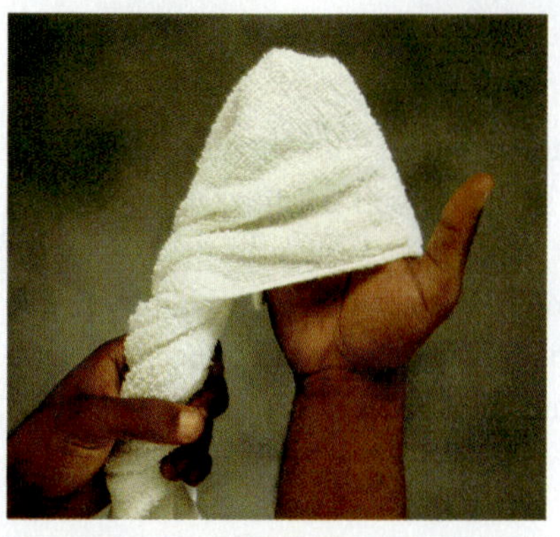
Figure 14-35 Draw towel over palm and twist the ends.

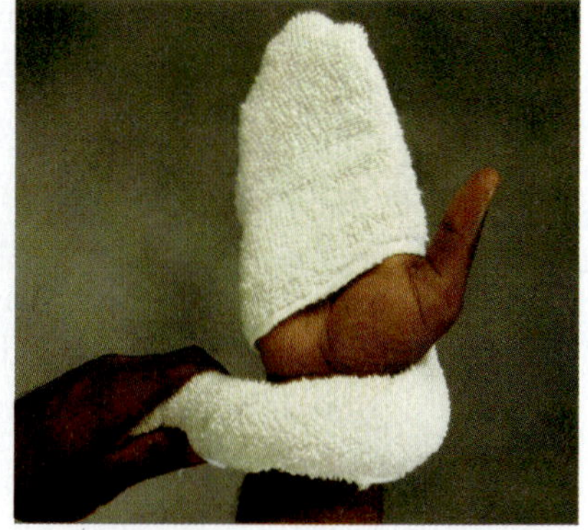
Figure 14-36 Wrap twisted towel ends around back of hand and across the wrist.

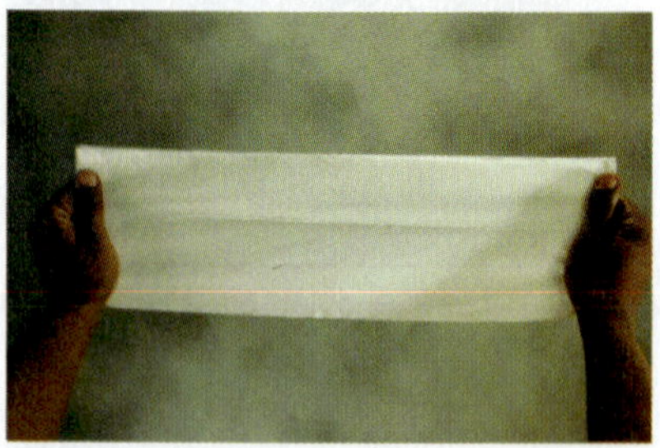
Figure 14-37 Grasp the towel lengthwise.

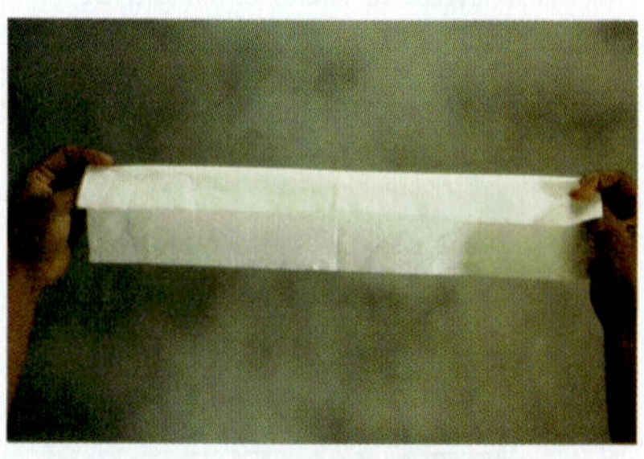
Figure 14-38 Fold down top third of towel.

Exercise No. 9:

TOWEL WRAP

Properly trained barbers and barber-stylists know how to wrap a towel around the hand with ease and skill for the purposes of:

1. Cleansing and drying the face.
2. Applying powder to the face.
3. Removing all traces of powder, lather, and loose hair from the face, neck, and forehead.

Barbering students should practice the towel-wrapping methods illustrated in Figures 14–34 to 14–44 before beginning a facial shave service. Figures 14–34 to 14–36 show one method of wrapping a cotton towel around the hand; Figures 14–37 to 14–44 illustrate wrapping with a paper barber's towel. Either wrapping method can also be used with a flat-weave cotton towel.

Cloth towel wrap: Grasp towel lengthwise (Figure 14–34). Holding your right hand in front of you, draw the upper edge of the towel across the palm

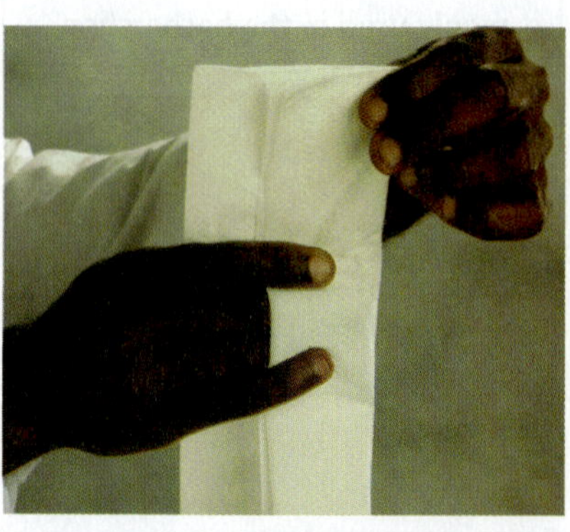
Figure 14-39 Insert two middle fingers into the fold.

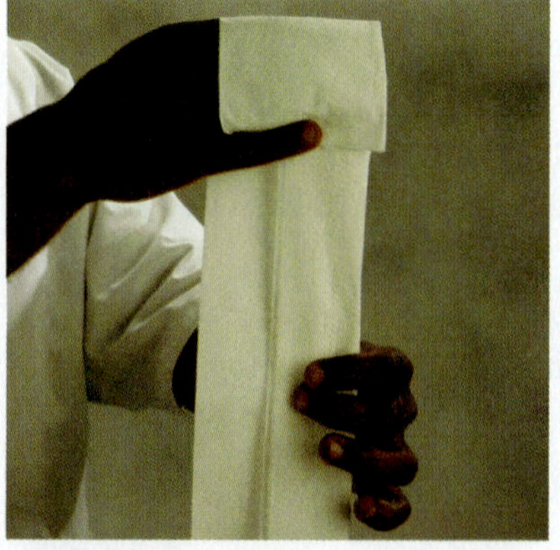
Figure 14-40a Bring top edge around hand and secure with fourth finger.

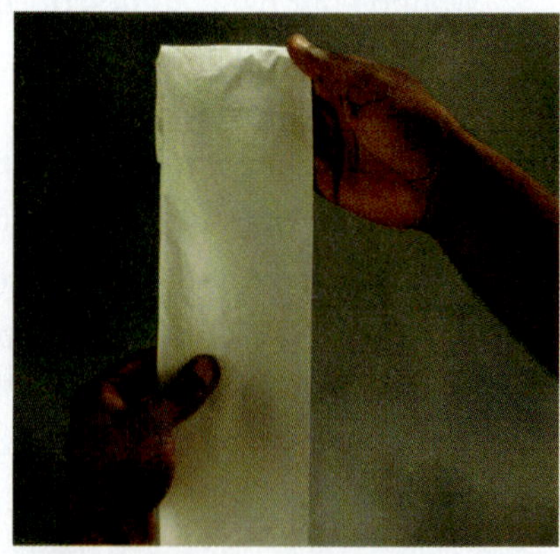
Figure 14-40b Front view.

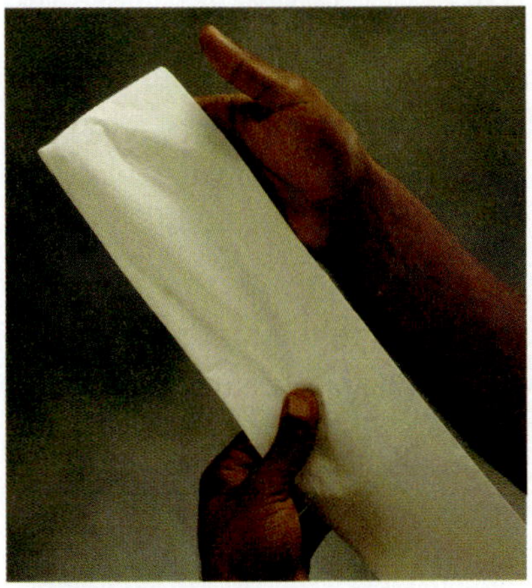

Figure 14-41 Reposition towel diagonally.

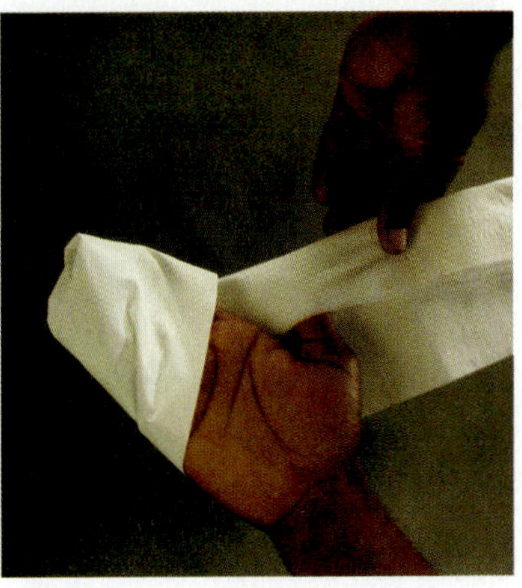

Figure 14-42 Wrap hand and insert thumb into fold.

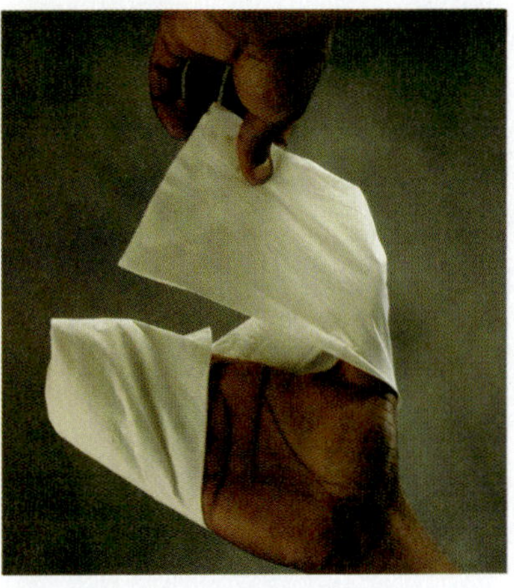

Figure 14-43 Wrap the thumb.

of the right hand; then grasp the towel ends and twist (Figure 14–35). Wrap the twisted ends of the towel around the back of the hand and bring over the inside of the wrist (Figure 14–36). Hold the ends of the towel while in use to prevent them from flapping in the client's face.

Paper towel wrap: Grasp the towel lengthwise (Figure 14–37). Fold down the top third of towel toward you (Figure 14–38). Holding the towel at one end, insert the two middle fingers into the fold (Figure 14–39); maintain your grip on the towel with the thumb, index finger, and fourth finger. Bring the top edge around the back of the hand and secure with the fourth finger (Figures 14–40a and 14–40b). Grasp the towel end and shift to a diagonal position (Figure 14–41). Wrap the remaining towel length around the back of the hand and insert thumb into the fold (Figure 14–42). Continue wrapping motion around the thumb (Figure 14–43). Tuck the towel end into wrap at the back of the hand (Figure 14–44).

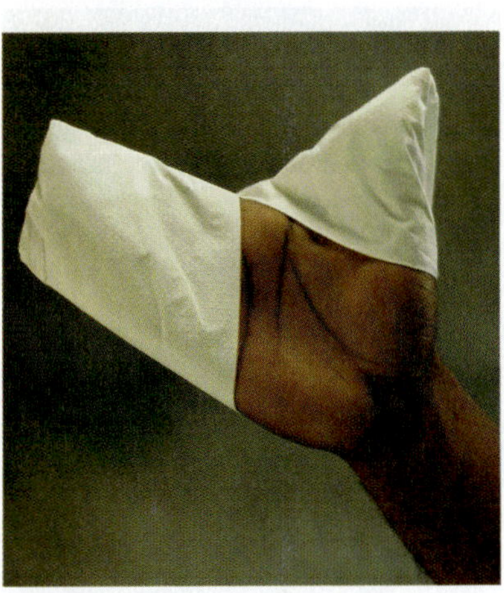

Figure 14-44 Tuck towel end into wrap at back of hand.

Exercise No. 10:

THE NECK SHAVE

The neck shave follows a haircut and involves shaving the neckline on both sides of the neck below the ears and across the nape if desired or necessary.

Raise the chair slowly to an upright position and tuck the towel around the back of the neck. Leave the drape and towel loose enough to facilitate access to the sides and bottom of the neckline. Tuck a neck strip or paper toweling into the neckline of the drape for wiping the blade of lather. Apply lather. Shave the neckline, first at the right side using a freehand stroke, and then at the left side using a reverse backhand stroke, as described in Exercise No. 4 (Figures 14–45 and 14–46). Use a freehand stroke to shave the nape area as desired (Figure 14–47).

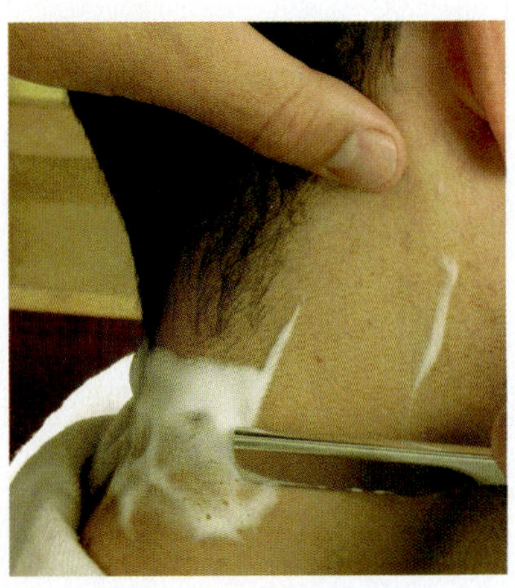

Figure 14-45 Neck shave on the right side with freehand stroke.

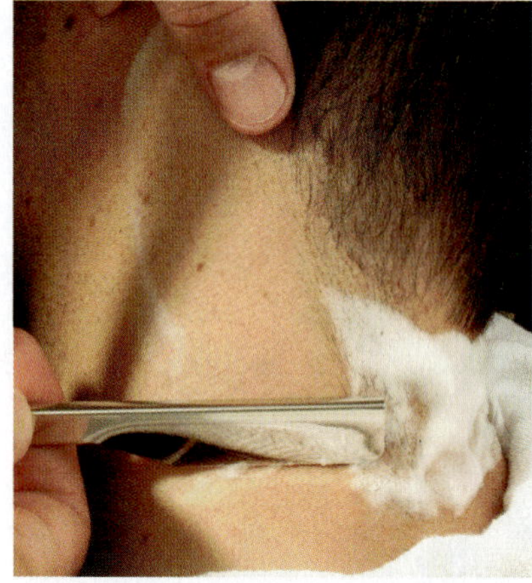

Figure 14-46 Neck shave on the left side with reverse backhand stroke.

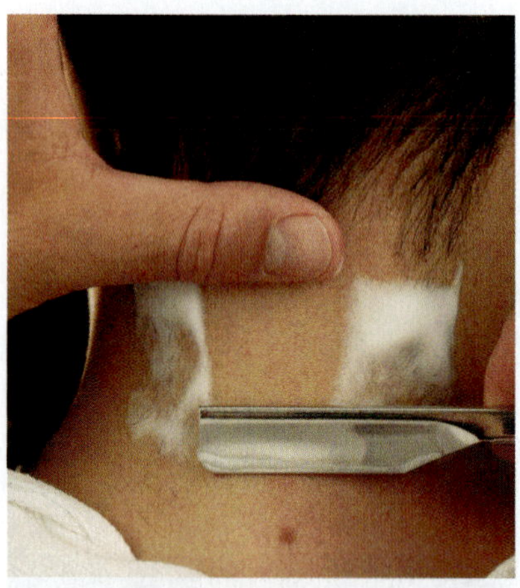

Figure 14-47 Neck shave in the nape area with freehand stroke.

14

FYI

Occasionally a client will request a neck shave following a facial shave in order to maintain a well-groomed appearance between haircuts.

Clean the shaven part of the neckline with toweling or a neck strip moistened with witch hazel, antiseptic, or warm water. Remove the towel from around the neck and dry thoroughly. (This is the time to suggest a leave-in scalp treatment or hair tonic.) Position yourself behind the chair, replace the towel around the client's neck, and comb or style the hair as desired by the client.

Take the towel from the back of the neck and fold it around the right hand. Remove all traces of powder and any loose hair. Discard the towel and remove the chair cloth from the client. Make out the price check and thank the client as it is handed to him. 5

Customer Satisfaction

While there are many reasons why a client may find fault with the shave procedure, the most common are as follows:

1. Dull or rough razors
2. Unclean hands, towels, or shaving cloth
3. Cold fingers
4. Heavy touch
5. Poorly heated towels
6. Lather that is either too cold or too hot
7. Glaring overhead lights
8. Unshaven hair patches
9. Scraping the skin and close shaving
10. Offensive body odor or foul breath of the barber

INTRODUCTION TO FACIAL HAIR DESIGN

In addition to cutting and styling hair, barbers and barber-stylists should be able to offer clients a full range of services for grooming facial hair. Unlike in the past, men do not have to wait for fashion trends to decide to grow their mustaches or beards. Because today's style is one of individuality, barbering students should become proficient, or even specialists, in the design and trimming of men's facial hair. The client that wears a mustache and/or beard will frequent a shop that can provide both haircutting and facial hair services.

THE MUSTACHE

The mustache is worn primarily for personal adornment rather than utility and the wearer is usually very particular about how it is designed and maintained. Care, artistry, and sensitivity to the client's preferences are required for this service. Corrective shaping or redesign of the mustache by the barber helps clients with their daily maintenance and trimming at home until the next visit to the barbershop.

In addition to knowing how to trim and shape mustaches, barbers and barber-stylists should be able to understand and apply certain principles of mustache design.

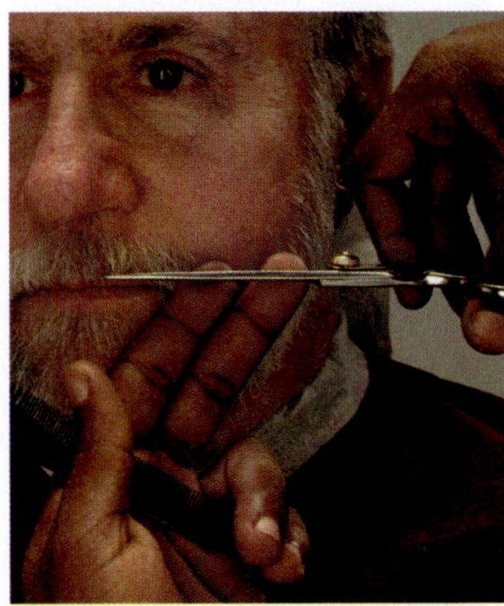

Figure 14-48 Trimming mustache length with shears.

Mustache Design

Choosing a suitable mustache design depends on the client's facial features, hair growth, and personal taste. As with hairstyling services, facial features are of primary importance in the selection process. The size of the mustache should correspond to the size of the features—such as a large design for heavy features, and a smaller design for fine, small facial features.

Important facial characteristics that help to determine the choice of mustache design include: the width of the mouth; size of the nose; shape of upper lip area; width of the cheeks, jaw, and chin; and the density of hair growth. As a general rule, be guided by the client's pattern of hair growth and avoid cutting into natural hairlines too deeply to minimize daily maintenance. Additional guidelines for mustache design and proportion are as follows:

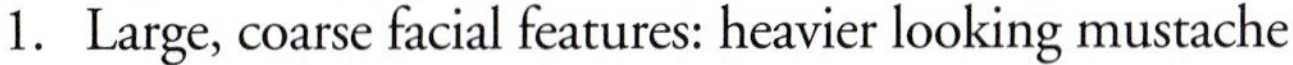

1. Large, coarse facial features: heavier looking mustache
2. Prominent nose: medium to large mustache
3. Long, narrow face: narrow to medium mustache
4. Extra-large mouth: pyramid-shaped mustache
5. Extra-small mouth: medium, short mustache
6. Smallish, regular features: smaller, triangular mustache
7. Wide mouth with prominent upper lip: heavier handlebar or large, divided mustache
8. Round face with regular features: semi-square mustache
9. Square face with prominent features: heavier, linear mustache with ends slightly curving downward

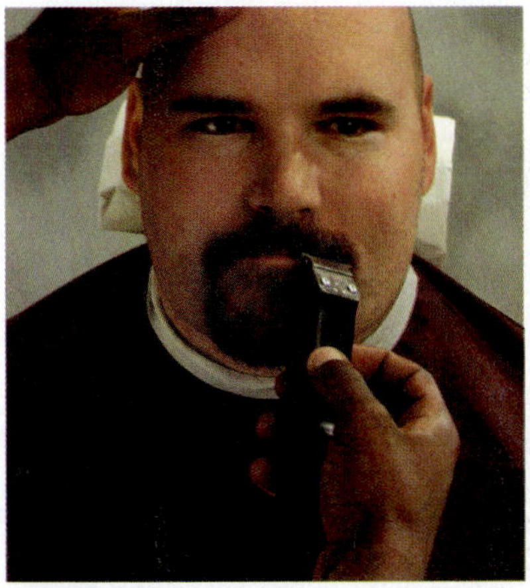

Figure 14-49 Trimming mustache length with outliner.

14

Procedure for Trimming a Mustache

1. Drape the client as for a haircut service.
2. Consult with the client regarding shape preferences.
3. Trim the mustache to the desired length with shears or outliner. Check for evenness of length at the corners of the mouth (Figures 14–48 and 14–49).
4. Remove bulk from the mustache using shears or shear-over-comb technique (Figures 14–50 and 14–51).
5. Shape the mustache with a razor or outliner (Figure 14–52).

Additional mustache services that may be offered with a mustache trim include waxing mustache ends, penciling with temporary color, or coloring for overall color evenness or compatibility with scalp hair color.

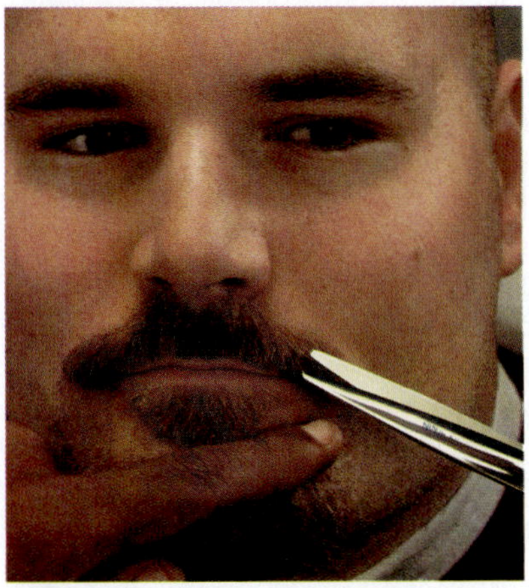

Figure 14-50 Removing bulk using shears.

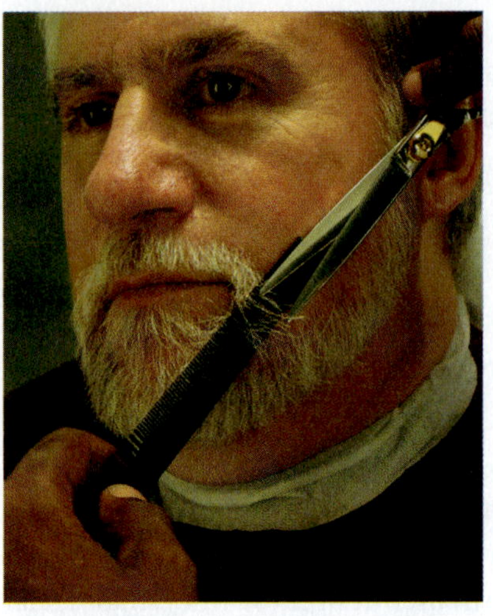

Figure 14-51 Removing bulk using shear-over-comb method.

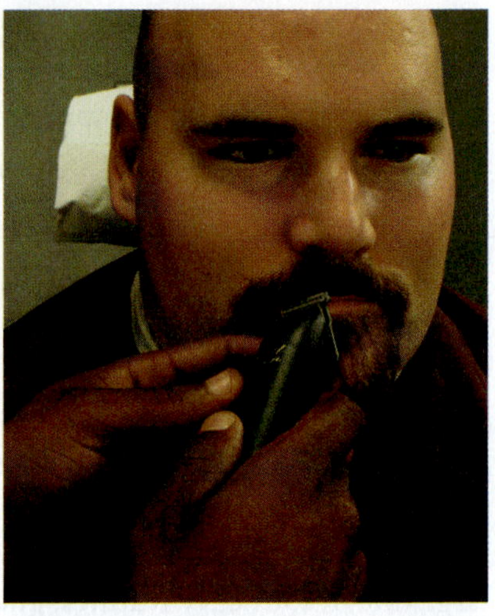

Figure 14-52 Shaping the mustache with outliner.

THE BEARD

The purpose of a beard or goatee is to balance the facial features and to correlate the proportions of face, head, and body. As with their mustaches, men are usually very particular about the design of their beards. Again, a careful approach, artistry, and sensitivity to the client's preferences are required for this service.

If the client is to receive a haircut service in addition to the beard trim, the decision must be made as to which service will be performed first. This is completely a matter of choice for the barber, as he or she will have his or her own reasons for doing so. Some barbers prefer to cut and style the hair prior to the beard trim so as to better balance the length and fullness of the beard with the hairstyle.

Beard Design

The correct shaping or redesign of the beard can emphasize pleasant facial features, minimize less desirable ones, and camouflage flaws. As with other hair design, it is important to develop a "good eye" for balance and proportion of the beard. Very few individuals have perfectly symmetrical face shapes, so barbers are usually challenged to create an illusion of symmetry. It may help the beginning barber to use an eyebrow pencil to draw the design and make any corrections prior to cutting the beard.

During the first trimming, it is advisable to leave the facial hair slightly longer than the desired end result. This helps to avoid cutting the hair too closely and leaves it long enough for retrimming toward the end of the

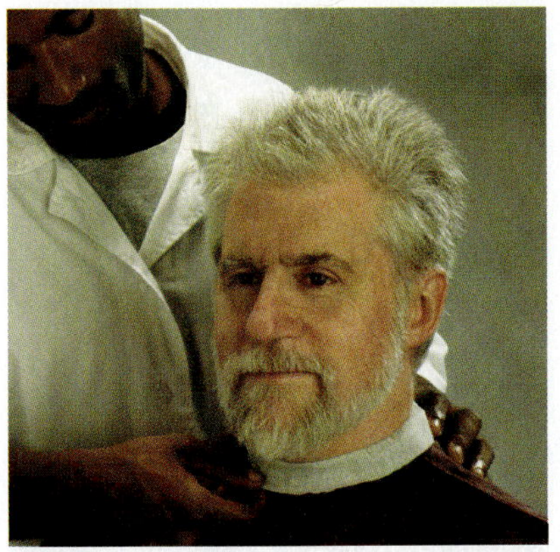
Figure 14–53a Drape for a haircut service.

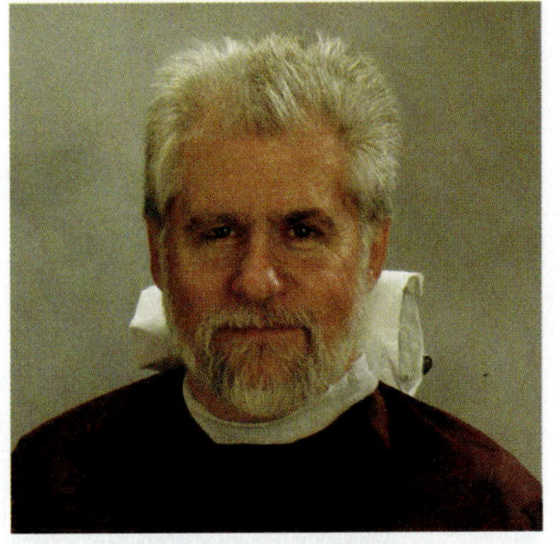
Figure 14–53b Client before beard trim.

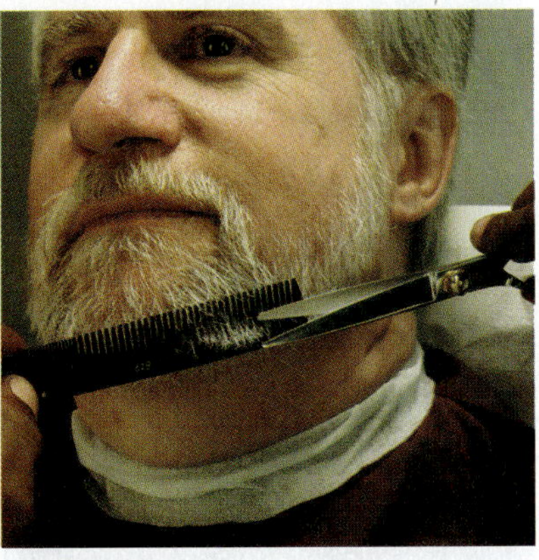
Figure 14–54 Trim excess hair.

beard design service. Beard design and trimming is usually performed with a combination of the shears, comb, outliner (and/or clippers), and razor.

Procedure for Trimming a Beard

1. Drape the client as for a haircut service (Figure 14–53a).
2. Consult with the client as to his desired design of the beard. Determine any preferences regarding length, density (thickness), and shape (Figure 14–53b).
3. With the client in an upright sitting position, use an eyebrow pencil to draw in the beard design (optional). Confer with the client as to his preferences and approval.
4. Adjust the headrest so the client's neck is supported while leaning his head back. The chair may also be reclined slightly or totally depending on your preference for reaching areas under the chin. Remember to check the proportion and shape of the beard when the client is returned to a sitting position.
5. Place a towel underneath the chin to protect the client's neck from stray hairs (optional).
6. Trim excess hair with shears and comb (Figure 14–54).
7. Create a design line with the outliner. Start in the center directly under the chin and outline the under part of the beard (Figure 14–55). Work to the right side of the face up to the sideburn and ear area, then repeat for the left side.
8. Outline the cheek and upper areas of the beard, blending with the sideburn area (Figure 14–56).
9. Using the shear-over-comb technique, taper and blend the beard from the outlined areas up to just under the bottom lip, mustache, and cheek areas (Figure 14–57).
10. Trim and blend the mustache (Figure 14–58).
11. Apply steam towel, lather areas to be shaved, shave carefully at the outline, and wipe clean.
12. Return client to sitting position.

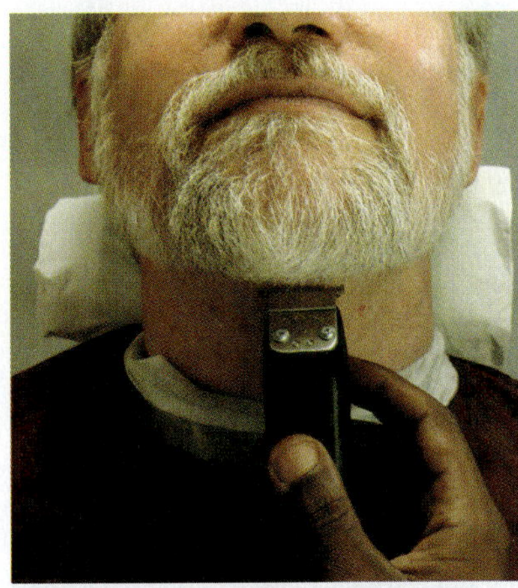
Figure 14–55 Create a design line with outliner.

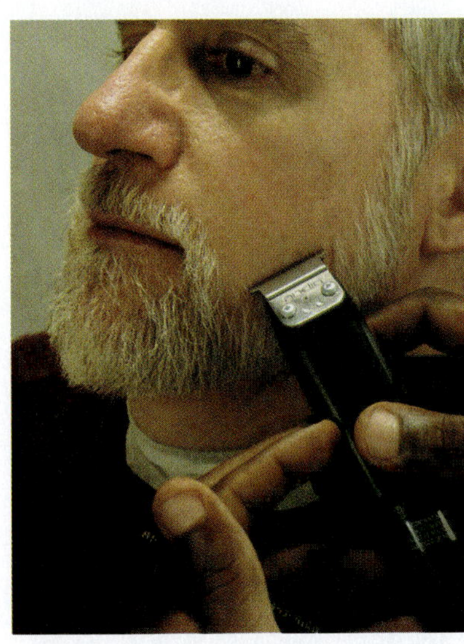
Figure 14–56 Outline the cheek areas of the beard.

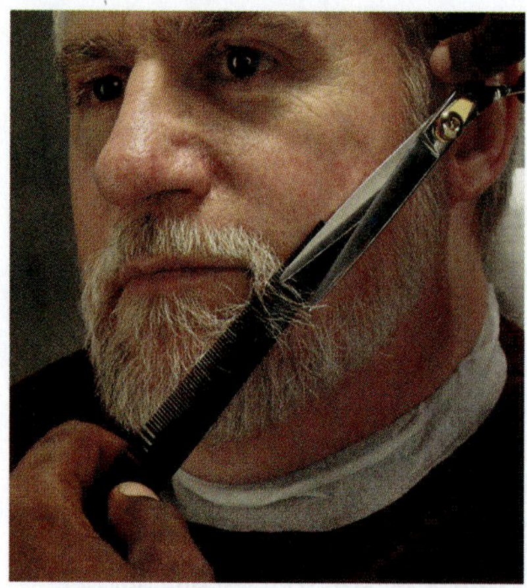

Figure 14–57 Blend from outlined areas to mustache.

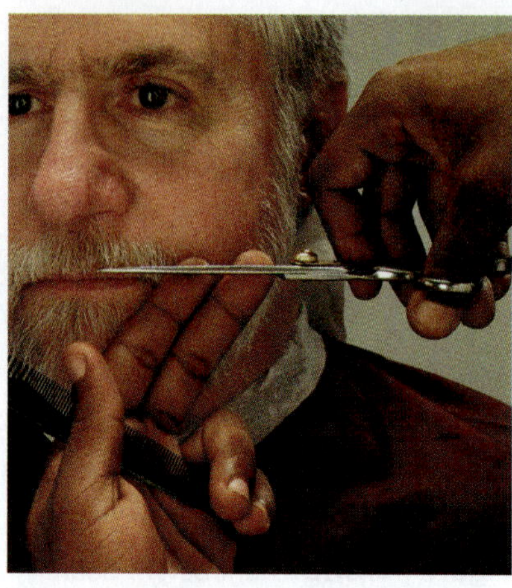

Figure 14–58 Trim mustache.

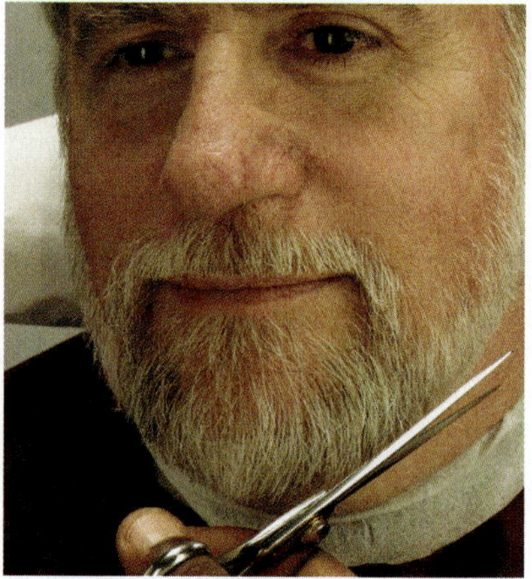

Figure 14–59 Complete detail finish work on beard with shears.

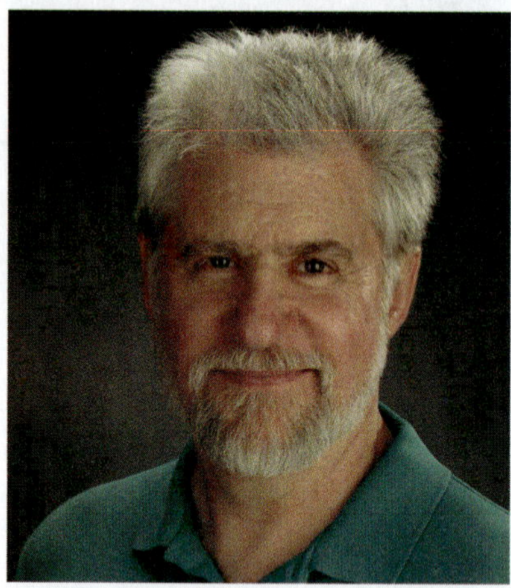

Figure 14–60 Completed beard trim.

13. Wipe off any remaining lather or pencil marks. Apply after-shave lotion.
14. Check and retouch the beard with shears and outliner wherever necessary (Figure 14–59).
15. Style or cut the hair as needed for a finished look (Figure 14–60).

In some cases, your client may desire more than a beard trim . . . he may desire a whole new look! Such a request requires the barber to create a new beard design that complements and balances the structure of the client's face. Figures 14–61 to 14–68 show the progression of creating a new mustache and goatee design. 6

Clippers, Comb, and Outliner Method

Clippers may also be used for beard trimming, especially if one overall length is desired. Clipper-cut beard trims are most successful on clients

14

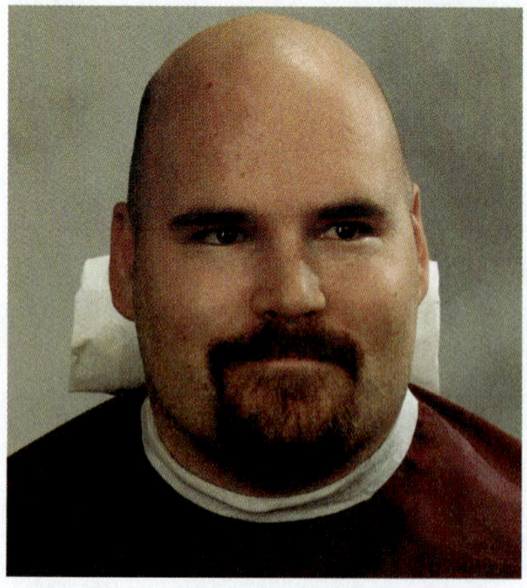

Figure 14–61 Client before beard design.

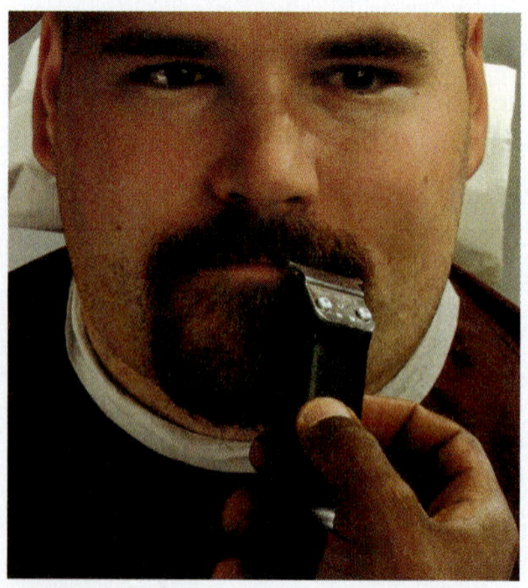

Figure 14–62 Establish mustache length.

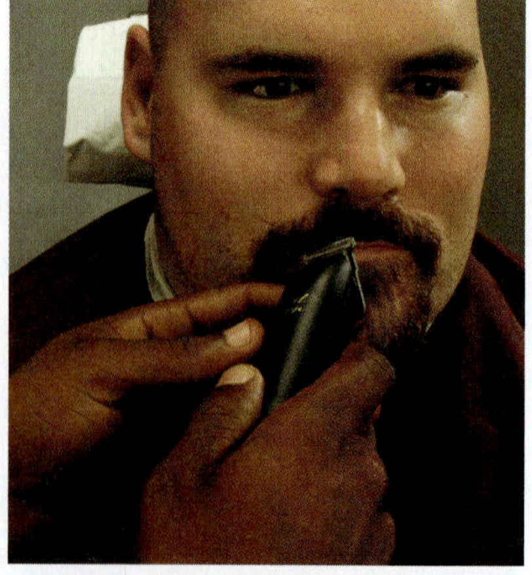

Figure 14–63 Shape mustache from center to corner.

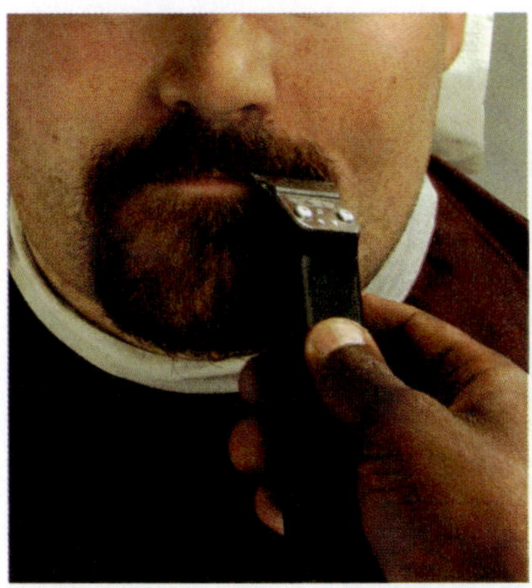
Figure 14-64 Shape corner and ends of mustache.

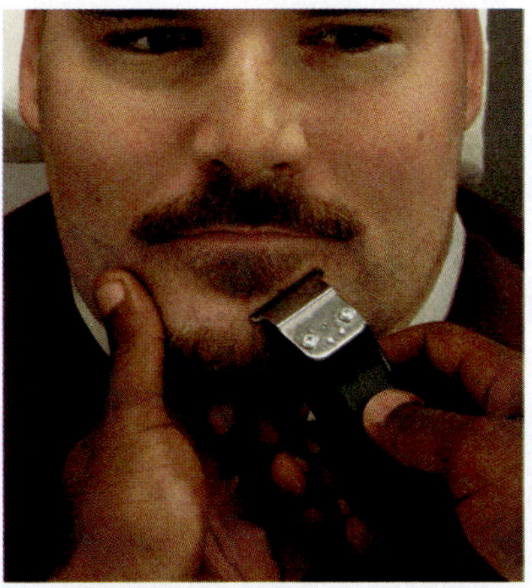
Figure 14-65 Shape patch area under bottom lip (optional).

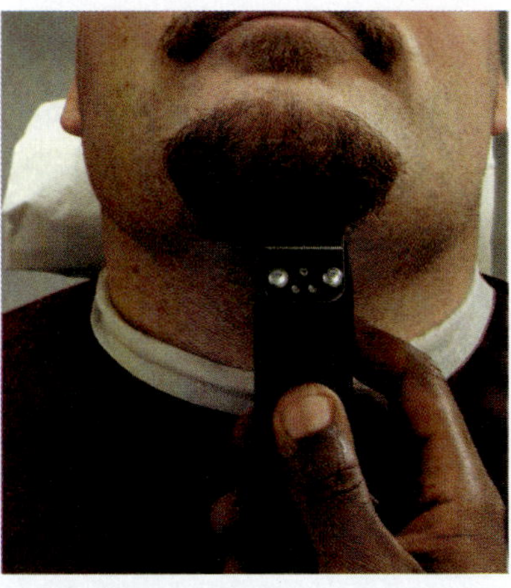
Figure 14-66 Establish goatee design line.

whose beards are of an even density and texture. This is important to note because sometimes all-over even cutting may produce whorls or patches, especially in wavy hair.

Many beard lengths will require the use of a clipper comb attachment. Follow steps 1 through 8 above. Then proceed by choosing a comb attachment close to the length of the client's beard. If more than a light trim is required, select the next shortest length comb attachment. Repeat as required until desired length is achieved. Always follow up with shears for the final trimming.

There is tremendous versatility in the designs of beards. The fact that the beard, in some form or another, has survived from the age of the caveman to the present day is testimony of its acceptance by men as a permanent part of facial grooming.

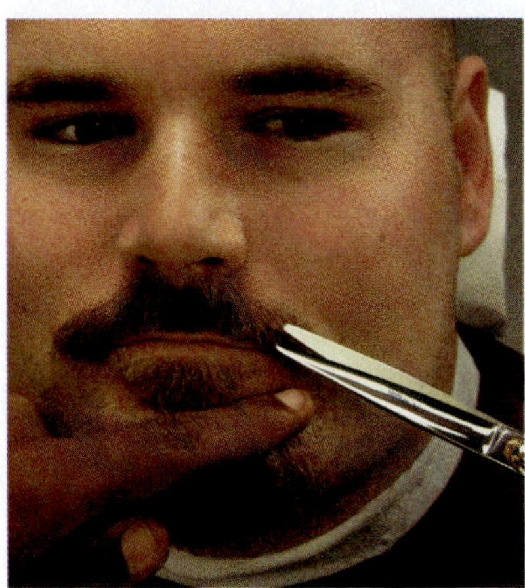
Figure 14-67 Complete detail finish work on mustache, patch, and goatee with shears.

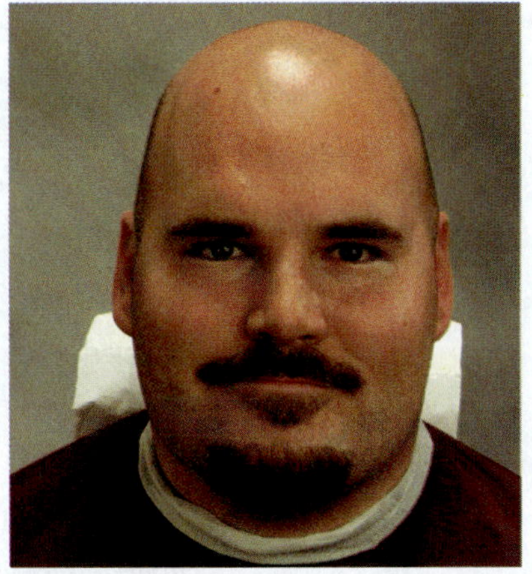
Figure 14-68 Finished mustache and goatee design.

spotlight on

The 44/20 Brand

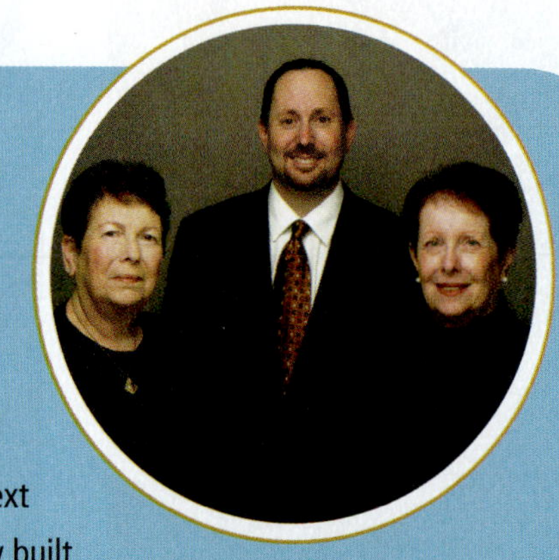

For almost a century, four generations of Harry Gomberg's family have been committed to supplying the industry with the finest quality barber and beauty products.

Family patriarch Harry Gomberg came to the United States at the age of fifteen and settled in Detroit in 1924. His uncle, "Mike" Derzaw, a partner in the E. Morris Manufacturing Company, manufactured for the barber and beauty industry. Harry apprenticed to his uncle and learned the business from the ground up. They worked together for 11 years.

As a young man, Gomberg had a gift for seeing something, whether a product or a machine, and knowing that he could make it better. He combined his passion for innovation with his experience. In 1938 Harry and his uncle started the Detroit Razor Strop Company. As the business grew and its products became well-known for their quality within the industry, the trademarked 44/20 brand was born. The name represented Derzaw's 44 years and Gomberg's 20 years of experience in the industry.

14

During World War II, Gomberg made precision mechanical parts for the government. With a foundation of success and the booming promise of the West Coast, Harry moved to California in 1947. He started a new company in Los Angeles and combined it with the existing company to create a new leader in the barber and beauty industry, the Economy Supply Company. Gomberg realized that the manufacturing process for thinning shears in the industry was not high quality. Once again, his passion for innovation and product improvement drove him to expand the industry's leading lines, which included professional haircutting scissors.

Over the next 30 years, Harry built the company on three simple guiding principles:

1. Take pride in creating the finest quality product.
2. Always achieve the highest levels of customer service.
3. Guarantee your work.

Thus, 44/20 became best known for its 44/20 Taper-Fine Tapering Shear along with its other scissors and a full selection of barber and beauty products. The 44/20 has been used by White House barbers, ensuring many presidents of the United States looked their best.

In 1978 Gomberg's daughters, Anne Mailman, Phyllis Waters, and Susan Gomberg, assumed leadership of the company. Anne and Phyllis continued the legacy of the company by following Harry's three business principles. They maintained deep customer relationships and 44/20 continued to be considered the #1 brand for professional scissors by barbers around the country.

Twenty-seven years later, Economy Supply Company is more vibrant and innovative than ever. The 44/20 family business is currently run by Michael Mailman, who, like his grandfather, learned the business from apprenticeship to journeyman. He is committed to maintaining and exceeding the high levels of customer service, product innovation, and quality that have been in the business for four generations. The company is proud of its long history, proclaiming that there is no substitute for quality and dedication to customer satisfaction, and it will continue to lead the way and to guarantee its work, just as Harry did.

chapter glossary

backhand stroke	razor position and stroke used in 4 of the 14 basic shaving areas: Nos. 2, 6, 8, and 9
close shaving	the procedure of shaving facial hair against the grain during the second-time-over
cutting stroke	the correct angle of cutting the beard with a straight razor
freehand stroke	razor position and stroke used in 6 of the 14 shaving areas: Nos. 1, 3, 4, 7, 11, and 12
neck shave	shaving the areas behind the ears, down the sides of the neck, and at the back neckline
once-over shave	single lather shave in which the shaving strokes are made across the grain of the hair
reverse backhand stroke	razor position and stroke used for making the left sideburn outline and shaving the left side behind the ear during a neck shave
reverse freehand stroke	razor position and stroke used in 4 of the 14 basic shaving areas: Nos. 5, 10, 13, and 14
second-time-over shave	follows a regular shave to remove any rough or uneven spots using water instead of lather; may be considered a form of close shaving
styptic powder	alum powder used to stop bleeding of nicks and cuts

chapter review questions

1. Identify three client characteristics that barbers should be aware of before beginning the shave service.
2. List the steps of client preparation for a shave.
3. List the effects shaving cream has on facial hair.
4. Describe the most effective way to rub lather into the beard.
5. Describe the effect of hot towels on facial hair.
6. List several reasons why a hot towel might not be applied to the face.
7. Identify the four standard positions and strokes used in shaving.
8. Explain the direction of the shaving strokes in respect to the grain of the hair.
9. Identify the number of shaving areas on the face.
10. Explain the difference between a standard shave and a once-over shave.
11. List the final steps to perform after shaving.
12. Explain at what step of the shave a facial might be suggested to the client.
13. Explain how a close shave differs from a standard shave.
14. Explain why a close shave may be considered undesirable.
15. Identify the primary reason that men wear mustaches.

16. List the important characteristics used to determine a mustache design.

17. List the steps for trimming a mustache.

18. List the tools used in mustache and beard design.

19. Explain why some barbers prefer to cut and style the hair before performing a beard trim service.

20. List the steps used to perform a beard trim with shears, comb, and outliner.

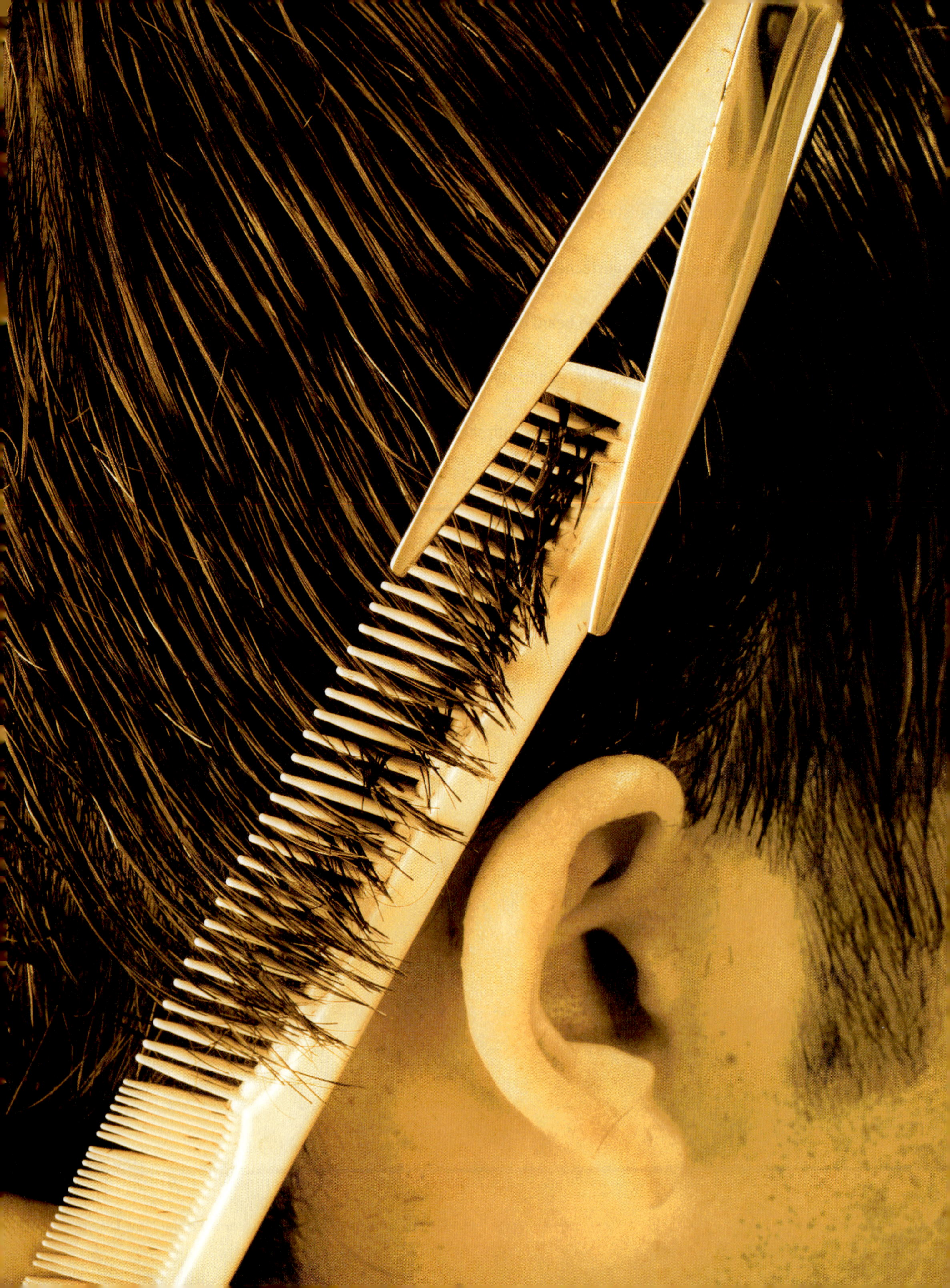

MEN'S HAIRCUTTING AND STYLING

Chapter Outline

- Do you prefer a similar style or are you looking for something new?
  The answer to this question can lead the barber directly to the cutting stage or to further discussion with the client about appropriate styles and options.
- What is your usual morning routine (shampoo, blow-dry, etc.)?
  The answer will indicate how much time the client is willing to spend on hair care.
- Are you having any particular problems with your hairstyle?
  This question provides an opportunity to open dialogue about specific hair-related issues such as problem areas, length, fullness, growth and wave patterns, hair texture, density, or color.

Additional consultation questions should lead to answers that help the barber to determine the length of the sideburns, the shape of the neckline, and whether or not the client desires a neck shave, eyebrow trim, etc. With practice and experience, barbers learn the questions to ask.

Envisioning is the process of picturing or visualizing in your mind the finished cut and style based on what the client has told you. With the information gained through the consultation, the barber is better able to visualize the client's expectations of the haircutting service. It is essential to achieve this understanding *before* beginning the haircut. 2

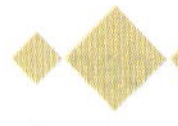

BASIC PRINCIPLES OF HAIRCUTTING AND STYLING

Each haircut is a representation and advertisement of the barber's work. Remember, a good haircut is the foundation of a good hairstyle.

Hairstyling has been defined as the artistic cutting and dressing of hair to best fit the client's physical needs and personality. Pay attention to details such as client comfort, sideburn lengths, outlines, balance, and proportion. The consultation should provide sufficient information about the client's lifestyle and personality to suggest a suitable style, but a study of facial shapes assists the barber in determining the *best* style for a client's features.

Facial Shapes

The **facial shape** of each individual is determined by the position and prominence of the facial bones. There are seven general facial shapes: oval, round, inverted triangular, square, pear-shaped, oblong, and diamond. In order to recognize each facial shape and then be able to give correct advice, the barber should be acquainted with the outstanding characteristics of each type. With this information, the barber can suggest a haircut and style that complements the facial shape in much the same way certain clothes flatter the body.

The following facial shapes should constitute a guide for choosing an appropriate style.

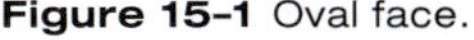

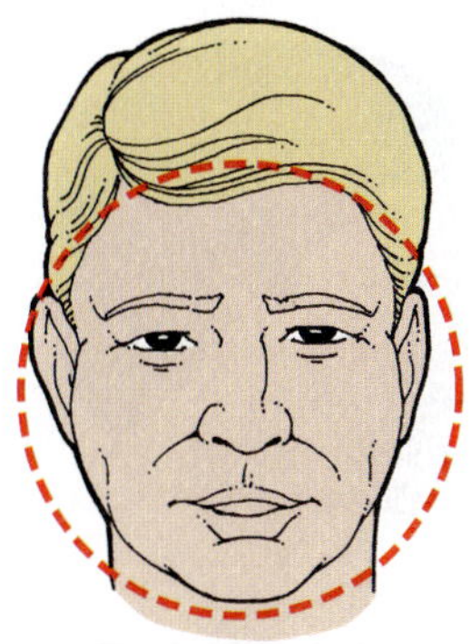

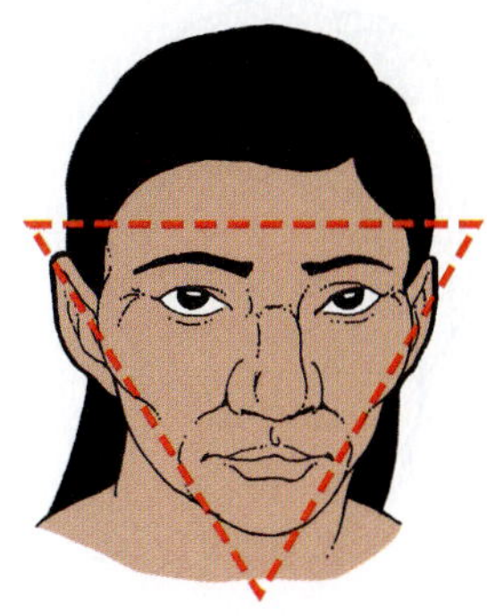

Figure 15-1 Oval face.

Figure 15-2 Round face.

Figure 15-3 Triangular face.

- *Oval:* The oval-shaped face is generally recognized as the ideal shape. Any hairstyle that maintains the oval shape is usually suitable (Figure 15–1). Try changing the part. Experiment, but keep in mind elements such as the client's lifestyle, comfort, and ease of maintenance.
- *Round:* The aim here is to slim the face. Hair that is too short will emphasize fullness, so create some height on the top to lengthen the look of the face (Figure 15–2). An off-center part and some waves at eye level will also help lessen the full appearance of the face. Beards should be styled to make the face appear oval.

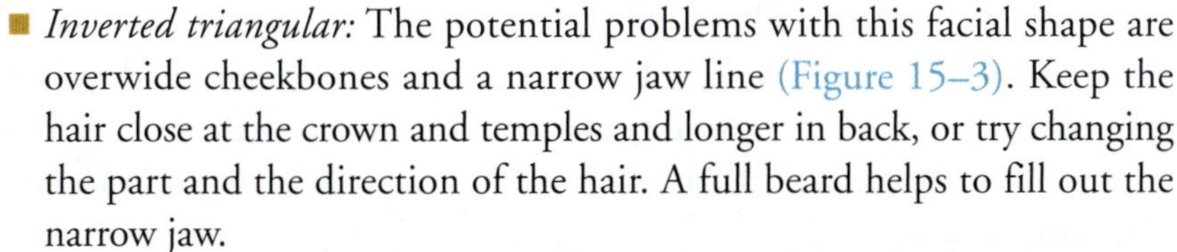

- *Inverted triangular:* The potential problems with this facial shape are overwide cheekbones and a narrow jaw line (Figure 15–3). Keep the hair close at the crown and temples and longer in back, or try changing the part and the direction of the hair. A full beard helps to fill out the narrow jaw.

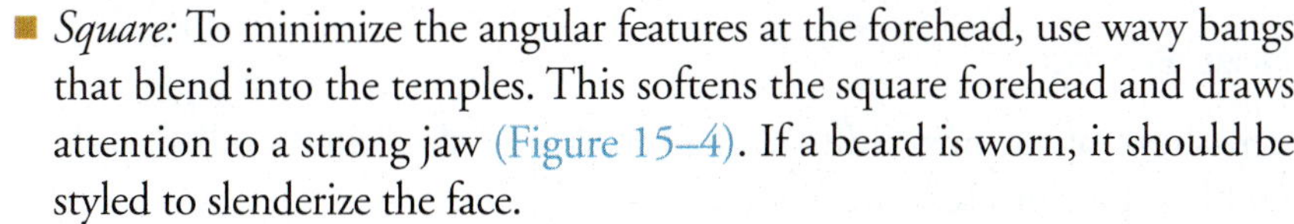

- *Square:* To minimize the angular features at the forehead, use wavy bangs that blend into the temples. This softens the square forehead and draws attention to a strong jaw (Figure 15–4). If a beard is worn, it should be styled to slenderize the face.

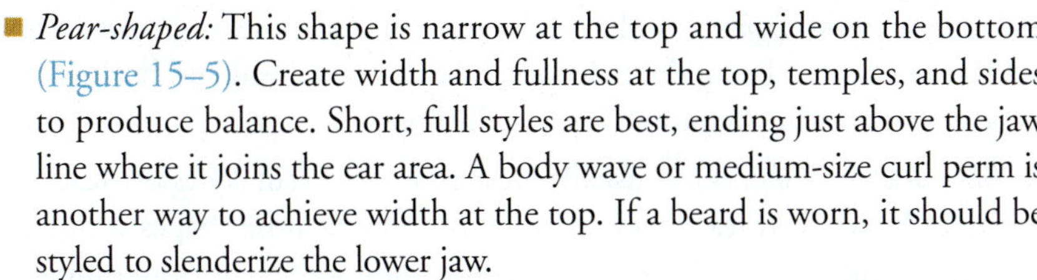

- *Pear-shaped:* This shape is narrow at the top and wide on the bottom (Figure 15–5). Create width and fullness at the top, temples, and sides to produce balance. Short, full styles are best, ending just above the jaw line where it joins the ear area. A body wave or medium-size curl perm is another way to achieve width at the top. If a beard is worn, it should be styled to slenderize the lower jaw.

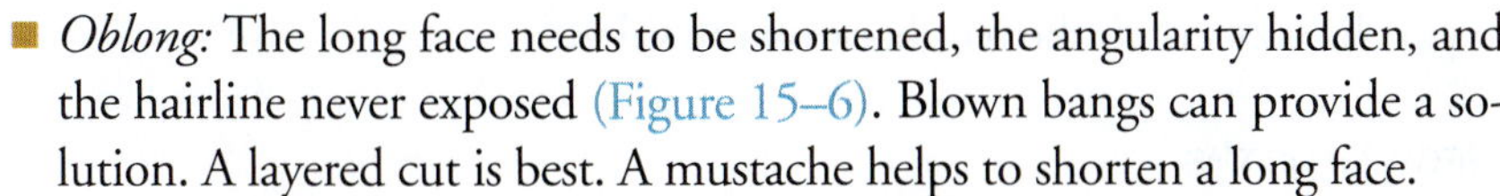

- *Oblong:* The long face needs to be shortened, the angularity hidden, and the hairline never exposed (Figure 15–6). Blown bangs can provide a solution. A layered cut is best. A mustache helps to shorten a long face.

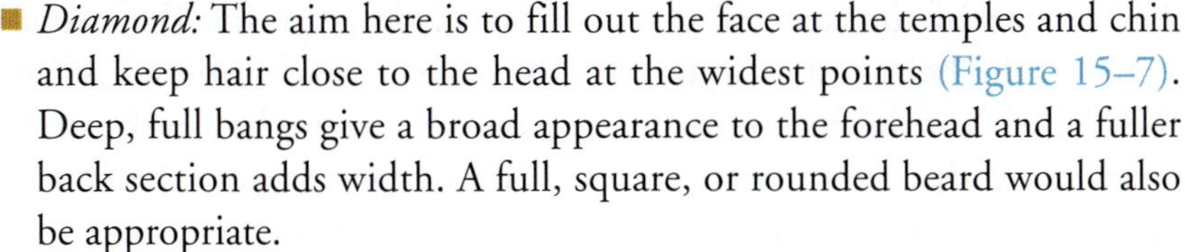

- *Diamond:* The aim here is to fill out the face at the temples and chin and keep hair close to the head at the widest points (Figure 15–7). Deep, full bangs give a broad appearance to the forehead and a fuller back section adds width. A full, square, or rounded beard would also be appropriate.

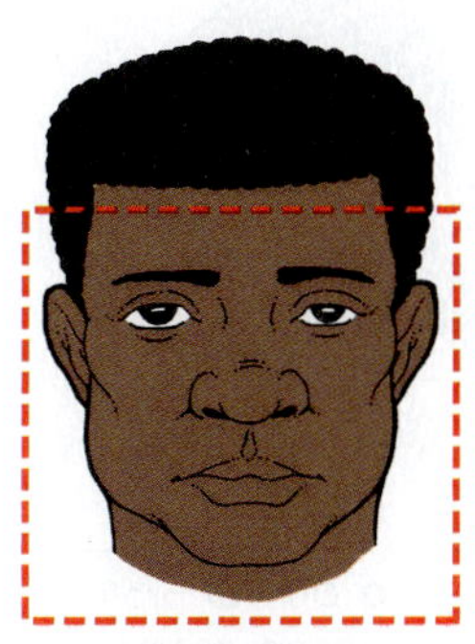

Figure 15-4 Square face.

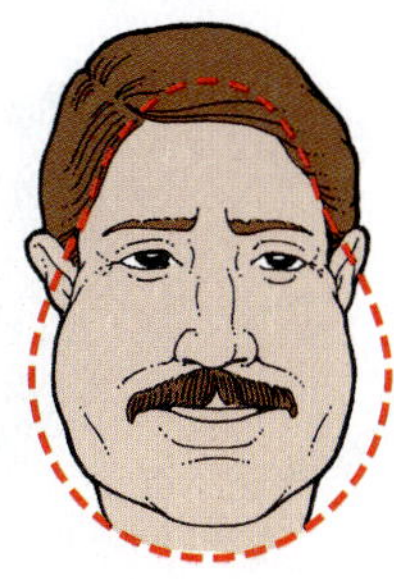

Figure 15-5 Pear-shaped face.

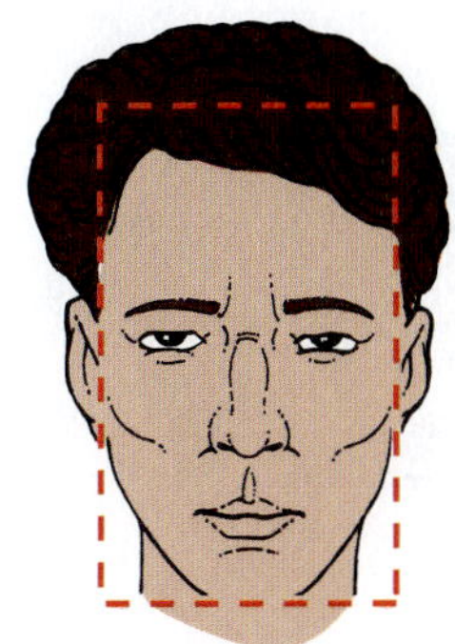

Figure 15-6 Oblong face.

15

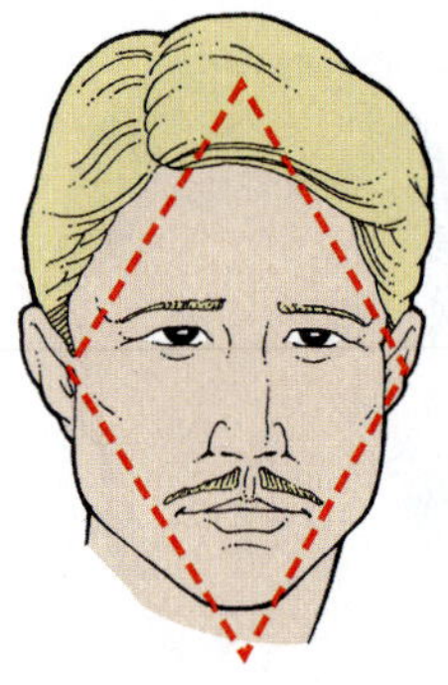

Figure 15–7 Diamond face.

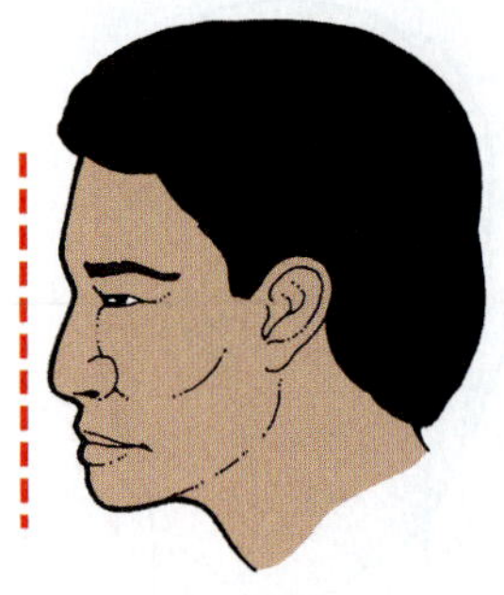

Figure 15–8 Straight profile.

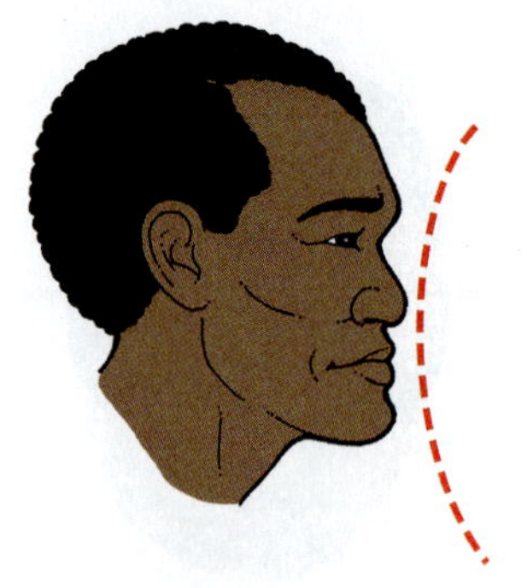

Figure 15–9 Concave profile (prominent forehead and chin).

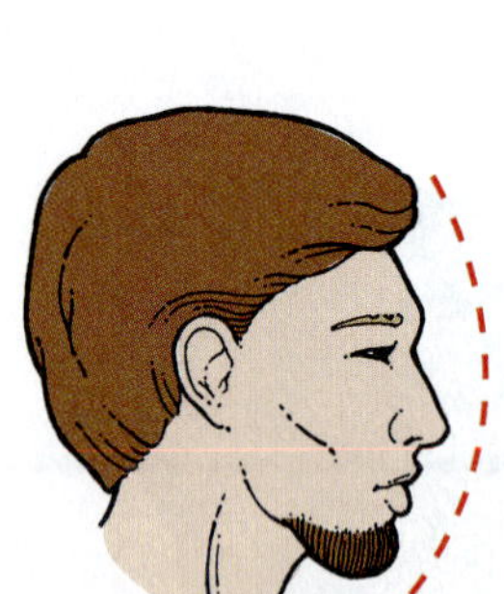

Figure 15–10 Convex profile (receding forehead, prominent nose, and receding chin).

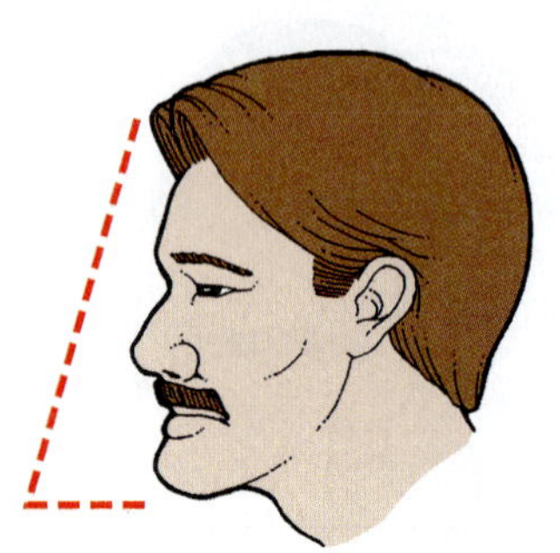

Figure 15–11 Angular profile.

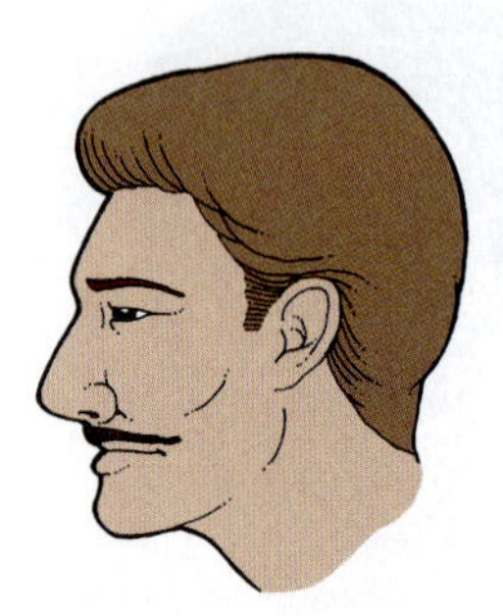

Figure 15–12 Prominent nose.

Profiles

Always be aware of the client's profile since it can influence the appropriateness of a haircut or style for that particular individual.

- *Straight profiles* tend to be the most balanced and can usually wear any hairstyle successfully (Figure 15–8).
- *Concave profiles* require a close hair arrangement over the forehead to minimize the bulge of the forehead (Figure 15–9).
- *Convex profiles* require some balance so arrange the top front hair over the forehead to conceal a short, receding forehead (Figure 15–10). A beard or goatee minimizes a receding chin.
- *Angular profiles* also have receding foreheads, but the chin tends to jut forward (Figure 15–11). Arrange the top front hair over the forehead to create more balance. A short beard and mustache help to minimize the protruding chin.

Nose Shapes

The shape of the nose influences a profile and should be studied both in profile and from a full-face view.

- *Prominent nose shapes* include a hooked nose, large nose, or pointed nose (Figure 15–12). Bring the hair forward at the forehead and back at the sides to minimize the prominence of the nose.
- *Turned-up nose shapes* can usually wear shorter haircut styles because the size or heavy features associated with prominent nose shapes is not an issue (Figure 15–13). Experiment with combing the hair from different part lines or comb the hair back on the sides.

Neck Lengths

The length of the neck is also a factor in determining the overall shape of the haircut and style. In most cases it is advisable to follow the client's natural hairline when designing a style; however, sometimes an overly long or very short neck limits the options. The length, density, growth pattern, and natural partings of the hair should be

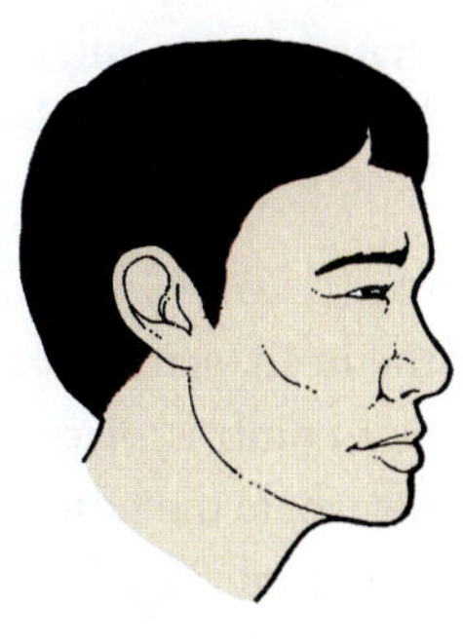

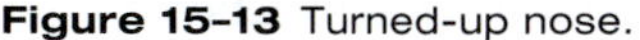

Figure 15-13 Turned-up nose.

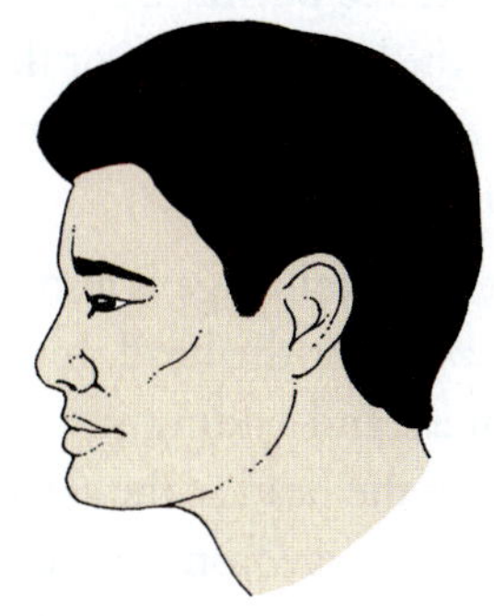

Figure 15-14 Long neck.

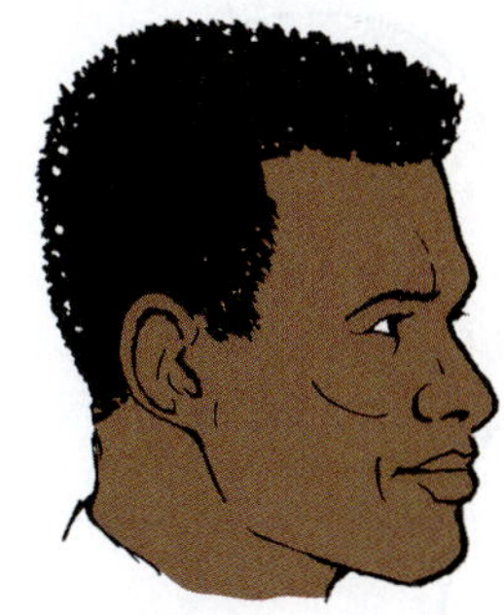

Figure 15-15 Short neck.

considered when deciding on a style that best complements the client's neck length.

Long necks are minimized when the hair is left fuller or longer at the nape (Figure 15–14).

Short necks are best served by leaving the neck exposed to create an appearance of length (Figure 15–15). Work with the natural hairline and perform a tapered cut that creates an illusion of a longer nape and neck area.

FUNDAMENTALS OF HAIRCUTTING

The fundamental principles of haircutting should be thoroughly understood. The same general techniques are used in cutting, shaping, tapering, and blending men's and women's hair. The differences between the two are usually evident in the overall *design line,* the contour or shape, which includes volume, and the finished style. The fundamental principles of haircutting include the head form, basic terms used in haircutting, and different haircutting techniques.

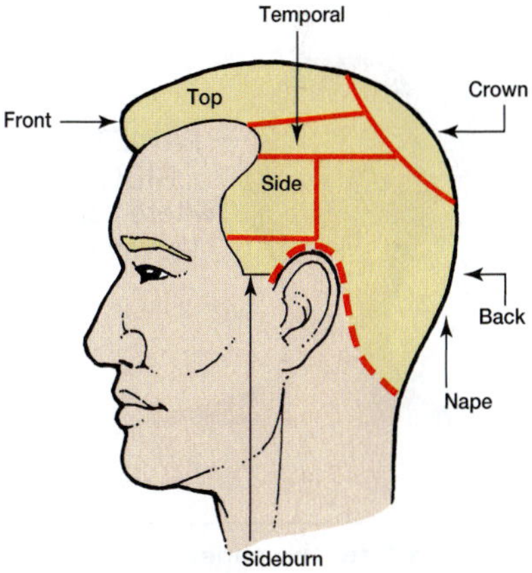

Figure 15-16 Diagram of sections of head, side view.

The Head Form

In order to create consistent and successful results in haircutting, it is necessary to understand the shape of the head. Hair responds differently in different areas of the head because of the curves and changes from one section to the next. The ability to visualize these sections will assist student barbers in the development of individual cutting patterns, help to eliminate technical mistakes, reduce confusion during the haircutting process, and facilitate easier checking of the final result.

When designing and cutting hair, the barber should envision the sections of the head as depicted in Figures 15–16 through 15–18. These sections include the front, top (apex), temporal, crown, sides, sideburns, back, and nape.

NOTE: The temporal section is part of the parietal ridge, which is also known as the crest, horseshoe, or hatband region of the head.

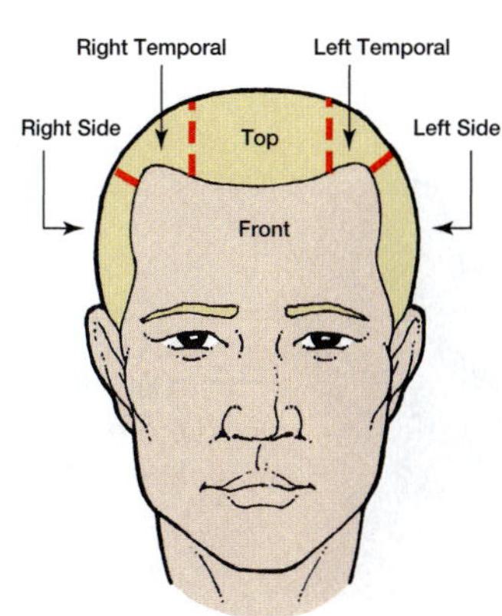

Figure 15-17 Diagram of sections of head, front view.

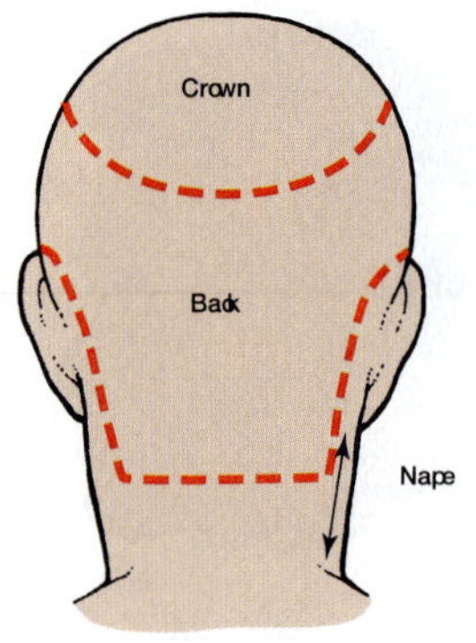

Figure 15-18 Diagram of sections of head, back view.

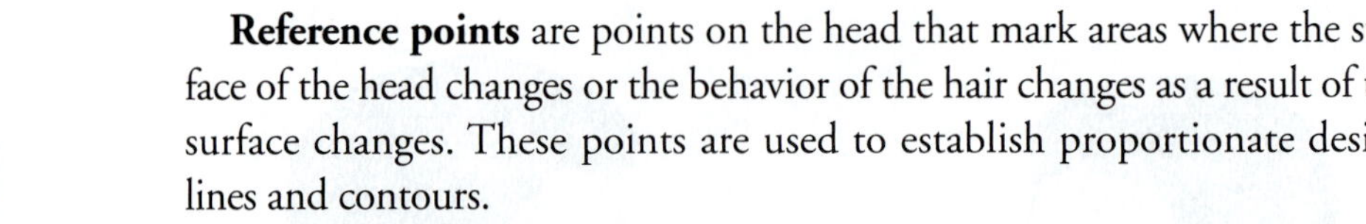

Reference points are points on the head that mark areas where the surface of the head changes or the behavior of the hair changes as a result of the surface changes. These points are used to establish proportionate design lines and contours.

- The **parietal ridge** is also known as the **crest**, *temporal, horseshoe,* or *hatband* area of the head. It is the widest section of the head, starting at the temples and ending just below the crown. When a comb is placed flat against the head at the sides, the parietal ridge begins where the head starts to curve away from the comb (Figure 15–19). The parietal ridge is one of the most important sections of the head when cutting hair because it serves as a transition area from the top to the front, sides, and back sections.
- The occipital bone protrudes at the base of the skull. When a comb is placed flat against the nape area, the occipital begins where the head curves away from the comb (Figure 15–20).
- The apex is the highest point on the top of the head (Figure 15–21). The four corners are located by crossing two diagonal lines at the apex (Figure 15–22). The lines will point to the front and back corners of the head. 4

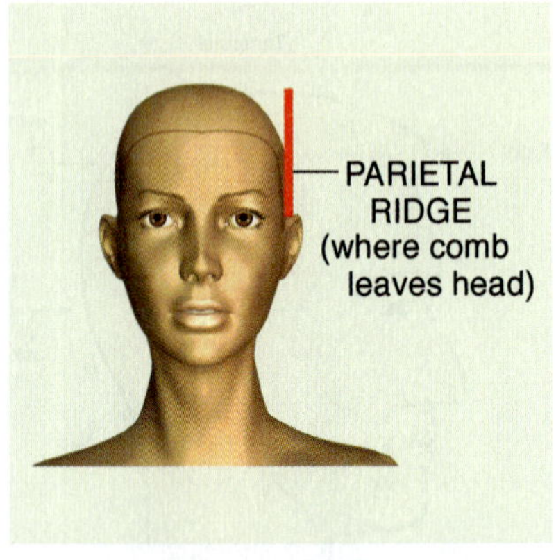

Figure 15-19 The parietal ridge.

Basic Terms Used in Haircutting

A *line* is simply a series of connected dots that result in a continuous mark. Straight and curved lines are used in haircutting to create the shape and direction from which the hair will fall (Figure 15–23). The three types of straight lines used in haircutting are the horizontal, vertical, and diagonal lines (Figure 15–24).

- **Horizontal** lines are parallel to the horizon or floor and direct the eye from one side to the other. Horizontal cutting lines build weight and are used to create a one-length look and low elevation or blunt haircut designs. These *weight lines* are usually created at the perimeter or at the occipital area of a haircut (Figures 15–25 and 15–26).
- **Vertical** lines are perpendicular to the floor and are described in terms of up and down. Vertical partings facilitate the projection of the hair at

15

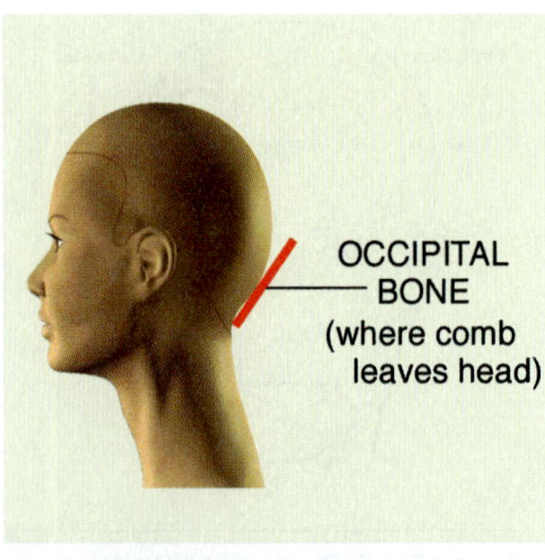

Figure 15-20 The occipital bone.

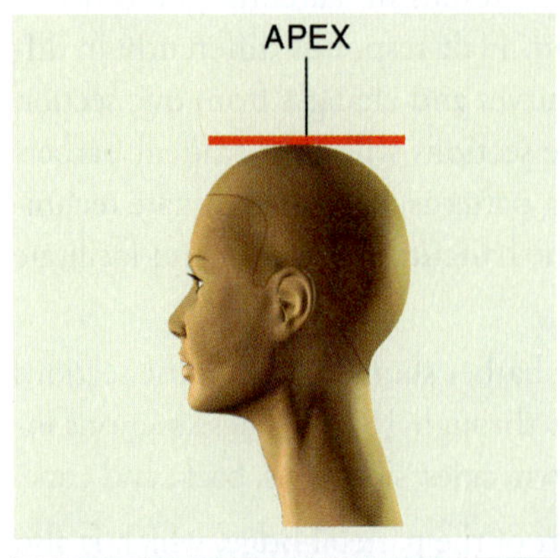

Figure 15-21 The apex.

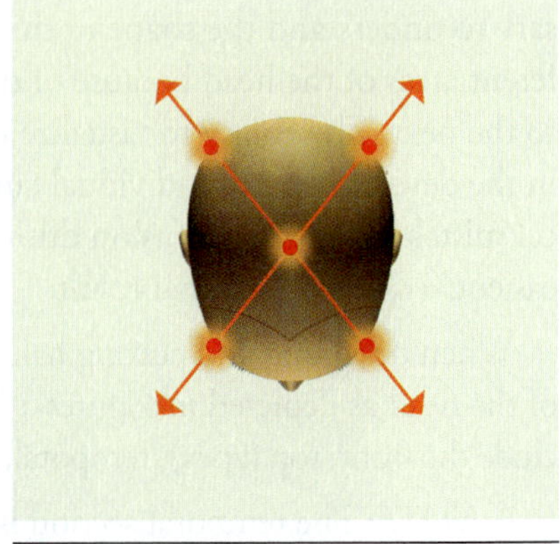

Figure 15-22 The four corners.

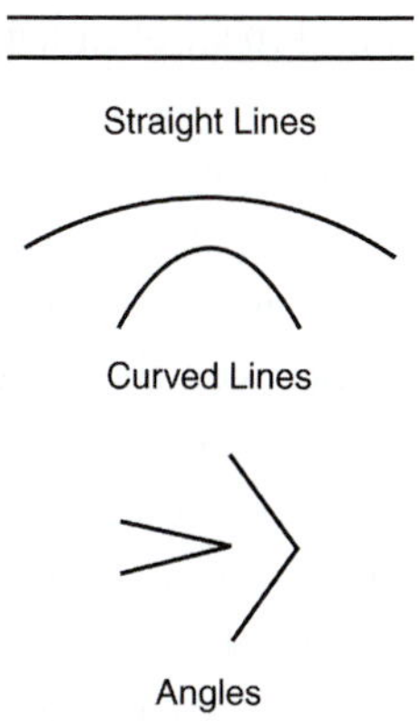

Straight Lines

Curved Lines

Angles

Figure 15-23 Lines and angles.

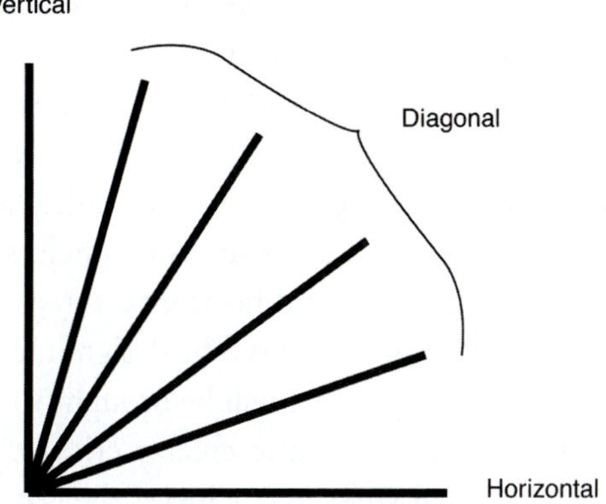

Figure 15-24 Horizontal, vertical, and diagonal lines.

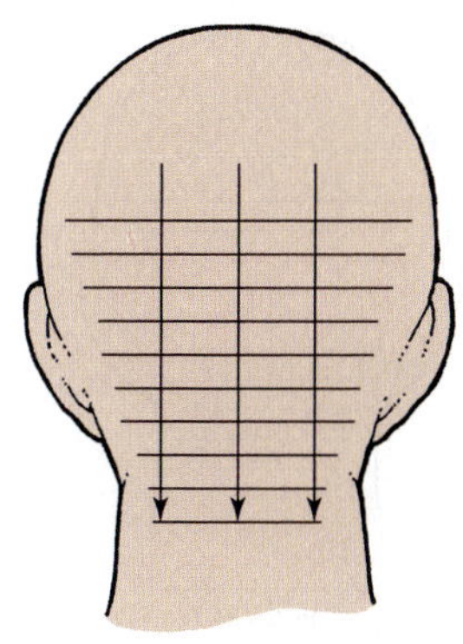

Figure 15-25 Weight line at perimeter.

higher elevations while cutting. Vertical cutting lines remove weight within the cut and create layers that may be used to cut from short to long, long to short, or uniformly depending on finger placement (Figure 15–27).

- **Diagonal** lines have a slanted direction and are used to create sloped lines at the perimeter on the design line (Figure 15–28). When used at the perimeter, these lines are often referred to as diagonal forward or diagonal back. Diagonal finger placement may also be used to create a stacked layered effect at the perimeter or to blend longer layers to shorter layers within a haircut.

An **angle** is the space between two lines or surfaces that intersect at a given point. Angles help to create strong, consistent foundations in haircutting and are used in two different ways. Angles can refer to the degree of elevation at which the hair is held for cutting or to the position of the fingers when cutting a section of hair (cutting line).

Elevation is the angle or degree at which a section of hair is held from the head for cutting, *relative from where it grows*. Elevation, also known as **projection**, is the result of lifting the hair section above 0 degrees or natural fall. This projection of the hair while cutting produces graduation or layers and is usually described in terms of degrees (Figure 15–29).

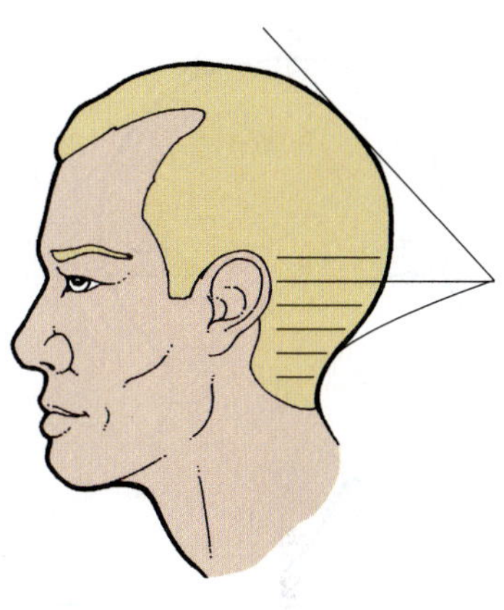

Figure 15-26 Weight line at occipital.

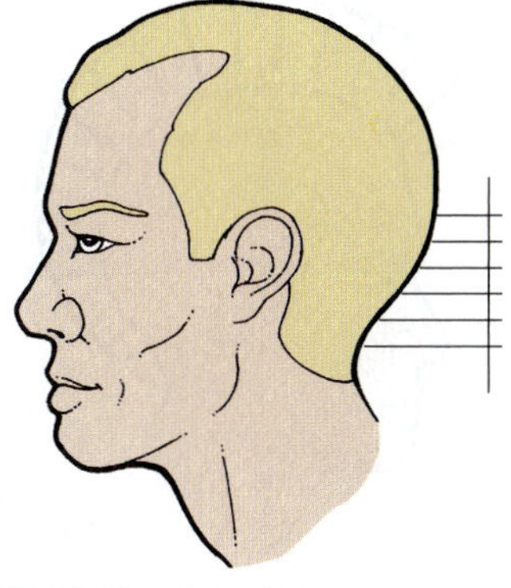

Figure 15-27 Vertical partings facilitate layering.

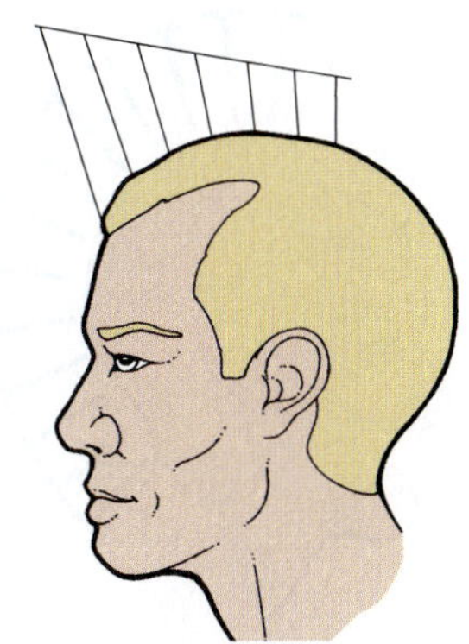

Figure 15-28 Diagonal line within top front sections.

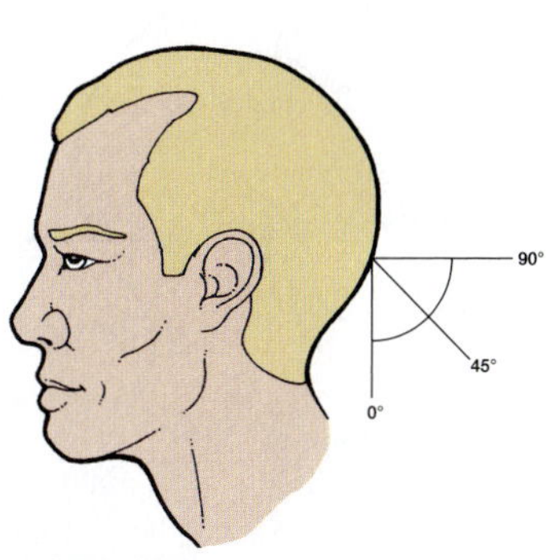

Figure 15-29 Elevations relative to the head form.

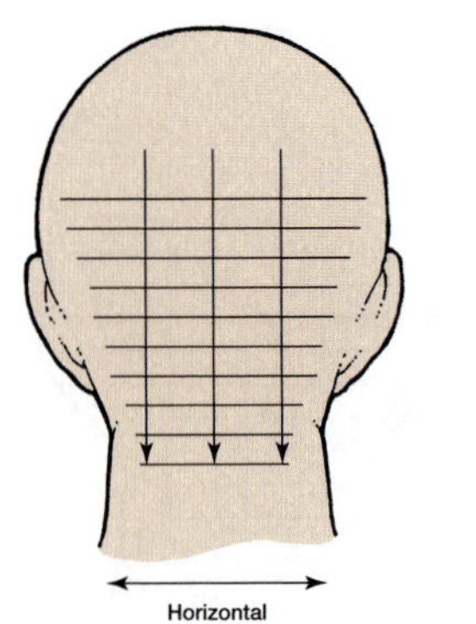

Figure 15-30 Horizontal, zero elevation.

- A low elevation of *0 degrees* produces weight, bulk, and maximum length at the perimeter of a hair design.

    To perform a 0-degree (zero elevation) cut, a *parting* is made in the section to be cut (Figure 15–30). After combing the hair straight down from where it grows, it is cut either against the skin (as in the nape or around-the-ear areas) or as it is held straight down between the fingers. Both stationary and horizontal traveling guides are used to create the design or perimeter line. The design line then serves as a guide for all subsequent partings that will be brought to the design (perimeter) line for cutting. This technique creates crisp, clean lines around the hairline on shorter hairstyles and achieves the standard "blunt cut" on longer hair.

- Holding the hair at *45 degrees* from where it grows is considered to be a medium elevation. Medium elevation or graduation creates layered ends or "stacking" within the parting of hair from the 0-degree distance to the 45-degree position. Movement and texture is created within the distance between the two degrees, depending on the length of the hair and the position of the angle in relation to the head form.

    Both stationary and horizontal traveling guides are used to achieve the graduated or stacked effect (Figure 15–31). Use of a vertical parting projected at 45 degrees, with the fingers holding the parting angled at a 45-degree diagonal, will create a *tapered* effect (Figure 15–32).

    A *90-degree* elevation is probably the most common angle used in men's haircutting. It produces layering, tapering, and blended effects. When using a 90-degree elevation, the hair is held straight out from the head from where it grows. This requires a traveling guide in order to move around the entire head. Lengths in various sections of the head can vary, but the hair will still be blended overall and considered to be a high-elevation cut. A 90-degree projection can be used to create uniform layers as depicted in Figure 15–33. Cutting each section of hair the same length creates *uniform* layers.

    To create a tapered effect as shown in Figure 15–34, the hair is held from a vertical parting and cut closer to the head form in the nape and around-the-ear areas at a 90-degree projection.

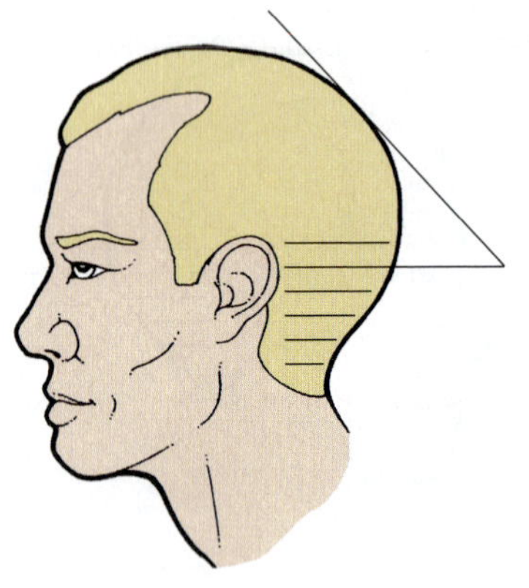

Figure 15-31 Horizontal, 45-degree elevation.

15

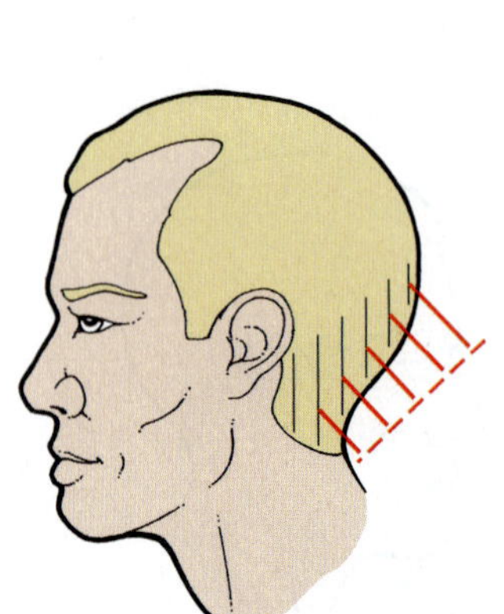

Figure 15-32 Vertical parting with 45-degree finger placement.

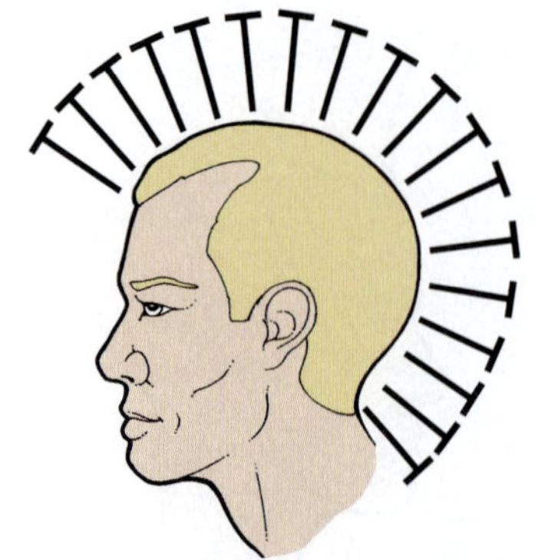

Figure 15-33 90-degree uniform layers.

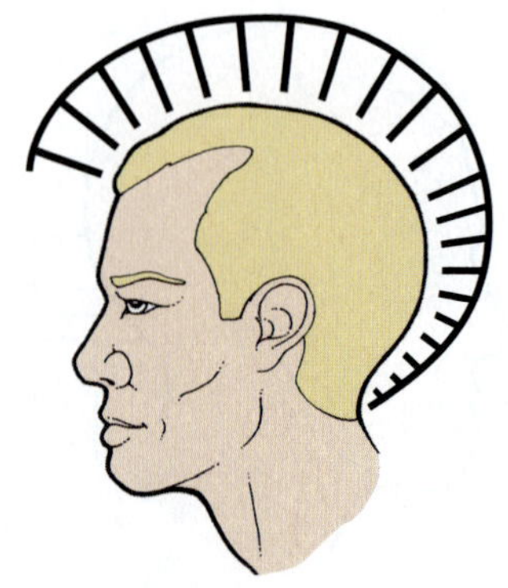

Figure 15-34 90-degree taper.

A **parting** is a smaller section of hair, usually ¼ to ½ inch thick, parted off from a larger section of the hair. The use of partings is essential to maintain control of the hair in manageable proportions while performing the haircut. Partings may be held horizontally, vertically, or diagonally depending on the desired effect with a usual projection range of 0 to 180 degrees.

The **design line** is the outer perimeter line of the haircut. It may act as a guide depending on the overall design of the haircut and the method the barber uses to achieve it.

A **guide**, also known as a guideline or guide strand, is a cut that is made by which subsequent partings or sections of hair will be measured and cut. Guides are classified as being either stationary or traveling. Both types may originate at the outer perimeter (design line) of the hair, or at an interior section, usually the crown area. Most haircuts are achieved by using a combination of the two types of guides.

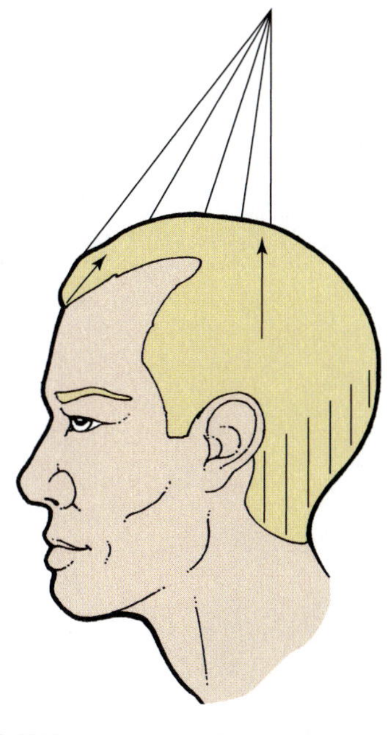

Figure 15-35 Stationary guide.

- A **stationary guide** is used for overall, one-length-looking designs at the perimeter, such as a solid-form blunt cut, or for maintaining the length of one section while subsequent partings are brought to it from other sections to meet it for cutting, producing either an overall long layered effect or extra length within a section (Figure 15–35).
- A **traveling guide** moves along a section of hair as each cut is made. Once the length of the initial guide has been cut, a parting is taken from in front of it or near it, combed with the original guide, and cut. Then, a new parting is taken, combed with the second parting of hair, and cut against that guide. It is this use of the previous guide to cut a subsequent parting of hair that makes it a traveling guide. Care must be taken not to recut the original or subsequent guides as the barber moves along the section. When performed properly, the traveling guide ensures even layering and blending of the hair from one section to another. Refer to Figures 15–33 and 15–34.

  Traveling guides are used internally within the cut to create blended layers; they are also used to finish perimeter designs after the hair is cut to the desired length from one section to another. For example, although a stationary guide is used when establishing the length at the perimeter, it becomes a traveling guide when subsequent cuts are made from left to right or right to left around the head form.

Layers are produced by cutting the interior sections of the hair; they can originate from the front, top (apex), crown, or perimeter (usually the design line). Layering can be angled (shorter on top and longer at the perimeter), uniform (even throughout), or fully tapered (longer on top and shorter at the perimeter). It creates blending, fullness, and/ or a feathered effect.

Tapered, or tapering, means that the hair conforms to the shape of the head and is shorter at the nape and longer in the crown and top areas. Blending of all of the hair lengths is extremely important in tapering (Figure 15–34).

A **weight line** refers to the heaviest perimeter area of a 0- or 45-degree cut. It is achieved by use of a stationary guide at the perimeter and may be cut in at a variety of levels on the head, depending on the style. In men's haircutting, a weight line is most often used in combination with a tapered nape area.

Texturizing is performed after the overall cut has been completed. Thinning or notching shears or razors can be used to create wispy or spiky effects within the haircut or along the perimeter.

Tension is the amount of pressure applied while combing and holding a section of hair for cutting. Tension ranges from minimum to maximum as a result of the amount of stretching employed when holding the hair between the fingers and the spacing between the teeth of the comb. For example, fine-toothed combs facilitate more tension while combing than wide-toothed combs.

- Use maximum tension on straight hair to create precise lines.
- Use minimal to moderate tension on curly and wavy hair as the hair may dry shorter than intended if maximum tension is used.

Thinning refers to removing excess bulk from the hair.

Outlining means marking the outer perimeter of the haircut in the front (optional, depending on hair texture), in front of and over the ears, and at the sides and nape of the neck.

Over-direction creates a length increase in the design and occurs when the hair is combed away from its natural fall position, rather than straight out from the head toward a guide.

Hairstyling involves arranging the hair in a particular style, appropriately suited to the cut, and may require the use of styling aids such as hair spray, gel, tonic, oil sheen, or mousse.

During the course of your barbering career, you will be introduced to a variety of haircutting terms. Terminology for the most part depends on who is presenting the information or technique and whether or not a new word has been created in place of former terminology. The same holds true for different style names and what the latest fashion trends are. As a barber you need to be aware that cutting the hair at certain angles and elevations creates specific effects and that hairstyle trends are cyclical in nature.

15

Variations of design will inevitably occur as history has a way of repeating itself in our industry. Crew cuts and boxed fades can be traced back to the years of World War II, finger waves were a hit in the 1920s, and braiding has been around since humans first walked the earth. This reinforces the fact that barbers must become proficient in the basic skills in order to adapt those skills and techniques to whatever the current trend may be. 5

HAIRCUTTING TECHNIQUES

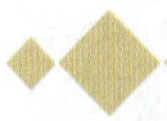

In Chapter 6, you were introduced to the correct holding position of the barber's basic tools, which include the comb, shears, clippers, and razor. These tools can be used in several different ways to cut hair and are classified as fingers-and-shear, shear-over-comb, freehand clipper cutting, clipper-over-comb, razor-over-comb, and razor rotation. It is important to note, however, that almost every haircutting procedure requires the use of a combination of techniques and tools. The most important factors that determine the tools chosen to achieve the haircut are the client's desired outcome, the texture and density of the hair, and the barber's personal preference. As a professional barber you should be comfortable and skillful with using all the tools of the trade.

Now it is time to begin your practical training in haircutting. Practice the following techniques and procedures to become familiar with different methods of using your tools.

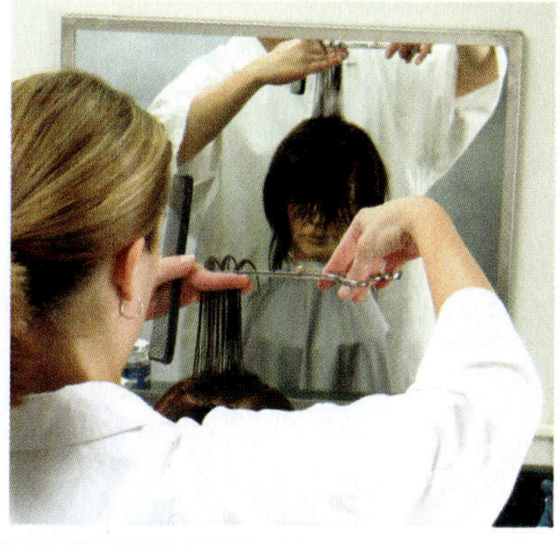

Figure 15-36 Cutting above the fingers.

The Fingers-and-Shear Technique

The **fingers-and-shear** technique may be used on many hair types from straight to curly. There are three basic methods for using the fingers-and-shear technique: cutting on top of the fingers, cutting below the fingers, and cutting palm-to-palm.

NOTE: The blades of the shears should rest flat and flush to the fingers for these positions. Angling the shear blades may cause injury.

- **Cutting above the fingers** is frequently used in men's haircutting to cut and blend layers in the top, crown, and horseshoe areas (Figure 15–36). It is also used when cutting hair that is held out at a 90-degree elevation from a vertical parting, such as the sides and back of the head form (Figure 15–37). Whether the barber's finger position is perpendicular to the floor or angled at 45 degrees in these sections, the cutting should be performed on the outside (on top of) the fingers.
- **Cutting below the fingers** is most often used to create design lines at the perimeter of the haircut (Figure 15–38).
- *Cutting palm-to-palm* may be preferred by some practitioners. Care must be taken not to bend the hair or to project it higher than intended from the head form when using this technique.

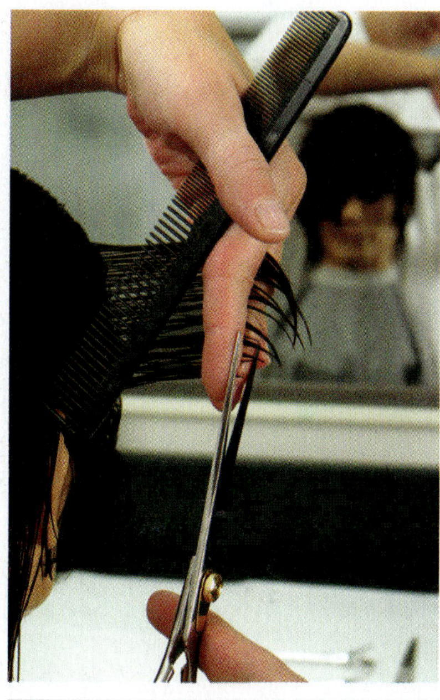

Figure 15-37 Cutting above the fingers using a vertical parting.

15

Practice Session #1:

FINGERS-AND-SHEAR TECHNIQUE WITH MIRROR: CUTTING ABOVE THE FINGERS HORIZONTALLY

1. Pick up shears and comb in dominant hand and face the mirror.
2. Palm the shears and pretend that there is a head of hair in front of you. With the teeth of the comb facing you, pretend to comb through a section of hair just below eye level at a 90-degree elevation. Position the first two fingers of the opposite hand underneath the comb and follow it up to eye level. The fingers and comb should be in a horizontal position parallel to the floor (Figure 15–36).

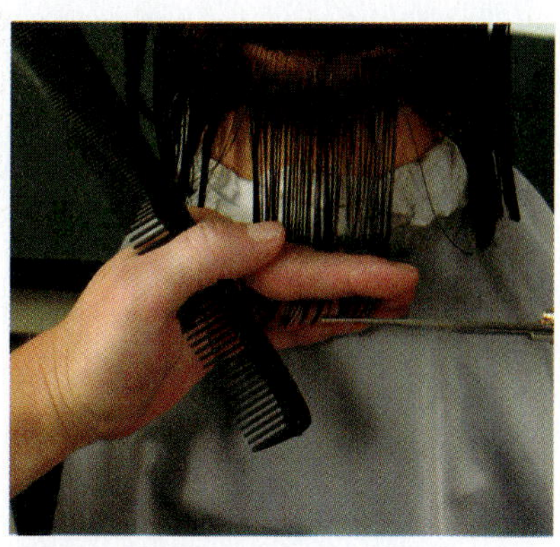

Figure 15-38 Cutting below the fingers at the perimeter.

3. Palm the comb in the opposite hand while simultaneously positioning the shears at the tip of the fingers holding the hair section. The fingers and shears should be at or near eye level and parallel to each other as the cutting begins. Practice opening and closing the shears along your fingers. This fingers-and-shear placement will be used to cut 90-degree layers within the sections of the head form.

Practice Session #2:

FINGERS-AND-SHEAR TECHNIQUE WITH MIRROR: CUTTING ABOVE THE FINGERS VERTICALLY

1. Pick up shears and comb in dominant hand and face the mirror.
2. Palm the shears and pretend that there is a head of hair in front of you. With the teeth of comb facing you in a vertical position, pretend to comb through a vertical section of side hair just below eye level at a 90-degree elevation. Position the first two fingers of the opposite hand underneath the comb and follow it out to the side with the tips of the fingers pointing downward and perpendicular to the floor. The fingers and comb should be in a vertical position perpendicular to the floor.
3. Palm the comb in the opposite hand while simultaneously positioning the tips of the shears on top of the tips of the fingers holding the hair section. The fingers and shears should be vertical and parallel to each other as the cutting begins (Figure 15–37). Practice opening and closing the shears along your fingers. This fingers-and-shear placement will be used to cut 90-degree vertical layers within sections of the head form using the perimeter for a guide (Figure 15–37).

Practice Session #3:

FINGERS-AND-SHEAR TECHNIQUE WITH MIRROR: CUTTING BELOW THE FINGERS

1. Pick up shears and comb in dominant hand and face the mirror.
2. Palm the shears and pretend that there is a head of hair in front of you. With the teeth of comb facing downward, pretend to comb through a section of hair that would end at just below your shoulder level at a 0-degree elevation. Position the first two fingers of the opposite hand just above the comb and follow it down no lower than chest level. The fingers and comb should be in a horizontal position.
3. Palm the comb in the opposite hand while simultaneously positioning the tips of the shears just below the finger tips holding the hair section. The fingers and shears should be horizontal and parallel to each other as the cutting begins (Figure 15–38). Practice opening and closing the shears along your fingers. This fingers-and-shear placement will be used to cut 0-degree projections along the perimeter or to create weight lines in sections of the head form.

Practice Session #4:

FINGERS-AND-SHEAR TECHNIQUE ON MANNEQUIN

Drape the mannequin and proceed as follows:

1. This practice session begins with learning how to cut *above the fingers.* Start at the front part of the crown and make a horizontal parting across the top of the head. Using the dominant hand, comb the parting of hair straight up at 90 degrees from where it grows. Use the first and second fingers of the other hand to secure the 90-degree parting in a position for cutting. Palm the comb and position the fingers and shears parallel to the horizontal parting. Cut the hair to the desired length (be guided by your instructor) along the top, or outside, of your fingers.

   Comb through the parting of hair to check for evenness and fine-tune as needed. When held between the fingers at 90 degrees, the cut hair section should represent a clean horizontal line. You have just created a 90-degree guide for the top section.

   NOTE: Make sure to palm the shears when using the comb, and palm the comb when cutting with the shears.

2. Part off a second parting, comb through it while picking up some of the previous parting, and comb into a 90-degree position. Remember that the hair you are going to cut should be held at 90 degrees. When holding two partings of hair, the first parting will be very slightly over-directed to facilitate using it for a guide for the subsequent parting, which should be at a true 90-degree elevation. The second parting should be thin enough to see the guide from the first parting. Cut the second parting along the horizontal line created with the first parting. Comb through, check, and fine-tune. You have just used the first parting as a traveling guide. This technique will be used to cut the entire top section during a haircut.

3. Next, practice *cutting below the fingers* as in Figure 15–38. Start at the nape or on one side of the mannequin. Create a ¼-inch to ½-inch thick parting at the hairline. Use a clip to secure excess hair out of the way. Comb the parting down at 0 degrees, follow the comb with your fingers, and secure the parting for cutting. Cut below your fingers to the desired length. Comb, check, and fine-tune the cut parting. You have just cut below the fingers and established a guide for the perimeter. Once completed, this perimeter will create the design line.

4. To practice cutting *above the fingers* on a *vertical parting,* start in the section just used to create the perimeter guide. Section off a ¼-inch-thick vertical parting from the crest to the perimeter if using a side section or from the occipital to the perimeter if working the back section. Comb the parting into a 90-degree projection, and straight out from the head form. Finger position should be vertical and perpendicular to the floor as in Figure 15–37.

   Using the perimeter as a guide, cut the hair extending beyond the fingers.

NOTE: The tips of the fingers should be positioned at the end of the perimeter guide as it is held out at 90 degrees from a vertical parting. When the perimeter length is used as a guide at 90 degrees, the hair that is cut above it should not influence the overall hanging length of the hairstyle. Note the layering that took place during this exercise. (You have just created layers by cutting above the fingers using the perimeter guide and vertical partings held at 90 degrees.)

When both horizontal and vertical fingers-and-shear cutting techniques have been practiced, refer to Haircutting Procedure #1 and Figures 15–129 through 15–158 to perform a complete haircut using these techniques. See Haircutting Procedure #2, Figures 15–159 and 15–160 for a variation of this method. Be guided by your instructor in learning other techniques.

NOTE: Traditionally, men's hair is not sectioned off with a hair clip unless the length of the hair warrants it. When working with long hair, there are three areas where a hair clip may be necessary to hold some of the hair out the way while cutting: the top section, at the sides, and at the nape when cutting in a design line.

The fingers-and-shear cutting method used in Haircutting Procedure #1 produces a well-balanced, evenly blended precision cut that is adaptable to almost any hair type. Some exceptions are excessively thick, bristly hair or very short, overly curly hair. The rule to follow is this: *If a parting can be made in the hair and picked up between the fingers to put into a position for cutting, precision layering can be performed.* The hair should be clean and uniformly moist to maintain control of the hair and to produce the most precise cut.

The Shear-over-Comb Technique

The **shear-over-comb** technique is used to cut the ends of the hair and is an important method used in tapering and clipper cutting. The comb is used to position the hair to be cut and is similar to holding a section of hair between the fingers. Most shear-over-comb cutting is performed in the nape, behind the ears, around the ears, and in the sideburn areas of a cut. An entire haircut, however, may also be accomplished using this method. Cutting in the nape and sideburn areas is facilitated by using vertical working panels. The cutting of areas both behind and around the ears usually requires some diagonal positioning of the comb for safety and easier access to the section. To learn the shear-over-comb technique, practice the following exercises in front of a mirror.

Practice Session #5:

SHEAR-OVER-COMB TECHNIQUE WITH MIRROR

1. Pick up the shears firmly with the right hand and insert the thumb into the thumb grip. Place the third finger into the finger grip and

leave the little finger on the finger-brace of the shears. Practice opening and closing the shears, using the thumb to create the movement.

2. Pick up the comb with the left hand and place the fingers on top of the teeth with the thumb on the backbone of the comb (Figure 15–39).

   NOTE: Students should start with the coarse teeth of the comb until competent at rolling the comb out and positioning the hair to be cut. After sufficient skill has been developed, use the fine teeth of the comb.

3. Practice aligning the still blade of the shears with the comb at the level where the teeth join the back as in Figure 15–39. The shears and comb should be parallel to each other. Next, move the comb upward, opening and closing the shears in tandem with the movement of the comb (Figure 15–40). After several cutting movements, roll the teeth of the comb away from you (as if you were combing a client's hair) by using the thumb and the first two fingers in a key-turning motion (Figure 15–41). Master these techniques before attempting to do an actual haircut.

   NOTE: The preceding procedures may be changed to conform to your instructor's technique.

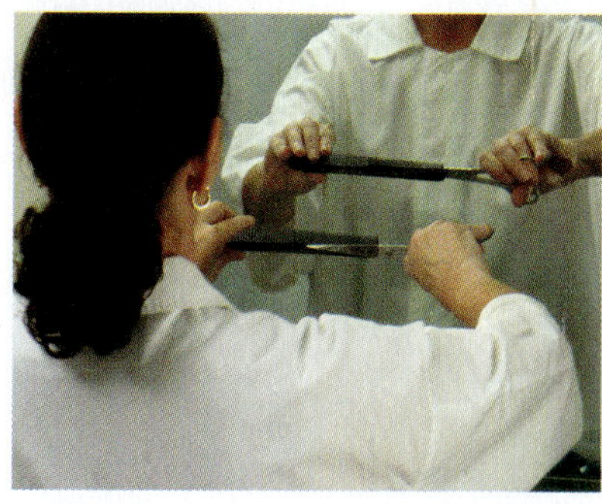

Figure 15–39 Positioning of comb and shears.

Practice Session #6:

SHEAR-OVER-COMB TECHNIQUE ON MANNEQUIN

Drape the mannequin and proceed as follows:

1. Start at the hairline in the center of the nape area.
2. With the teeth of the comb pointing upward, comb into a section of hair at the hairline, rolling the comb out toward you (Figure 15–42a). When performed correctly, the hair should protrude from the teeth of the comb and be in a position for cutting. This is called **rolling the comb out.**
3. Hold the comb parallel with the still blade of the shears, as practiced in Figure 15–39, and control the movement of the cutting blade with the thumb.
4. While manipulating the shears, move both the shears and the comb slowly upward at the same time, cutting the hair in the process. Stop at the occipital area.
5. Turn the teeth of the comb down when combing the hair down toward the hairline, as practiced in Figure 15–41.
6. Begin the next working panel by including some hair from the center section with the hair to the right or left of center. There should now be two lengths of hair in the comb: shorter hair from the center section and longer hair from the second section. The shorter hair from the center section becomes the guide for the second panel (Figure 15–42b). Finish one vertical strip at a time before proceeding with the next section.

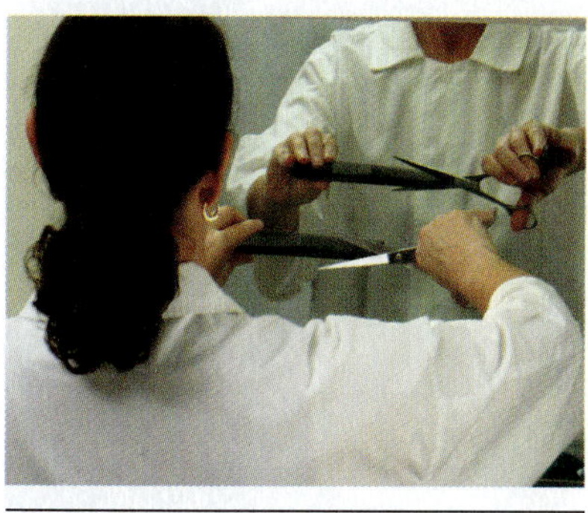

Figure 15–40 Open and close the shears in tandem with the upward movement of the comb.

15

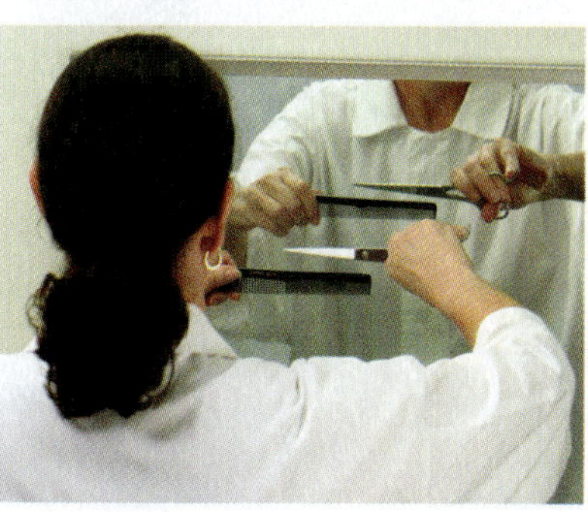

Figure 15–41 Roll the comb using a key-turning motion.

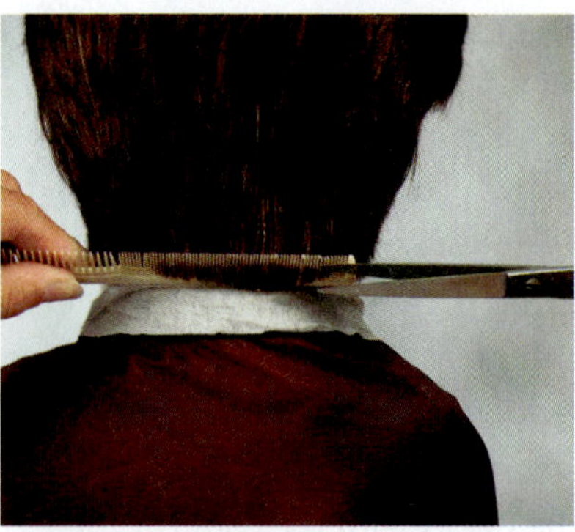

Figure 15-42a Position the hair to be cut by rolling the comb out.

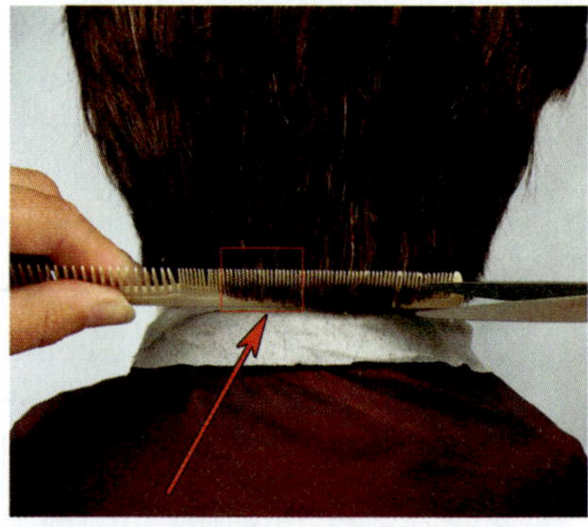

Figure 15-42b Center point, cut to guide.

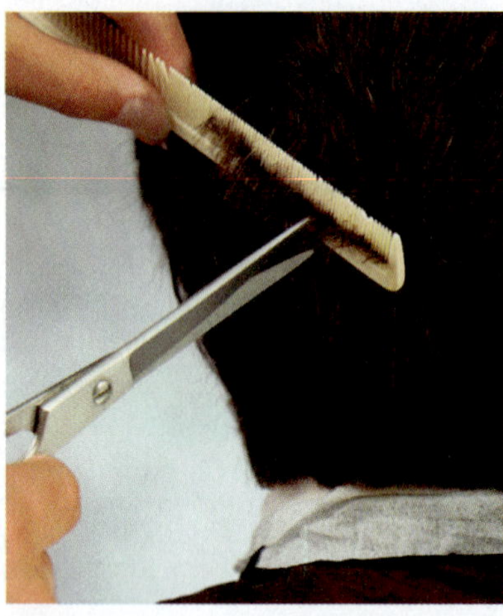

Figure 15-43 Shear-point taper in back section.

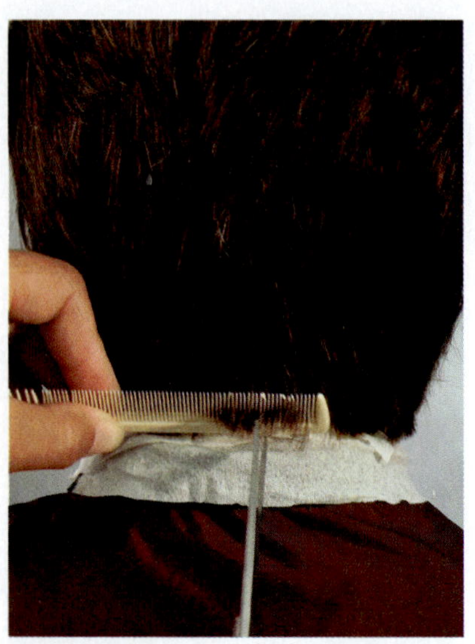

Figure 15-44 Shear-point taper in nape area.

7. To practice cutting along the sides of the neck, position the comb diagonally behind the ear parallel to the hairline. Proceed to trim the hair as described for the nape area.
8. Continue to practice the shear-over-comb technique in front of and around the ear. Make sure to blend the hair from the nape section to the sides of the neck and the around-the-ear areas.

Once the shear-over-comb technique has been practiced on the mannequin, refer to Haircutting Procedure #3 on page 395, Figures 15–161 through 15–172 to perform a haircut using this method.

Be guided by your instructor to learn other variations of this method, such as beginning on the right or left sides.

Shear-Point Tapering

Shear-point tapering is a useful technique for thinning out difficult areas of the hair caused by hollows, wrinkles, whorls, and creases in the scalp. Dark and ragged hair patches on the scalp can be minimized by this special technique. The shear-point taper is performed with the cutting points of the shears (Figures 15–43 and 15–44). Only a few strands of hair are cut at a time and then combed out. Continue cutting around the objectionable spot until it becomes less noticeable and blends in with the surrounding hair or hairline.

The Arching Technique

The **arching technique** is a way of marking the outer border of the haircut along the hairline at the bottom of the sideburn, in front of the ears, over the ears, and down the sides of the neck. This outlining technique is accomplished with the points of the shears or an outliner and is part of the finish work of most haircuts.

As with the other techniques in this text, the following practice session is simply one method of performing the procedure. Be guided by your instructor for variations in the method.

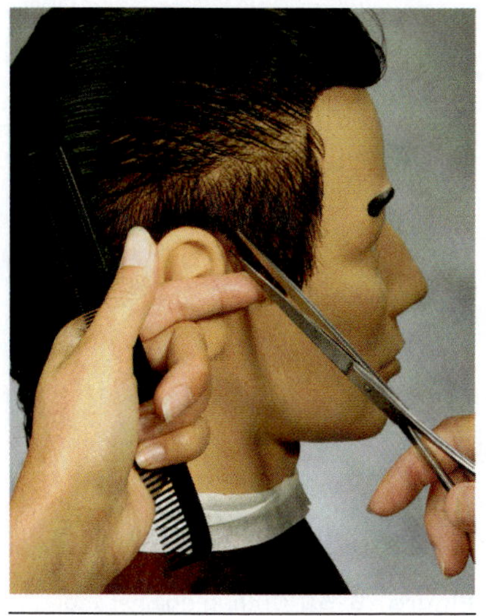

Figure 15-45 Steady the points of the shears.

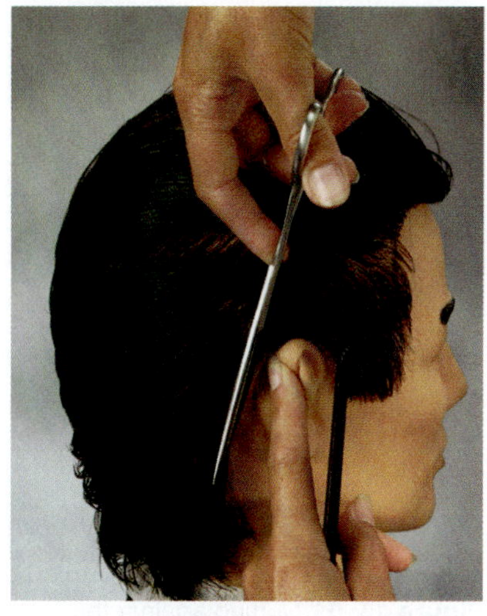

Figure 15-46 Cut a continuous line around the ears and down the sides of the neck.

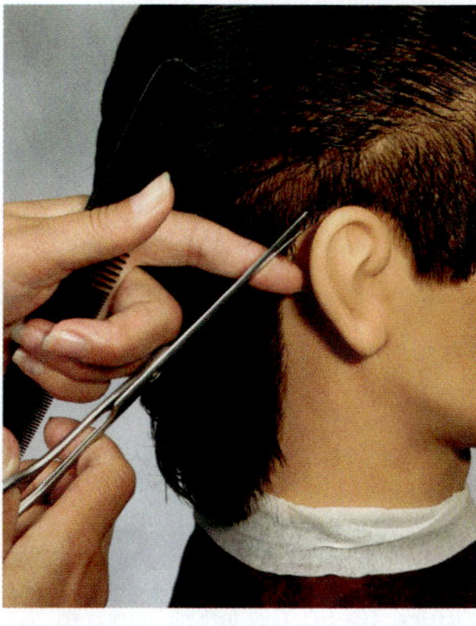

Figure 15-47 Reverse the direction of arching.

Practice Session #7:

ARCHING TECHNIQUE ON MANNEQUIN

1. Holding the shears with the right hand.
   a) Pick up the shears and insert the thumb in the thumb grip. Place the third finger into the finger grip and the little finger on the brace of the shears.
   b) Use the most convenient fingertip of the left hand to steady the point of the shears.
2. Arching the right side.
   a) Always make an outline around the ear as close to the natural hairline as possible.
   b) Start in front of the ear and cut a continuous outline around the ear and down the side of the neck (Figures 15–45 and 15–46).
   c) Reverse the direction of arching back to the starting point (Figure 15–47).
   d) Continue arching around the ear until a definite outline is formed.
   e) Square off and establish the length of the right sideburn (Figure 15–48).
3. Arching the left side.
   a) Start in front of the left ear and cut a continuous outline with the shears over the left ear and down the side of the neck (Figure 15–49).
   b) Reverse the direction of the shears and return to the starting point. Continue arching around the ear until a definite outline is formed.

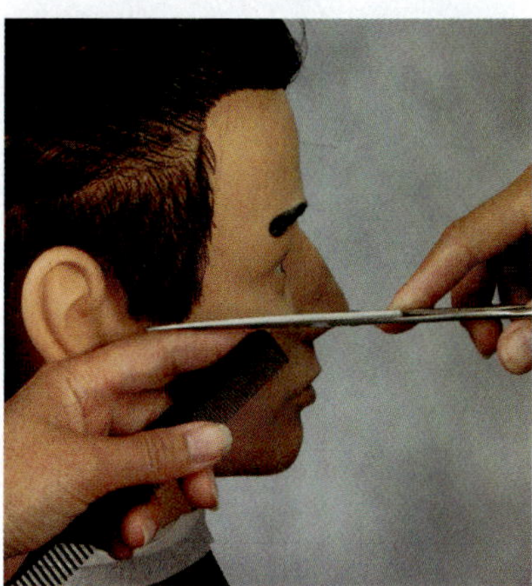

Figure 15-48 Establish length of right sideburn.

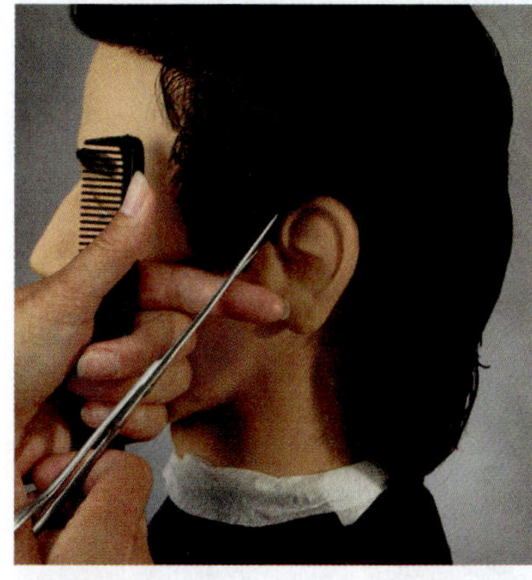

Figure 15-49 Cut a continuous outline over the left ear and sides of the neck.

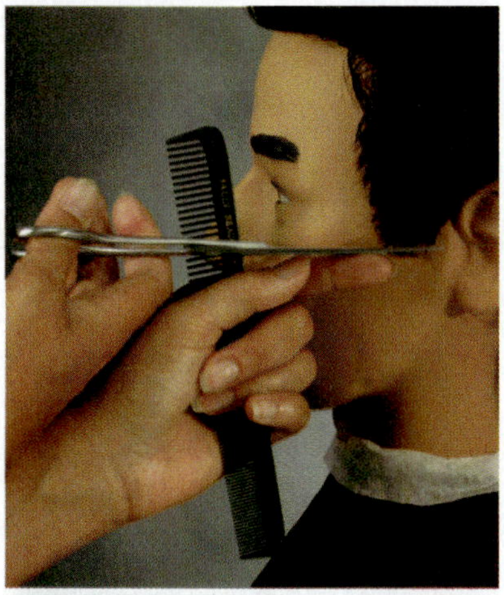

Figure 15-50 Cut left sideburn to match the right sideburn.

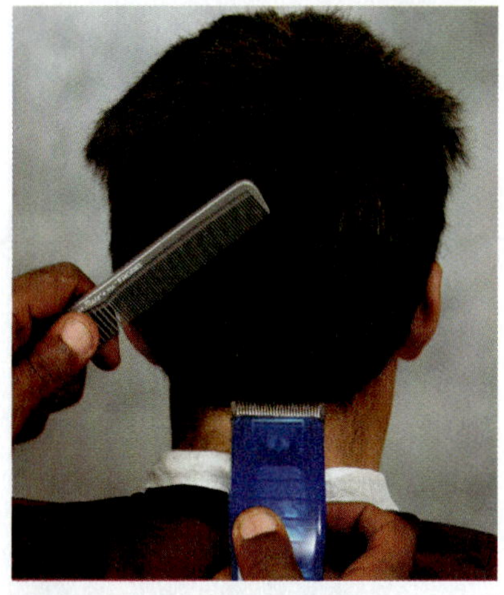

Figure 15-51 Cutting against the grain on straight hair.

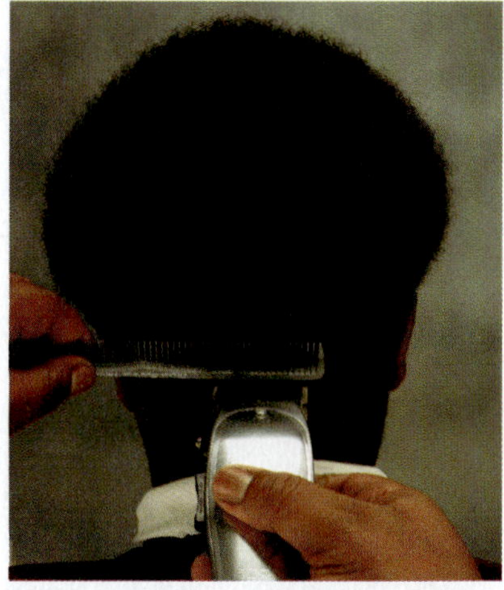

Figure 15-52 Cutting against the grain on curly hair.

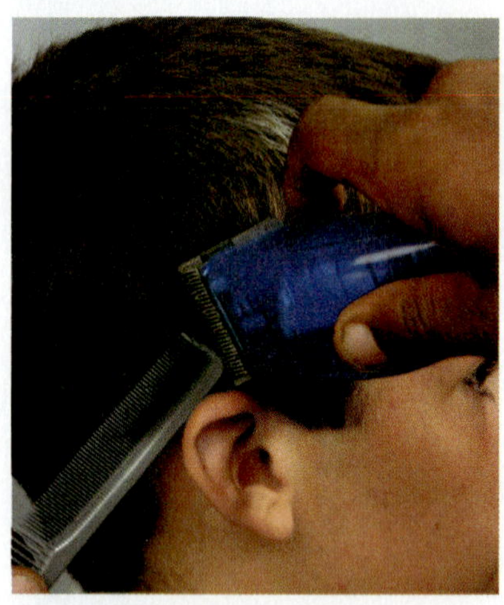

Figure 15-53 Cutting with the grain on straight hair.

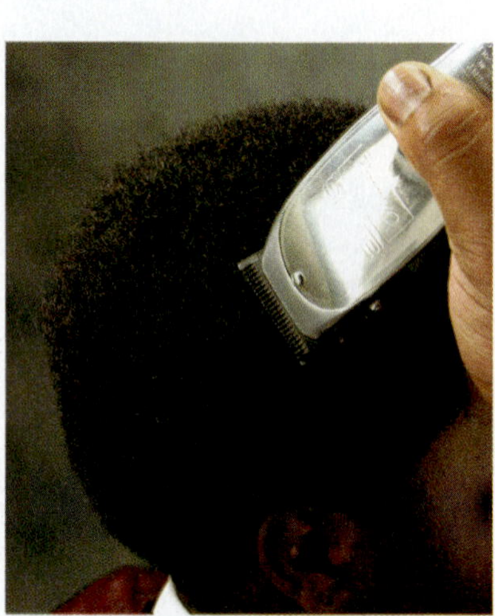

Figure 15-54 Cutting with the grain on curly hair.

c) Square off of the left sideburn to match the right sideburn (Figure 15–50).

NOTE: Before beginning the arching procedure, check to determine if one sideburn is longer than the other. Start on the side with the shortest sideburn to avoid unnecessary repetition of the procedure.

Clipper Cutting

Clippers are versatile tools that can be used in several ways to produce a variety of haircut textures and styles. The standard techniques are **freehand clipper cutting** and **clipper-over-comb** cutting. As a general rule, clipper cutting is followed up with shear and comb work to fine-tune the haircut and/or to perform the arching technique.

Directional Terms Used in Clipper Cutting

Cutting and tapering the hair with clippers can be accomplished in the following ways:

- Cutting *against the grain* is accomplished by cutting the hair in the opposite direction from which it grows (Figures 15–51 and 15–52). Taper the hair by gradually tilting the clipper until it rides on its heel.
- Cutting *with the grain* means the cutting is performed in the same direction in which the hair grows (Figures 15–53 and 15–54). When using a clipper on hair that has a tight curl formation, try to cut with the grain or growth pattern. Cutting tight, curly hair against the grain clogs up the clipper blades and may leave patches or spots in the haircut.
- When cutting *across the grain* with clippers, the hair is cut neither with nor against the grain. This direction in cutting is usually performed on transition areas in the crest or side regions. (Figures 15–55 and 15–56).

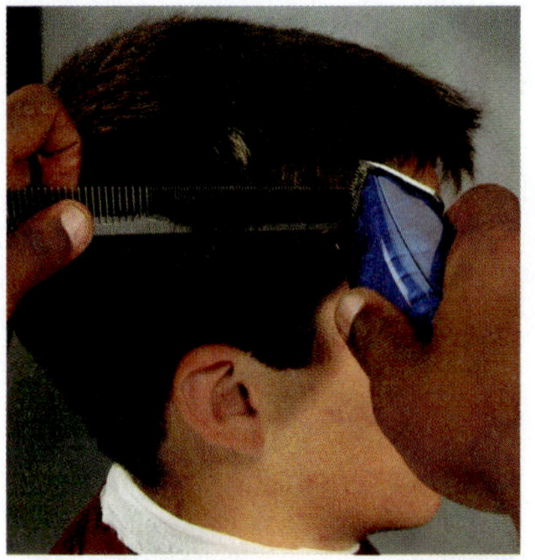

Figure 15-55 Cutting across the grain on straight hair.

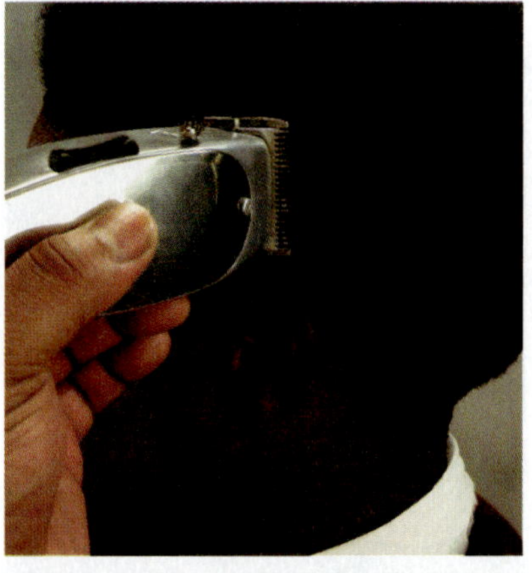

Figure 15-56 Cutting across the grain on curly hair.

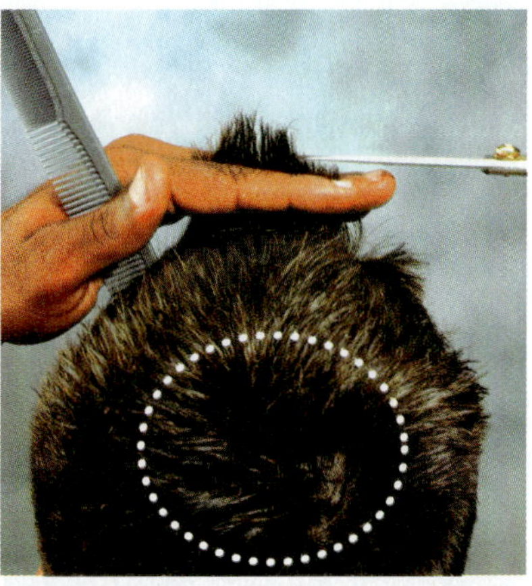

Figure 15-57 Whorl in crown area in straight hair.

- In whorl areas, or in places where the hair does not grow in a uniform manner (Figure 15–57), cutting the hair in a *circular motion* using clippers is advisable.

Arching with a Clipper

Many barbers prefer to use an outliner or trimmer with a fine cutting edge to square off sideburns and perfect the outline around the ears and down the sides of neck. This method of arching is efficient and precise due to the maneuverability of the smaller cutting head of the tool. If the desired result can be accomplished with the standard clipper, that method is equally acceptable (Figures 15–58 and 15–59).

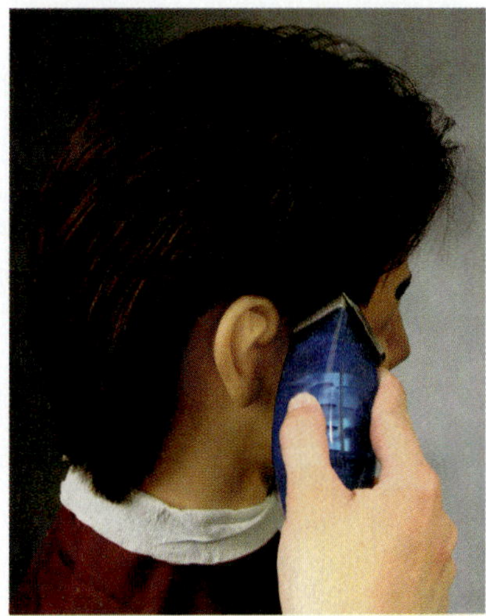

Figure 15-58 Arching with clipper in front of the ear.

Freehand and Clipper-Over-Comb Cutting

Freehand clipper cutting requires a steady hand and consistent use of the comb or hair pick while cutting. The use of the comb or pick is important for two reasons: first, both implements put the hair into a position to be cut, and second, both implements help to remove the excess hair cut from the previous section. This provides the barber with a clear view of the results of the previous work and any areas that may need reblending.

A true freehand clipper cutting technique tends to be used on two extremes of hair length: (1) very short straight, wavy, and curly lengths in which little clipper-over-comb work is performed, and (2) longer, very curly hair lengths that require more sculpting (Figures 15–60 and 15–61).

For short hair styles, clippers with detachable blades range from size 0000 (close to shaving) to size 3½, which leaves the hair almost ½ inch long. Detachable blades should not be confused with clipper attachment combs, most commonly known as *guards*. Guards are placed on top of a clipper blade, allowing for more hair length to remain while cutting.

NOTE: The use of guards is not considered to be a form of freehand clipper cutting, nor are guards generally acceptable for state board practical examinations.

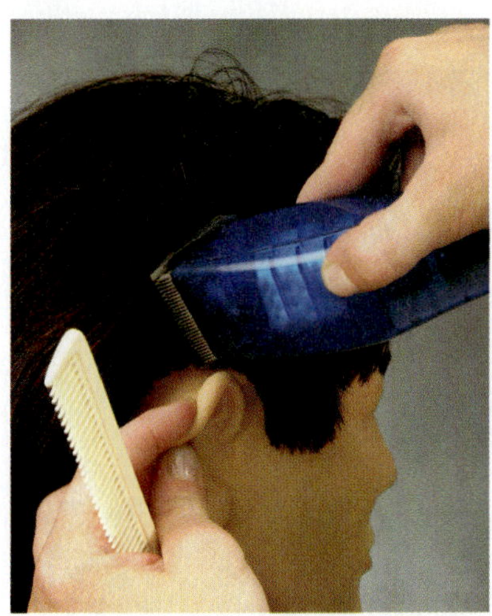

Figure 15-59 Arching with clipper around ear.

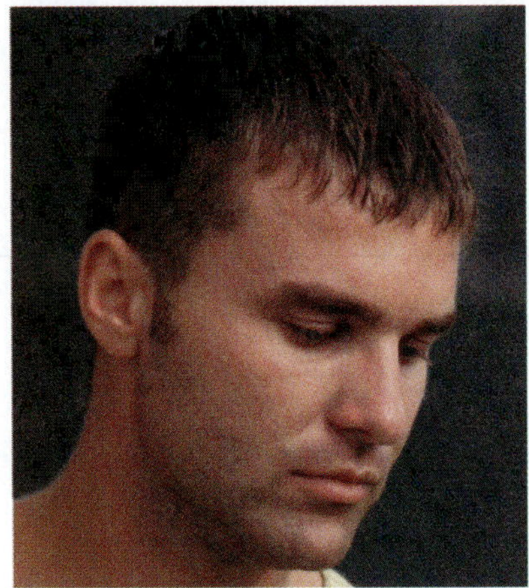

Figure 15–60 Finished freehand clipper cut on straight hair.

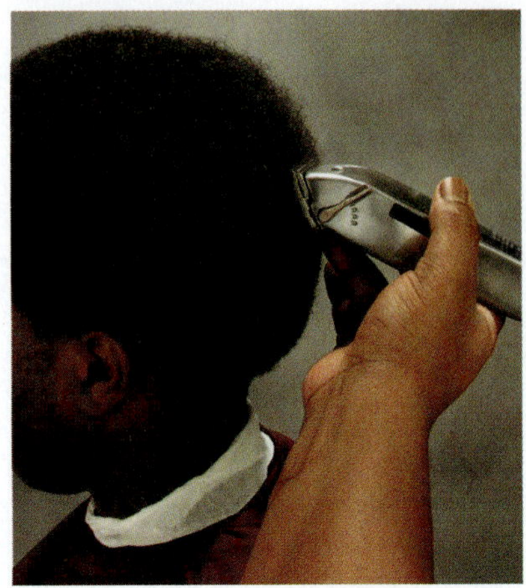

Figure 15–61 Freehand clipper cutting.

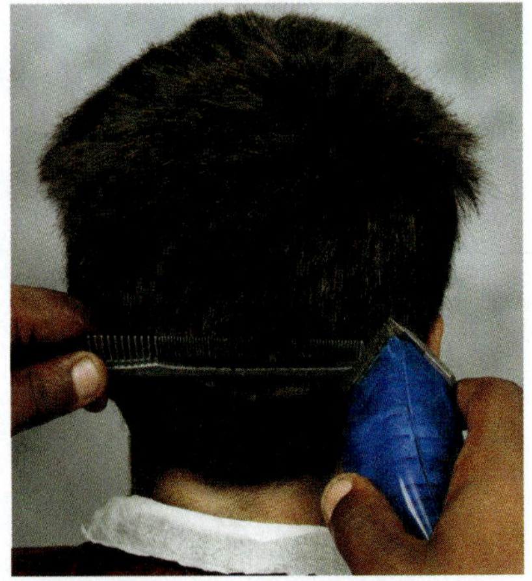

Figure 15–62 Clipper over comb on straight hair.

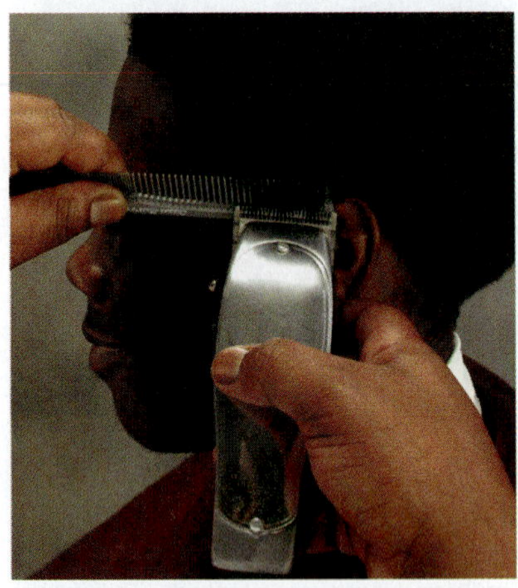

Figure 15–63 Clipper over comb on curly hair.

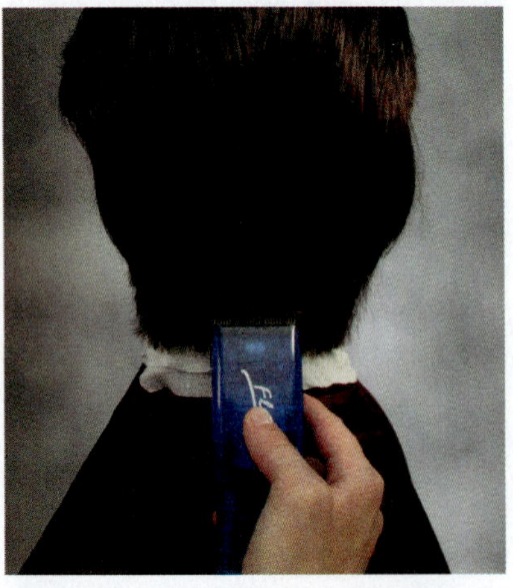

Figure 15–64 Hold clipper to permit freedom of wrist movement.

Freehand clipper cutting is also used for tightly curled hair when a natural look is the desired result. Because most tightly curled hair grows up and out of the scalp, rather than falling to one side or another as with straighter hair types, the hair texture lends itself to being picked out and put into position for freehand clipper cutting. Cutting this type of hairstyle requires a keen eye for haircut balance, shape, and proportion as the hair is sculpted into the desired form.

Clipper-over-comb cutting can be used to cut the entire head or to blend the hair from shorter tapered areas to longer-haired areas such as the top, crest, or occipital. Much like the shear-over-comb technique, the comb places the hair in a position to be cut and utilizes the same blending principles (Figures 15–62 and 15–63). Freehand clipper cutting, clipper-over-comb, and fingers-and-shear work are techniques frequently used to perform a single haircut.

Practice Session #8:

CLIPPER CUTTING ON STRAIGHT-HAIRED MANNEQUIN

This practice session will involve clipper-over-comb cutting and standard freehand clipper cutting using an all-purpose comb.

1. How to hold the clipper and comb for *clipper-over-comb cutting.*
   a) Pick up the clipper with the dominant hand.
   b) Place the thumb on the top left side and fingers underneath along the right side of the clipper. Hold it firmly, but lightly, to permit freedom of wrist movement (Figure 15–64).
   c) Use the largest numbered detachable clipper blade or fully open the adjustable blade clipper.

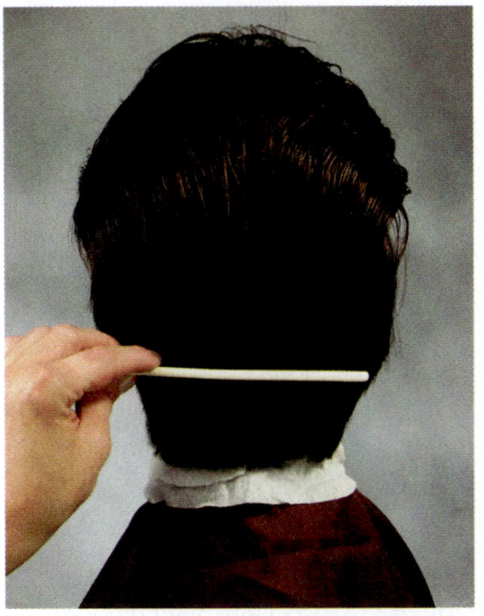

Figure 15-65 Comb the hair down.

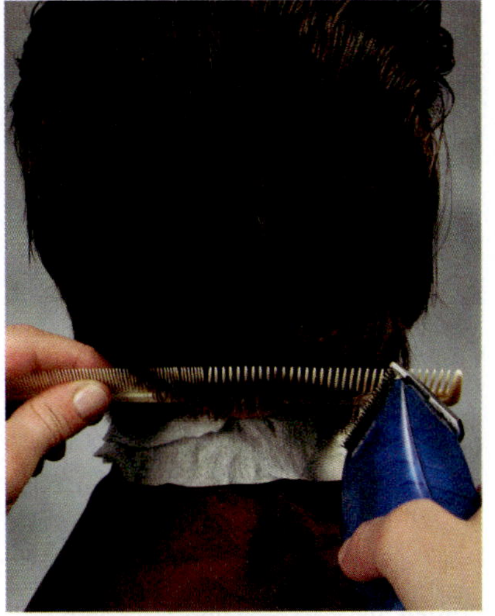

Figure 15-66 Roll the comb out to put the hair in a position to be cut.

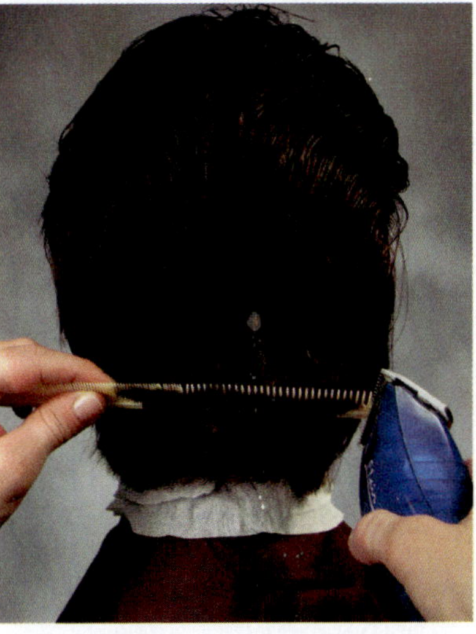

Figure 15-67 Continue clipper-over-comb cutting to the occipital area.

   d) Begin in the center of the nape area and comb the hair down with the opposite hand (Figure 15–65).
   e) With the teeth of the comb pointing upward, comb into a section of hair at the hairline, rolling the comb out toward you as in Figure 15–66.
   f) Use the clipper to cut the hair section to the desired length. Comb through, check, and begin the next section to the right or left of center.

2. Clipper-over-comb: cutting the nape area
   a) For a gradual, even taper from shorter to longer in each section of hair, roll the comb out to put the hair in a position to be cut.
   b) Gradually taper the hair from the hairline to an inch or two above the hairline. Do not taper higher than the occipital for this exercise, or cut into the hair along the sides of the neck at this point (Figure 15–67).
3. Clipper-over-comb: cutting the sides
   a) Begin in the front of the ear and position the comb parallel to the hairline. Roll the hair out at about a 45-degree projection and cut (Figure 15–68). Follow the forward curve of the hairline around the ear.
   b) Bend the ear forward and use the same projection technique to continue cutting along the hairline to meet the hairline at the topmost part at the back of the ear.
4. Clipper-over-comb: cutting behind the ears
   a) The guide around the ears and at the corner of the neck should be visible.
   b) Place the comb parallel to the hairline on a diagonal, roll the comb out, and blend from the guide at the back of the ear to the nape corner (Figures 15–69a and 15–69b). The hair in the tapered areas should blend from the nape to the side of the neck, and around the ear.

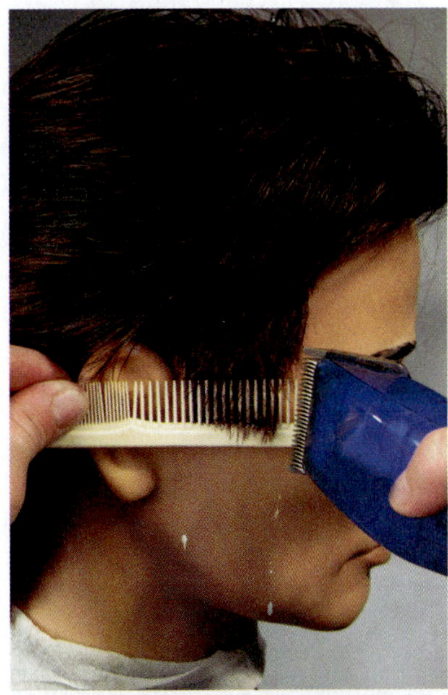

Figure 15-68 Position the comb at the hairline and roll out to 45 degrees.

15

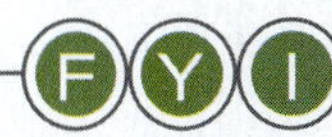

When tapering with the clipper-over-comb technique, be sure to tilt the comb away from the head to create a blended taper from shorter to longer sections.

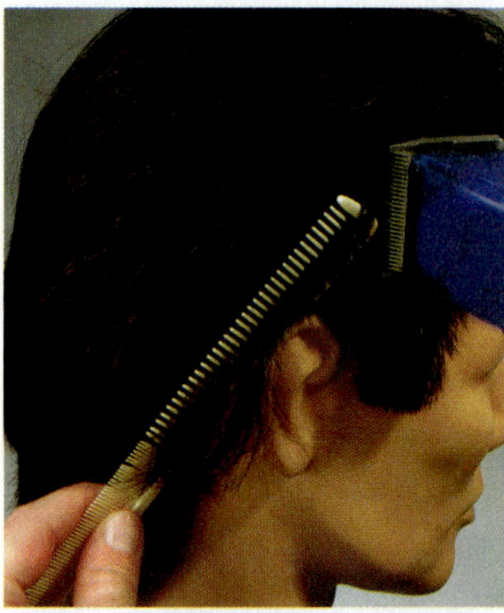

Figure 15-69a Position the comb parallel to the hairline.

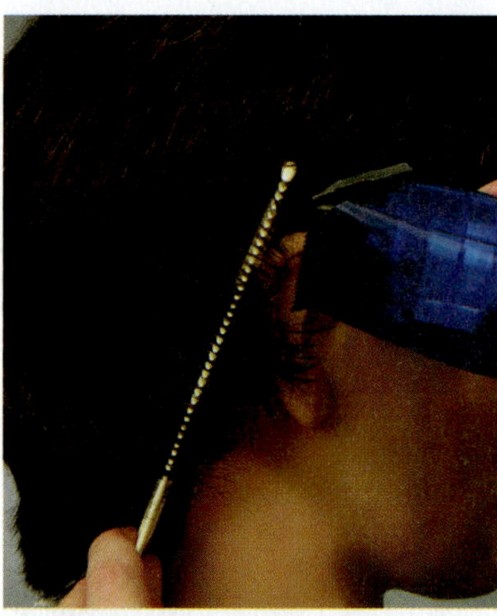

Figure 15-69b Continue cutting to the corner of the nape.

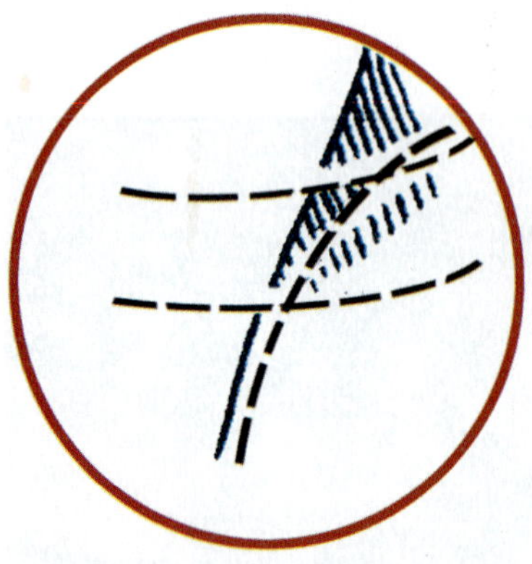

Figure 15-70 When tapering with a clipper, be sure to tilt the comb away from the head to create a blended taper from shorter to longer sections.

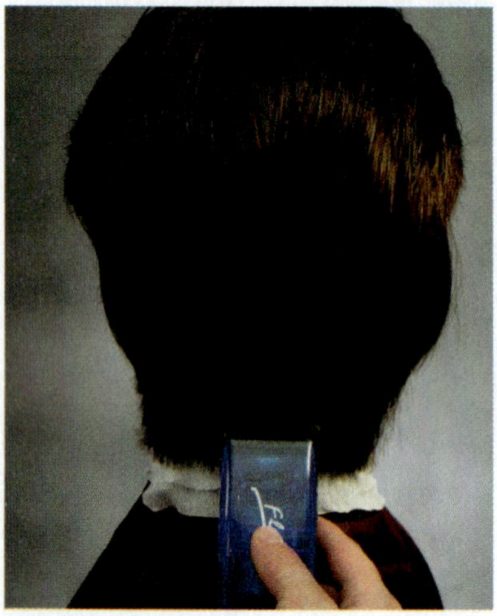

Figure 15-71 Guide the clipper blades through the ends of the hair.

5. How to hold the clipper for freehand clipper cutting.
   a) Pick up the clipper with the dominant hand.
   b) Place the thumb on the top left side and fingers underneath along the right side of the clipper. Hold it firmly, but lightly, to permit freedom of wrist movement. Depending on the section of the head form being cut, the holding position will change for comfort and access to the area.
   c) Use the largest-numbered detachable clipper blade or fully open the adjustable blade clipper.
   d) Begin in the center of the nape area and comb the hair down with the opposite hand.
   e) Palm the comb and steady the clipper with the tip of the index finger of the opposite hand.
6. Freehand clipper cutting: the nape area
   a) Begin with the clipper blades open. With the teeth of the bottom blade placed flat against the skin at the center of the nape hairline, lightly guide the clipper upward into the hair ¼ to ½ inch above the hairline (Figure 15–71). Remember, this is just a practice session to become familiar with the clippers, so avoid removing too much hair.
   b) For a gradual, even taper from shorter to longer hair, gradually tilt the blade away from the head so that the clipper rides on the heel of the bottom blade (Figure 15–72). Do not taper higher than the occipital for this exercise. Gradually taper the hair only an inch or two above the hairline.

   NOTE: The style will determine the point on the head at which the tapered area is blended into longer hair. Very short styles, such as butch and crew cuts, have a high taper and are blended in the crest areas; longer styles may be blended at or just below the occipital. There are as many variations as there are heads of hair to cut.

   c) Do not move the clipper into the hair too fast as it may have a tendency to jam the clipper blades and pull the hair.

d) After tapering one short strip of hair, comb it down, check the results, and start tapering the section to the right or left of center. Be guided by your instructor.

7. Freehand clipper cutting: the sides
   a) Begin at the front of the ear at the hairline and comb the hair down. Tilt the clipper at about a 45-degree angle so that the first few teeth of the blades will be used for cutting the curve around the ear.
   b) Bend the ear forward and continue cutting along the hairline, meeting the top of the hairline at the side of the neck.
8. Freehand clipper cutting: behind the ears
   a) The guide around the ears and at the corner of the neck should be visible.
   b) Comb the hair down and blend from the nape corner to the guide at the back of the ear. The hair in the tapered areas should blend from the nape to the side of the neck and around the ear.

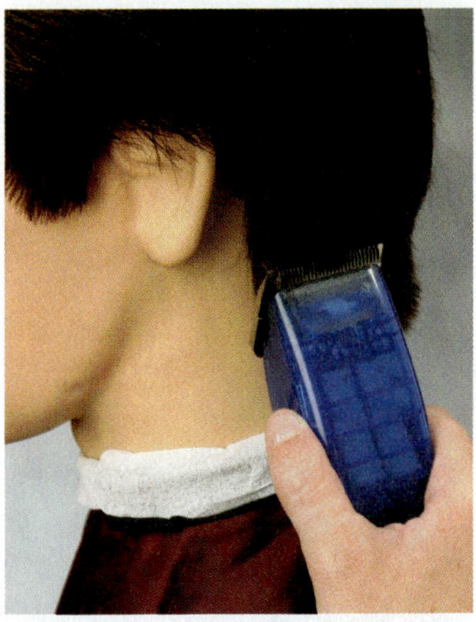

Figure 15–72 Gradually tilt the clipper blades away from the head.

When the clipper-over-comb and freehand techniques have been practiced on the mannequin, refer to Haircutting Procedure #4 on page 397, Figures 15–173 through 15–185, to perform a medium-length haircut using these methods. Be guided by your instructor to learn other variations, such as beginning on the right or left sides.

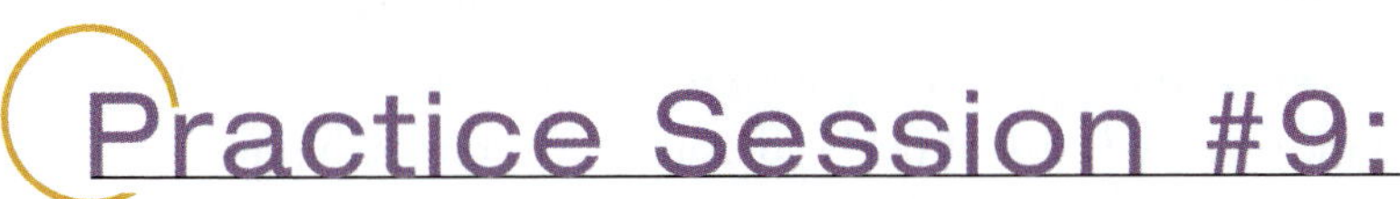

Practice Session #9:

CLIPPER CUTTING ON MANNEQUIN WITH TIGHTLY CURLED HAIR

1. Hold the clipper as for freehand clipper cutting.
2. Use a pick or Afro comb to comb the hair up and outward from the scalp.
3. If the hair is too thick or too tightly curled to use an all-purpose comb while cutting, use a wide-tooth comb to practice the clipper-over-comb technique as performed on the model in Figure 15–63.
4. When the clipper-over-comb technique has been completed, practice the freehand clipper cutting method in Figure 15–61.

Be guided by your instructor as to where to begin the clipper cut and the order of the subsequent sections. Some barbers prefer to start in the center of the nape area, while others work from right to left or left to right. As long as the hair is tapered evenly, all methods are equally correct.

Once the clipper-over-comb and freehand clipper cutting techniques have been practiced on the mannequin, refer to Haircutting Procedure #5 on page 400, Figures 15–186 through 15–198, to perform a medium-length haircut on tightly curled hair using these methods. Be guided by your instructor to learn other variations of this method.

15

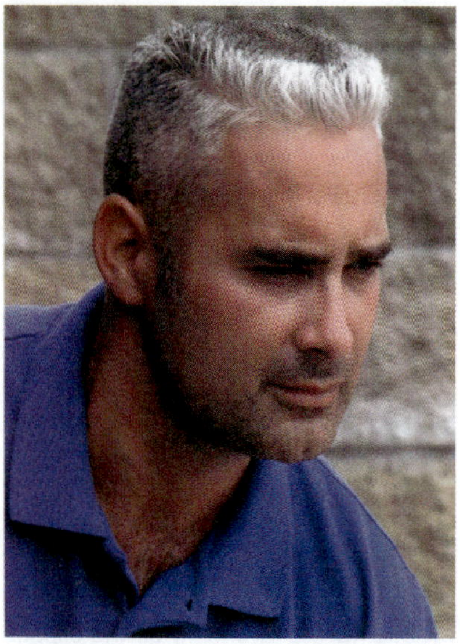

Figure 15–73 Flat-top style.

Clipper Cut Styles

Variations of the basic clipper cut styles have been around since the hand clipper was invented. Flat tops, crew cuts, and the Quo Vadis are three of the most popular styles that have stood the test of time and cyclical haircut trends.

Flat tops are very short on the sides and in the back areas, as are crew cuts. Flat tops are traditionally slightly longer in the front and crest sections and flat across the top of the head form. The top of the crest area should look squared off when viewed from the front. Variations of the style and length of the top section will be determined by the client's preference, hair texture, and hair density. Clippers or shears or use of both tools may be used to cut a flat top (Figure 15–73).

Suggested procedures for cutting the flat top are as follows:

1. Stand behind the client. The hair at the crown is cut flat to about ¼ to ½ inch in length, 1 inch in depth, and 2 to 3 inches in width.
2. Stand in front of the client. Position the comb flat across the front center area, cutting the hair to a length of 1 to 1½ inches, depending on the client's preference. This cutting area will span the width of the client's top section. Cut straight across from side to side.
3. Ask the client if the front hair is the desired length. If it is not, then cut the hair to the desired height.
4. Complete all finish work such as arching and the neck shave.

Crew cuts are also referred to as the *short pomp* or *brush cut.* The length of hair on the sides and back of the head usually determines the crew cut style, as described in the following list.

- Short sides and back: short crew cut.
- Semishort sides and back: medium crew cut.
- Medium sides and back: long crew cut.

15

Generally, the back and sides are cut first and relatively high to the bottom of the crest area. The hair on top is then combed from front to back to make it stand up, followed by blending the tapered area to the crest and top sections. Since the top section should be smooth and almost flat, use a wide-toothed comb to provide a level guide. Begin cutting in the front to the desired length and cut back toward the crown. This section should be graduated in length from the front hairline to the back part of the crown. Repeat the procedure until the top section has been cut. When viewed from the front, the top section should blend with the top of the crest, with a slight curvature to conform to the contours of the head. Use the shears and comb to smooth out any uneven spots left by the clipper work.

The brush cut is a variation of the crew cut and popular with young men as it requires the least attention. The sides and back areas are cut as for a short crew cut, but the hair on top is cut the same length all over, about ¼ to ½ inch, and follows the contours of the head.

The Quo Vadis is a popular haircut style that is suitable for very curly hair. The main objective with this haircut is to achieve an even and smooth cut over the entire head. Since the hair is cut close to the scalp, clipper lines and patches are readily noticeable. Be guided by the natural hair growth pattern and cut with the grain to avoid gaps. Outline and taper the nape area with a #000 clipper blade and then use a #1 clipper blade over the rest of the head.

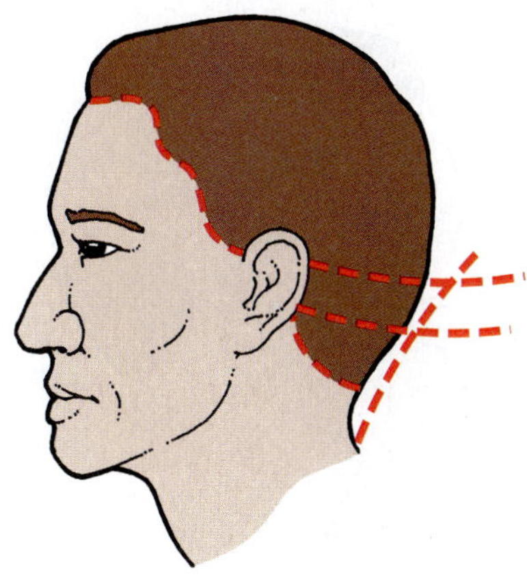
Figure 15–74 Taper area for longer hair style.

Basic Tapering and Blending Areas

To simplify the clipper or shear cutting procedures, the primary tapering and blending areas of haircut styles may be identified as belonging to one of four basic classifications: long cuts and trims, medium lengths, semishort lengths, and short cuts. A variety of hairstyles, such as the fade and bilevel, can be created from these basic classifications to suit the client's tastes and desires.

Long haircut styles and trims usually require the least amount of clipper tapering. Tapering is performed from the nape hairline to just above the bottom of the ear and below the occipital using the fingers-and-shear, shear-over-comb, or clipper-over-comb techniques (Figure 15–74). An outliner or trimmer is used to remove fine hair at the nape and along the sides of the neck. Sideburns and over-the-ear areas are shortened using the shear-over-comb method along the natural hairline and then outlined with trimmers and/or razor.

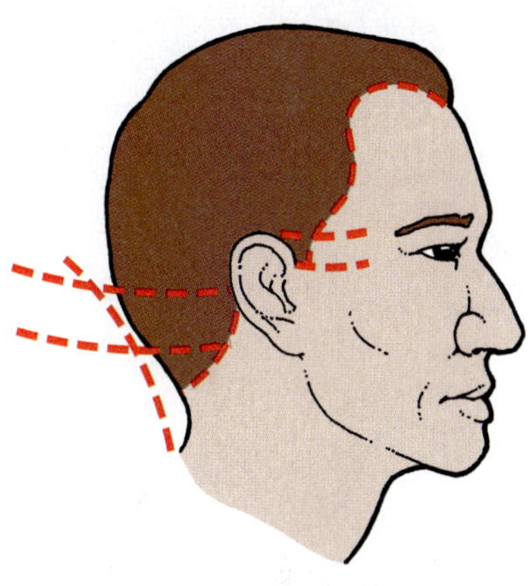
Figure 15–75 Taper area for medium-length style.

Medium-length styles do not usually have a scalped appearance, although the hair is cut closer to the head than in longer styles (Figure 15–75). Clipper cutting in the nape should be performed with the clipper tilted on its heel until reaching a point about midway to the ears. In the sideburn areas, the taper should end no higher than the tops of the ears. An outliner or razor is used at the nape hairline.

Semishort styles usually require tilting the clipper back off the hair when the top of the ear areas are viewed from the back section. The hair in the back may be left slightly longer than on the sides. In the sideburn areas, the clipper tapers out at about the top of the ears. When cutting around the ears, remove about ½ inch from the hairline, then use an outliner to trim the sideburns and around the ear areas (Figure 15–76).

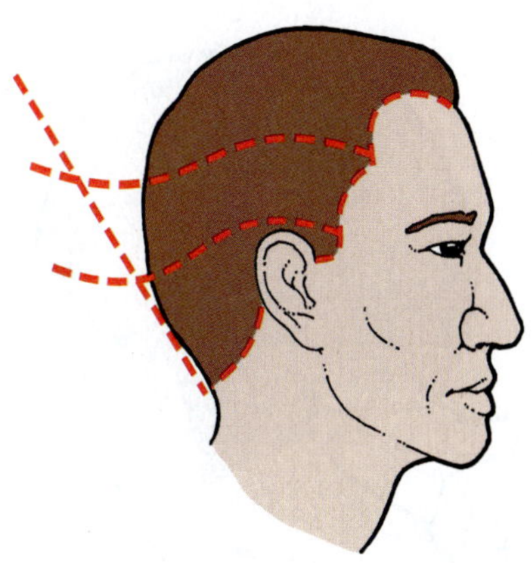
Figure 15–76 Taper area for semi-short style.

Short haircut styles usually require cutting up to the crest area and then gradually tilting the heel of the clipper back as the clipper is brought up until it runs off the curve of the head. This movement is repeated all the way around the head form. An outliner is used to taper the sideburns and nape (Figure 15–77).

The *fade style* derives its name from the fact that the hair at the nape and sides is cut extremely close, becoming gradually longer in the crest and lower crown areas and longest at the top. Hence, it fades to nothing at the hairline.

This cut requires close cutting from the nape to the bottom of the crest or horseshoe area. The sides are cut to the temporal region using the

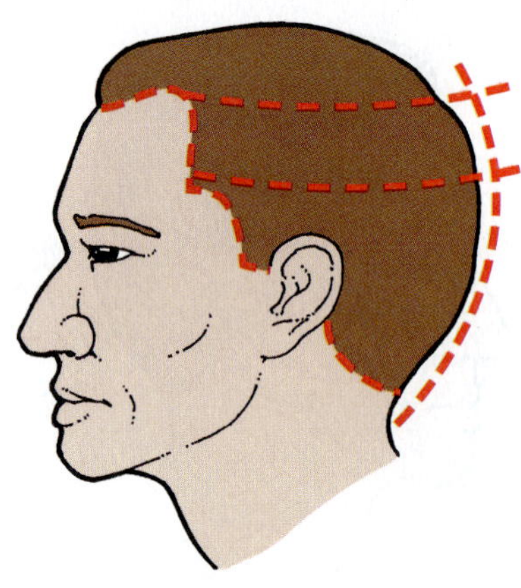

Figure 15-77 Taper area for short styles.

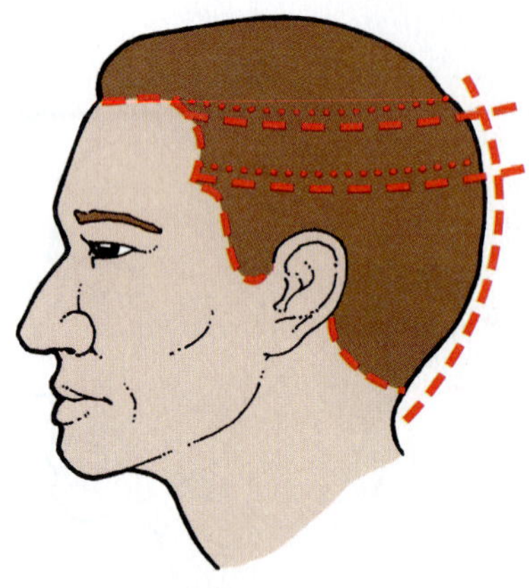

Figure 15-78 Taper area for a fade style.

next-longer clipper blade, or one that will taper in the crest area to the top section. The top section is cut and blended to the crest (Figure 15–78). To gradually blend the fine clipper taper with the longer clipper taper, tilt the heel of the clippers, moving with and across the grain as necessary.

A *bilevel style* cut is most often achieved with clippers and shears. The clipper is used to cut the nape and sides to the desired length (Figure 15–79). The top is either layered and texturized or cut to one length using a weight line. The weight line may vary in style lengths.

For a medium-length style, the top, crown, and crest area hair is sectioned off and secured with a hair clip. Clipper cutting is performed up to the occipital area in the back and on the sides to the bottom of the crest. A horizontal parting is taken from the secured hair to establish a design/guide line. The hair is cut at 0 degrees until all the partings are cut. Using the design line as a guide, the hair is projected at 45 or 90 degrees to produce layers if desired. Clipper cutting for a shorter length, bilevel style usually requires cutting higher into the temporal region with slight blending to the top section.

Popular Sideburn Lengths

When trimming or redesigning the length of sideburns, every effort should be made to make sure that the sideburns appear even in length. When seen in profile, the client's ear, eye, or other anatomical feature may be used as a general guide for trimming the sideburns. However, *always check the length of both sideburns by facing the client toward the mirror.* No one's face is truly symmetrical and differences will be noticed when viewing the client from the front. In addition, check to see that the thickness (density) of the sideburns complements the facial shape and hairstyle (Figures 15–80 through 15–84).

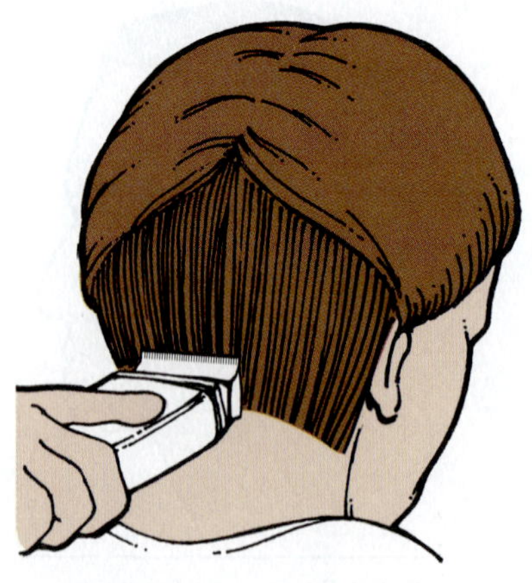

Figure 15-79 Taper area for a bilevel style.

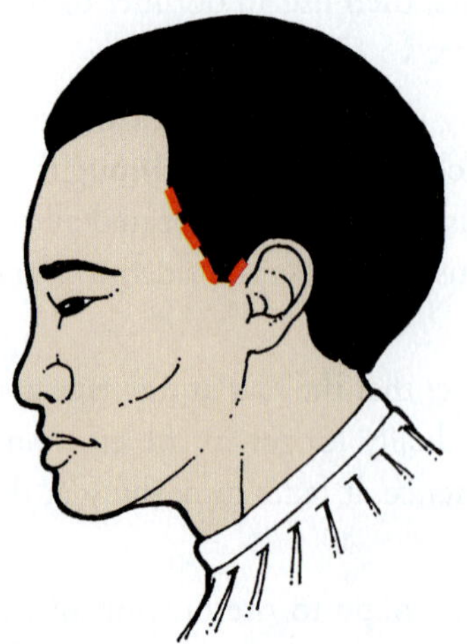

Figure 15-80 Short sideburn.

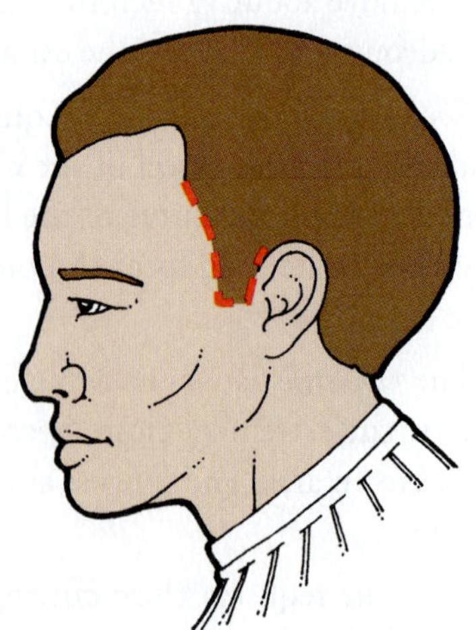

Figure 15-81 Medium sideburn.

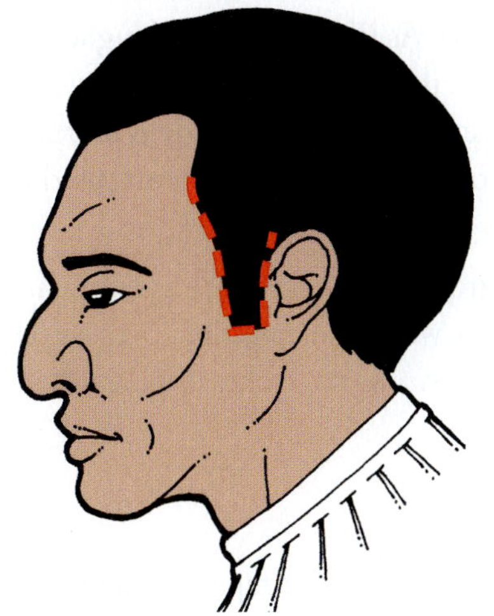
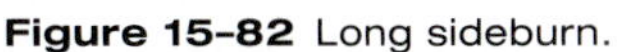

Figure 15-82 Long sideburn.

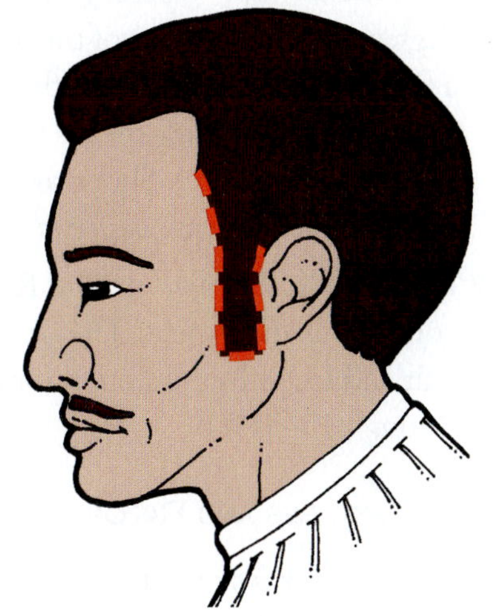

Figure 15-83 Extra-long sideburn.

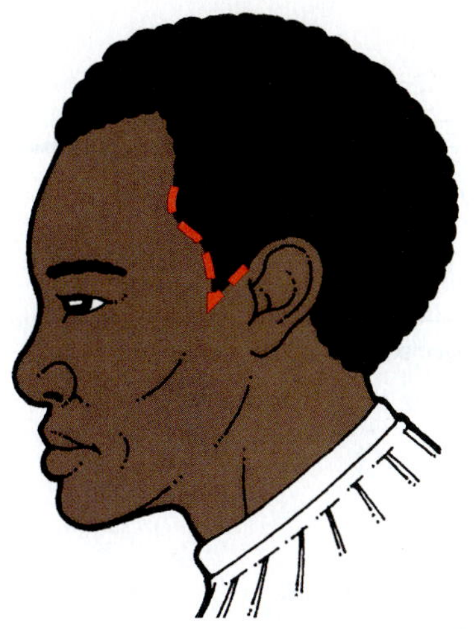

Figure 15-84 Pointed sideburn.

Razor Cutting

Razor cutting provides an opportunity for the barber to create a variety of different effects in the hair (Figure 15–85). It is especially suitable for thinning, shortening, tapering, blending, or feathering specific areas and can help make resistant hair textures more manageable. For client comfort and a precise cut, the hair should always be clean and damp. As always, the barber must consider the client's styling wishes, features, head shape, facial contour, and hair texture. The technique of handling a razor should be mastered completely before attempting to use it to cut a client's hair. CAUTION: The use of a razor with a safety guard is recommended for the beginner. Once proficient in the techniques, the razor may be used without a safety guard.

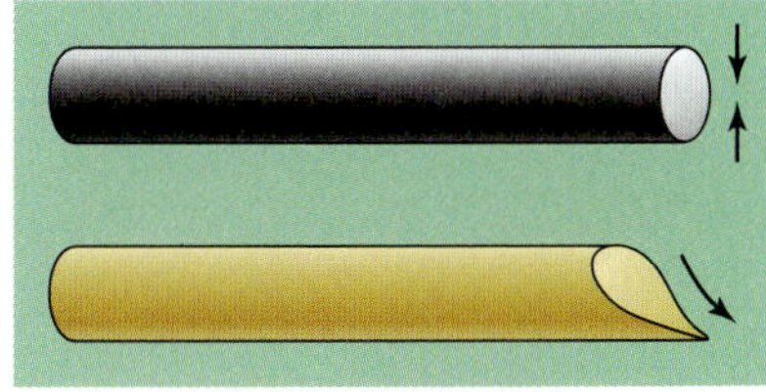

Figure 15-85 Shear cut and razor cut strands.

Razor Stroking and Combing

Proper stroking of the razor and combing during the tapering process are of utmost importance in razor cutting. It is better to taper a little at a time than to taper too much.

- *Arm and hand movements:* Some barbers prefer the arm movement, in which the razor stroking and combing is done with stiff arms, using the elbows as a hinge. Others use both wrist and arm movements. This is a matter of preference. The barber should develop a technique best suited to the individual and that gives the desired results.
- *Razor taper-blending:* Razor cutting is thought by some barbers to be the best technique to use for tapering and blending the hair. The cutting action of the razor permits a smoother blend than that usually accomplished with shears and/or clippers.

  Light taper-blending requires that the razor is held almost flat against the surface of the hair. Note the small amount of hair that is cut when the blade is only slightly tilted and very little pressure is used (Figure 15–86).

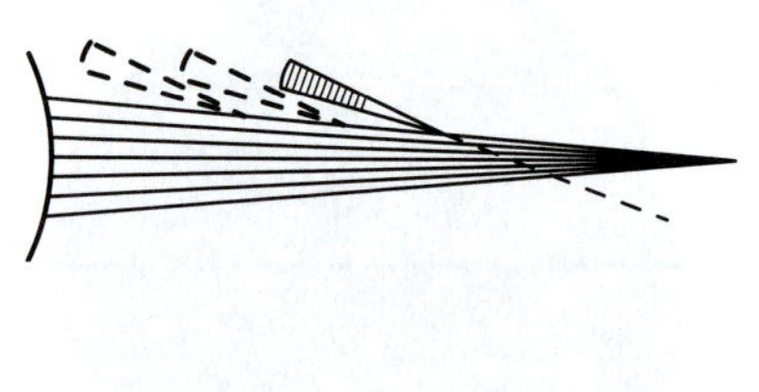

Figure 15–86 Light taper-blending.

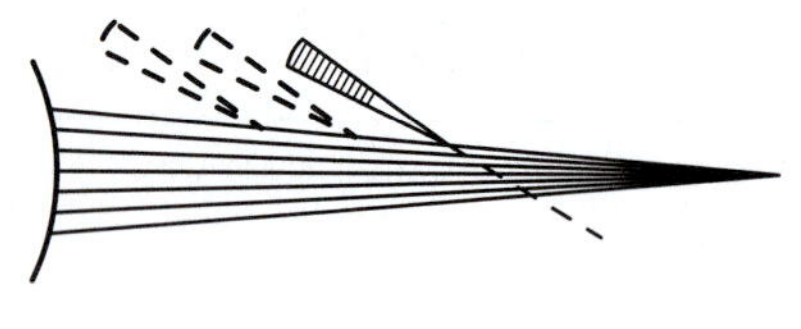

Figure 15–87 Heavier taper-blending.

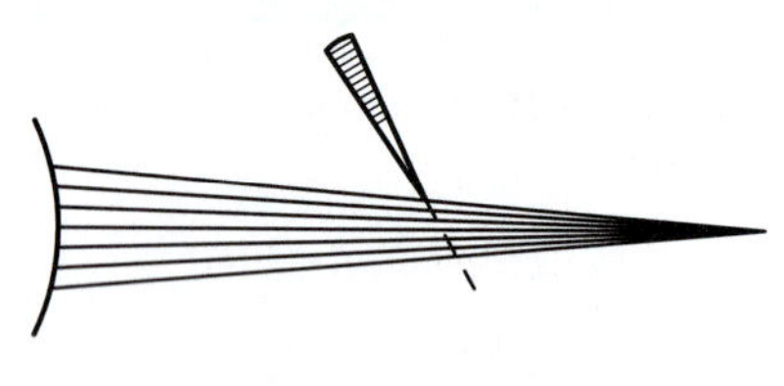

Figure 15–88 Terminal blending.

Heavier taper-blending is performed with the razor held up to 45 degrees from the surface of the hair strand. As the razor is tilted higher and a little more pressure is used, the depth of the cut increases (Figure 15–87).

Terminal blending means that the angle of the razor blade is increased to almost 90 degrees. Short sawing strokes are used. Other terms used for terminal blending are *hair-end tapering* and *blunt cutting* (Figure 15–88).

- *Razor and comb coordination:* Razor stroking and combing are done in a continuous movement. The razor tapers while the comb removes the cut hair and recombs the section for the next stroke or strokes (Figures 15–89 through 15–91).

Hair Textures and Razor Cutting

- *Coarse, thick hair* requires more strokes and heavier tapering than other textures. The first strip of hair is combed, followed by three razor strokes and followed again with the comb. The comb removes the cut hair and recombs the hair, allowing the barber to see how much hair has been cut. It also helps to keep the guide in view for use in tapering the next strip (Figures 15–92 through 15–94).
- *Medium-textured hair* requires fewer razor strokes and lighter pressure than coarse, thick hair as pictured in Figures 15–95 through 15–98.
- *Fine hair* typically does not have any bulk to remove; however, the razor may be used to blend hair ends to achieve a particular hairstyle. Stroking of the razor is usually lighter than that used for medium-textured hair.

Terms Associated with Razor Cutting

Removing weight can be accomplished by holding a parting of damp hair out from the head with the fingers positioned at the end of the section. Place the razor flat to the hair and gently stroke the razor to remove a thin sheet of hair from the section. This technique tapers the ends of the hair (Figure 15–99).

15

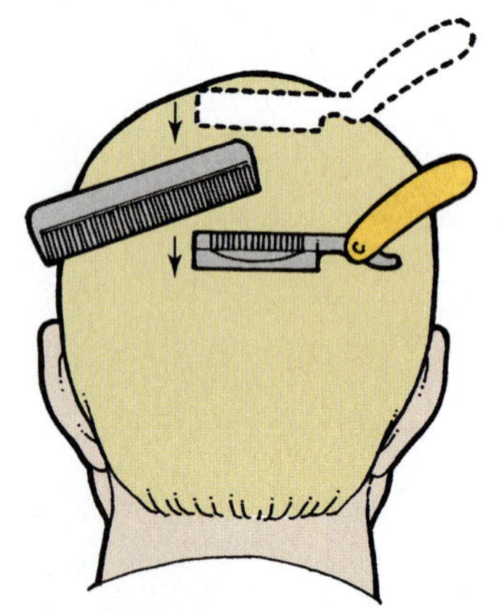

Figure 15–89 Crown area: razor and comb coordination.

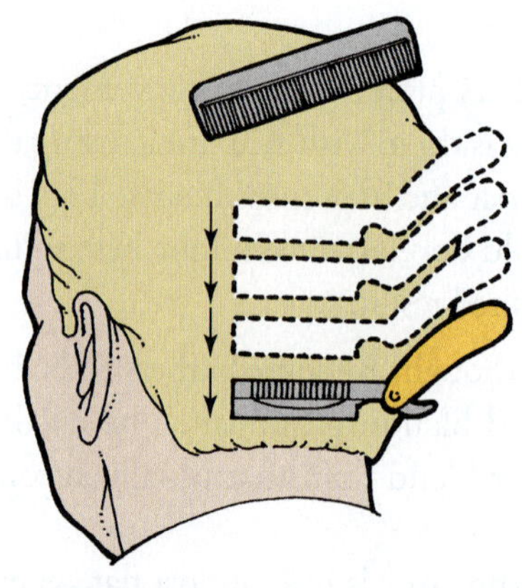

Figure 15–90 Nape area: razor and comb coordination.

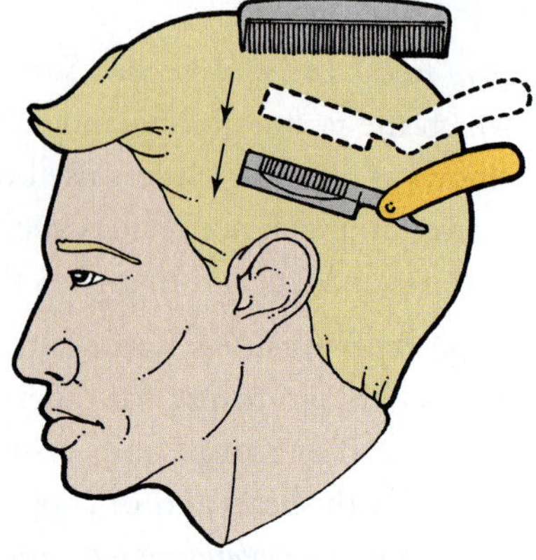

Figure 15–91 Side areas: razor and comb coordination.

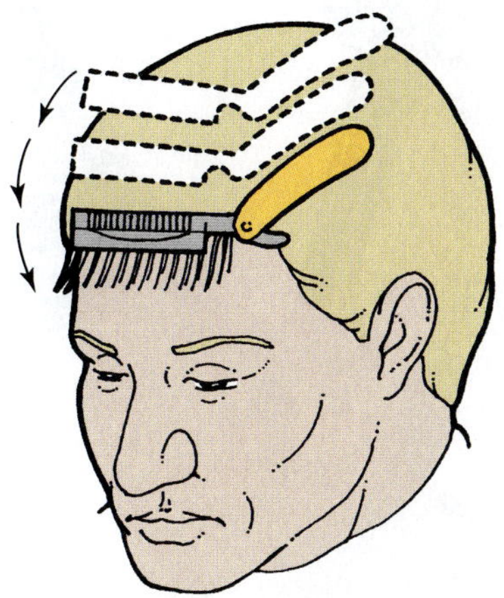

Figure 15-92 Top area. Consideration must be given to the hairstyle to be created. The stroking and the pressure of the razor largely depend upon the amount of hair to be removed to achieve the finished hairstyle.

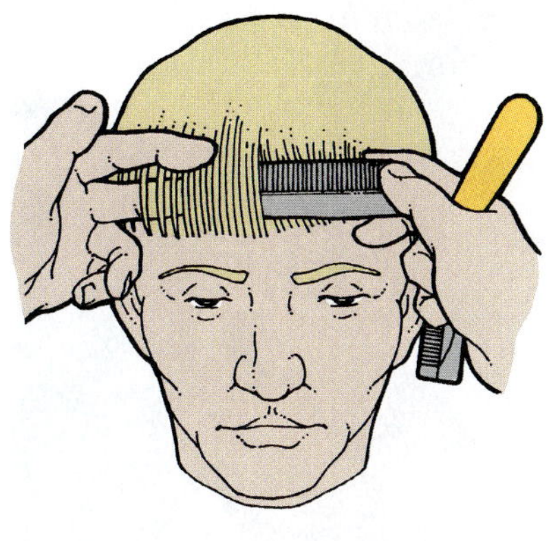

Figure 15-93 Front hair. To equalize the length of long and uneven front hair, pick up the hair with the comb in the right hand. Hold the hair straight out between the middle and index fingers of the left hand.

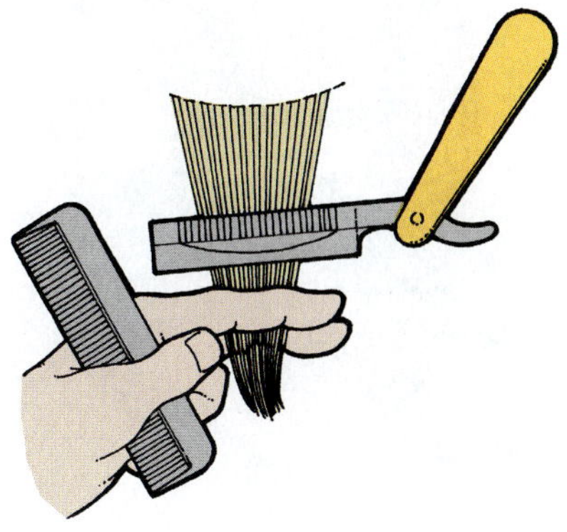

Figure 15-94 Palm the comb to the left hand. Hold the razor at an angle, and with short, sawing strokes cut the hair to the desired length.

Freehand slicing can be used in the midshaft of a section or at the ends of the hair. The hair is combed out from the head and held between the fingers where the tip of the razor will be used to slice out pieces of hair. This technique releases weight from the subsection and allows for more movement within the hairstyle. When used to cut the design line, freehand slicing the ends helps to create soft perimeters (Figures 15–100 and 15–101).

Razor-over-comb cutting is slightly different from shear or clipper-over-comb techniques in which the comb is used to project the hair into a position for cutting. In razor-over-comb cutting, the razor is held in the freehand position and situated just above the comb as it follows the comb's downward direction through the hair (Figure 15–102). Short, precise strokes with medium pressure are applied to the surface of the hair. This technique is often used to taper nape areas or to soften weight lines.

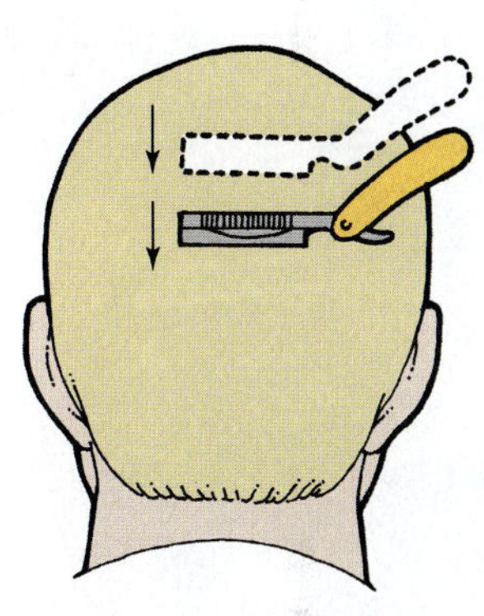

Figure 15-95 Crown area: two long strokes are used.

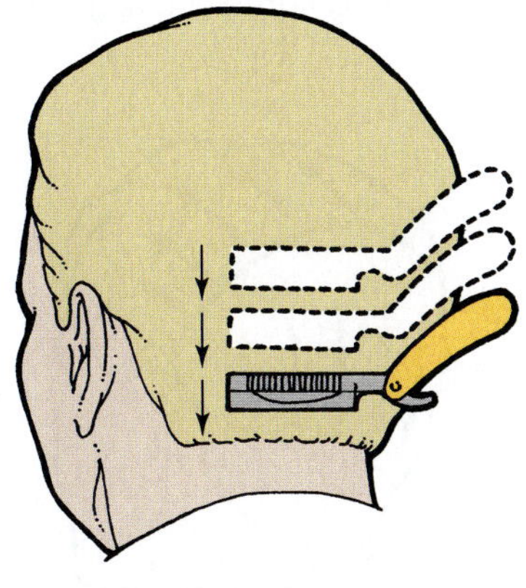

Figure 15-96 Nape area: three short strokes are used.

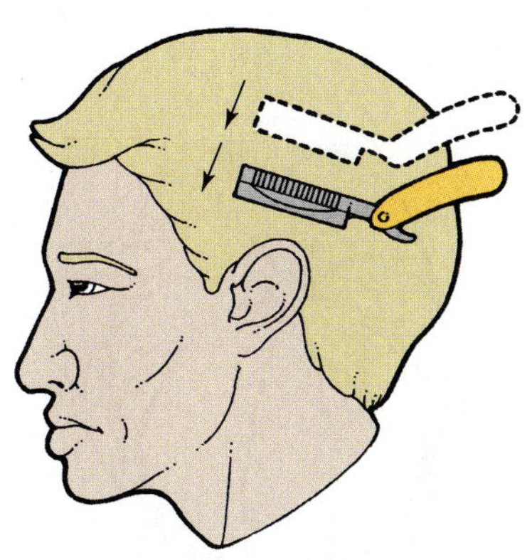

Figure 15-97 Left and right sides of the head: two short strokes may be used.

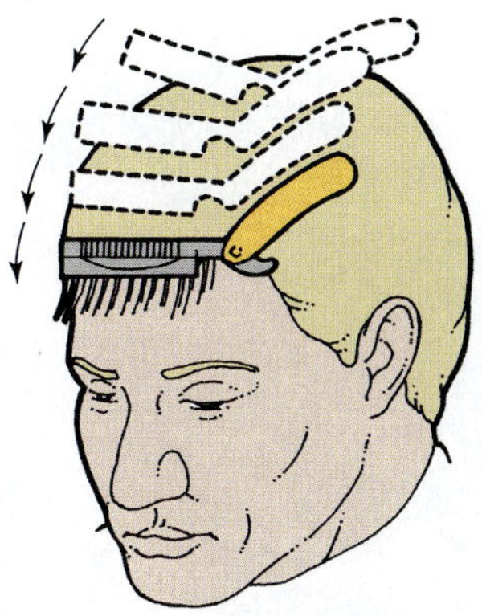

Figure 15-98 Top area: the stroking and pressure of the razor in this area are the same as for the sides and back area.

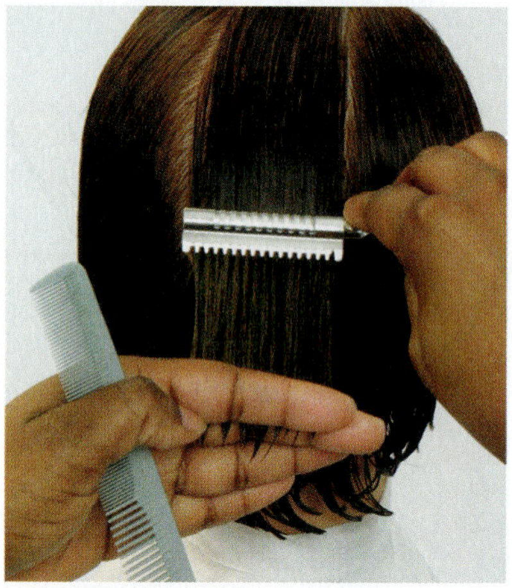

Figure 15-99 Removing weight with freehand slicing.

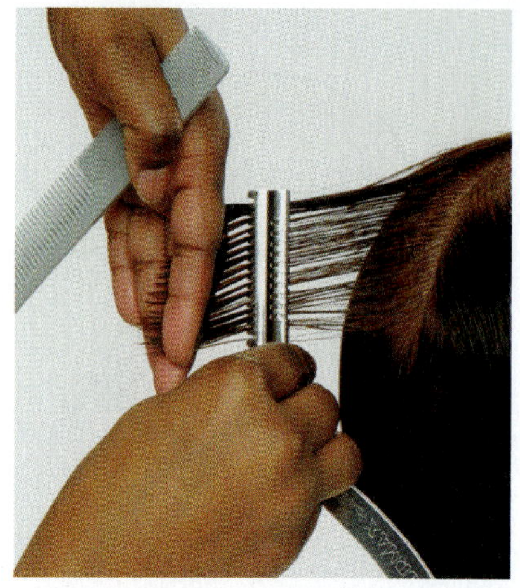

Figure 15-100 Releasing weight from a subsection.

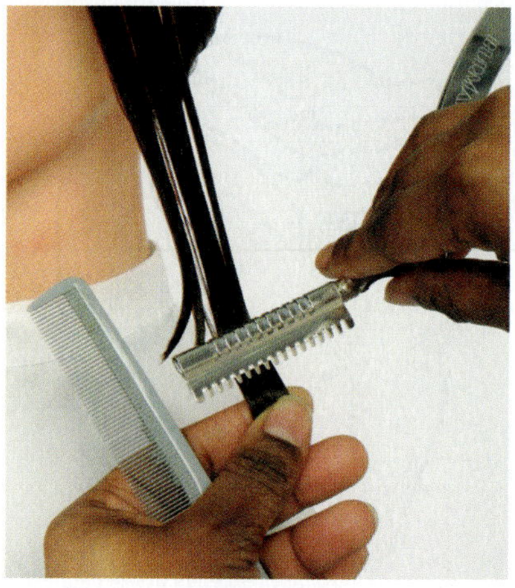

Figure 15-101 Establishing a design line at the perimeter.

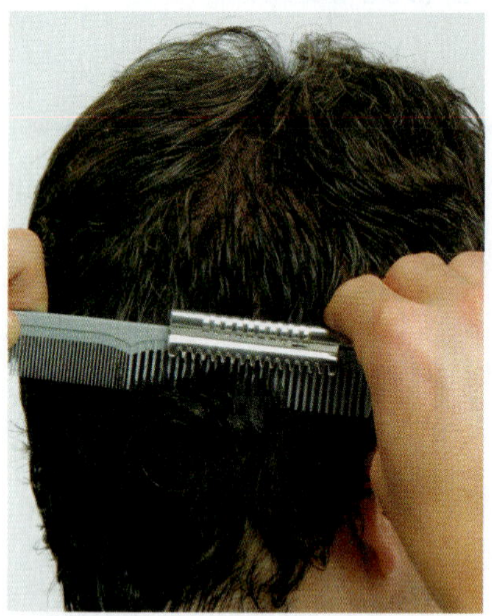

Figure 15-102 Razor-over-comb technique.

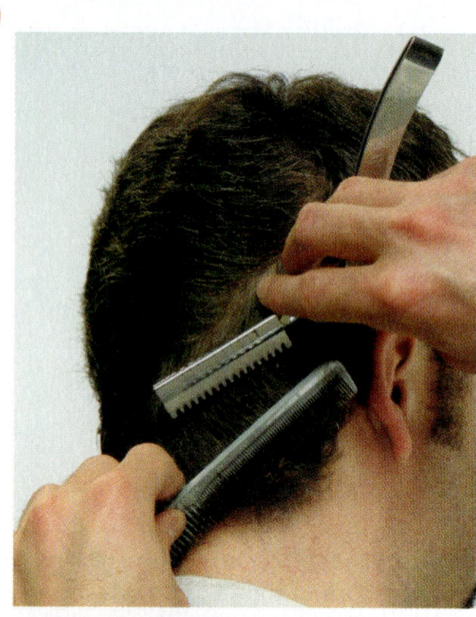

Figure 15-103 Razor rotation.

Razor rotation is performed by using a rotating motion with the comb and razor as the hair is being cut. In the first movement, the razor follows the comb through the hair. Then the comb follows the razor and so on (Figure 15–103).

Hair Sectioning for Razor Haircutting

There are several effective ways to section the hair for razor cutting. These include the two-section, three-section, four-section, and five-section methods. All methods begin by combing the hair into the umbrella effect, which is created by combing the hair into natural directions from the crown (Figure 15–104). Be guided by your instructor.

- *Two sections.* First, part the hair from ear to ear across the crown. All hair in front of the part is combed forward. All hair behind or below the part is combed down (Figure 15–105).
- *Three sections.* First, part the hair from ear to ear across the crown. All top and side hair is combed forward. Then make a vertical part from the crown to the nape. Each of these subsections is combed toward the sides. In the nape area where there is no part, comb the hair down (Figure 15–106).

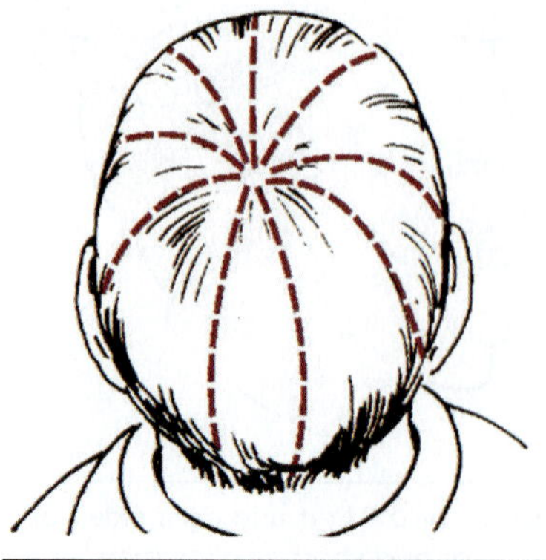

Figure 15-104 Umbrella effect.

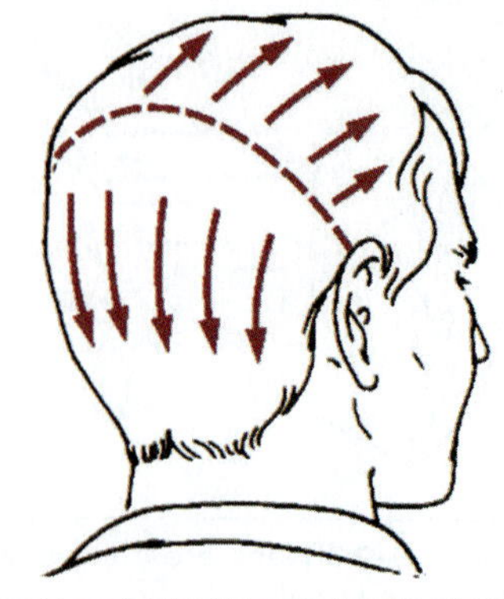

Figure 15-105 Two sections.

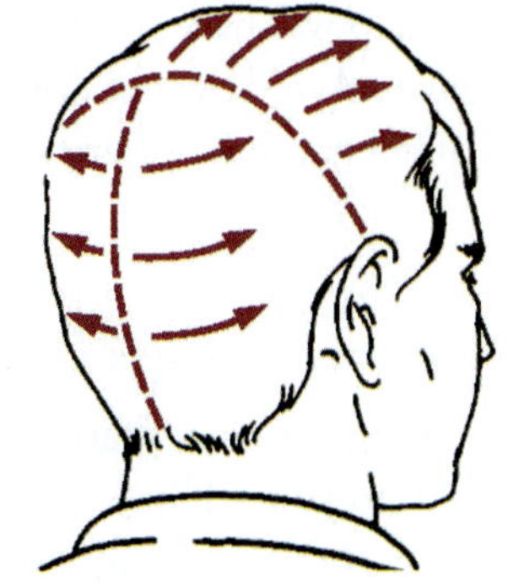
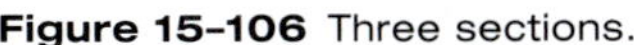

Figure 15–106 Three sections.

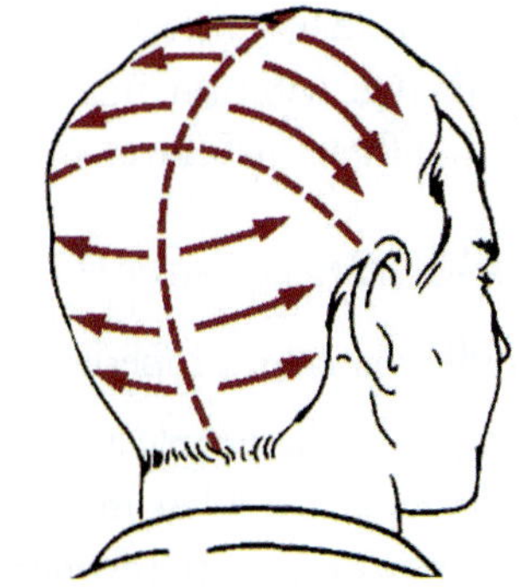

Figure 15–107 Four sections.

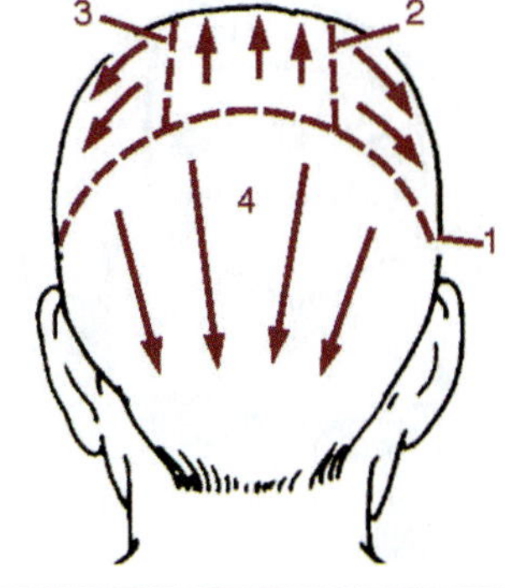

Figure 15–108 Four sections (alternate method).

- *Four sections.* Add one more section to the previous three sections. Make a top center part and comb each side down (Figure 15–107).
- *Four sections, alternate method.* First, part the hair from ear to ear across the crown. Second, section the right side from the center of the right eyebrow to the crown and comb down. Make another section on the left side from the center of the left eyebrow to the crown and comb down. Comb all back hair down (Figure 15–108).
- *Five sections.* Sectioning is the same as the alternate four section, except that the back section is divided in two and combed as indicated by the arrows in Figure 15–109.

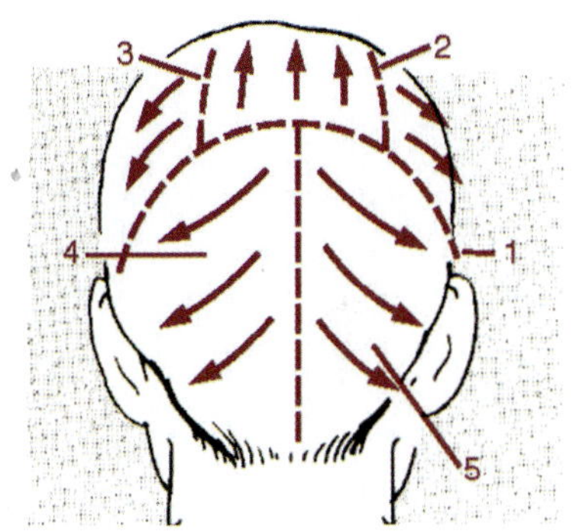

Figure 15–109 Five sections.

A *pattern for cutting* needs to be established by the barber so that there is a plan to follow. In this text, one basic plan is followed. Other procedures may be different, but equally correct. Be guided by your instructor.

1. Back part of head (Figure 15–110)
   a) Downward
   b) Top right to left, downward
   c) Top left to right, downward
2. Right side of head (Figure 15–111)
   a) Downward
   b) Toward the back
   c) Toward the face
3. Left side of head
   a) Downward
   b) Toward the back
   c) Toward the face
4. Top hair (Figure 15–112)
   a) Crown to forehead
   b) Top left side
   c) Top right side

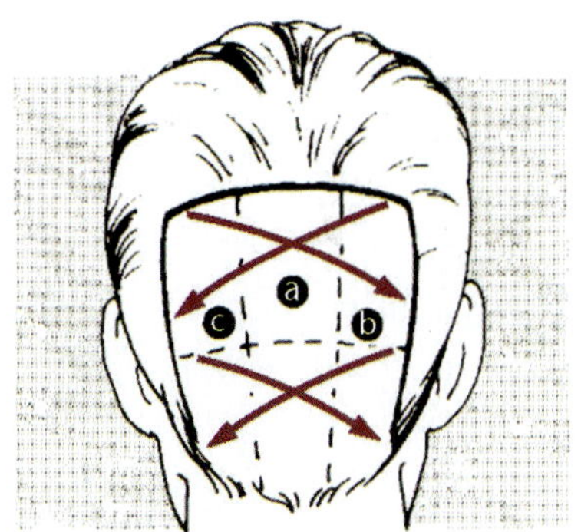

Figure 15–110 Back.

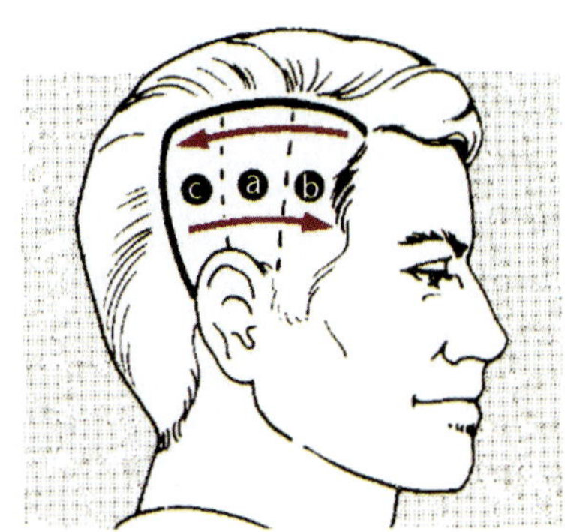

Figure 15–111 Sides.

For the best results in razor cutting the hair must be clean and damp. Avoid tapering too close to the hair part or the scalp. Tapering the hair too closely to the hair part will cause the hair to stand up, making the part look

15

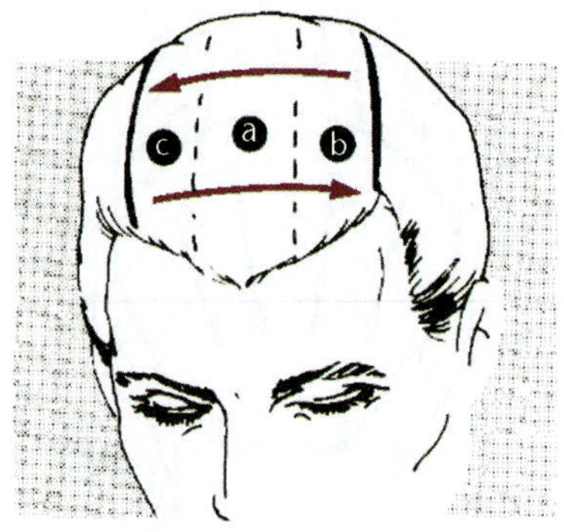

Figure 15–112 Top.

ragged. Coarse hair that is cut too closely to the scalp will have short, stubby hair ends that will protrude through the top layer. Avoid overtapering the hair; it is difficult to correct a haircut after too much hair has been removed.

Razor-Cutting Safety Precautions

- Handle the razor properly, keeping it closed whenever not in use.
- Be aware of the people around you when working with any sharp tool or implement. A careless motion can cause injury to yourself or others. Do not annoy or distract anyone who is in the process of performing a service.
- Purchase and use only good-quality haircutting implements.
- Use changeable-blade razors and dispose of used blades in a sharps container.
- Replace dull razor blades, during a cut if necessary, as a dull blade will pull the hair and cause pain or discomfort to the client. Dull blades will also influence the quality of the haircut.

Practice Session #10:

RAZOR CUTTING ON A MANNEQUIN

1. Pick up the razor (with guard) with the dominant hand.
2. Comb hair into the umbrella effect.
3. Position yourself behind the mannequin.
4. Hold the razor in a freehand position.
5. Use the freehand slicing technique to create a design line in the nape area.
6. Use the razor-over-comb technique to taper the nape area.
7. Use the razor rotation method to blend the hair at the occipital with the nape area.

Once the razor-cutting techniques have been practiced on the mannequin, refer to Haircutting Procedure #6, Figures 15–211 through 15–223 to perform a haircut using these methods. Be guided by your instructor to learn other variations of this method. 6

Hair Thinning and Texturizing

Hair thinning is used to reduce the bulk or weight of the hair. The barber can use thinning (serrated) shears, regular shears, clippers, or a razor for this purpose. Regardless of the tool used to perform the procedure, some general rules to follow when removing bulk from the hair are as follows:

1. Make a careful observation of the hair to determine the sections that require some reduction in bulk or weight and cut accordingly.
2. Avoid cutting top surfaces of the hair where visible cutting lines can be seen.

15

Figure 15–113 Removing bulk midshaft with thinning shears.

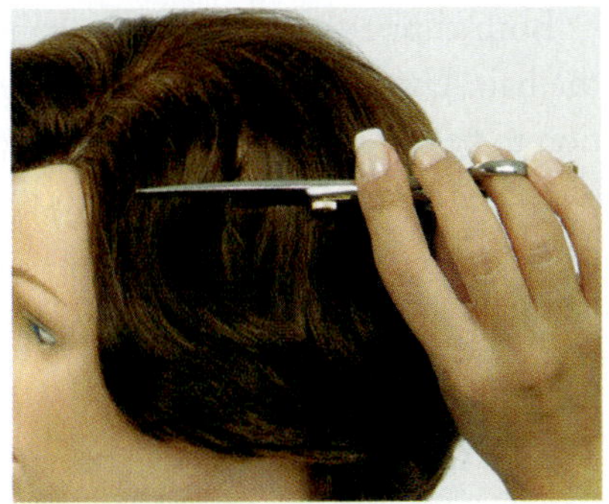

Figure 15–114 Slicing on hair surface to remove bulk.

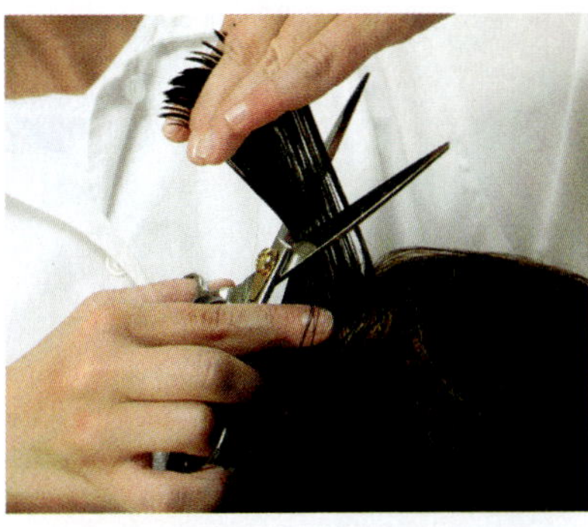

Figure 15–115 Carving with shears to remove bulk.

3. Part off and elevate the hair to be cut to avoid cutting too deeply into the section.
4. Avoid cutting too closely to the scalp or part lines.

Removing Bulk

When thinning with serrated shears the hair parting is combed and held between the index and middle finger. The shears are placed about midshaft on the strands and a cut is made (Figure 15–113). If another cut is necessary it should be made about 1 inch from the first cut. Do not cut twice in the same place.

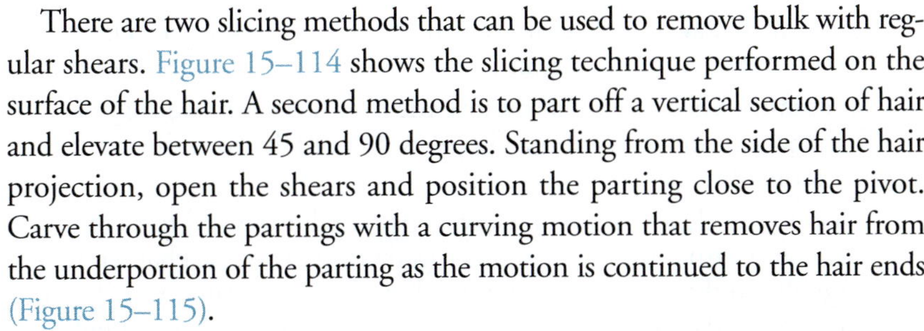

There are two slicing methods that can be used to remove bulk with regular shears. Figure 15–114 shows the slicing technique performed on the surface of the hair. A second method is to part off a vertical section of hair and elevate between 45 and 90 degrees. Standing from the side of the hair projection, open the shears and position the parting close to the pivot. Carve through the partings with a curving motion that removes hair from the underportion of the parting as the motion is continued to the hair ends (Figure 15–115).

Another method that can be used to remove bulk with regular shears involves *slithering*. In this procedure a thin parting of hair is held between the fingers. The shears are positioned for cutting and an up-and-down sliding motion along the parting is combined with a slight closing of the shears each time they are moved toward the scalp (Figure 15–116).

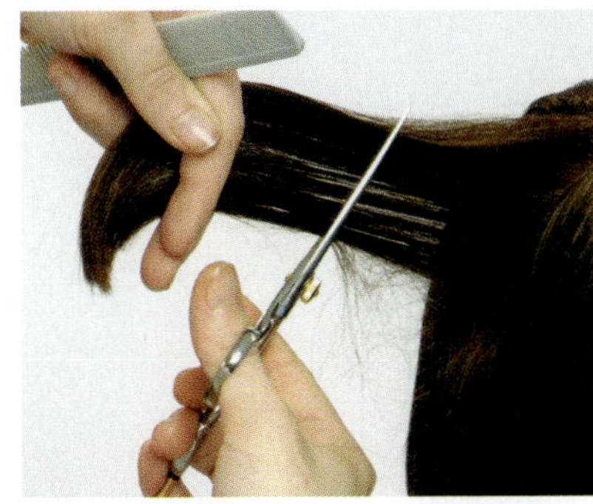

Figure 15–116 Slithering midshaft to remove bulk.

Removing Weight from the Ends

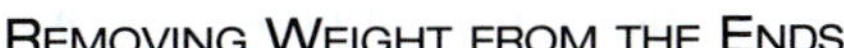

Removing weight from the ends helps to taper the perimeter of graduated and blunt haircuts. This can be accomplished using thinning shears by elevating the section and placing the shears at an angle as the cuts are made or by using the comb to put the hair into position for cutting (Figure 15–117).

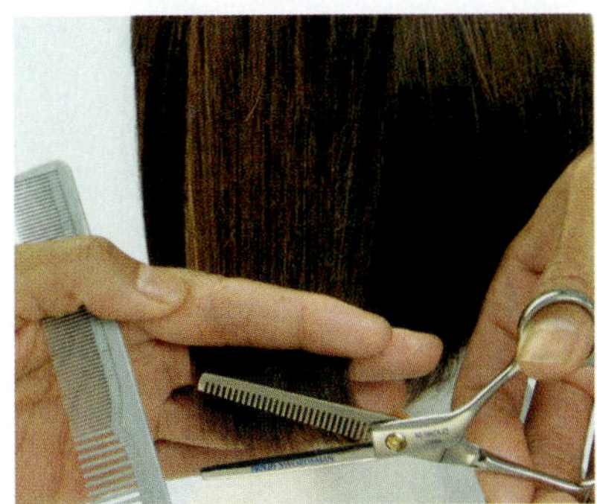

Figure 15–117 Removing weight from the ends.

To remove weight with regular shears, *point cutting* or *notching* can be used to reduce weight in the ends of the hair. For either technique, a parting is held between the fingers and the tips of the shears are used on a vertical angle to create points or notches in the hair (Figure 15–118).

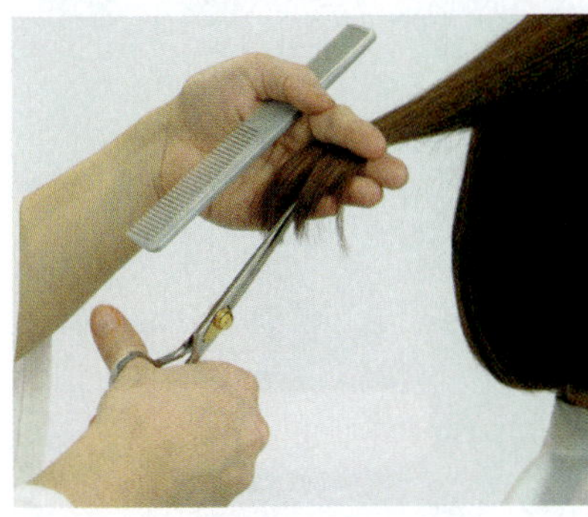

Figure 15–118 Notching.

Both clippers and razors can be used to remove weight from the ends of the hair. Use a clipper-over-comb technique to put the hair ends in a position to be cut and position the clipper blades under the ends of the hair. Use a *reverse* rotation technique with the clipper to comb through and cut the ends from one section to another. The razor-over-comb technique should be used when lightening hair ends with a razor.

Haircut Finish Work: Shaving the Outline Areas

The performance of a neck shave and the shaving of the outline areas as a feature of the haircut service contribute to the appearance of the finished cut and provide the client with a true barbershop experience. At one time, it was the barber's standard operating procedure to finish a haircut with these shaving services. Yet, while many traditionally oriented barbers still perform neck and outline shaves, others in the industry have exchanged razors for outliners or trimmers on a more or less permanent basis. This is a trend that should be changed by today's barber as the rebirth of traditional barbering services are once more being sought by consumers.

The traditional *neck shave* consists of shaving the sides of the neck and across the nape with a razor (see Figures 14–45 through 14–47 in Chapter 14). The *outline* consists of the sideburn areas and around the ears and nape area; with African-American styles, the front hairline is often included (Figures 15–120 through 15–128). The following preparation steps should be used in the performance of these shaving services:

1. Remove all cut hair from around the head and neck with a clean towel, tissues, or hair vacuum.
2. Loosen the chair cloth and remove the neck strip used during the haircut. Be careful that loose clippings do not fall down the client's neck or shirt.
3. Pick up the chair cloth at the lower edge, fold it upward to the top edge, and gather the four corners together. Remove the chair cloth carefully so that cut hair does not fall on the client. Turn away from the chair and drop the lower edge of the chair cloth, giving a slight shake to dislodge all cut hair.
4. Replace the chair cloth, resting it a few inches away from the neck so that it does not touch the client's skin.
5. Spread a terry cloth or paper towel straight across the shoulders and tuck it loosely around the client's neck. Secure the chair cloth and fold the towel over the neckband. The drape should be loose enough to permit easy access to the neck area. Tuck a towel or neck strip into the neckband of the drape for wiping the razor. (Figure 15–119).

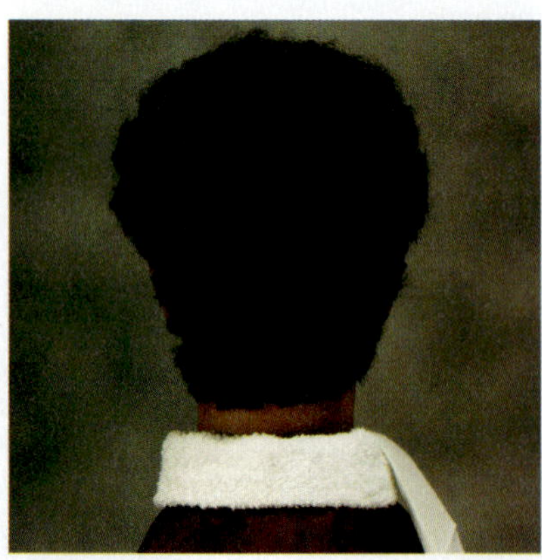

Figure 15-119 Draping for outline shave.

Practice Session # 11:

SHAVING THE OUTLINE AREAS ON A MANNEQUIN

Preparation: To avoid ruining the mannequin, apply a thin *bead* of colored glue around the hairline and dry thoroughly before shaving, or, practice

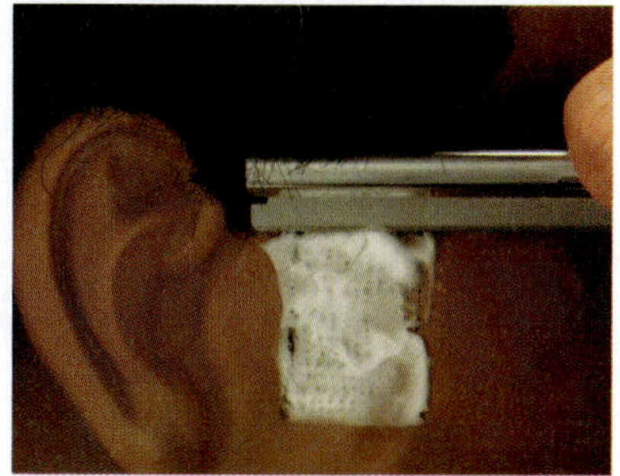

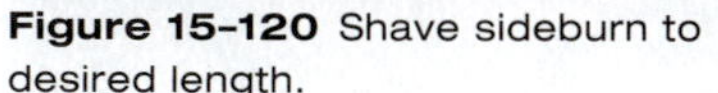

Figure 15–120 Shave sideburn to desired length.

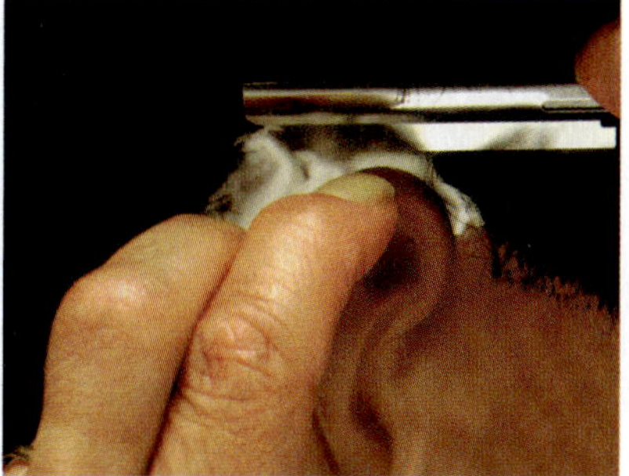

Figure 15–121 Shaving around the ear.

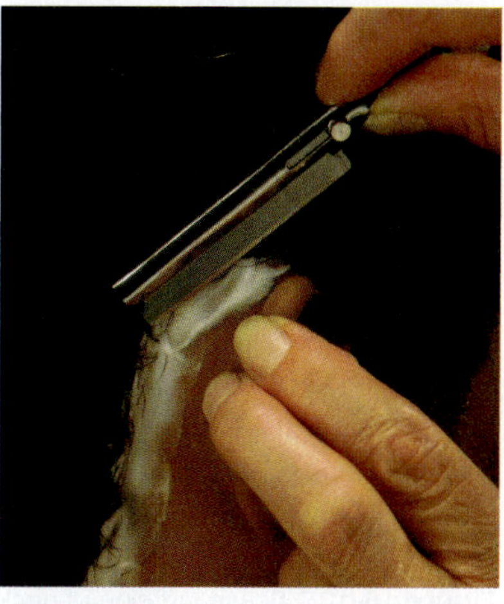

Figure 15–122 Shaving in back of the ear.

without a blade in the razor to master the position of the shaving strokes.

1. Apply a light coating of lather at the hairline of the sideburns, around and over the ears, the front hairline, down the sides of the neck, and across the nape. *Apply lather to the back of the neck and/or the front hairline of the client only if these areas are to be shaved.* Rub the lather in lightly with the balls of the fingers or thumb.
2. Shaving the right side
   a) Hold the razor for a freehand stroke.
   b) Place the left thumb on the scalp above the point of the razor and pretend to stretch the skin under the razor.
   c) Shave the sideburn to the desired length (Figure 15–120).
   d) Shave around the ear at the hairline and straight down the side of the neck, using the freehand stroke with the point of the razor. Be careful not to shave into the hairline at the nape of the neck (Figures 15–121 through 15–123).
3. Shaving the left side
   a) Hold the razor as in the reverse backhand stroke.
   b) Place the left thumb on the scalp above the razor point, and pretend to stretch the skin under the razor.
   c) Shave the sideburn to the proper length using reverse-backhand stroke (Figure 15–124).
   d) Shave around the ear at the hairline, using the freehand stroke.
   e) Shave the side of the neck below the ear, using the backhand stroke with the point of the razor (Figure 15–125). Hold the ear away with the fingers of the left hand. If the stroke is done with one continuous movement, a straight line will be formed down the side of the neck.
   f) Shave the nape area with a freehand stroke (Figure 15–126).
4. Front hairline
   a) Start in the center of the front hairline and work toward the corners using a freehand stroke to the client's right side and a backhand stroke to the client's left side (Figure 15–127).
   b) Follow the natural hairline shaving the outline through the temporal (crest, horseshoe, etc.) area to the front corner of the sideburns (Figure 15–128).

Be guided by your instructor to learn other variations of this method.

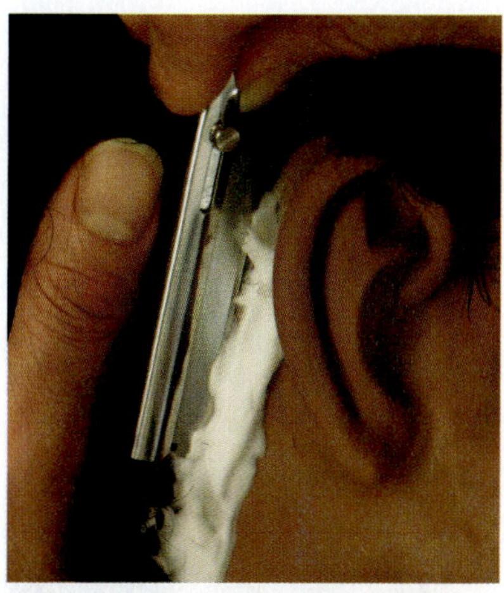

Figure 15–123 Shaving behind the ear to the nape corner.

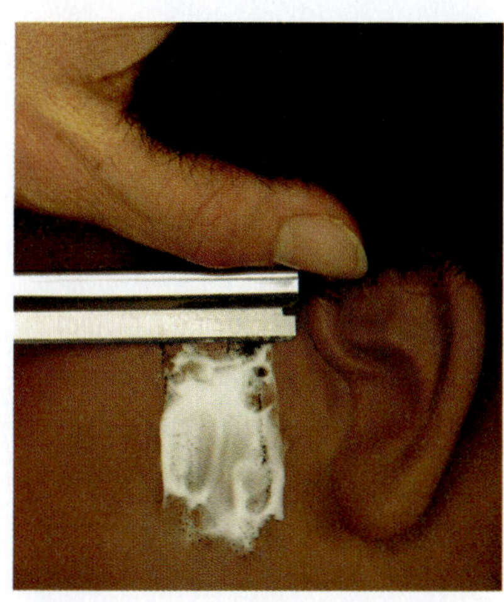

Figure 15–124 Shave the left sideburn using reverse backhand stroke.

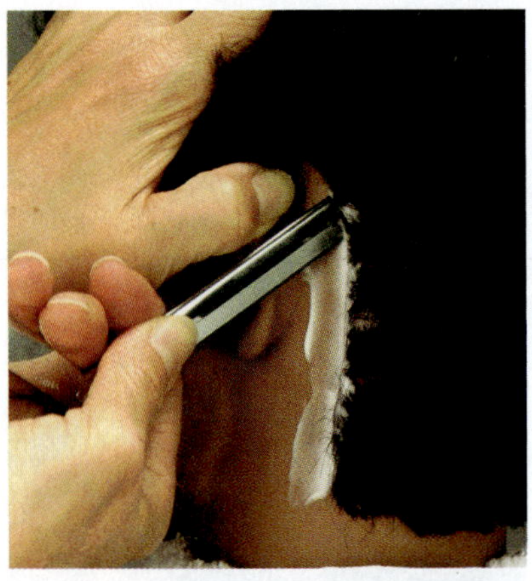

Figure 15–125 Shave left side of neck to nape using the backhand stroke.

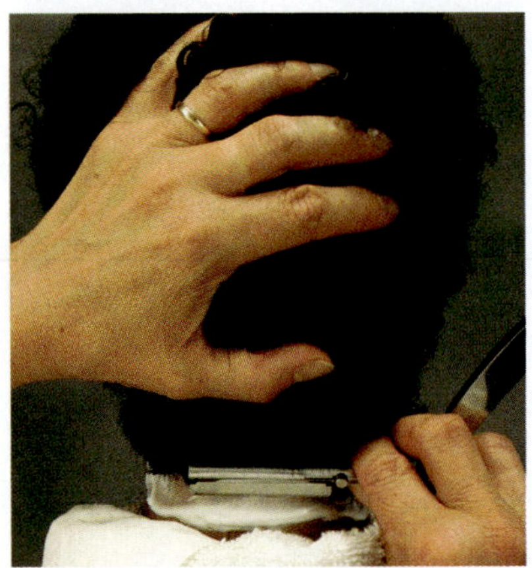

Figure 15–126 Use the freehand stroke to shave the nape area.

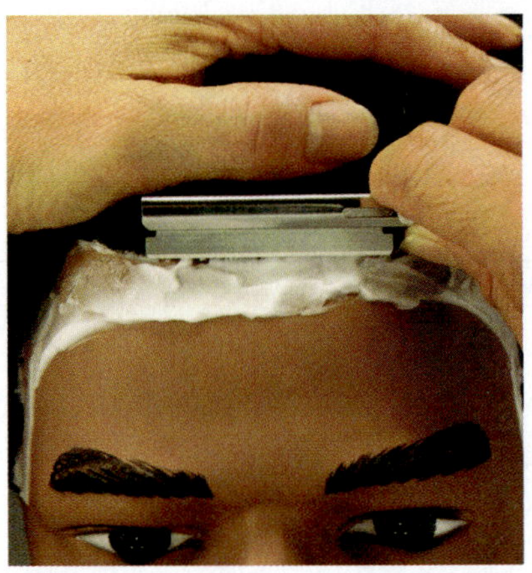

Figure 15–127 Start at center of front hairline and shave toward corners.

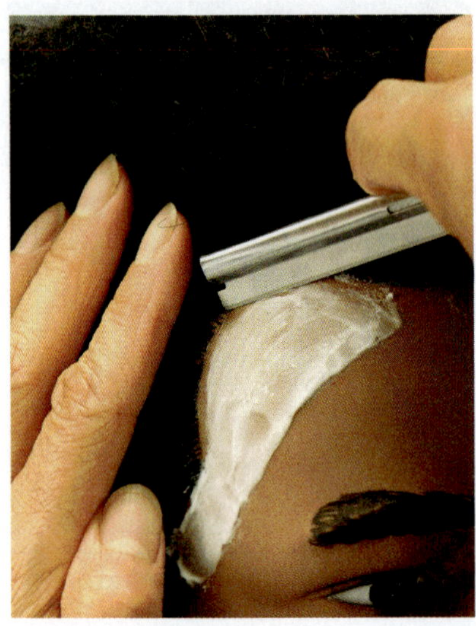

Figure 15–128 Follow the natural hairline to the sideburns.

15

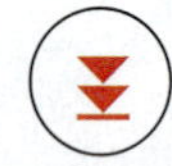

Here's a tip:

To assist you in developing a rhythm for using a traveling guide, say the following to yourself as you go through the procedure in Step 1, # 4: part on 1; comb forward on 2; pick up on 3; and cut on 4.

Haircutting Procedure #1: Fingers-and-Shear Technique on Model

Preparation

1. Conduct model consultation.
2. Drape the model for wet service.
3. Shampoo and towel dry hair.
4. Remove the waterproof cape and replace it with a neckstrip and haircutting chair cloth.
5. Face the model toward the mirror and lock the chair.

Reminder: Maintain uniform moisture throughout the haircutting procedure.

Step 1

1. Comb the hair down in front, sides, and back. Standing behind the model, take a ¼- to ½-inch parting (depending on the density of the hair) at the forward-most part of the crown.
2. Comb the parting straight up at 90 degrees and hold it between the fingers of the left hand.
3. Bend the parting from right to left to determine at what length the hair will bend (bending point) to lie down smoothly (usually between 2 and 3 inches). When this length has been determined, recomb the parting and, using the fingers of the left hand as a level, cut the hair that extends beyond the fingers (Figure 15–129). This cut establishes the traveling guide for the top section.
4. Pick up a second parting, retaining the guideline, comb, and cut. (The guideline should be visible and parallel to the top of the fingers.) A rhythm will soon develop: part hair for parting (1); comb hair in front of parting forward (so it doesn't interfere with first parting) (2); comb parting, retaining previous guide (3); and, cut hair that extends past the guideline (4).
5. Complete the top section of hair, moving forward toward the front with each parting and cut. Remember to hold each parting that is to

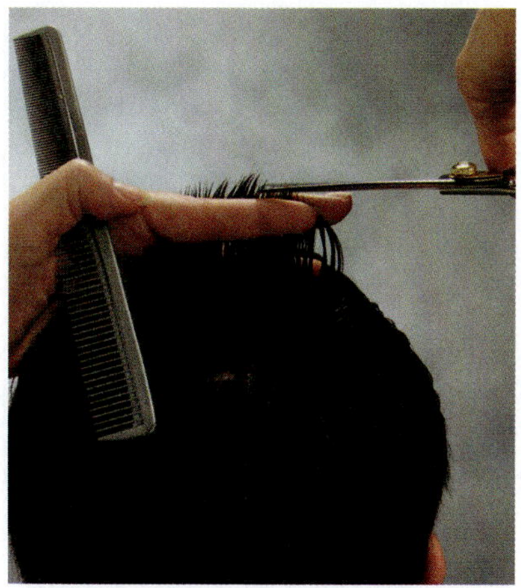

Figure 15–129 Step 1. Establish guide for top section.

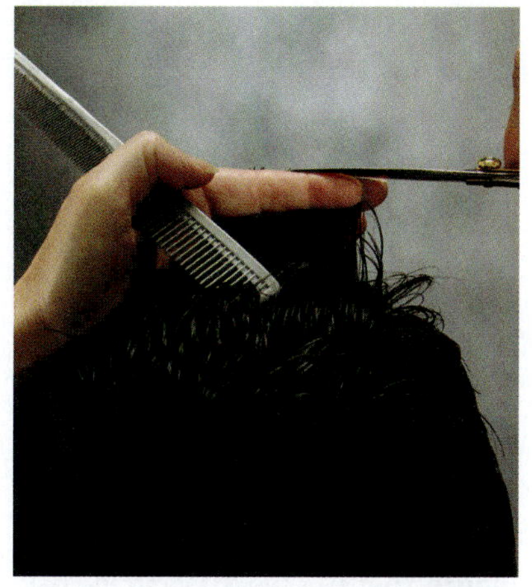

Figure 15–130a Hold each parting at a 90-degree elevation while working toward the front.

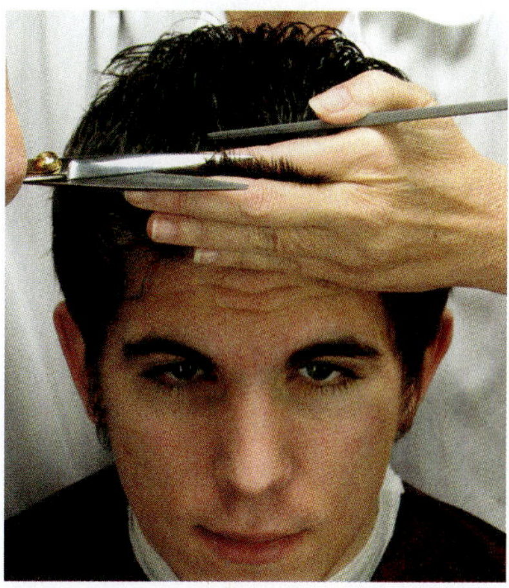

Figure 15–130b Front view of last 90-degree parting in top section.

be cut at a 90-degree elevation from where it grows (Figures 15–130a and 15–130b).

STEP 2

1. Comb the top section back (Figure 15–131). Move to the model's left side. Starting at the forehead, part off the top section of hair, front to back, with the thumb and middle finger.
2. Hold the original guideline and a ½-inch parting at the crown at 90 degrees, and cut (Figure 15–132). This establishes the guide for the crown and back sections.
3. Work forward, still maintaining a side-standing position. Following the arc and contour of the head, even off any length that does not blend with the traveling guide (Figure 15–133). If Step 1 was performed correctly, no more than ¼ inch of hair should need to be evened or blended. Step 2 is a checkpoint for your work in the top section (Figure 15–134).

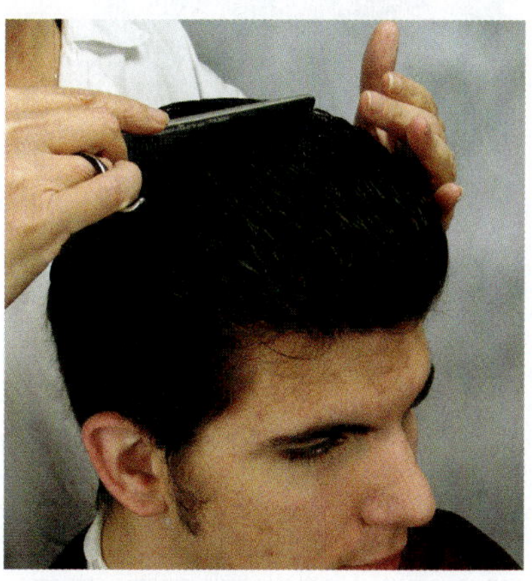

Figure 15–131 Step 2. Comb the top section back.

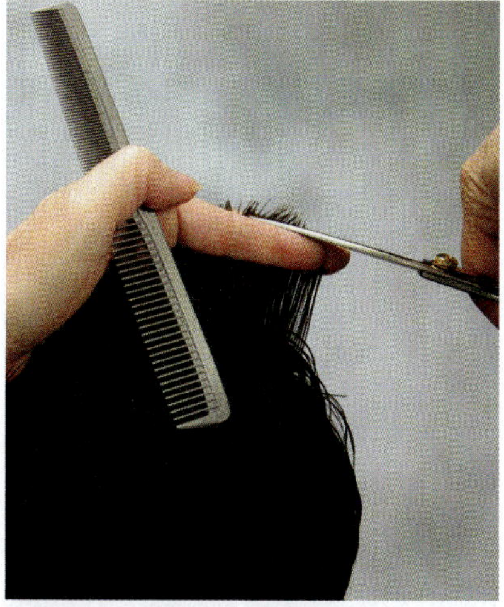

Figure 15–132 Hold the original guide and 1/2-inch section of hair at the crown.

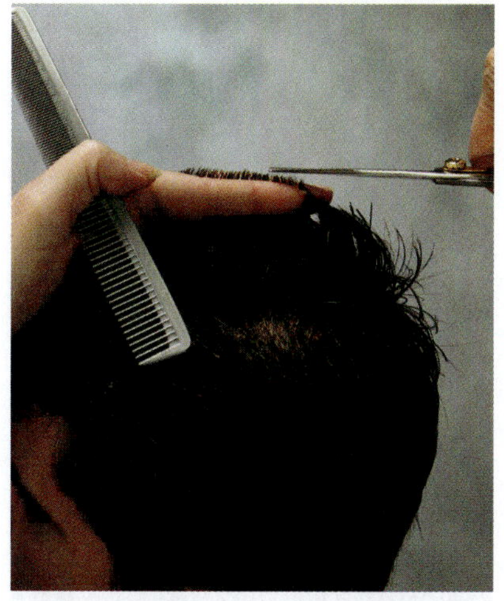

Figure 15–133 Follow the arc of the head, trimming strands that do not blend with the traveling guide.

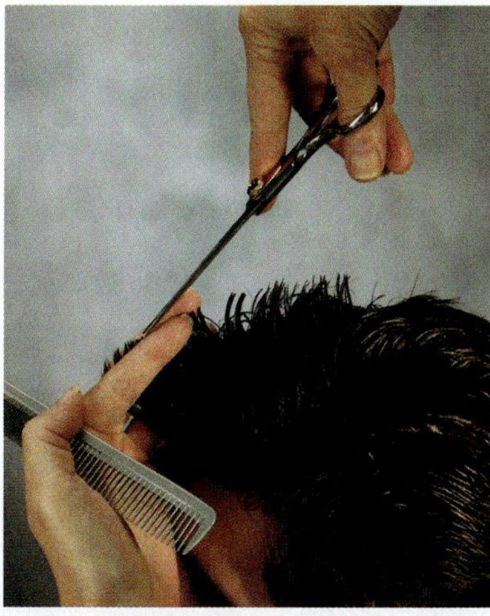

Figure 15–134 Step 2 is checkpoint for work in the top section.

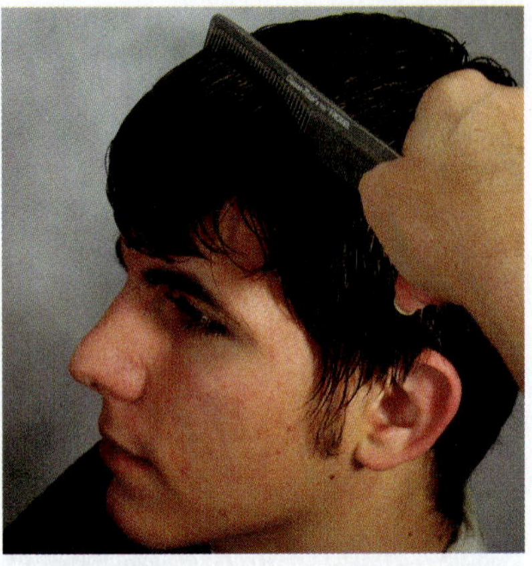

Figure 15-135 Step 3. Comb the hair forward.

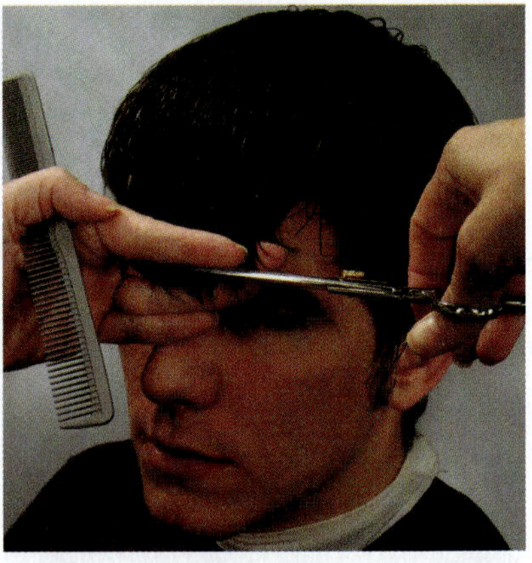

Figure 15-136 Establish front design line.

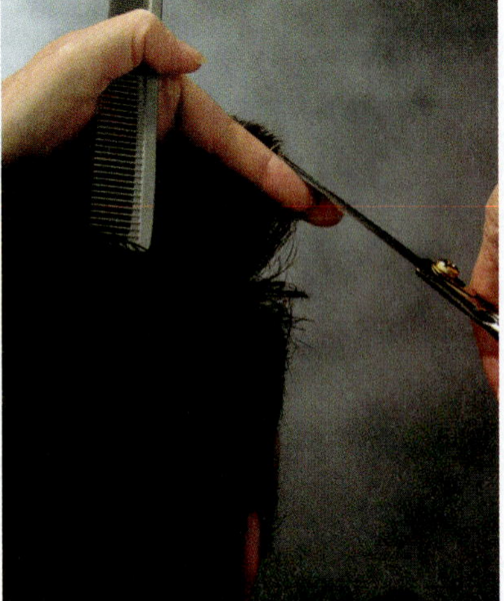

Figure 15-137a Step 4. Hold front temporal section at 90 degrees and cut to the top guide.

Step 3

1. Comb the hair forward and move in front of the model (Figure 15–135). Holding the front hair section between the fingers of the left hand at 0 degrees, begin in the center and cut to the desired length to establish the front design line (Figure 15–136). Cut right, and then left of the center to the ends of the width of the eyebrows, or to include the temporal area. The front and temporal design line has just been completed and will act as a traveling guide for the temporal area.

Step 4

1. Move behind the model.
2. Beginning on the right side, pick up the front hair of the temporal/crest region. A small amount of the previously cut top hair should be visible.
3. Hold the hair at 90 degrees and cut to the top guide (Figures 15–137a and 15–137b).
4. Continue cutting the crest area, working back to the center of the crown area (Figures15–138a and 15–138b). Cut hair only from the

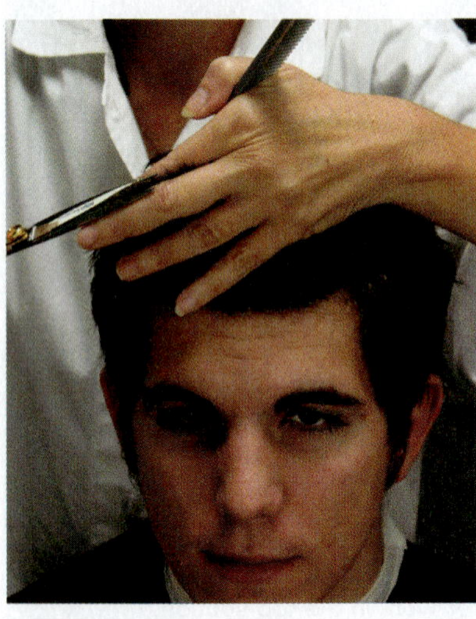

Figure 15-137b Front view of cutting right temporal section.

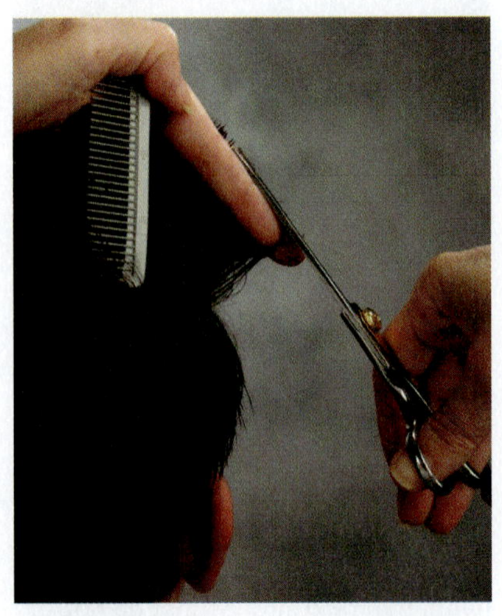

Figure 15-138a Continue cutting through the crest (temporal) area.

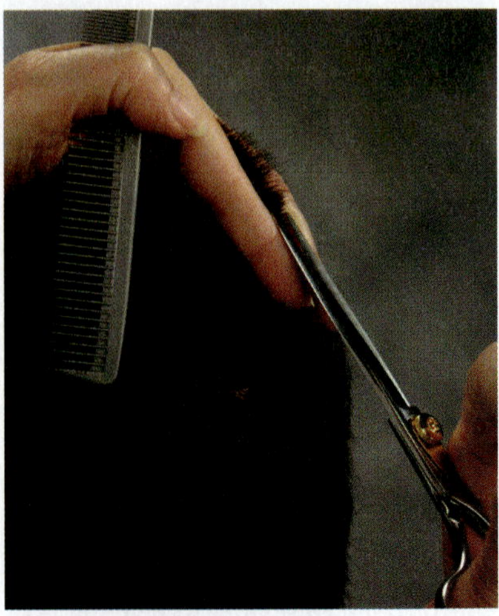

Figure 15-138b Work back to the center of the crown.

temporal region; do not pick up side hair. When approaching the crown area, reposition yourself so as to move toward the model's left, but not as far as the side of the model.

Step 5

1. Repeat Step 4 procedure on the left side of the model's hair. Cuts will be made *from* the top guide through the temporal region, rather than *to* the top guide. If the front design line was cut correctly, the excess hair in the front temporal region should not exceed 1 to 1½ inches. The crown hair from the right and left sides should meet upon completion of Step 5 (Figures 15–139a and 15–139b).
2. The top, temporal, and crown areas are now cut.
3. Comb the hair for Step 6.

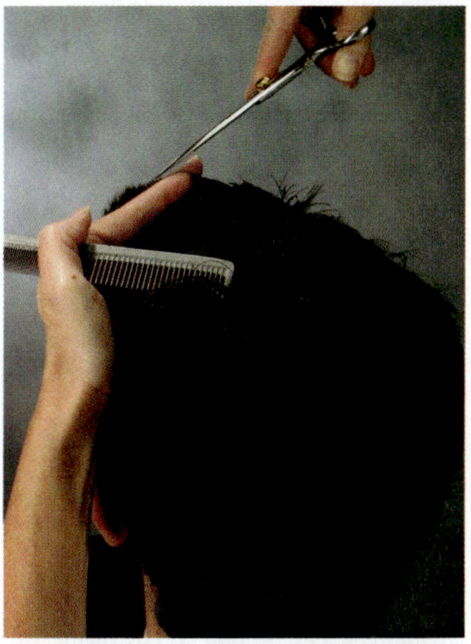

Figure 15–139a Step 5. Repeat Step 4 on left side.

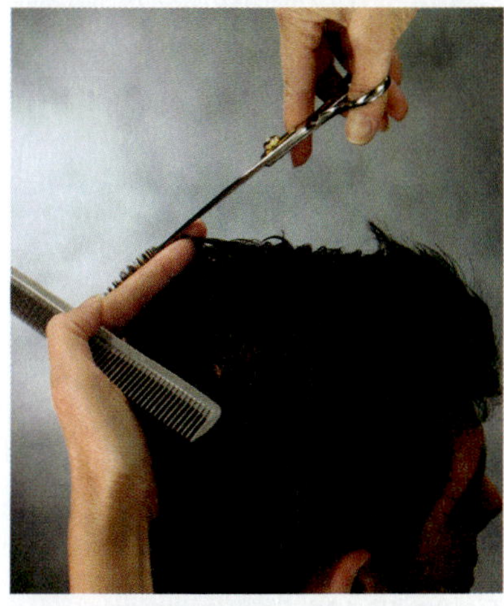

Figure 15–139b The crown hair from the right and left should meet.

Step 6

1. Moving to the right of the model, comb the hair straight down on the sides.
2. Take a ¼- to ½-inch horizontal parting at the hairline, from the top of the ear to the sideburn area, and a diagonal parting of the same thickness from the right temple to the sideburn (Figure 15–140).
3. Comb the remaining hair back or secure it with a hair clip.
4. Cut the design line either around the ears or to cover part of the ears at the desired length (Figure 15–141). If cutting around the ear, gently bend or slightly tug the ear down out of the way (Figure 15–142).
5. Move toward the front of the model, facing the temporal and side areas.
6. Using the front and side design lines (which are acting as guides), cut the hair between these two points at 0 degrees against the skin, cutting along the natural hairline (Figure 15–143).
7. Holding the hair between the fingers at 0 degrees, check the design line cut.
8. Proceed cutting the remaining side hair section, repeating the partings as the density of the hair requires.

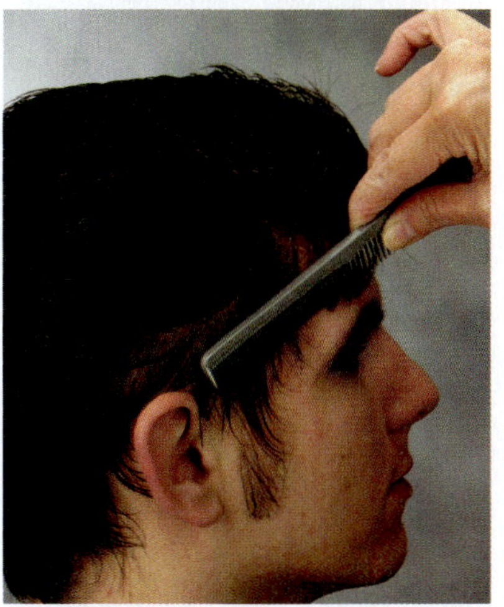

Figure 15–140 Step 6. Comb down parting from hairline.

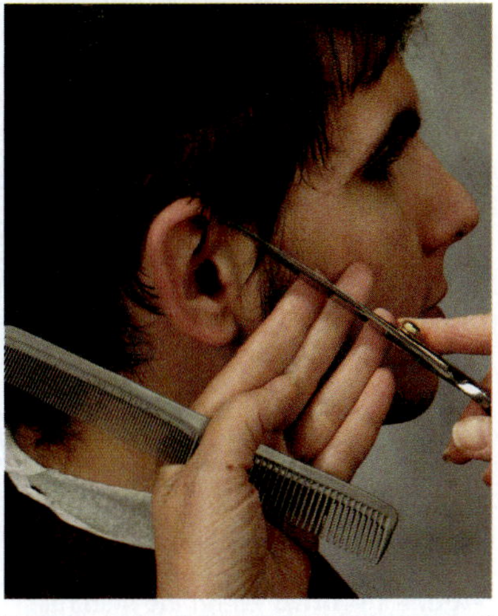

Figure 15–141 Cut side hair to desired length.

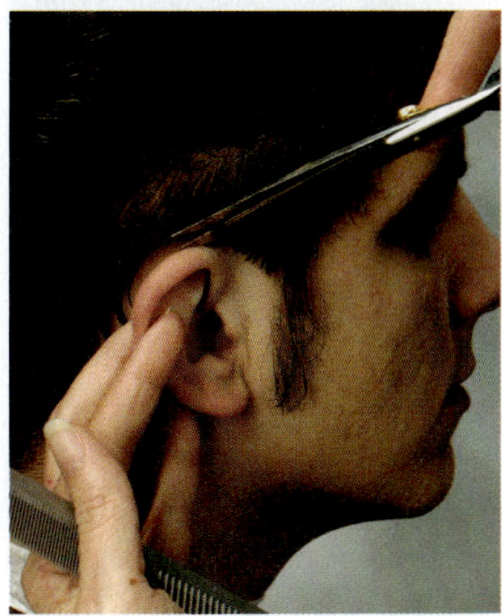

Figure 15–142 Gently tug the ear down.

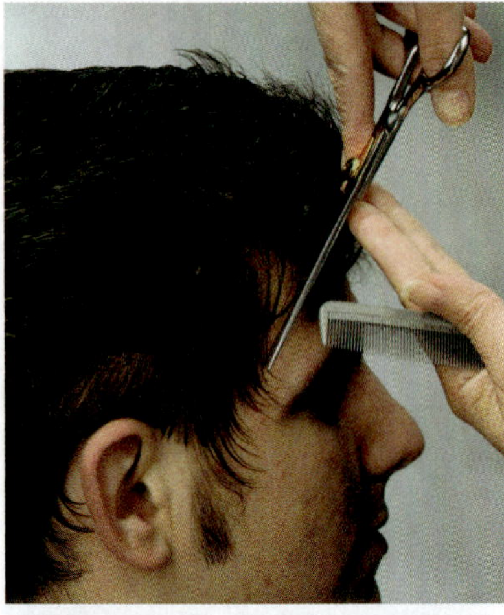

Figure 15-143 Use the front and side design lines as guides to cut along the natural hairline.

9. Repeat this procedure on the left side, then check the length of the sides in the mirror for evenness.
10. Move behind the model. Pick up the hair in vertical partings, holding it straight out to the side at 90 degrees. The design/guide line should be visible at the tips of the fingers when working on the right side of the model's head (Figure 15–144).
11. Make a straight, vertical cut from the design/guide line, cutting off any hair that extends past the guide.
12. Continue cutting partings of hair while following the contour of the head until reaching the temporal/crest region (Figures 15–145a and 15–145b). The hair lengths should meet and blend. Check the procedure by checking the blend of hair from the side design/guide line to the top section guide.
13. Proceed until all the side hair is cut. Stop at the topmost point behind the ear. Repeat for the left side. You may be positioned facing the client in order to work from the design/guide line up when blending the hair, or may prefer to remain behind the model.
14. The front, top, temporal, crown, and side areas are now cut.

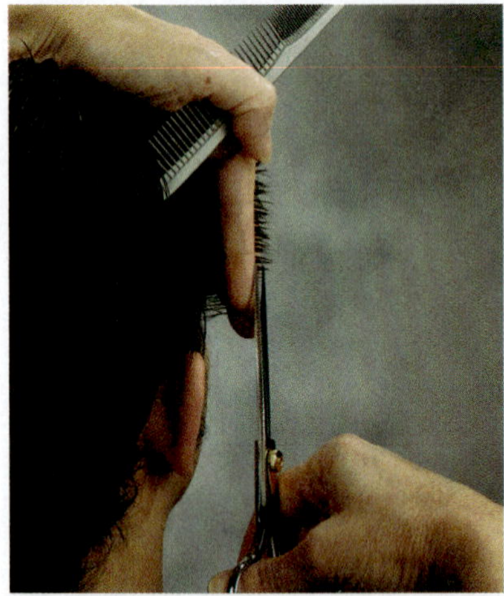

Figure 15-144 Pick up vertical partings at 90 degrees.

Step 7

1. Move behind the model. Section off a ¼- to ½-inch horizontal parting at the nape of the neck (Figure 15–146). Secure excess hair with a clip if necessary.
2. Starting in the center of the nape, cut the hair to the desired length; cut left and then right, to the corners of the nape area (Figure 15–147). Check the design line cut.
3. Move to the model's right side. Part off a ¼- to ½-inch section along the hairline. Cut hair in a downward direction from the side design line guide to right nape corner (Figure 15–148).
4. Comb and check the cut. Repeat for the left side. A backhand shear cutting position is required to cut downward on the model's left side (Figure 15–149).

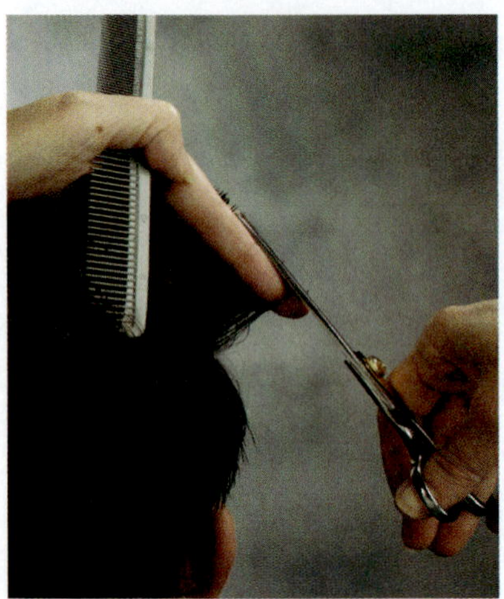

Figure 15-145a Follow the contour of the head.

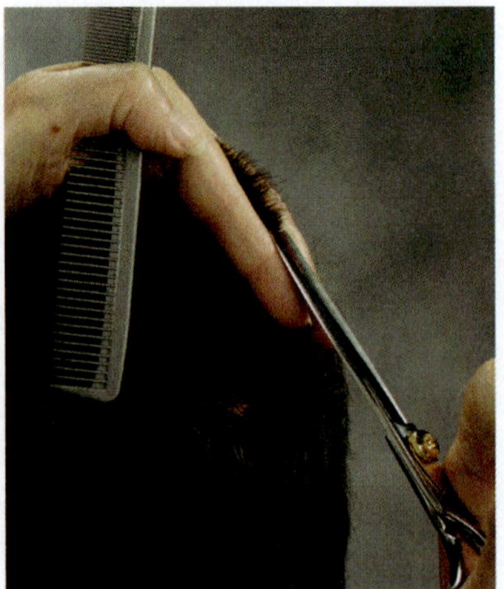

Figure 15-145b Blend the side hair to the crest.

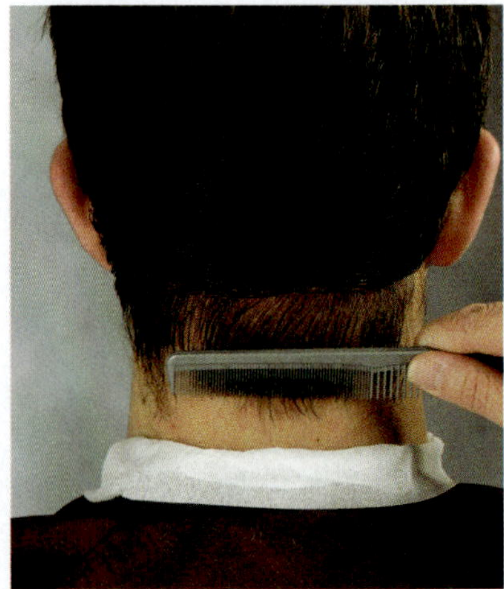

Figure 15-146 Step 7. Section off a parting from the nape.

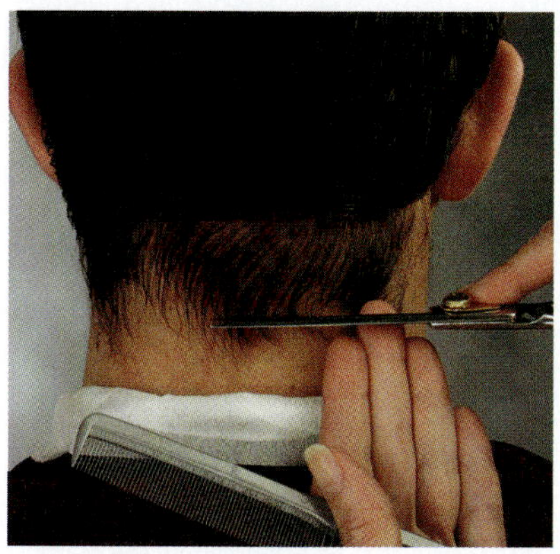

Figure 15-147 Begin back design line at center of nape; cut to corners.

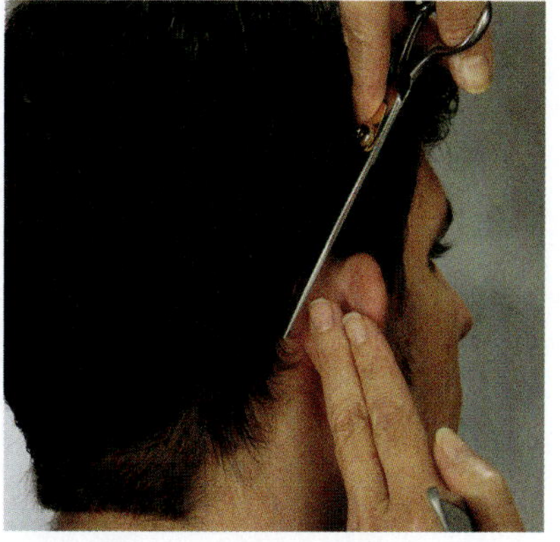

Figure 15-148 Cut from side guide to nape corner along hairline.

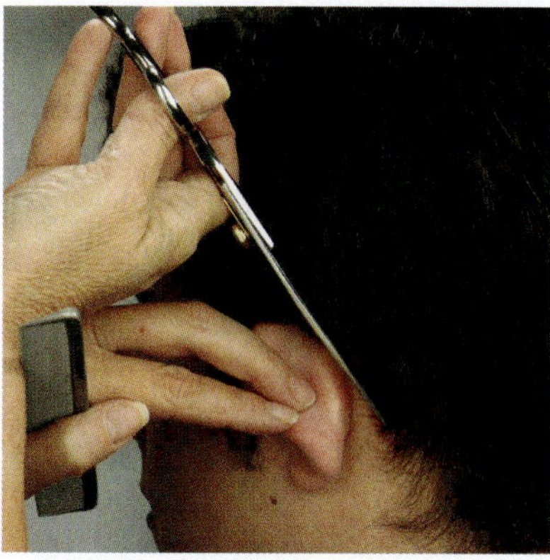

Figure 15-149 Repeat Step 7 on the left side.

5. Part off a subsequent parting and comb hair down. Holding the design/guide line and parting between the fingers, cut hair at 0 degrees (Figure 15–150). Complete 0-degree cutting at the nape and behind-the-ear areas as density requires (Figure 15–151).
6. Pick up the hair in vertical partings at 90 degrees; blend through the back section up to meet the guides in the crown and crest areas (Figures 15–152 and 15–153).
7. Proceed until the entire back section is cut and sides are blended to the back (Figure 15–154).
8. Check the entire haircut by combing the hair up in 90-degree sections, making sure that the hair blends from one section to another.
9. Perform a neck shave and shave outline areas as desired.

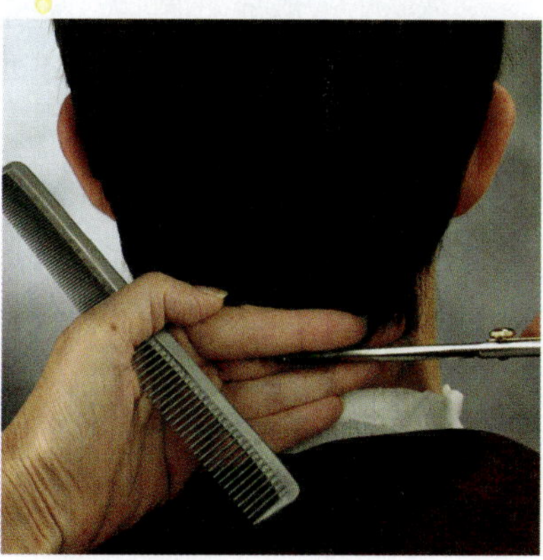

Figure 15-150 Cut subsequent nape partings at 0 degrees.

Step 8

1. Dry the model's hair in a free-form style. This method requires the barber to move the dryer briskly from side to side while drying the hair. Begin at the nape, using a brush or comb in the left hand to hold midsection hair out of the way while drying the underneath hair first. The nozzle of the dryer should be pointing downward,

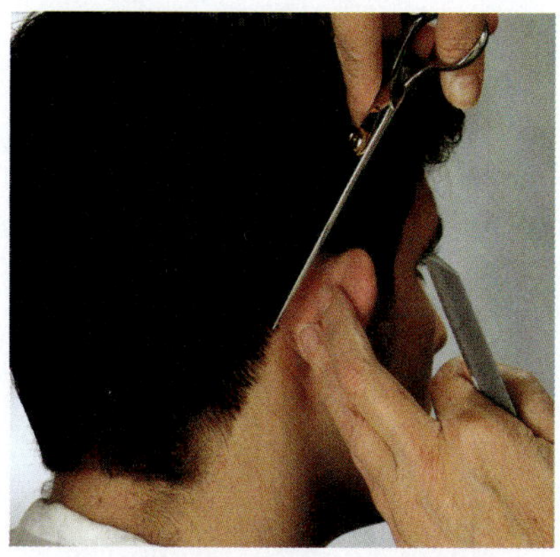

Figure 15-151 Complete 0-degree cutting behind the ears to the nape.

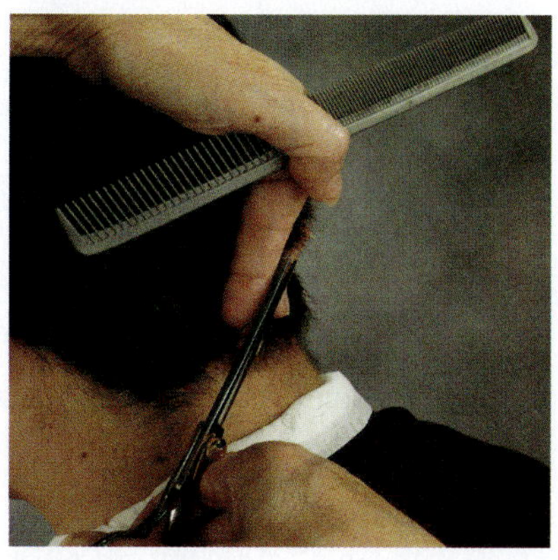

Figure 15-152 Pick up vertical parting at 90 degrees and blend through back section.

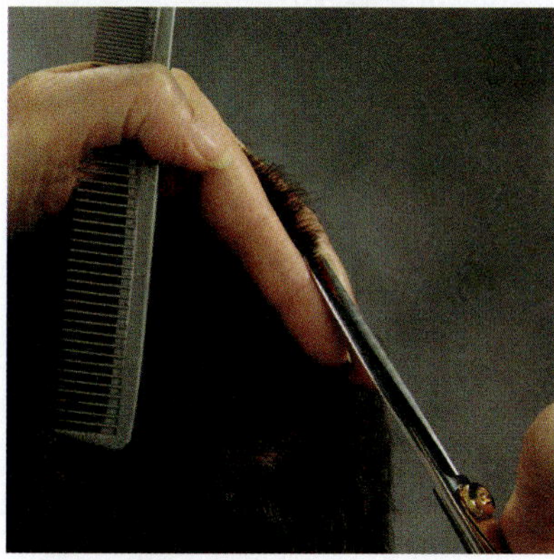

Figure 15-153 Blend back section to meet crown and crest areas.

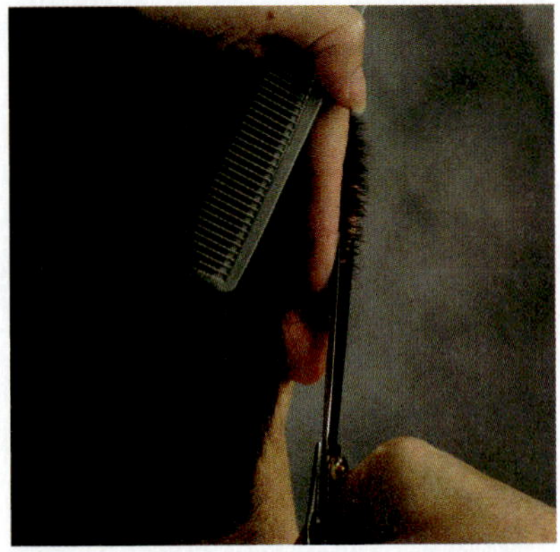

Figure 15-154 Blend sides to the back.

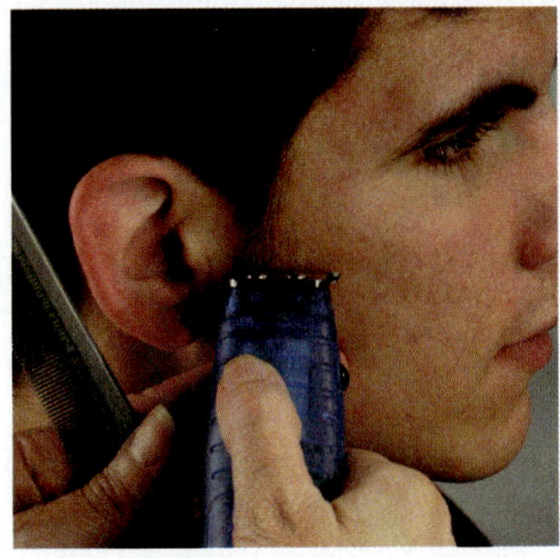

Figure 15-155 Step 8. Trim the sideburns.

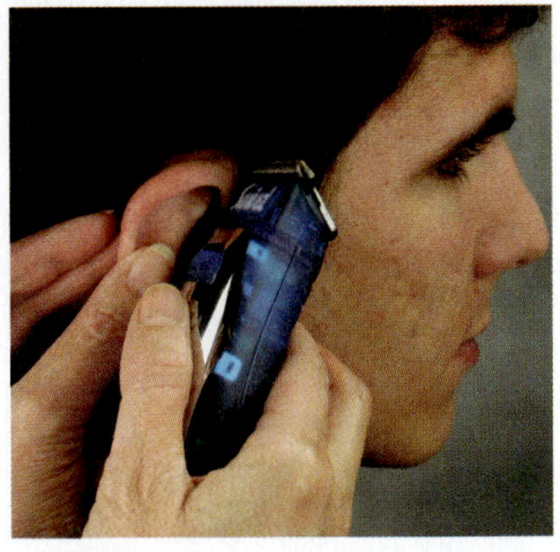

Figure 15-156 Trim around the ears.

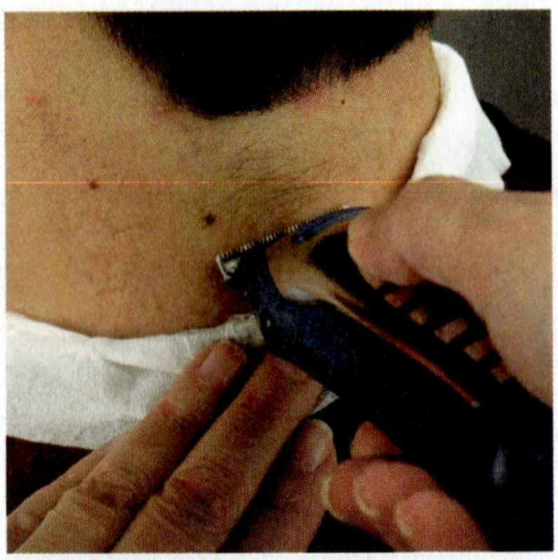

Figure 15-157 Trim and clean up the nape.

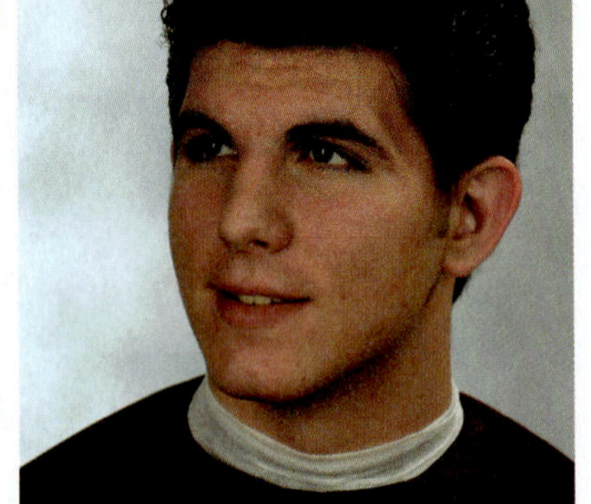

Figure 15-158 Finished style.

6 to 10 inches away from the hair. As the hair dries, check the cut for blending qualities. Proceed to dry the sides and top.

2. Brush the hair into place using a directional nozzle, if needed.
3. Use a trimmer (outliner) to clean up sideburns, sides (in around-the-ear styles), and nape (Figures 15–155, 15–156, and 15–157). Check the behind-the-ear area for any difference in hair length or design. Complete finish work by performing a neck shave after outlining the bottom of the sideburn and around-the-ear areas with a razor.
4. Recomb the hair into the finished style (Figure 15–158).
5. Consult with the client regarding the use of a styling aid.
6. The haircut and style are now complete. Dust or vacuum stray hairs, making sure none remain on the client's face or neck.

Haircutting Procedure #2: Alternative Fingers-and-Shear Technique

Some barbers prefer to begin fingers-and-shear cutting in the front section or with a side part established in the hair. Be guided by your instructor.

Preparation

1. Conduct model consultation.
2. Drape the model for wet service.
3. Shampoo and towel dry hair.
4. Remove the waterproof cape and replace it with a neckstrip and haircutting chair cloth.
5. Face the model toward the mirror and lock the chair.

Reminder: Maintain uniform moisture throughout the haircutting procedure.

Step 1

Comb model's hair into desired style with a side part. Start at the front hairline and project a parting of hair to 90 degrees. Cut to desired length and use as a traveling guide to cut back toward the crown (Figure 15–159).

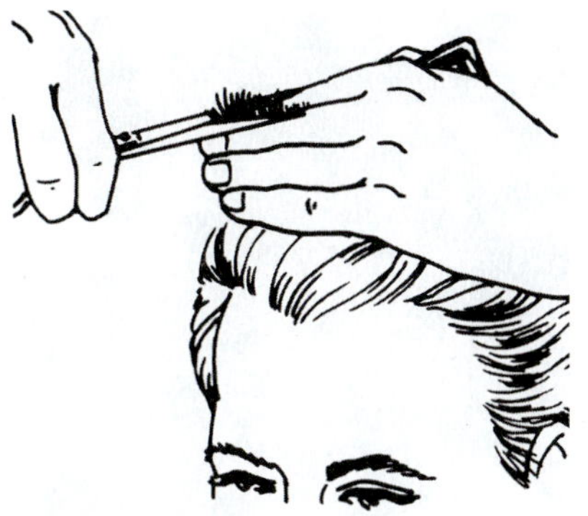

Figure 15-159 Establish 90-degree guide in front top section.

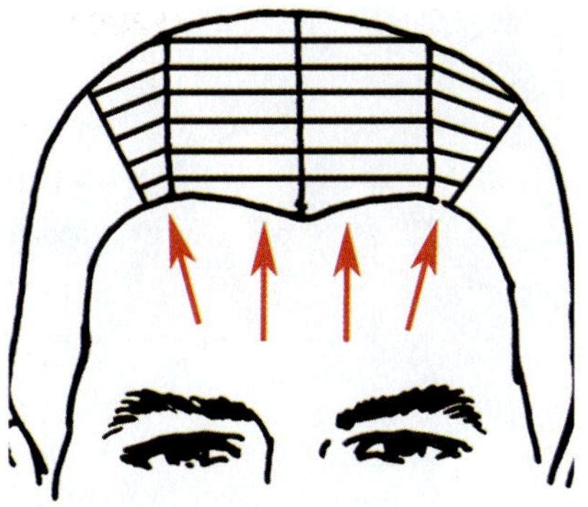

Figure 15-160 Diagram for alternate fingers-and-shear technique.

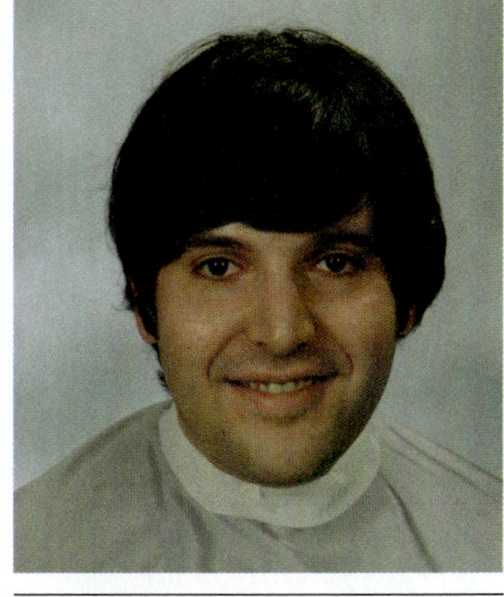

Figure 15-161a Before shear-over-comb techique.

Step 2

Pick up hair from the front temporal/crest area using the same procedure as in Step 1 to cut back toward the crown (Figure 15–160). Continue cutting all around the crest area through to the left side; or, stop at the center of the crown and repeat procedure on the left side, working from the front to the crown. Continue with Steps 6–8 of Haircutting Procedure #1.

Haircutting Procedure #3: Shear-over-Comb Technique on Model

Preparation

1. Conduct model consultation.
2. Drape the model for wet service.
3. Shampoo and towel dry hair. Blow-dry hair if dry cutting is preferred.
4. Remove the waterproof cape and replace it with a neckstrip and haircutting chair cloth.
5. Face model toward the mirror and lock the chair (Figure 15–161a).

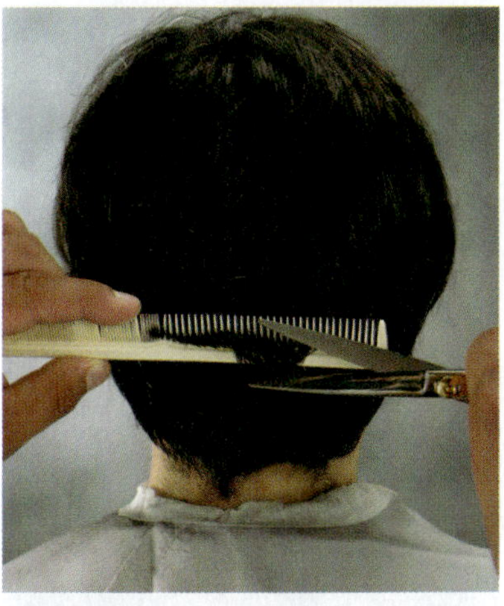

Figure 15-161b Start in nape area and cut to the occipital.

Step 1

Comb the hair. Start cutting in the nape area, trimming hair to the desired length and thickness up to the occipital (Figure 15–161b).

Step 2

Move to right side and begin shear-over-comb cutting from the sideburn hairline into the side section (Figure 15–162).

Step 3

Continue technique over and behind the right ear (Figure 15–163).

Step 4

Using a diagonal comb position, blend the hair behind the ear to the hair at the right corner of the nape along the hairline (Figure 15–164).

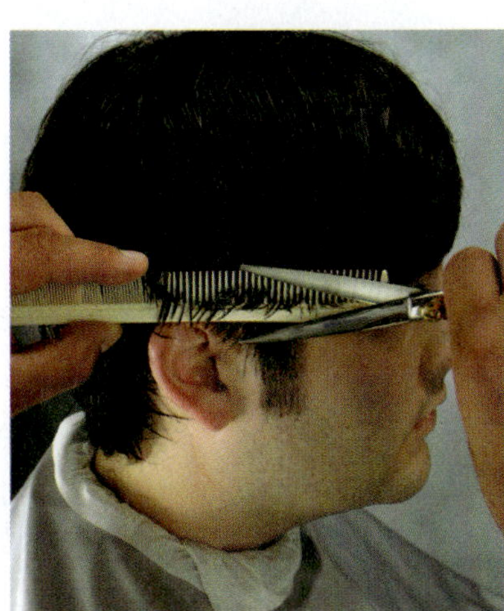

Figure 15-162 Cut from the sideburn into side section.

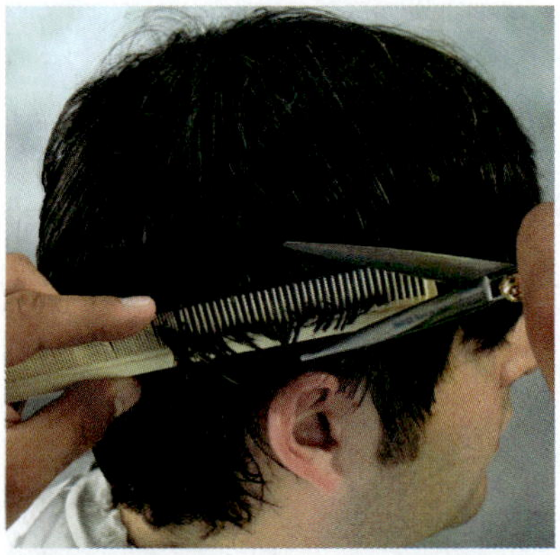

Figure 15-163 Continue cutting over and behind the ear.

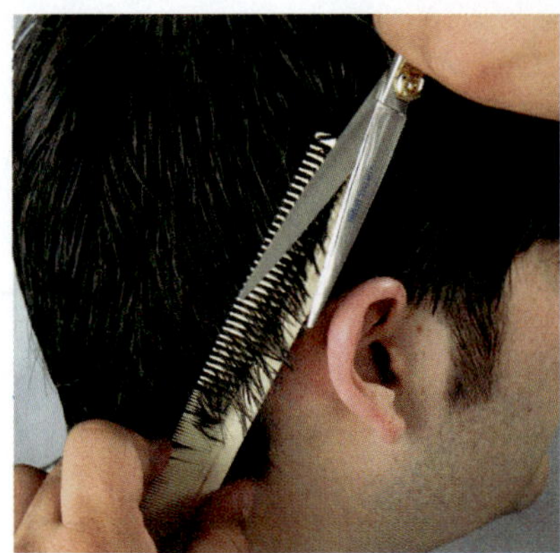

Figure 15-164 Use a diagonal comb position from side to nape corner.

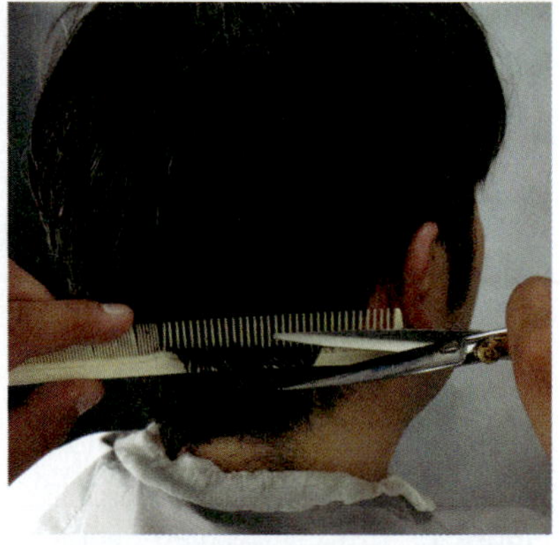

Figure 15-165 Blend hair into back section.

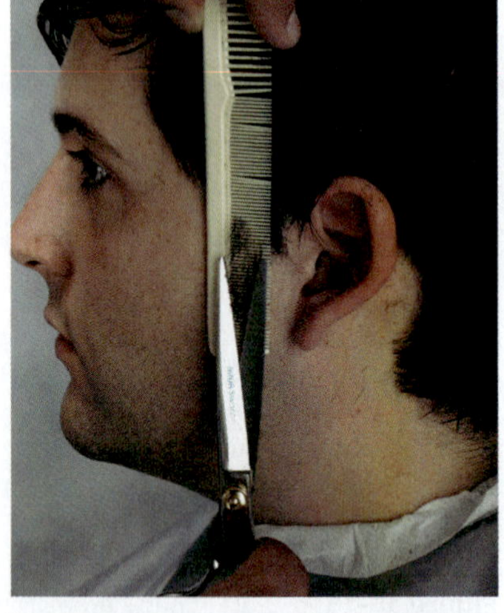

Figure 15-166 Repeat sideburn and side section cutting on left side.

STEP 5

Blend hair at the side of the neck into the back section (Figure 15–165).

STEP 6

Move to left side and repeat shear-over-comb cutting from the sideburn hairline into the side section (Figure 15–166).

STEP 7

Continue technique over and in back of the left ear.

STEP 8

Using a diagonal comb position, blend the hair behind the ear to the hair at the left corner of the nape along the hairline (Figure 15–167).

STEP 9

Blend hair at the side of the neck into the back section (Figure 15–168).

STEP 10

Blend hair from the occipital to the crown (Figure 15–169).

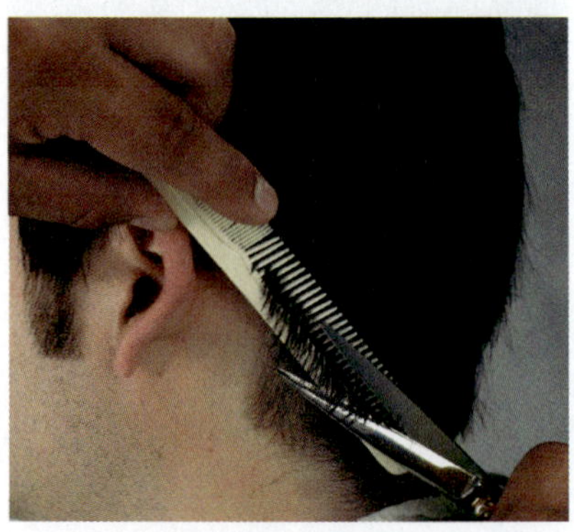

Figure 15-167 Blend hair behind ear to left nape corner.

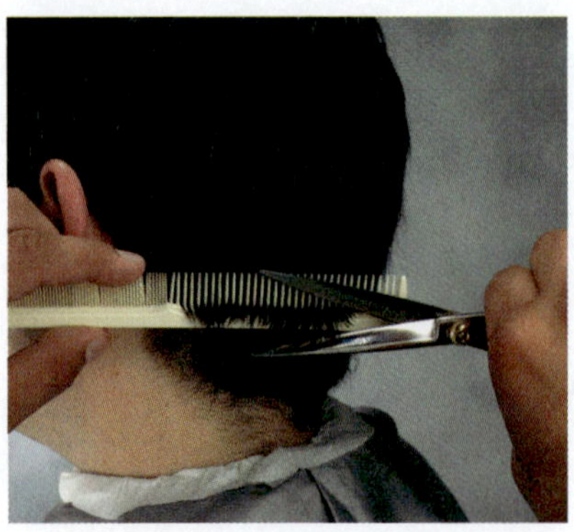

Figure 15-168 Blend hair at side of neck into back section.

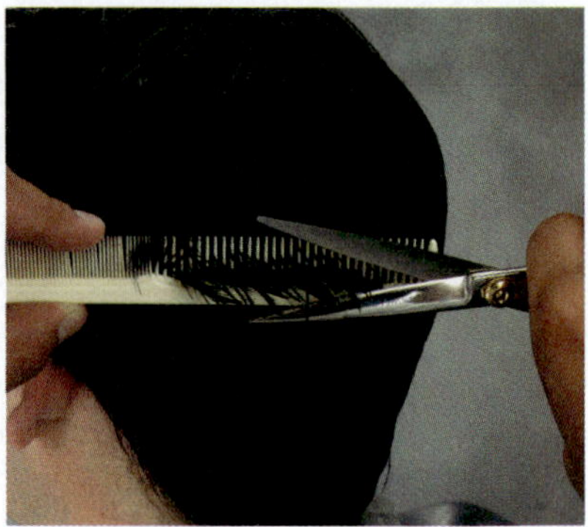

Figure 15-169 Blend hair from occipital to crown.

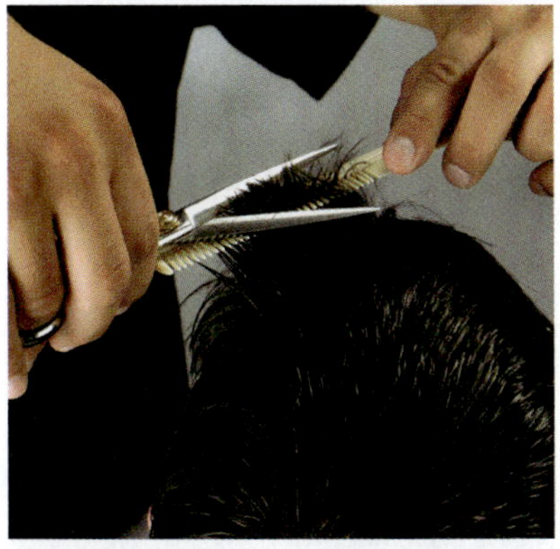

Figure 15-170 Blend hair from crown through crest and top areas.

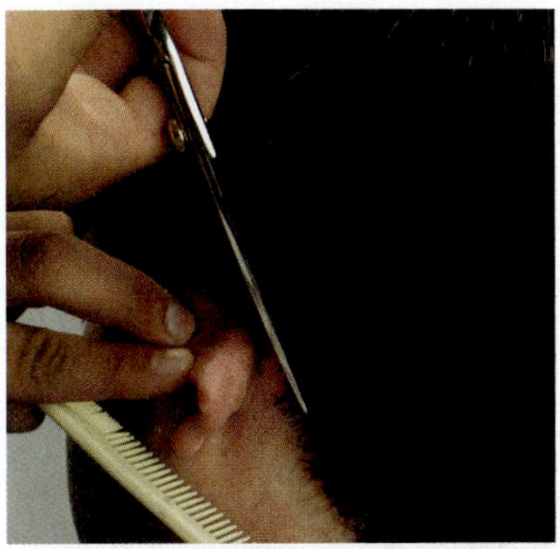

Figure 15-171 Outline with shears, followed by the trimmer.

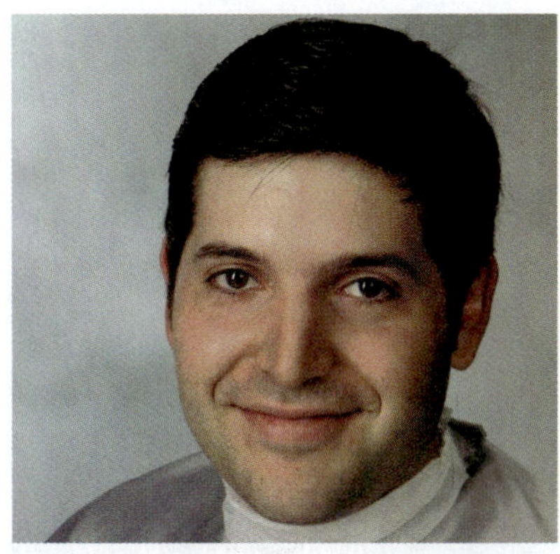

Figure 15-172 Finished shear-over-comb cut.

STEP 11

Blend hair from the crown through the right and left crest areas into the top section (Figure 15–170). Trim front section to an appropriate length for blending with the top and crest.

STEP 12

Outline sideburns, around the ear, and behind-the-ear areas with shears, followed by the trimmer (Figure 15–171). Finish the haircut with a neck and/or outline shave as the client desires. Also consult with the client regarding the use of a styling aid. Style the hair as desired. The haircut and style are now complete (Figure 15–172). Dust or vacuum any stray hairs on the client's face or neck.

Haircutting Procedure #4: Freehand and Clipper-over-Comb Technique on Model with Straight Hair

PREPARATION

1. Conduct model consultation.
2. Drape the model for wet service.
3. Shampoo and towel dry hair. Blow-dry hair if dry cutting is preferred.
4. Remove the waterproof cape and replace it with a neckstrip and haircutting chair cloth.
5. Face model toward the mirror and lock the chair.

STEP 1

Comb the hair. Start in nape area and freehand taper the first inch or so of hair. Proceed with clipper-over-comb cutting to the occipital and lower crown areas (Figures 15–173a and 15–173b).

STEP 2

Move to right side and establish the length of the sideburn (Figure 15–174a). Begin clipper-over-comb cutting from the sideburn hairline into the side section (Figure 15–174b).

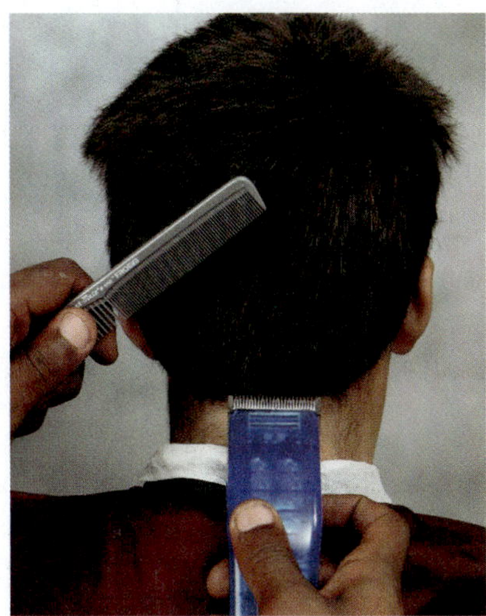

Figure 15-173a Step 1. Start in the nape area.

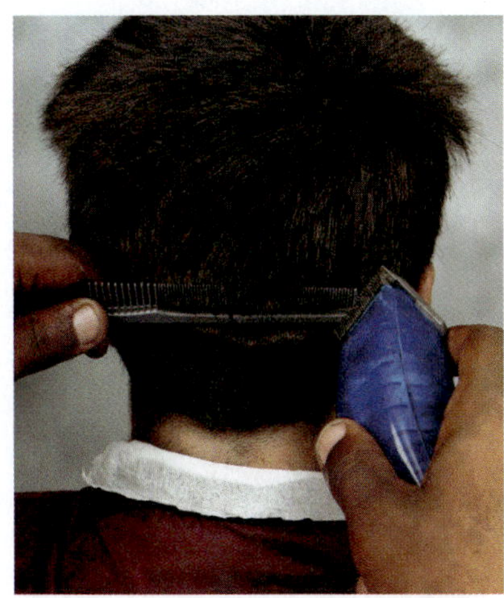

Figure 15-173b Cut to the occipital.

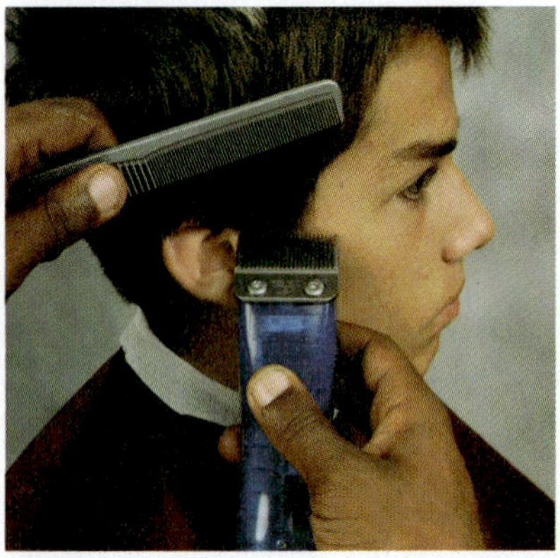

Figure 15-174a Step 2. Establish the length of the sideburn.

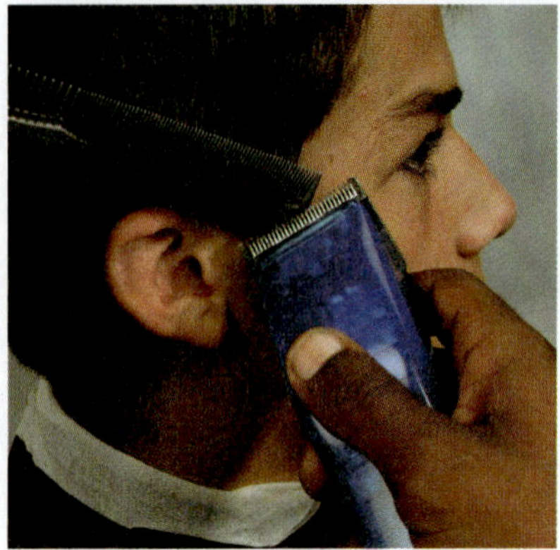

Figure 15-174b Blend from the sideburn into the side section.

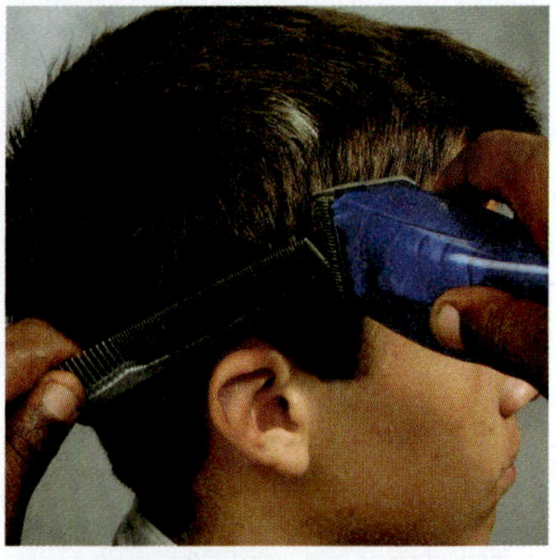

Figure 15-175a Step 3. Blend hair above the right ear.

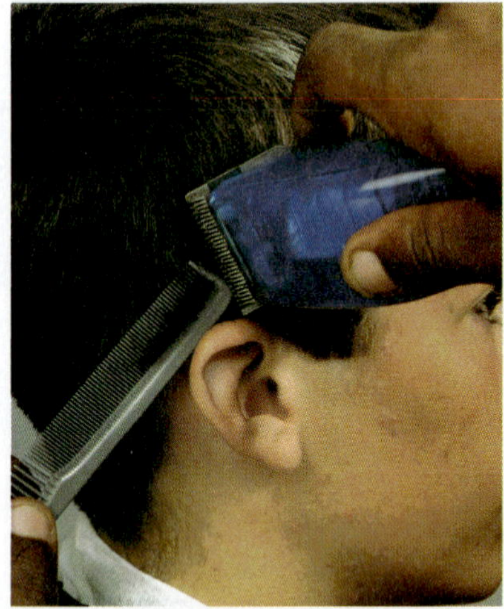

Figure 15-175b Blend hair in back of right ear.

STEP 3

Continue technique above and in back of the right ear (Figures 15–175a and 15–175b).

STEP 4

Using a diagonal comb position, blend the hair behind the ear to the hair at the right corner of the nape along the hairline (Figure 15–176a).

STEP 5

Blend hair on the right side of the neck into the back section (Figure 15–176b).

STEP 6

Move to left side, establish sideburn length and begin clipper-over-comb, cutting into the side section (Figure 15–177).

STEP 7

Continue technique above and in back of the left ear (Figure 15–178).

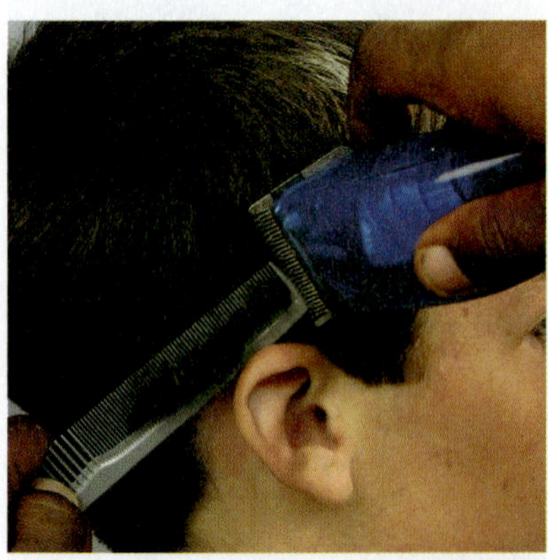

Figure 15-176a Step 4. Position comb diagonally to blend behind the ear.

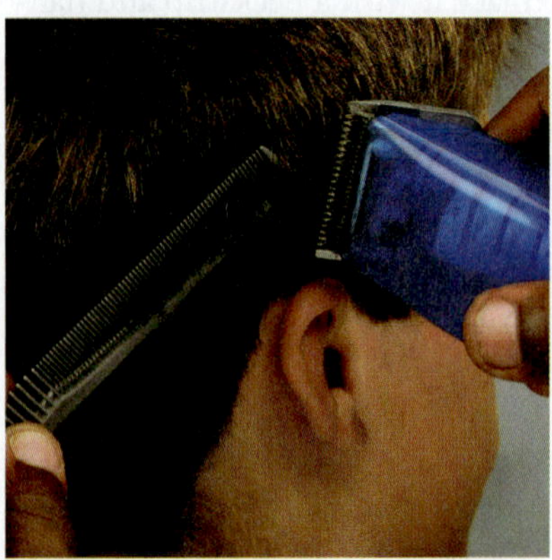

Figure 15-176b Blend to back section.

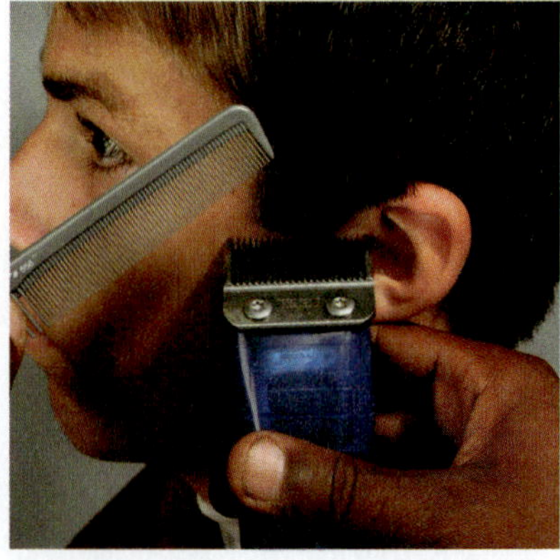

Figure 15-177 Step 6. Establish sideburn length and cut side section.

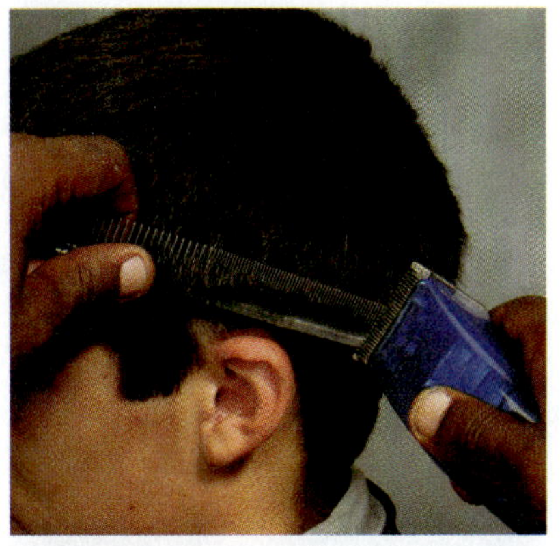

Figure 15-178 Step 7. Blend around the ear.

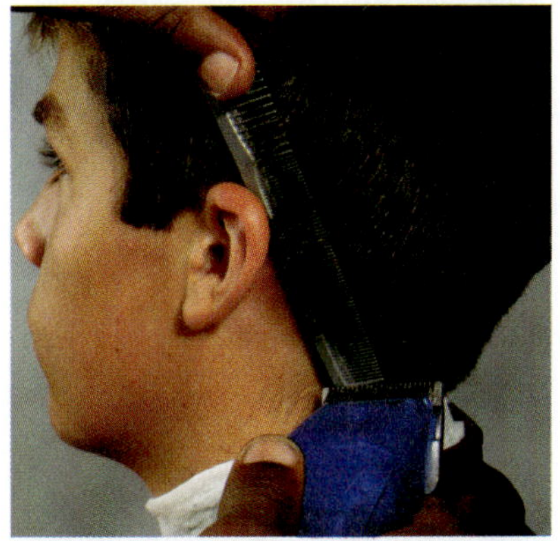

Figure 15-179 Step 8. Blend sides to left nape corner.

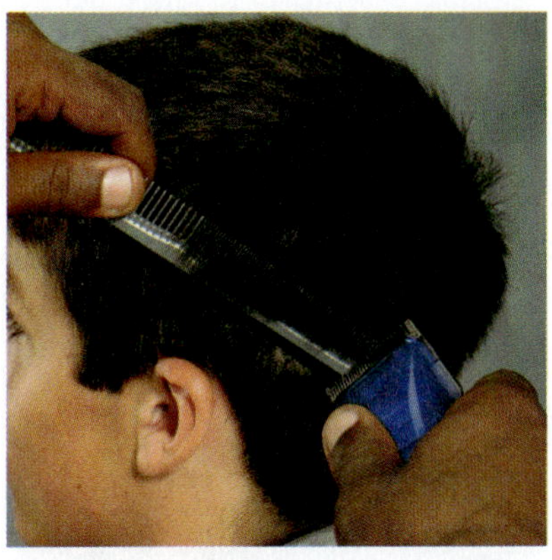

Figure 15-180 Steps 5 through 9. Blend sides to back section.

Step 8

Using a diagonal comb position, blend the hair behind the ear to the hair at the left corner of the nape along the hairline. (Figure 15–179).

Step 9

Blend hair at the side of the neck into the back section (Figure 15–180).

Step 10

Blend hair from the occipital to the crown (Figure 15–181).

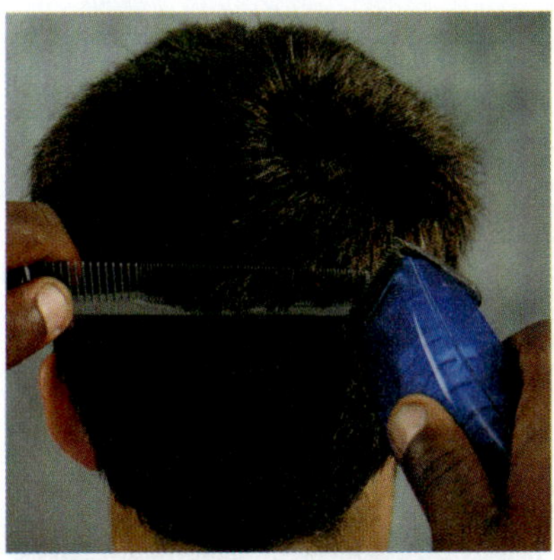

Figure 15-181 Step 10. Blend from occipital to crown.

Step 11

Blend hair from the crown through the right and left crest areas to meet the side sections. (Figure 15–182). Trim top section using fingers-and-shear method to achieve the desired length (Figures 15–183). Check blending and fine-tune using fingers-and-shear method (Figure 15–184).

Step 12

Outline sideburns, around the ear, back of the ear areas, and nape with shears and then trimmer. Complete finish work by performing a neck shave

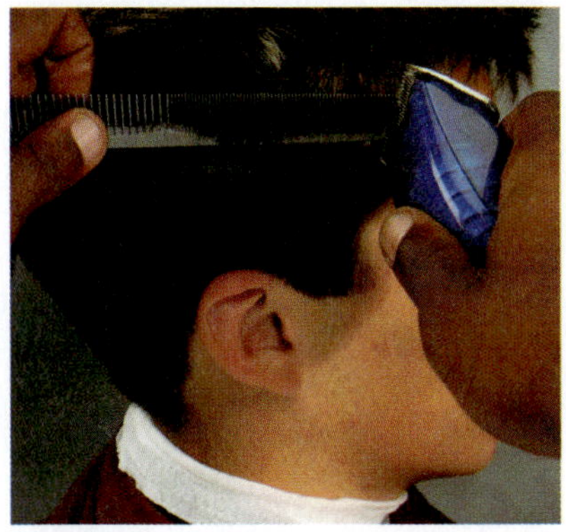

Figure 15-182 Step 11. Blend crest and side.

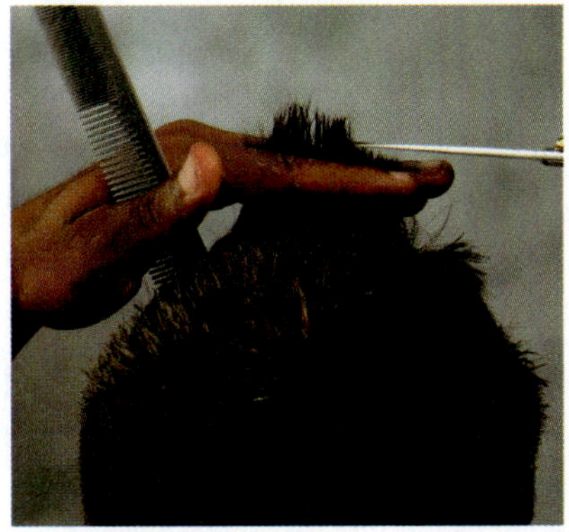

Figure 15-183 Trim top section.

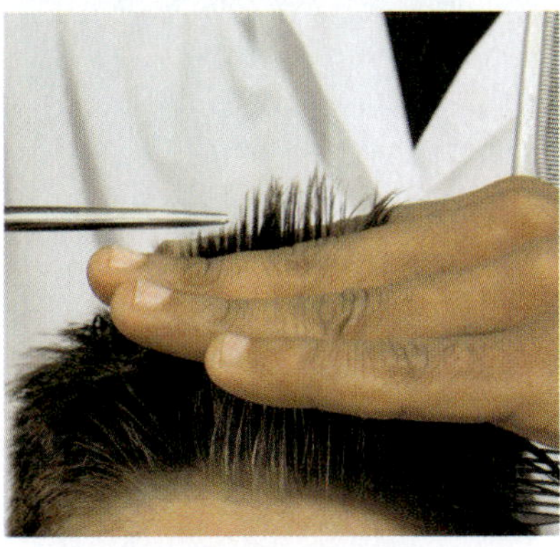

Figure 15-184 Check for evenness and blending.

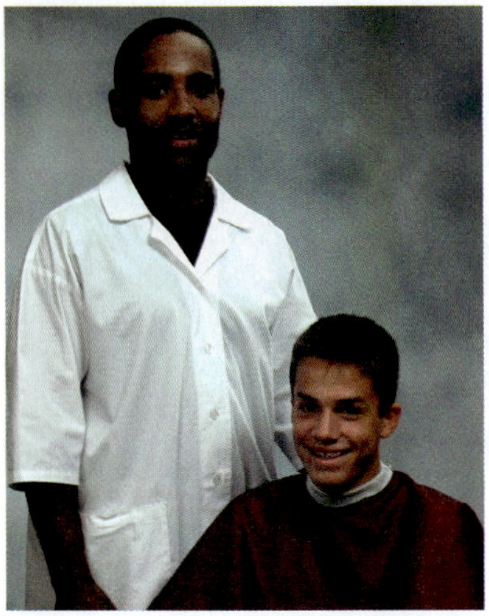

Figure 15-185 Finished style.

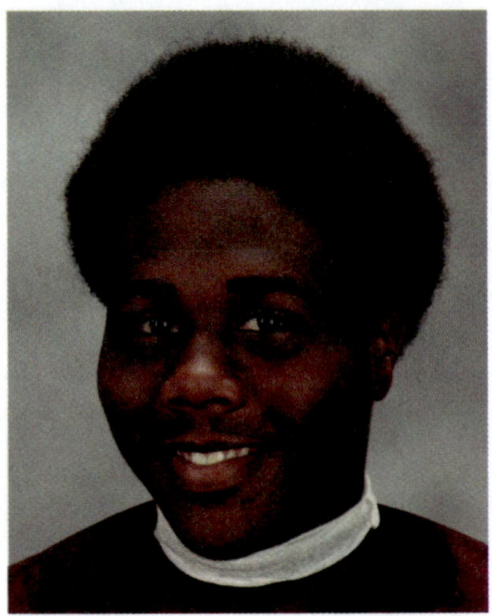

Figure 15-186a Model before haircut.

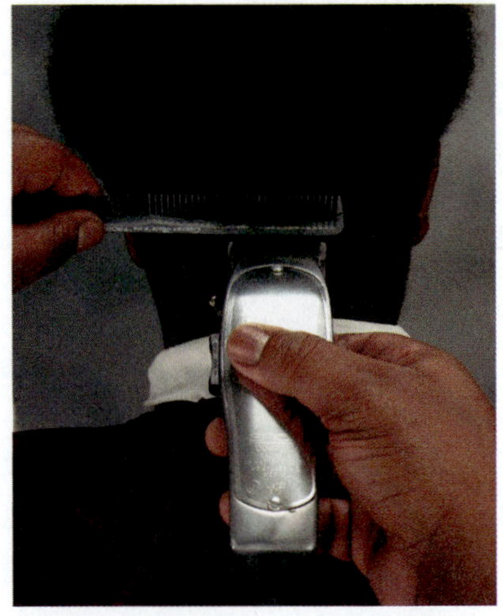

Figure 15-186b Step 1. Clipper-over-comb taper (or freehand taper) nape to occipital.

after outlining the bottom of the sideburn and around-the-ear areas with a razor. Consult with the client regarding the use of a styling aid, then style the hair as desired. The haircut and style is now complete (Figure 15–185). Dust or vacuum any stray hairs from the client's face or neck.

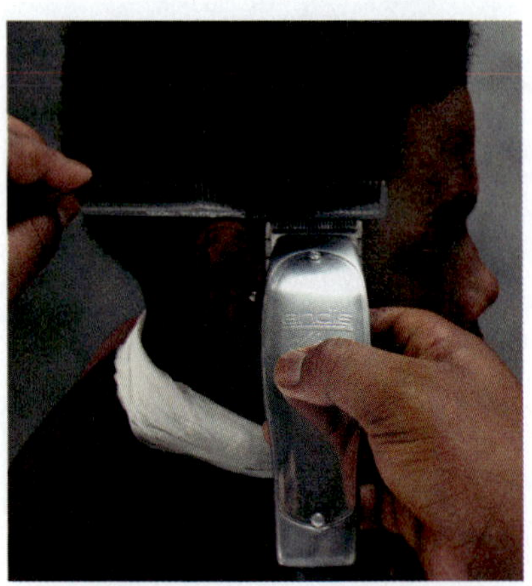

Figure 15-187 Step 2. Cut and blend to the crest.

Haircutting Procedure #5: Freehand and Clipper-over-Comb Technique on Model with Tightly Curled Hair

1. Conduct model consultation.
2. Drape the model for wet service.
3. Shampoo and towel dry hair. Blow-dry hair if dry cutting is preferred.
4. Remove the waterproof cape and replace it with a neckstrip and haircutting chair cloth.
5. Face model toward the mirror and lock the chair (Figure 15–186a).

Step 1

Comb or pick the hair out. Start in nape area and freehand taper or clipper-over-comb taper the first inch or so of hair (Figure 15–186b). If hair density allows, proceed with clipper-over-comb cutting to the occipital area. If the hair is thick, freehand clipper cut to the occipital area.

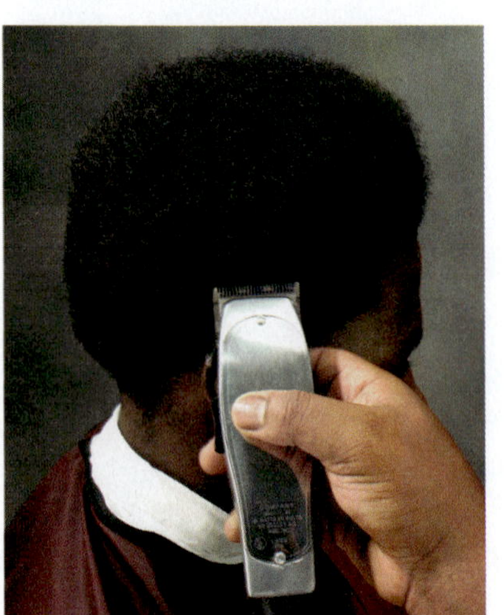

Figure 15-188 Step 3. Blend above and in back of ear.

Step 2

Move to right side and use freehand or clipper-over-comb to cut and blend from the sideburn hairline up to the crest (Figure 15–187).

Step 3

Continue technique above and in back of the right ear (Figure 15–188).

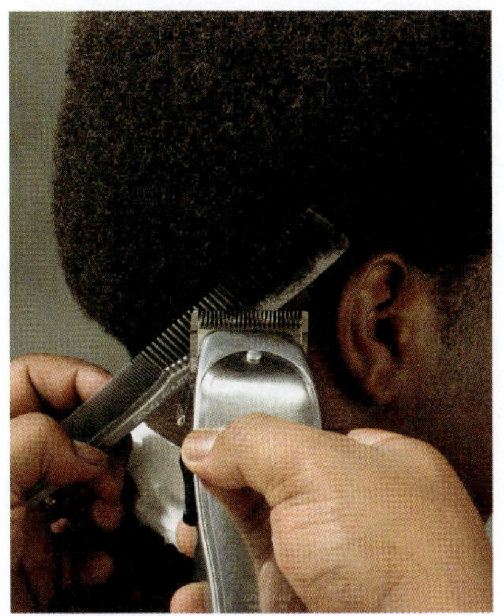

Figure 15–189 Step 4. Blend from side to nape corner.

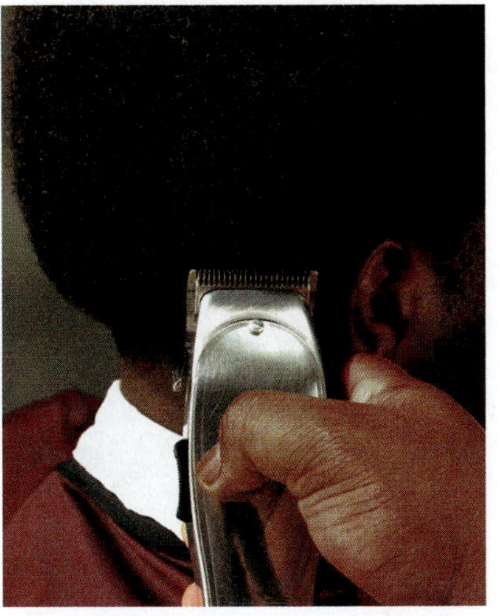

Figure 15–190 Step 5. Blend into back section.

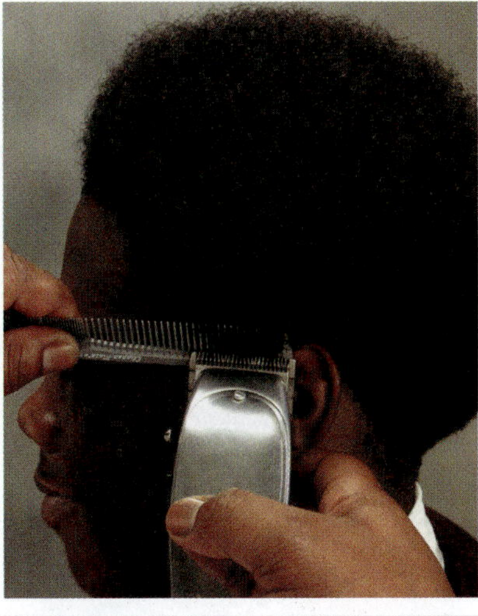

Figure 15–191 Step 6. Cut from sideburn to crest.

Step 4

Using a diagonal comb position, blend the hair behind the ear to the hair at the right corner of the nape along the hairline; or, freehand the entire section (Figure 15–189).

Step 5

Blend hair at the side of the neck into the back section (Figure 15–190).

Step 6

Move to left side and begin freehand or clipper-over-comb cutting from the sideburn hairline to the crest (Figure 15–191).

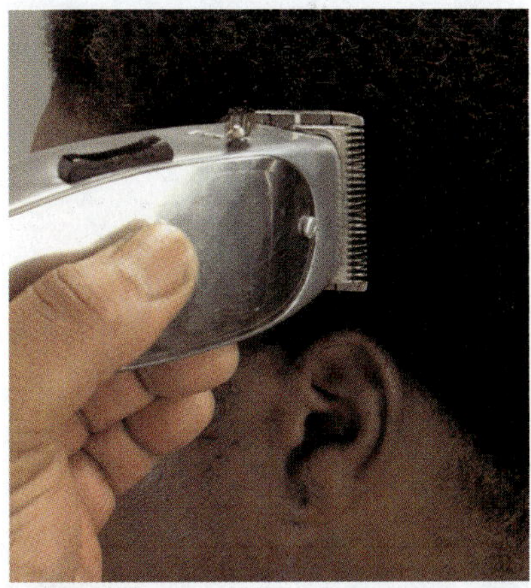

Figure 15–192 Step 7. Cut above and in back of left ear.

Step 7

Continue technique above and in back of the left ear (Figure 15–192).

Step 8

Using a diagonal comb or freehand position, blend the hair behind the ear to the hair at the left corner of the nape along the hairline (Figure 15–193).

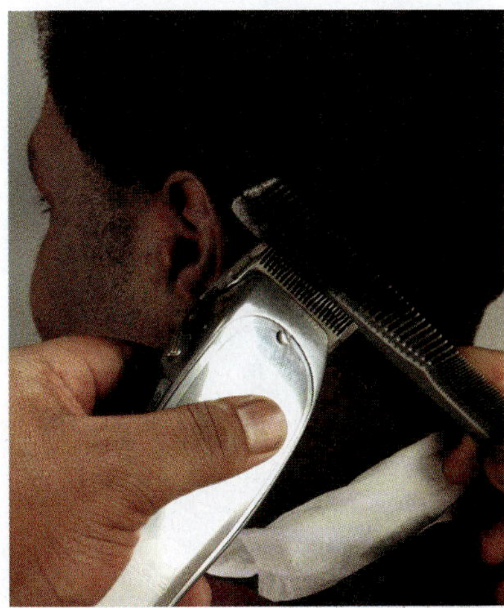

Figure 15–193 Step 8. Blend behind ear to nape corner.

Step 9

Blend hair at the side of the neck into the back section (Figure 15–194).

Step 10

Establish guide in front center of top section and cut back to crown area (Figure 15–195).

Figure 15-194 Step 9. Blend hair into back section.

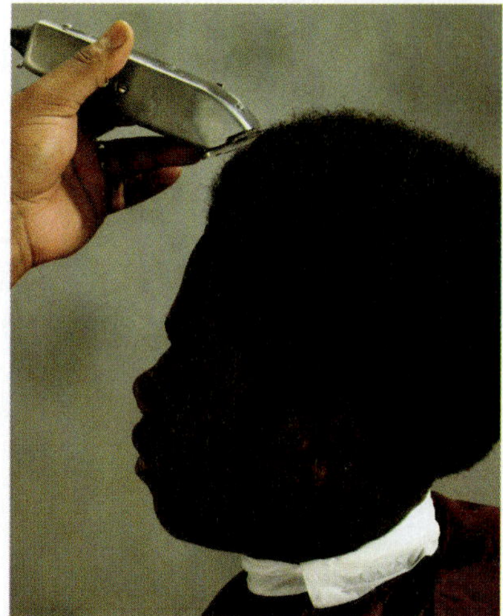

Figure 15-195 Step 10. Establish guide in front center section, cut back to crown.

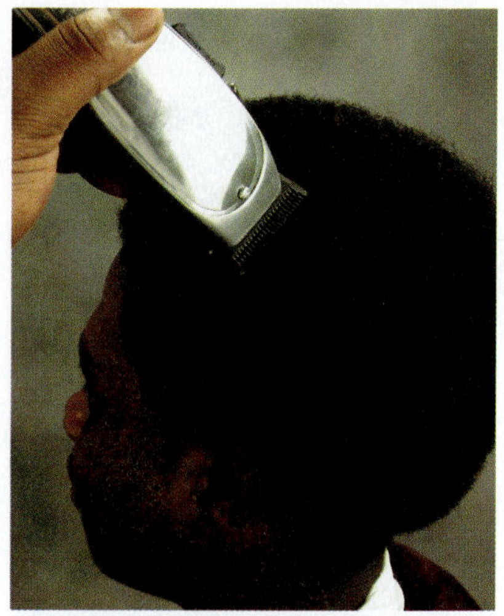

Figure 15-196 Step 11. Blend crest to top guide.

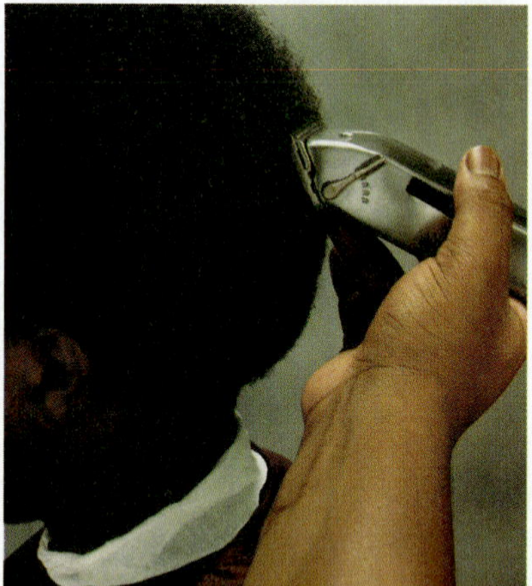

Figure 15-197 Step 12. Blend occipital area to crest. Check blending to top section.

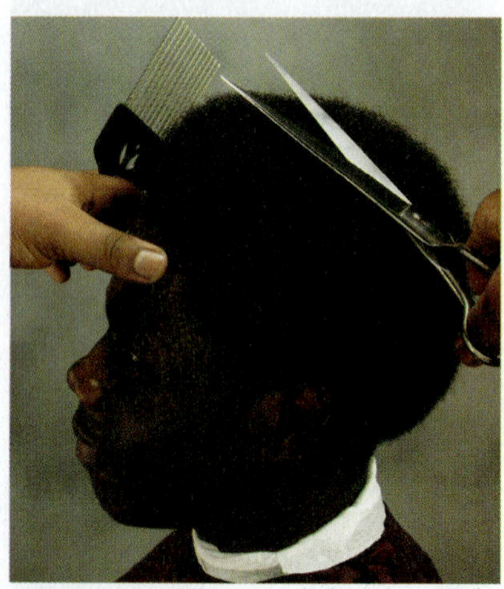

Figure 15-198 Step 13. Fine-tune with shears.

STEP 11

Blend crest to top guide around the entire head (Figure 15–196).

STEP 12

Blend occipital area to crest, then check the blend to the top section (Figure 15–197).

STEP 13

Comb or pick hair out. Fine-tune with shears (Figure 15–198).

STEP 14

Outline sideburns, around the ear, and back of the ear areas with clippers or trimmers. Consult with the client regarding the use of a styling aid and style the hair as desired. The haircut and style portion of the service is now complete. Finish with the neck and outline shaving procedure shown in Haircut Finish Work: Procedure #6. Dust or vacuum stray hairs from the model's face and neck.

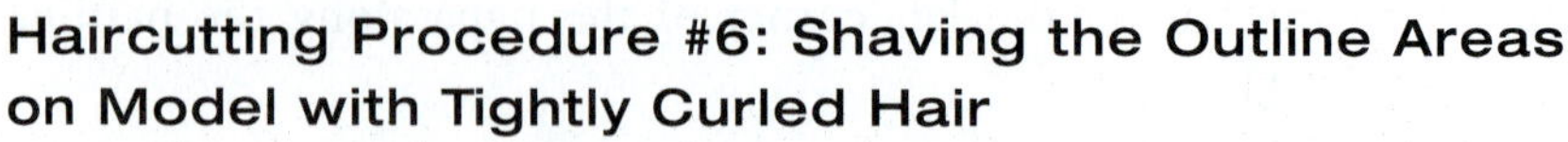

Haircutting Procedure #6: Shaving the Outline Areas on Model with Tightly Curled Hair

1. Model should still be draped from the haircut service.
2. Loosen chair cloth and apply towel to neckline, leaving it loose enough for access when securing the drape.

STEP 1

Apply a light coating of lather at the hairline of the areas to be shaved (sideburns, around and over the ears, front hairline, sides of the neck, and across the nape). Rub the lather in lightly with the balls of the fingers or thumb (Figure 15–199).

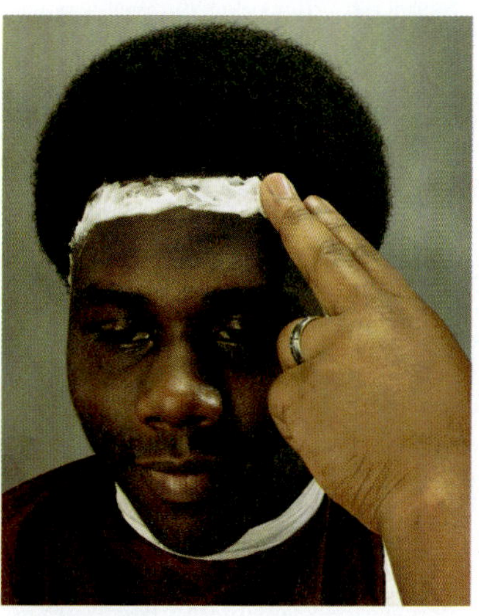

Figure 15-199 Step 1. Apply lather around hairline.

Step 2

Move to the model's right side. Stretch the skin in the sideburn area. Using a freehand stroke, shave the sideburn to the desired length (Figure 15–200). Next, shave around the ear at the hairline in front of the ear, around the ear, and straight down the side of the neck, using the freehand stroke with the point of the razor. Hold the ear away with the fingers of the left hand as necessary for safety (Figures 15–201 through 15–203). Be careful not to shave into the hairline at the nape of the neck.

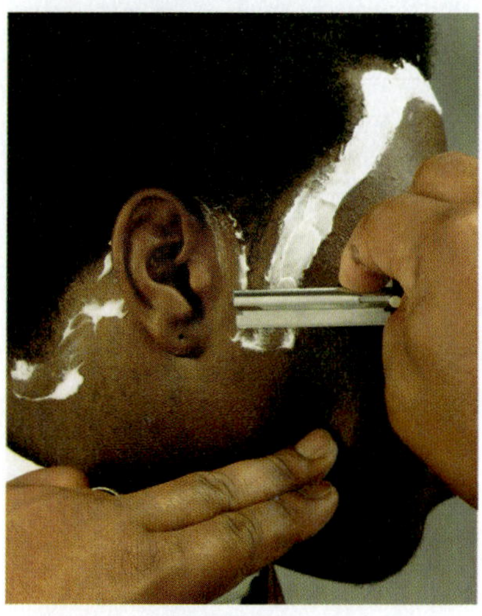

Figure 15-200 Step 2. Shave sideburn to desired length.

Step 3

Move to the model's left side. Stretch the skin in the sideburn area. Use a freehand or backhand stroke to shave the sideburn to the appropriate length (Figure 15–204). Next, use the freehand stroke to shave around the ear at the hairline. Hold the ear away with the fingers of the left hand as necessary for safety and use the backhand stroke to shave down the side of the neck with the point of the razor (Figures 15–205 through 15–206b). Be careful not to shave into the hairline at the nape of the neck.

Step 4 (Optional)

Shave the nape area with a freehand stroke (Figure 15–207).

Step 5 (Optional)

Use a freehand stroke to shave the front hairline. Start in the center and work toward the right temple corner, then the left (Figures 15–208 and 15–209). Follow the natural hairline, shaving the outline through the temporal (crest, horseshoe, etc.) area to the previously shaved front corners of the sideburns. Clean up model's hairline with a warm moist towel. Apply astringent, moisturizing cream, talc, or after-shave lotion as desired. Figure 15–210 shows the finished haircut and outline shave.

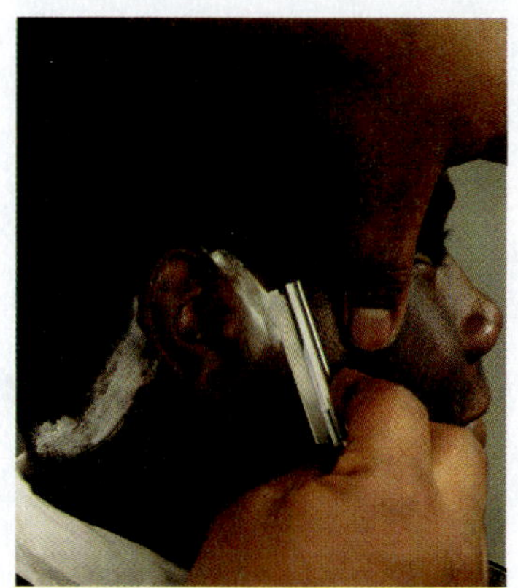

Figure 15-201 Stretch skin and shave in front of ear.

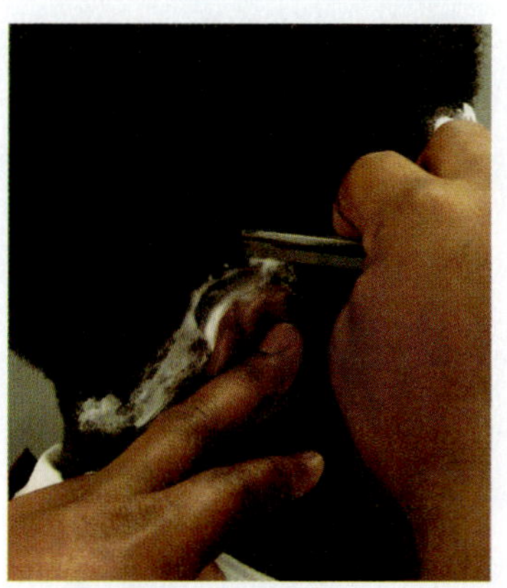

Figure 15-202 Shave around the ear.

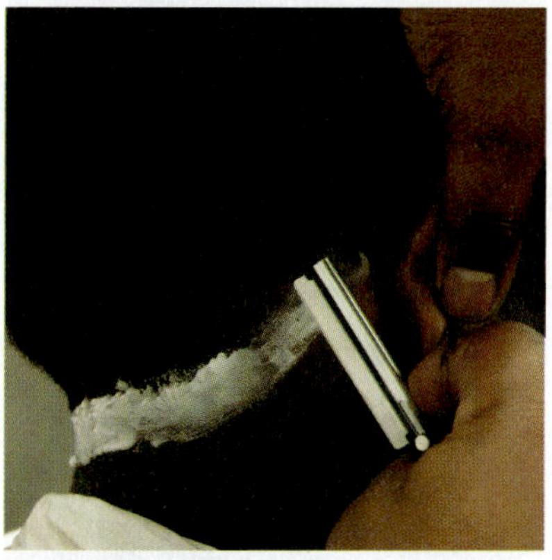

Figure 15-203 Shave down the side of the neck.

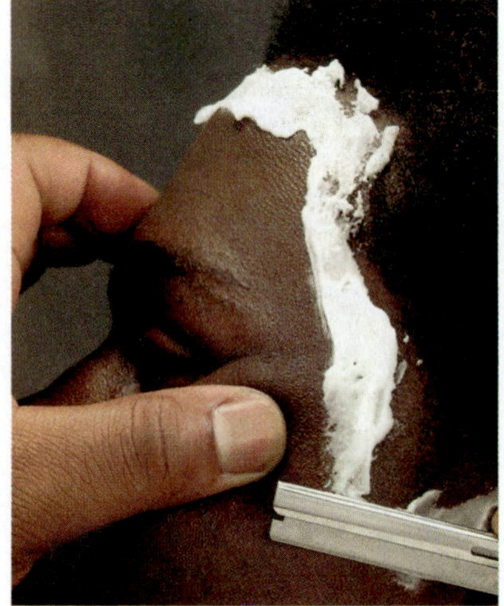

Figure 15-204 Step 3. Shave sideburn to appropriate length.

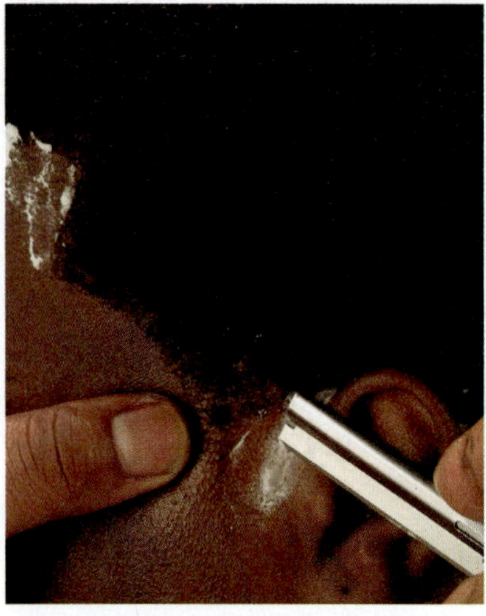

Figure 15-205 Shave in front of ear.

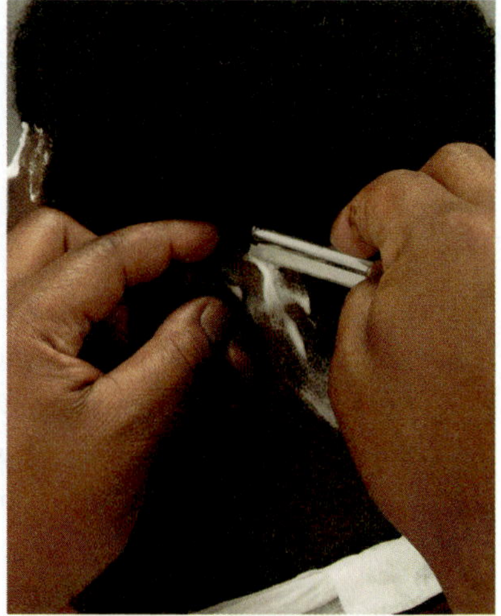

Figure 15-206a Shave around ear.

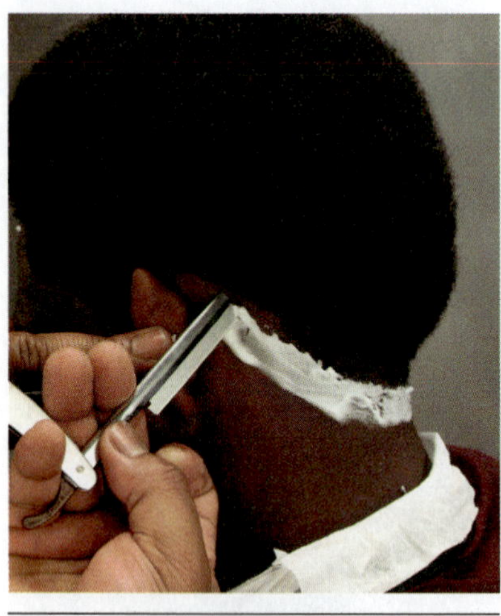

Figure 15-206b Shave behind the ear to the nape corner.

Haircutting Procedure #7: Razor Cutting on Model

1. Conduct model consultation.
2. Drape the model for wet service.
3. Shampoo and towel dry hair.
4. Remove the waterproof cape and replace it with a neckstrip and haircutting chair cloth.
5. Face model toward the mirror and lock the chair

Step 1

Section the hair into four sections from crown to nape, crown to front, and crest to sides. Subdivide the back section into three subsections (Figure 15–211).

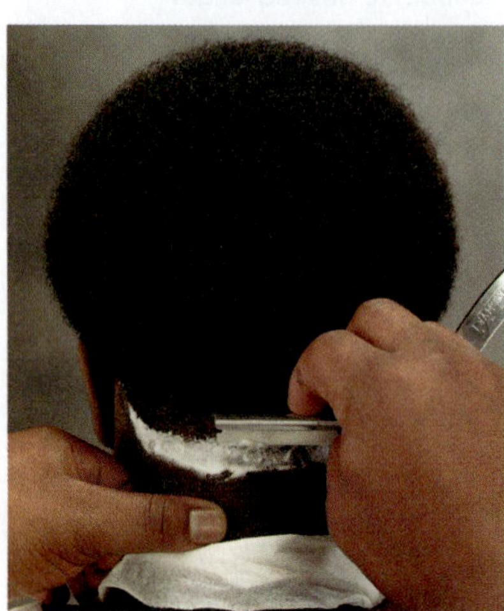

Figure 15-207 Shave the nape area (optional).

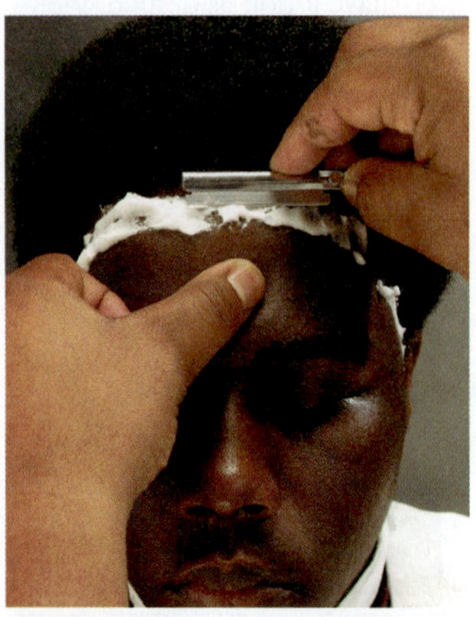

Figure 15-208 Step 5 (optional). Start at the front hairline and shave in the center.

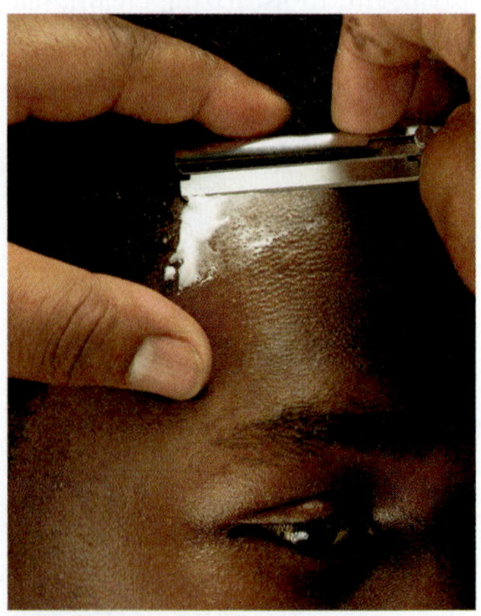

Figure 15-209 Shave to temple corner.

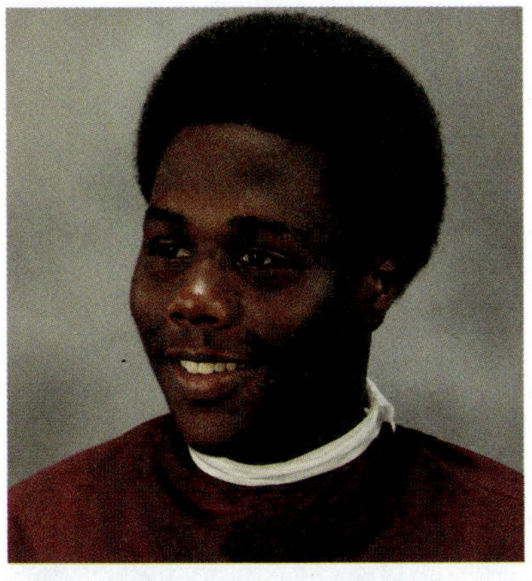

Figure 15-210 Finished haircut and outline shape.

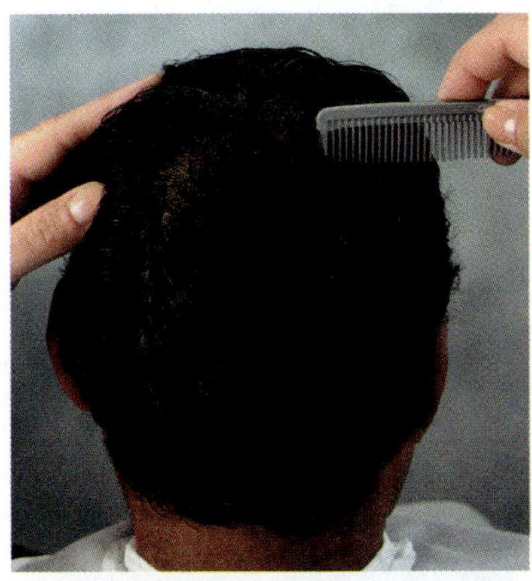

Figure 15-211 Step 1. Sectioning for razor cut.

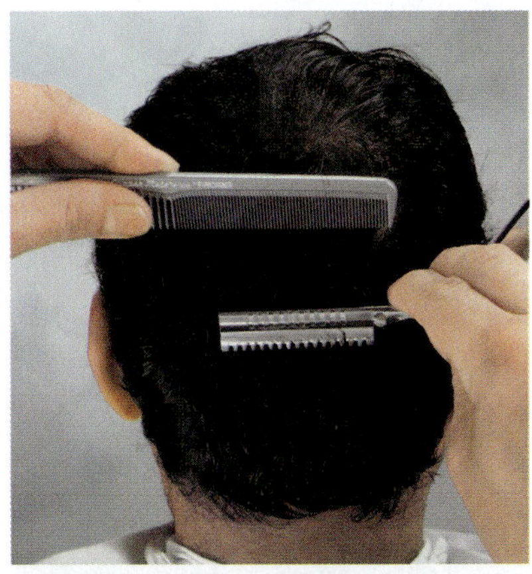

Figure 15-212 Step 2. Begin razor rotation.

Step 2

Begin in the center section just below the crown. Taper the hair using the razor rotation technique, one strip at a time in a downward direction to the hairline. Blend each new cut with the hair previously trimmed. Use short, even razor strokes to avoid ridges, lines, or any appearance of unevenness (Figure 15–212).

Step 3

Comb the hair downward from the top right side toward the left midsection in the back. Lightly taper from right to left in the top section (Figure 15–213). Taper the lower section to blend with the nape hair (Figure 15–214).

Step 4

Comb the hair downward from the top left side toward the right. Repeat the procedure used in Step 3 (Figure 15–215).

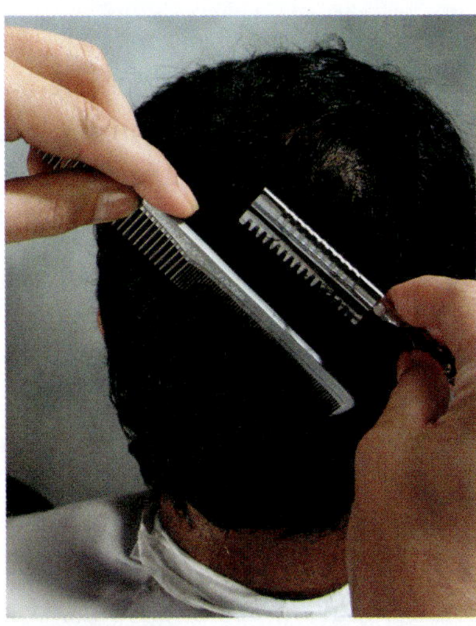

Figure 15-213 Step 3. Lightly taper from top right to left midsection.

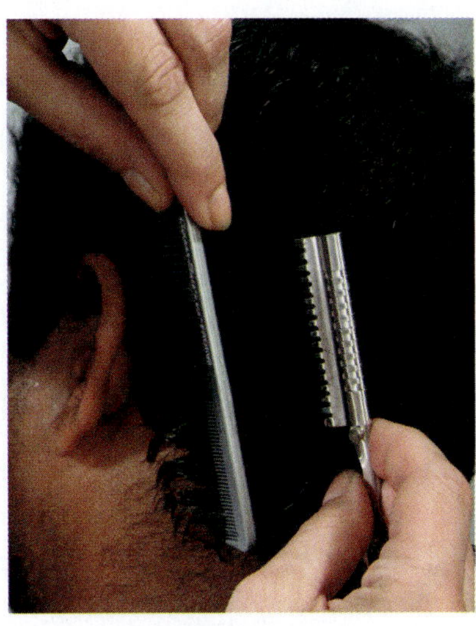

Figure 15-214 Continue tapering through lower left section.

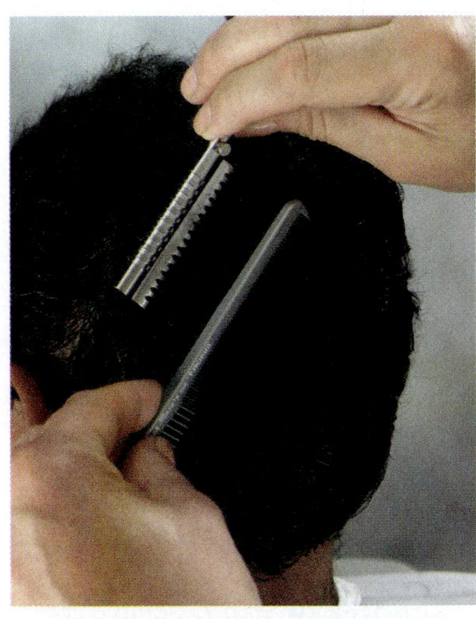

Figure 15-215 Step 4. Repeat Step 3, working from left to right.

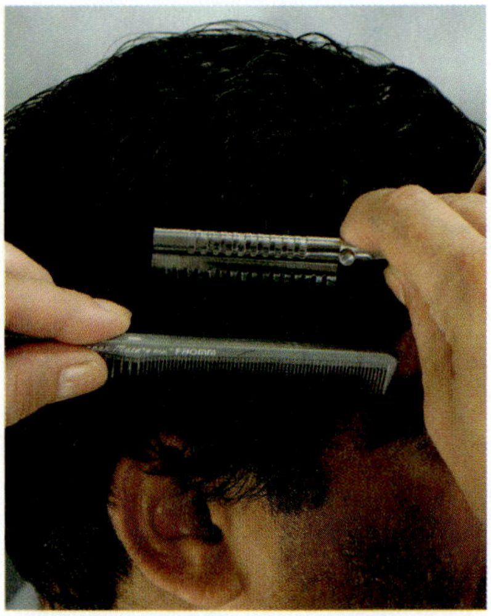

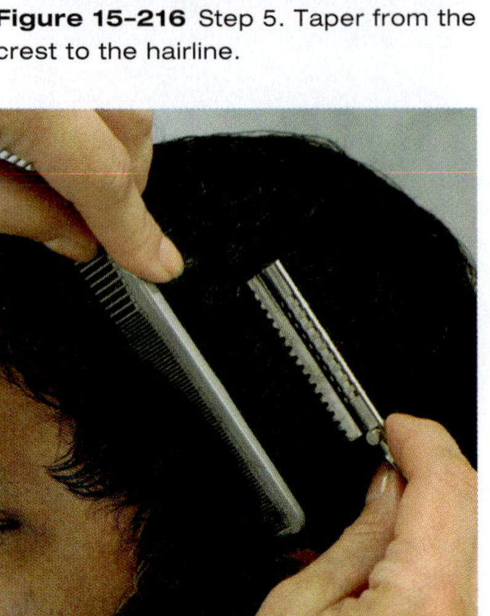

Figure 15-216 Step 5. Taper from the crest to the hairline.

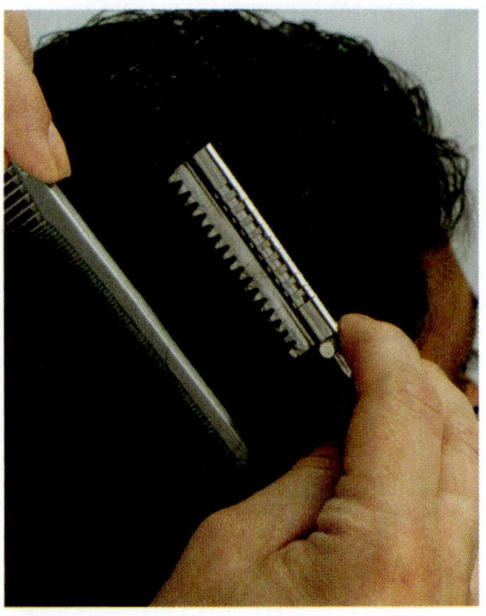

Figure 15-217 Lightly taper side to blend with back section.

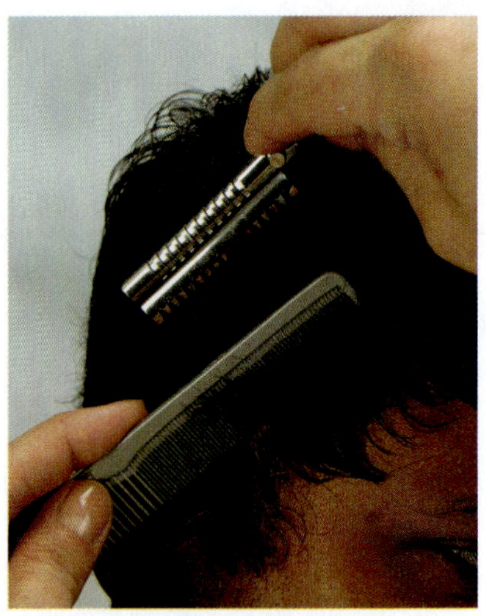

Figure 15-218 Lightly taper toward the face. Trim design line as needed.

Step 5

Comb side hair downward and subdivide it into three vertical partings. Begin tapering about ¾ of an inch from the crest. Taper downward through the three sections to the hairline (Figure 15–216). Comb the hair toward the back and taper lightly in that direction, then blend with the back section (Figure 15–217). Comb the hair forward and taper lightly toward the face, trimming the perimeter (design) line as needed (Figure 15–218).

Step 6

Repeat Step 5 procedures on left side of head (Figure 15–219).

Figure 15-219 Step 6. Repeat Step 5 procedures on left side.

15

Step 7

Comb top hair forward with even distribution over the head form (Figure 15–220).

Start tapering, just forward of the crown, in the top section (Figure 15–221). Work toward the forehead on the right side. Repeat on the left side then taper the center section. Make sure to blend all three sections. Hold the front section at 0 degrees and trim using the freehand slicing technique (Figure 15–222).

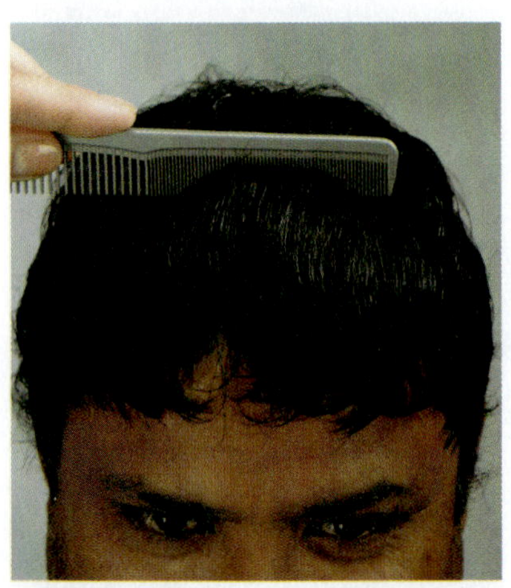

Figure 15-220 Step 7. Comb hair forward with even distribution.

Step 8

Comb through the cut, redistributing the sections in a variety of directions to check for blending and evenness. Consult with the client regarding a neck shave, outline shaving, and the use of styling aids. Style the hair as desired. The haircut and style are now complete (Figure 15–223). Dust or vacuum stray hairs, making sure none remain on the client's face or neck.

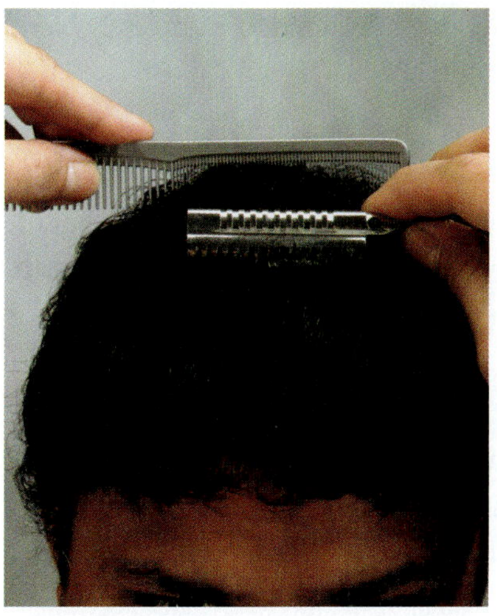

Figure 15-221 Start tapering in top section.

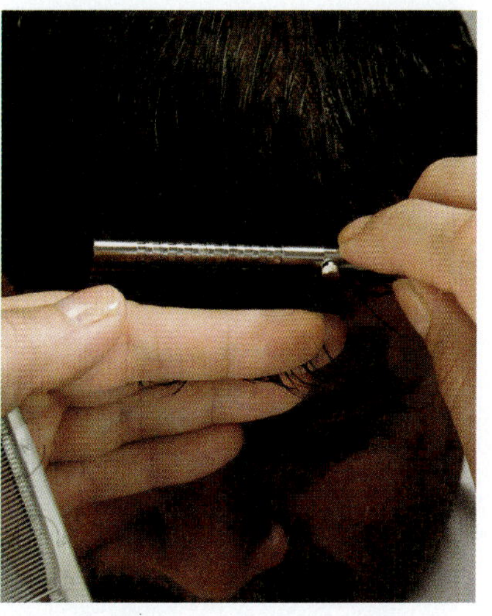

Figure 15-222 Trim front length using freehand slicing movement.

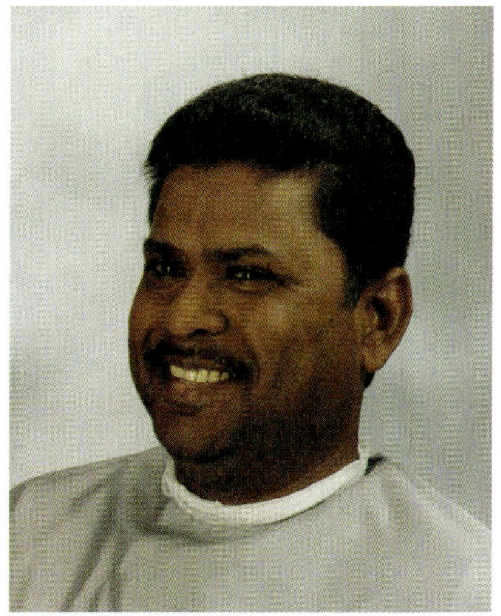

Figure 15-223 Finished cut and style.

Haircutting Procedure #8: Fade Cut

The standard characteristics that apply to the many variations of fade cuts today include a close, tight cut at the sides and back; blending at the occipital and crest areas; and a customized design at the temples and front sections. To facilitate blending, the clipper blades are opened or closed based on the hair's density and curl pattern.

Reminder: Cutting against the grain achieves a closer cut than cutting with the grain. The following procedure offers one method to achieve a close fade cut. Be guided by your instructor for technique and fade style variations.

Step 1

Set the clipper blade in the closed position to achieve a close cut. Start at the center of the nape, cutting to just below the occipital (Figure 15–224). Cut the sections right and left of center.

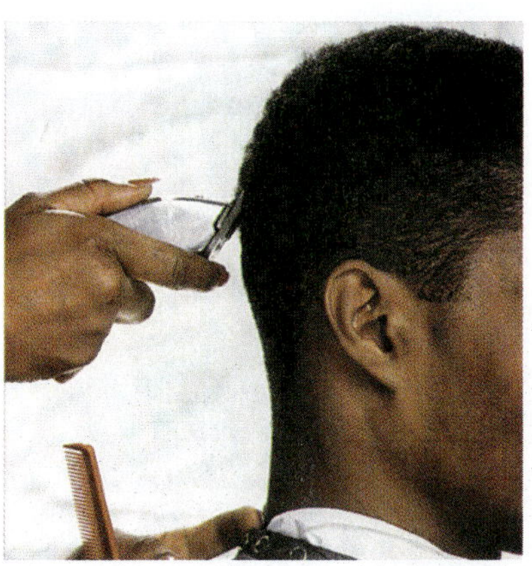

Figure 15-224 Start at center of nape cutting to just below occipital.

Step 2

Move to the right side (or left, depending on preference) and cut from the hairline to the top, middle, or bottom of the crest area as desired by the client (Figure 15–225). Cut around the ear and into the previously cut back section, cutting up and/or across as the growth pattern allows. Complete cutting the left side in the same manner.

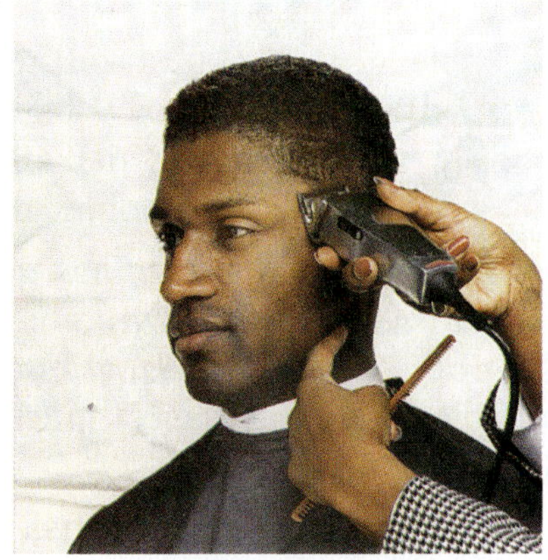

Figure 15-225 Cut the side section to the crest.

Step 3

When the back and sides are completed, open the clipper blades (one-quarter of the way for fine hair; almost one-half for thick hair) to begin blending a ¼-inch horizontal section at the point you stopped cutting at the crest. Continue cutting only the ¼-inch section from the right side, across the back, and into the left side area. Option: You may choose to stop at the center back and

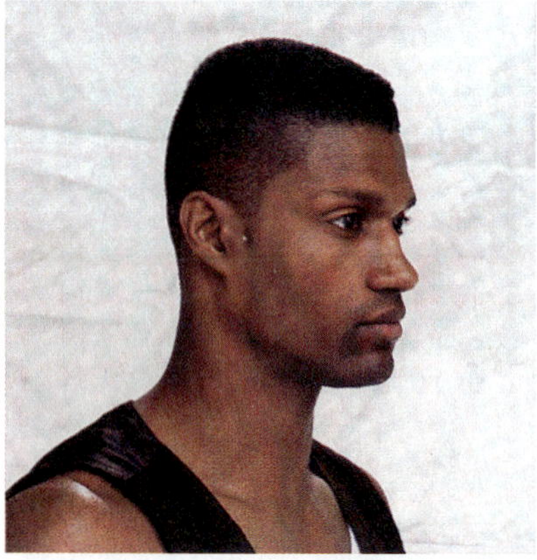

Figure 15-226 Finished fade style.

cut *from* the left side to the center back. Repeat as required to completely blend that section of the crest area around the entire head.

STEP 4

Open the blade another quarter and repeat the procedure in Step 3, cutting another ¼-inch section above the one previously cut. Repeat a third time.

STEP 5

Place a #1 guard on the clipper blades and position the lever halfway open. The guard will facilitate blending into the longer lengths of the top section. When complete, remove the guard and use a clipper-over-comb technique all around the head for final blending.

STEP 6

Layer the top section uniformly and blend with previously cut hair in the crest areas. Finish with the trimmer and/or outline shave to define the hairline (Figure 15–226).

Haircutting Procedure #9: Head Shaving

The shaved head is one of today's current fashion trends that is chosen by many men regardless of the density or growth pattern of their hair. A head shave should be performed with a changeable-blade or conventional straight razor. CAUTION: Do not adjust outliner blades flush with each other to accomplish the service instead of using a razor, as doing so may cause serious injury to the client's skin. The following is one method used to perform a head shave.

STEP 1

Examine the scalp for any abrasions, primary or secondary lesions, or scalp disorders.

STEP 2

Remove excess hair length with the clippers. Use a balding clipper blade if available. Shampoo the remaining hair and reexamine the scalp.

STEP 3

Apply shaving cream or gel and lather. Next, apply two or three steam towel treatments to soften the remaining hair.

STEP 4

Start at the back and use a freehand stroke to shave with the grain of the hair from the crown to the nape. Use the opposite hand to stretch the skin taut as needed for each area to be shaved. Follow the curve of the head, taking short strokes with the first half of the blade from its point to midsection.

STEP 5

Move in front of the client and tip his head forward slightly. Continue shaving from the crown to the front hairline, reapplying lathering agent as needed.

NOTE: Keep the skin moist to facilitate shaving.

STEP 6

When the top section is completed, work down the sides. Just below the crest, hold the ear out of the way with the left hand, finish shaving the side, and carefully shave in front of and around the ears.

STEP 7

Upon completion of the head shave, check for any missed areas. Remove remaining lather with a warm towel, apply witch hazel or toner, and follow with a cool towel application for two to three minutes.

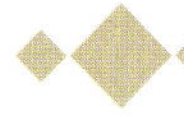

INTRODUCTION TO MEN'S HAIRSTYLING

Hairstyling is the art of arranging the hair into an appropriate style following a haircut or shampoo. Today, many haircuts require minimal hairstyling techniques due to the quality of the cuts and the availability of effective styling aids such as gels, mousses, and styling sprays. Other haircuts require more styling attention, such as blow-drying or picking the style into place. In some cases, even finger-waving techniques are used to create the final style, so it is important that barbers are versatile in all the techniques.

Blow-Dry Styling

Blow-dry styling—the technique of drying and styling damp hair in one operation—has revolutionized the hair care industry. While most men may not wish to do more than to comb the hair into place, the use of a blow-dryer offers some options for speed-drying and special-effects styling.

The main parts of a blow-dryer are the handle, nozzle, fan, heating element, speed/heat and sometimes cooling buttons. The nozzle is a directional feature that helps to direct the airstream to a more concentrated area. A diffuser attachment disperses the airflow to a larger area, creating a softer stream while still allowing the heat for drying purposes (Figure 15–227).

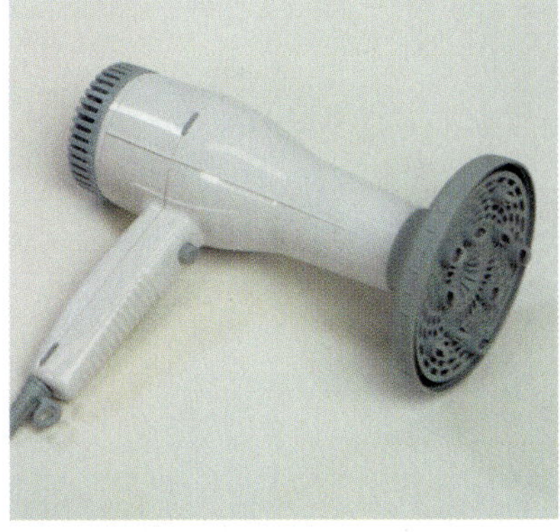

Figure 15-227 Blow-dryer and diffuser.

The implements most often used to style men's hair with a blow-dryer are combs, picks, and a variety of brushes. Some barbers prefer a narrow brush with wire or hard plastic bristles. Others prefer vent or grooming

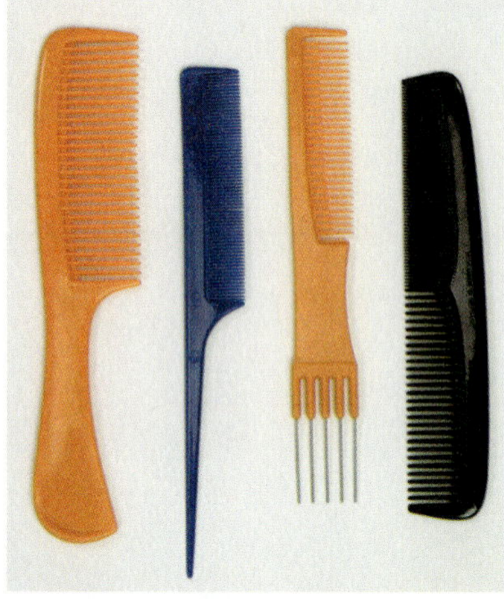

Figure 15-228 Combs.

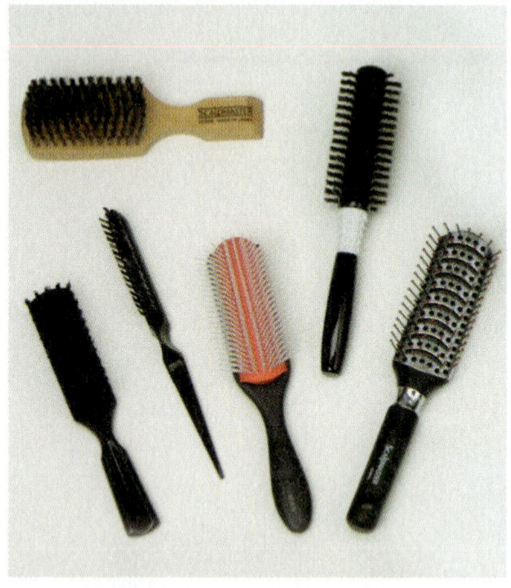

Figure 15-229 Brushes.

brushes. In most cases, the texture of the hair and the desired effect will dictate the type of implement to use (Figures 15–228 and 15–229).

There are three general blow-drying techniques used in men's hairstyling: free-form, stylized, and diffused.

Blow-Drying Techniques

Free-form blow-drying is a quick, easy method of drying the client's hair. This technique can build fullness into the style while allowing the hair to fall into the natural lines of the cut. Some barbers choose this method for the following reasons:

- It shows the client the ease with which the style can be duplicated.
- It demonstrates the quality of the haircut as the hair falls into place.
- The blow-drying service is accelerated.
- It allows the barber to check the accuracy of the work as the hair falls into place.

Stylized blow-drying creates a more styled appearance because each section is dried in a definite direction with the aid of a comb or brush. It may be performed with or without styling products applied to damp hair.

Diffused drying is used when the client desires to maintain the natural wave pattern of the hair, as opposed to temporarily straightening it with the blow-dryer and brush. Diffused drying is an effective option to use when arranging or picking out very curly hair textures, manipulating sculpting and styling products, or employing scrunching techniques.

Building Volume

Occasionally extra volume is needed in the crown, crest, or top (apex) areas of a style to create a more proportionate look. To build volume and/or to create an even contour throughout the hairstyle, use the dryer and brush in the following manner:

1. Lift the hair with a brush, bending the section as the blow-dryer is directed at the base of the section and followed through to the ends. Avoid burning the scalp.
2. Follow the same procedure to build fullness on the sides. Use horizontal partings if the hair is to be styled down on the sides and vertical or diagonal partings if the hair will be brushed back.

Practice Session #12:

BLOW-DRYING MANNEQUIN FROM PRACTICE SESSION #4

Free-Form Blow-Drying

1. After completing the mannequin haircut performed in Practice Session #4, moisten and comb the hair into the basic style.

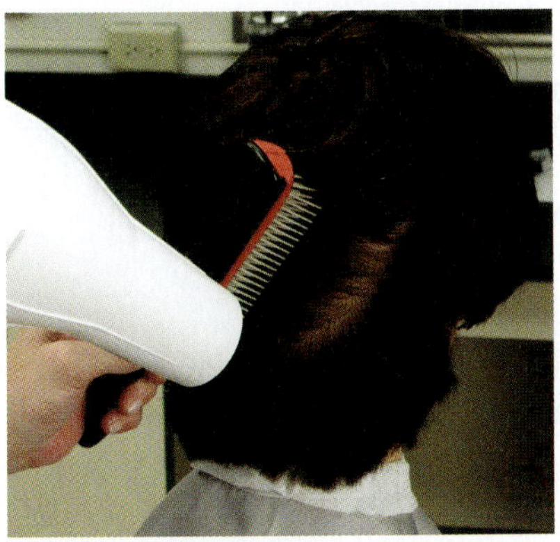
Figure 15-230 Free-form blow-drying nape and back secions.

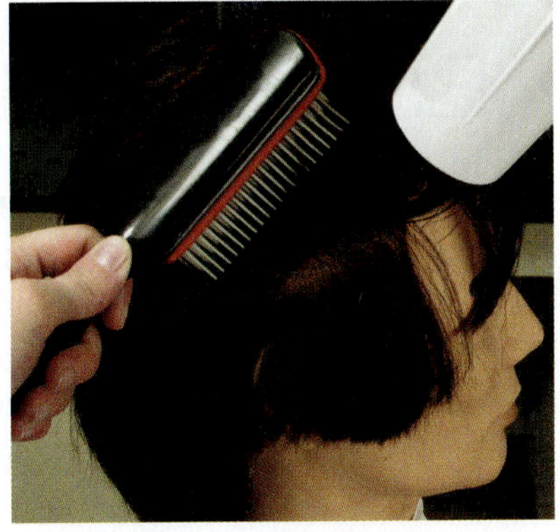
Figure 15-231 Drying the side section.

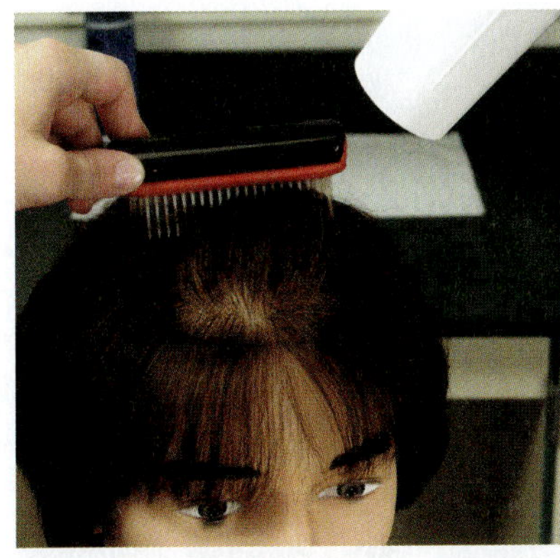
Figure 15-232 Drying the front section.

2. Hold the blow-dryer in the dominant hand. The dryer should be held 6 to 10 inches from the area being dried, at an angle with the nozzle pointing downward on the hair, and should be moved briskly from side to side as it dries the hair.
3. Beginning at the nape area, hold the hair above the hairline out of the way with a brush or comb in the opposite hand (Figure 15–230). As the hair underneath is dried, the brush or comb releases the next layered section for drying. Comb or brush the hair down after each section is dried.
4. Dry the sides in the same manner (Figure 15–231).
5. The top should be dried loosely and then brushed in to the desired style, followed by the dryer (Figure 15–232).
6. Apply different styling aids such as mousses, gels, and hairsprays to compare and contrast the effects.

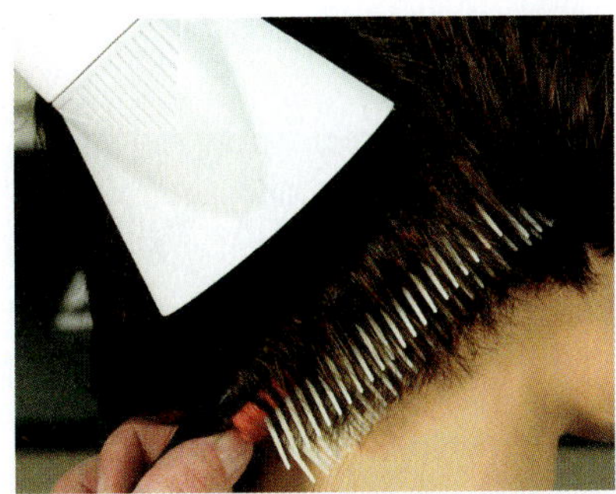
Figure 15-233 Follow the brush with concentrated heat from the dryer.

Stylized Blow-Drying

1. Remoisten the mannequin hair. Begin in the back section and lift a section of hair with the comb or brush. While combing or brushing through the parting, follow the movement with the dryer to apply a concentrated stream of heated air to the section. Repeat the process until the hair is dry in that section and continue the process with subsequent partings or sections of hair (Figure 15–233).
2. Dry the sides in the same manner.
3. To create lift or direction in the top section, work from the natural part, parting off a section with the comb or brush. Elevate for desired fullness and follow with the blow-dryer.
4. To create a definite direction in the front section, the comb or brush can be used on top of a section of hair along the hairline. Insert the comb/brush about 1½ inches from the hairline, first drawing the comb/brush a little to the back and then toward the hairline in one motion. This will create a ridge or bend in the hair that will "set it" in a different direction (Figure 15–234a). Lift the hair for volume (Figure 15–234b). Adjust the blow-dryer to hot and direct the hot air back and forth until a soft ridge has been formed. Repeat, following these instructions, for subsequent sections in the top and crest areas.
5. Apply a suitable styling aid to finish the styling service.

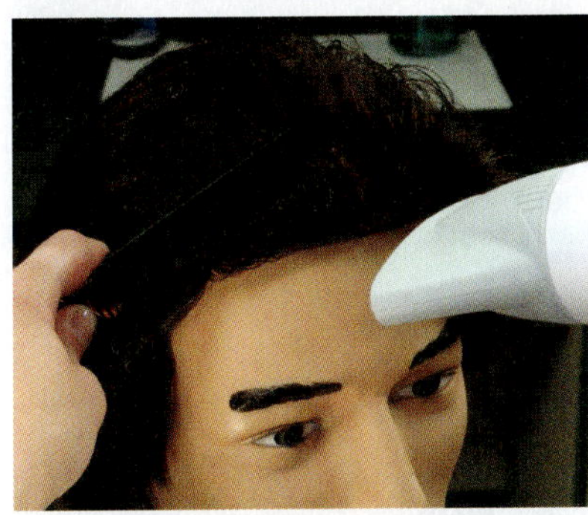
Figure 15-234a Create a ridge or bend in the hair with the comb.

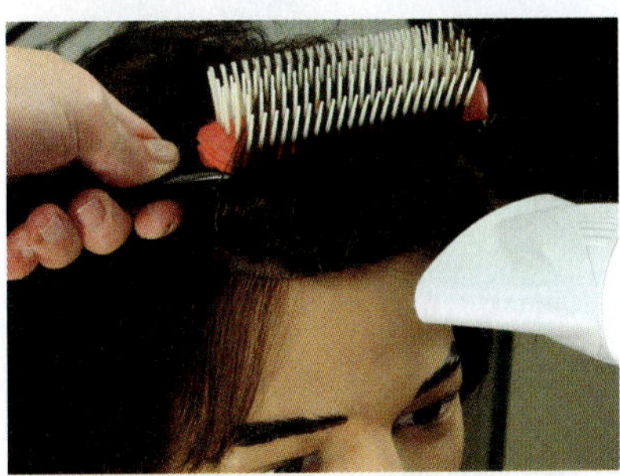
Figure 15-234b Lift the hair for volume.

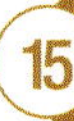

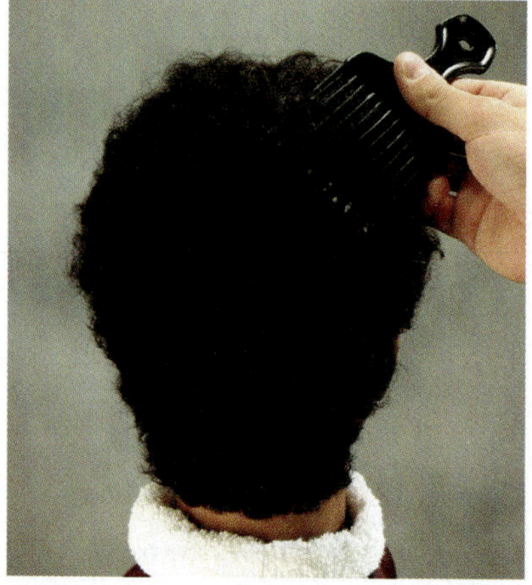

Figure 15-235 Pick out the hair.

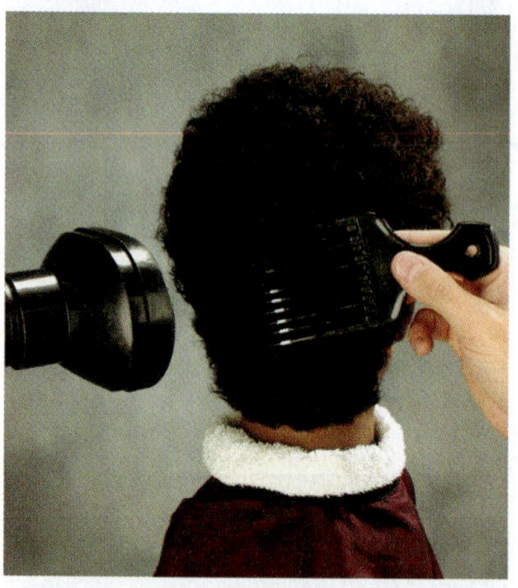

Figure 15-236 Begin drying in the back section.

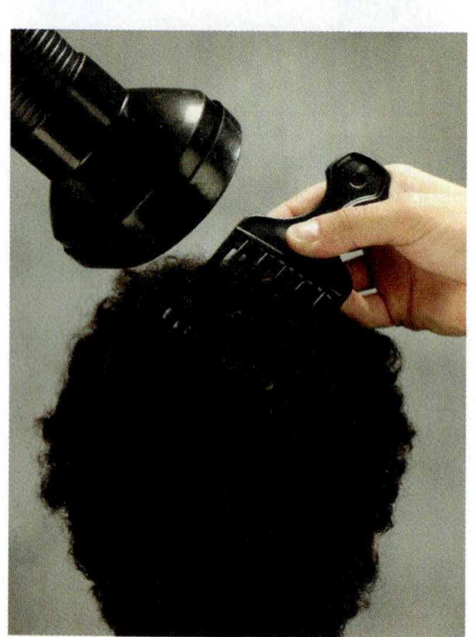

Figure 15-237 Dry top section.

Practice Session #13:

DIFFUSED DRYING WITH MANNEQUIN FROM PRACTICE SESSION #9

1. After completing the mannequin haircut performed in Practice Session #9, moisten the hair in preparation for combing or detangling.
2. Pick the hair out into the basic shape of the desired style (Figure 15–235).
3. Begin drying in the back section working toward the crown and sides. Gently pick the hair out as the dryer is moved from section to section (Figure 15–236).
4. Dry the sides in the same manner.
5. Dry the top section forward from the crown, picking the hair out as each area is dried (Figure 15–237).
6. Apply a suitable styling aid to complete the styling service.

Braids and Locks

The techniques associated with styling the hair into braids and locks is a form of *natural hair care* that originated in Africa thousands of years ago. Natural hair care has gained such popularity that an entirely new division of the hair care industry has developed. As a recognized professional segment of our industry, natural hair care is an active and exciting division that is currently involved in education, licensing, and legislative changes to meet the needs of its educators, practitioners, and clients.

Braids

While there are many variations of braids and braiding styles, *on-the-scalp cornrows* is one of the most popular styles chosen by men today (Figure 15–238). If the client has very short hair, you will be working close to the scalp across the curves of the head. The braid may begin at the nape, top, or sides depending on the desired finished result.

Figures 15–239 through 15–244 illustrate the underhand braiding method used to create cornrows.

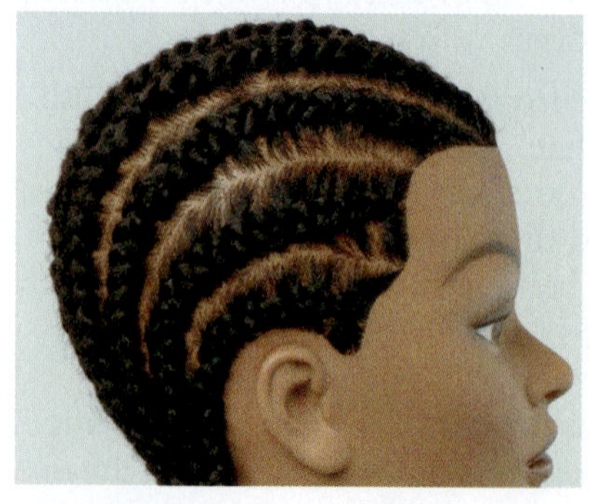

Figure 15-238 Cornrows.

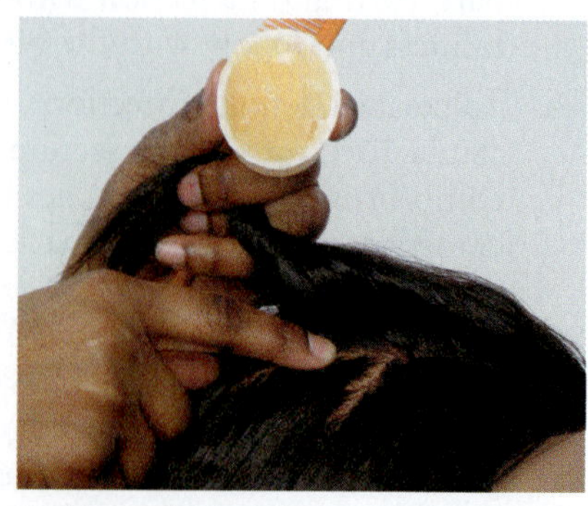

Figure 15-239 Massage essential oil through hair.

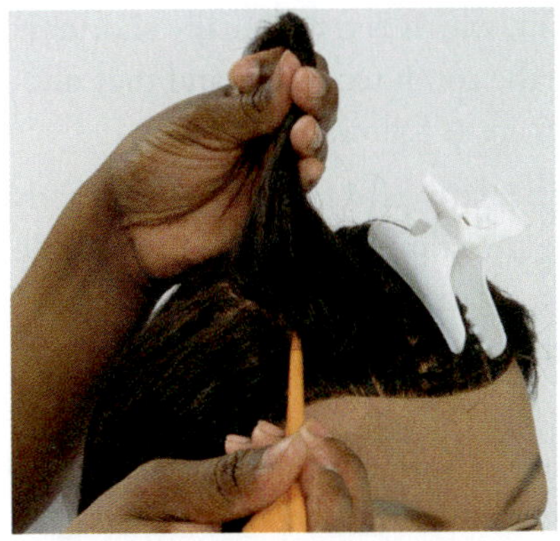

Figure 15-240 Part out a panel.

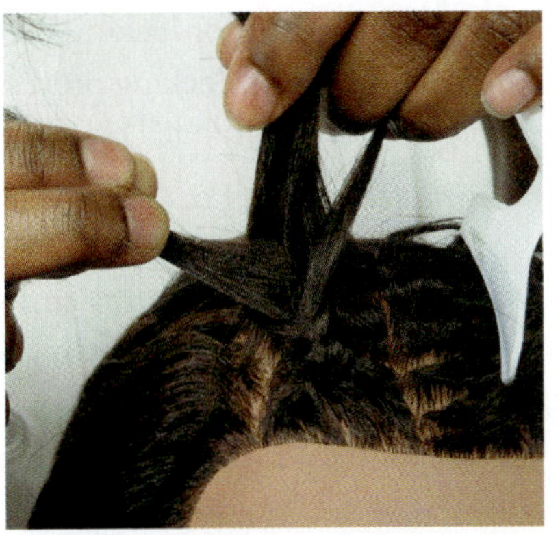

Figure 15-241 Pass left strand of hair under center strand.

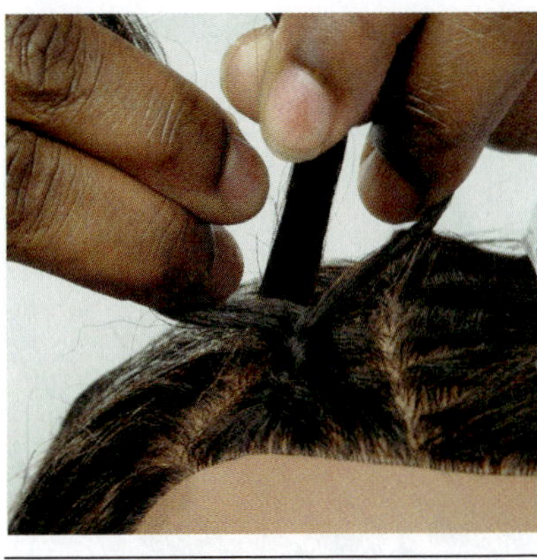

Figure 15-242 Pass right strand under center strand.

1. Apply and massage essential oil to the scalp (Figure 15–239). Determine the correct size and direction of the cornrow base. Create two parallel partings to form a neat row for the cornrow base (Figure 15–240).
2. Divide the parting into three strands. Place fingers close to the base and cross the left strand under the center strand (Figure 15–241).
3. Cross the right strand under the center strand (Figure 15–242).
4. With each crossing under, pick up hair from the base of the panel and add it to the outer strand before crossing it under the center strand (Figures 15–243 and 15–244).
5. Braid subsequent panels in the same manner. Finish with oil sheen or an appropriate styling aid for a finished look.

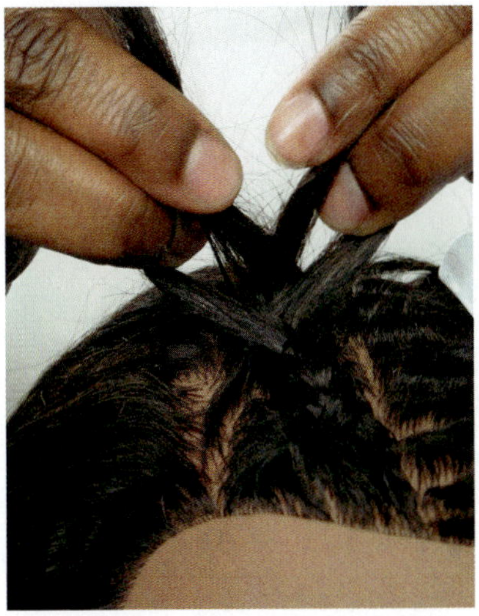

Figure 15-243 Add hair to left outer strand.

Locks

Locks, also known as dreadlocks, are created from natural textured hair that is intertwined together to form a single network of hair. **Hairlocking** is the process that occurs when coily hair is allowed to develop in its natural state without the use of combs, heat, or chemicals. The more coil revolutions within a single strand, the faster the hair will coil and lock.

Cultivated locks are those that are intentionally guided through the natural process of locking. There are several ways to cultivate locks such as twisting, braiding, and wrapping. The preferred and most effective technique is palm or finger rolling, depending on the length of the hair.

When consulting with the client who is considering locks, it is important to stress the following:

- Once locked, the locks can be removed only by cutting them off.
- The hair locks in progressive stages that can take from six months to a year to complete.
- General maintenance includes regular shop visits for cleaning, conditioning, and rerolling. Once the hair locks into compacted coils, it may be shampooed regularly and managed with a non-petroleum-based oil. Heavy oils should be avoided.

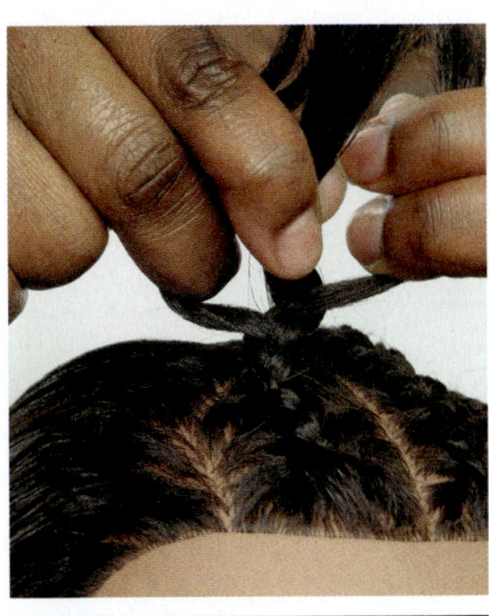

Figure 15-244 Add hair to right outer strand.

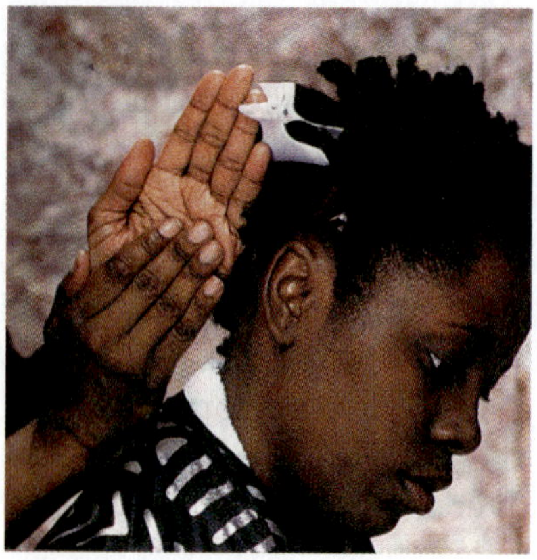

Figure 15–245 Palm rolling.

Two basic methods for locking men's hair, which is traditionally shorter at the beginning of the locking process, are the comb technique and the palm- or finger-rolling method. The procedures are as follows:

- *Comb technique.* This method is particularly effective during the early stages of locking and involves placing the comb at the base of the scalp and spiraling the hair into a curl with a rotating motion. With each revolution, the comb moves down along the strand until it reaches the end of the hair shaft.
- *Palm or finger rolling.* This method takes advantage of the hair's natural tendency and ability to coil. Rolling begins with shampooed and conditioned hair. Next, part the hair in horizontal rows from the nape to the front hairline and divide the rows into equal subsections. Apply gel to the first subsection to be rolled. Begin rolling at the nape by using the index finger and thumb to pinch the hair near the scalp; then twist the strands in one full clockwise revolution. Use the fingers or palms to repeat the clockwise revolutions down the entire strand (Figure 15–245). Maintain a constant degree of moisture by spraying with water as needed. Once all the hair has been rolled, place the client under a hood dryer set on low heat. When the hair is completely dry, apply a light oil to add sheen to the hair.

Finger Waving Men's Hair

Finger waving is the technique of creating hairstyles with the aid of the fingers, comb, waving or styling lotion or gel, hairpins or clips, and a styling hair net. The best results in developing soft, natural waves are obtained in hair that has a natural or permanent wave.

Finger waves are usually performed with styling lotion and a comb. The styling lotion makes the hair pliable and keeps it in place while creating the waves. As with other products, the styling lotion or gel should be chosen based on the texture and condition of the client's hair. A good styling lotion is harmless to the hair and should not flake after drying. Hard rubber combs with both fine and coarse teeth are recommended for the finger-waving procedure.

Practice Session #14:

FINGER WAVING USING MANNEQUIN FROM PRACTICE SESSION #4

The finger wave may be started on either side of the head. In this presentation, the work will begin on the top right side of the mannequin head.

1. The mannequin should be freshly shampooed and left damp.
2. Comb the hair and arrange it into the basic shape of the desired style. Apply styling lotion and distribute throughout the hair with the comb. Avoid using excessive amounts of styling lotion.

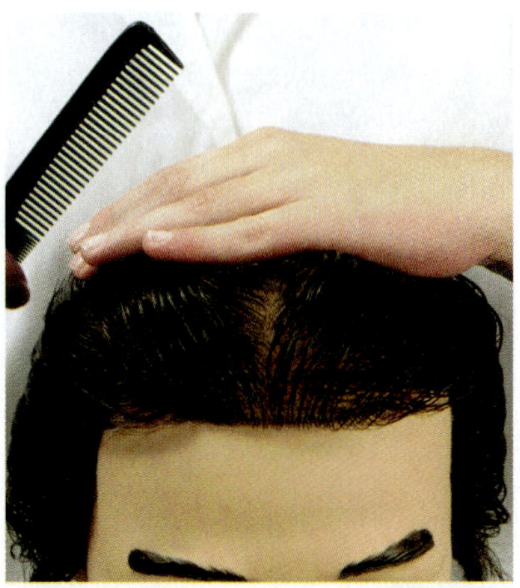

Figure 15-246 Locate the natural part line.

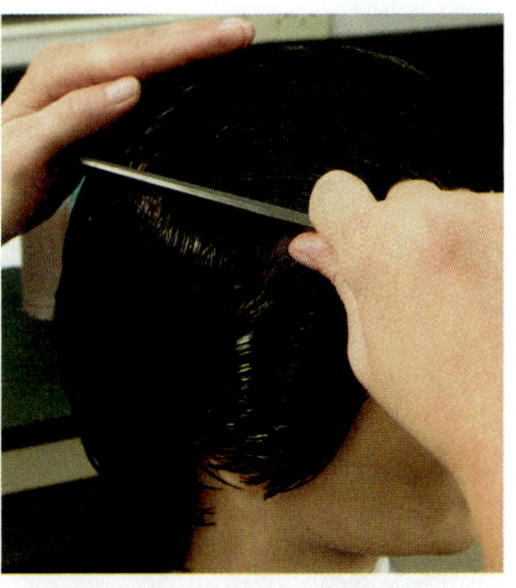

Figure 15-247 Shape top section with a circular movement.

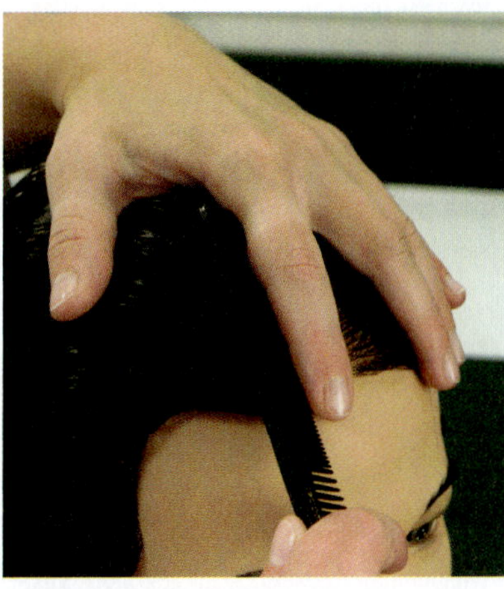

Figure 15-248 Flatten comb to hold ridge in place.

3. Locate the direction of the natural part line by combing the hair away from the face, then pushing it forward with the palm of the hand (Figure 15–246).
4. Shape the top section using a circular movement starting at the front hairline and work toward the back until the crown has been reached (Figure 15–247).
5. Place the index finger of the left hand directly above the position for the first ridge. With the teeth of the comb pointing slightly upward, the comb is inserted directly under the index finger. Draw the comb forward about 1 inch along the fingertip. With the teeth still inserted in the ridge, flatten the comb against the head to hold the ridge in place (Figure 15–248).
6. Remove the left hand from the head and place the middle finger above the ridge and the index finger on the teeth of the comb. Emphasize the ridge by closing the two fingers with pressure (Figure 15–249).
7. Without removing the comb, turn the teeth down and comb the hair in a right semicircular motion to form a dip in the hollow part of the wave (Figure 15–250). This procedure is followed section by section until the crown area has been reached. The ridge and wave of each section should match evenly without showing separations in the ridge and hollow part of the wave.
8. Form the second ridge at the front of the crown area (Figure 15–251). The movements are the reverse of those followed in forming the first ridge. The comb is drawn back from the fingertip to direct the formation of the second ridge. All movements are followed in a reverse pattern until the hairline is reached and the second ridge is completed (Figure 15–252).

   NOTE: If an additional ridge is required, the movements are the same as for the first ridge.
9. Place a net over the hair and set under hairdryer.

   NOTE: Protect the client's forehead and ears with cotton or gauze. Allow the hair to dry thoroughly.
10. Remove the hair net and comb the hair into natural waves.

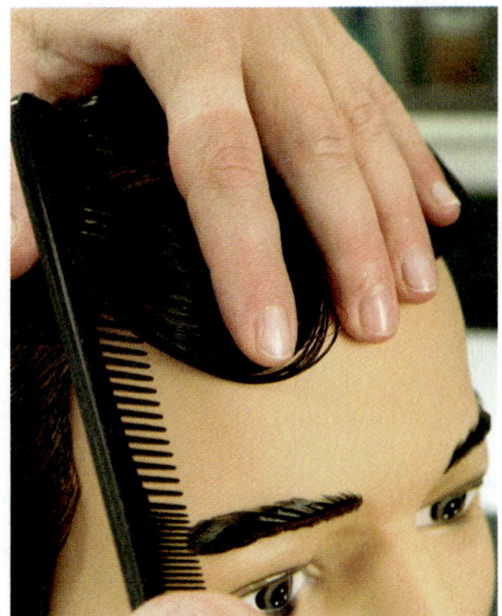

Figure 15-249 Close fingers to emphasize the ridge.

15

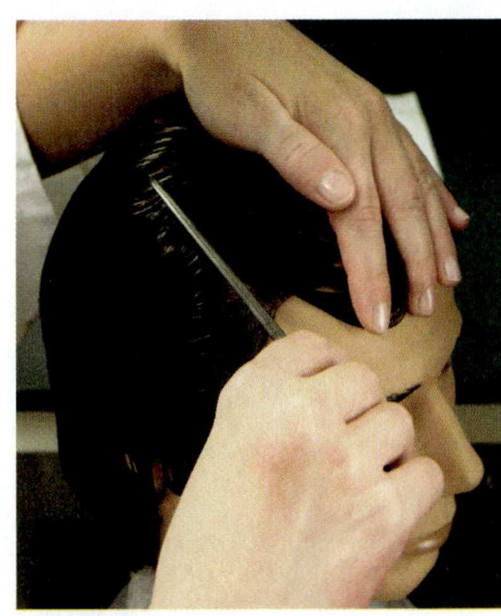

Figure 15-250 Form a dip in the wave.

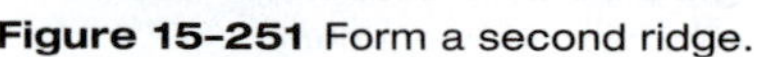

Figure 15-251 Form a second ridge.

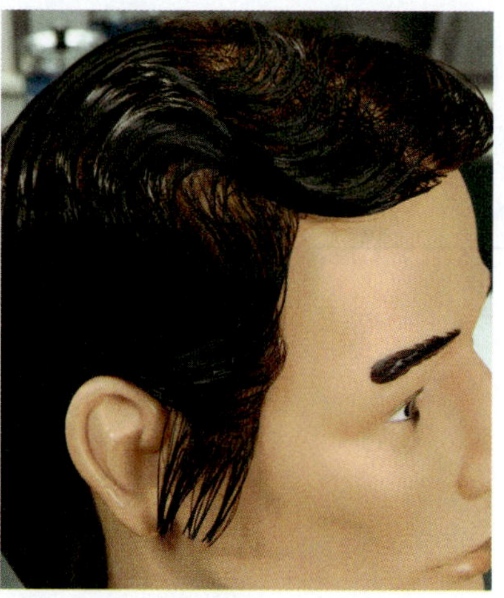

Figure 15-252 Completed second ridge.

Shadow Waving

Shadow waving is recommended for the sides, and sometimes the back of the head form. The wave is made in exactly the same manner as in finger waving, except that the ridges are kept low.

Finger-Waving Guidelines

- Avoid using excessive amounts of styling lotion.
- Locate the natural wave in the hair before beginning the finger wave.
- To emphasize the ridges of a finger wave, press and close the fingers, holding the ridge against the head with pressure.
- To create a longer-lasting finger wave, mold the waves in the direction of the natural hair growth.
- Make sure the hair is thoroughly dried before combing out.
- Use a net to protect the setting pattern while the hair is being dried.

Safety Precautions for Haircutting and Styling

- Use all tools and implements in a safe manner.
- Properly sanitize and store tools and implements.
- Avoid applying dryer heat in one place on the head for too long.
- Keep metal combs away from the scalp when using heat.
- Keep work area clean and sanitized.

chapter glossary

angle	the space between two lines or surfaces that intersect at a given point; in haircutting, the hair is held away from the head to create an angle of elevation
arching technique	method used to cut around the ears and down the sides of the neck
blow-dry styling	one-step operation for drying and styling the hair
clipper-over-comb	cutting over a comb with the clippers
crest	widest area of the head, also known as the parietal ridge, temporal region, hatband, or horseshoe
cutting above the fingers	method of holding the hair section between the fingers so that cutting can be performed on the outside of the fingers; used with horizontal or vertical 90-degree projections of hair
cutting below the fingers	method of holding the hair section between the fingers so that cutting can be performed on the inside of the fingers; used in 0- and 45-degree elevation cutting
design line	usually the perimeter line of the haircut
diagonal	lines positioned between horizontal and vertical lines
elevation	angle or degree at which a subsection of hair is held, or elevated, from the head when cutting; also referred to as projection
envisioning	the process of visualizing a procedure or finished haircut style
facial shape	oval, round, inverted triangular, square, oblong, diamond, and pear-shaped
finger waving	the process of shaping and directing the hair into a pattern of "S"-shaped waves through the use of the fingers, combs, and waving lotion
fingers-and-shear	technique used to cut hair by holding the hair into a position to be cut
freehand clipper cutting	generally interpreted to mean that guards are not used in the cutting process
freehand slicing	method of removing bulk from a hair section with the shears
guide	section of hair, located at either the perimeter or the interior of the cut, that determines the length the hair will be cut; also referred to as a guideline; usually the first section that is cut to create a shape
hairlocking	the process that occurs when coily hair is allowed to develop in its natural state without the use of combs, heat, or chemicals
horizontal	lines parallel to the horizon
layers	graduated effect achieved by cutting the hair with elevation or over-direction; the hair is cut at higher elevations, usually 90 degrees or above, which removes weight
outlining	finish work of a haircut with shears, trimmers, or razor

over-direction	combing a section away from its natural falling position, rather than straight out from the head, toward a guideline; used to create increasing lengths in the interior or perimeter
parietal ridge	widest area of the head, also known as the crest, hatband, horseshoe, or temporal region
parting	a line dividing the hair of the scalp that separates one section of hair from another or creates subsections; a subsection from a larger section of hair
projection	angle or elevation that hair is held from head for cutting
razor-over-comb	texturizing technique in which the comb and the razor are used on the surface of the hair
razor rotation	texturizing technique similar to razor-over-comb, done with small circular motions
reference points	points on the head that mark where the surface of the head changes or the behavior of the hair changes, such as ears, jaw line, occipital bone, apex, etc.; used to establish design lines that are proportionate
rolling the comb out	a method used to put the hair into position for cutting by combing into the hair with the teeth of the comb in an upward direction
shear-over-comb	haircutting technique in which the hair is held in place with the comb while the shears are used to remove the lengths
shear-point tapering	haircutting technique used to thin out difficult areas in the haircut, such as dips and hollows
stationary guide	guideline that does not move, but all other hair is brought to it for cutting
tapered	haircuts in which there is an even blend from very short at the hairline to longer lengths as you move up the head; "to taper" is to narrow progressively at one end
tension	amount of pressure applied when combing and holding a section, created by stretching or pulling the section
texturizing	removing excess bulk without shortening the length; changing the appearance or behavior of hair, through specific haircutting techniques, using shears, thinning shears, clippers, or a razor
thinning	removing bulk from the hair
traveling guide	guideline that moves as the haircutting progresses, used when creating layers or graduation; also referred to as moving or movable guidelines
vertical	lines that are straight up and down
weight line	a visual "line" in the haircut, where the ends of the hair hang together; the line of maximum length within the weight area: heaviest perimeter area of a 0-degree (one-length) or 45-degree (graduated) cut

chapter review questions

1. List the characteristics of the art of haircutting.
2. Explain what a good hairstyle should accomplish.
3. List the physical considerations that help to determine the best haircut and style for an individual.
4. Explain the process of envisioning.
5. List the haircutting areas of the head used in men's haircutting.
6. List and define the basic haircutting terms.
7. List the haircutting techniques used in men's haircutting.
8. Explain shaving the outline areas.
9. Explain why the hair should be in a damp condition for razor cutting.
10. Describe the razor rotation technique.
11. Explain the differences between free-form blow-drying and stylized blow-drying techniques.
12. Explain the braiding techniques used to create cornrows.
13. Define hairlocking.
14. Define finger waving.

with a doubled base material for increased strength and a more exact fit. Double-knotted hair in the hairpiece ensures that the hair remains intact through use and cleaning. Conversely, single-knot hairpieces may come untied during the cleaning process due to alcohol-based solvents, which can weaken the hair. Plastic or nylon-mesh bases resist shrinkage and wrinkling when cleaned in water-based solutions or shampoos.

New construction techniques with more natural-looking materials are constantly evolving in the manufacture of hairpieces. Some of the standard types of construction are as follows:

- **Wefted** hairpieces are usually machine-made. Wefts are strips of material or thread to which the hair is sewn. Most wefts are spaced for balance and proper hair distribution when sewn onto a mesh cap.
- Handmade, **hand-tied** hairpieces are costly because each hair strand is sewn in individually. These pieces are usually ventilated and comfortable to wear.
- **Lace-front** hairpieces consist of a silk gauze foundation with a lace-edged front; they are suitable for pompadour or parted hairstyles that are combed away from the face.
- **Hard-base** hairpieces are made of plastics and resins into which the hair is positioned before the material hardens. Although the hair is rooted in a specific design and direction, this style of hairpiece is less flexible than some other types.
- **Soft-base** hairpiece materials usually consist of silk gauze, nylon mesh, or plastic mesh.

Stock and Custom Hairpieces

Hairpieces are available from manufacturers and distributors in stock sizes and colors, which allows the barber to maintain an inventory of these products. Stock hairpieces can be used as samples to show prospective hairpiece clients how a toupee may look, or may be customized by the barber to fit the client.

Custom hairpieces are obviously more tailored to each client's head shape and hair replacement needs because the barber creates a pattern and color matching for the supplier to use as a guide in the production of the hairpiece.

A pattern or contour analysis should be done prior to fitting any hairpiece. This analysis will help to determine whether the client has the option of purchasing a stock product or requires a custom-made hairpiece.

Supplies for Hairpiece Services

Most barbershops will already have many of the implements and supplies required for hairpiece services (Figure 16–2). The few that may not be standard items can be obtained from a barber or hairpiece supply company. Be guided by the following checklist when purchasing hairpiece service supplies.

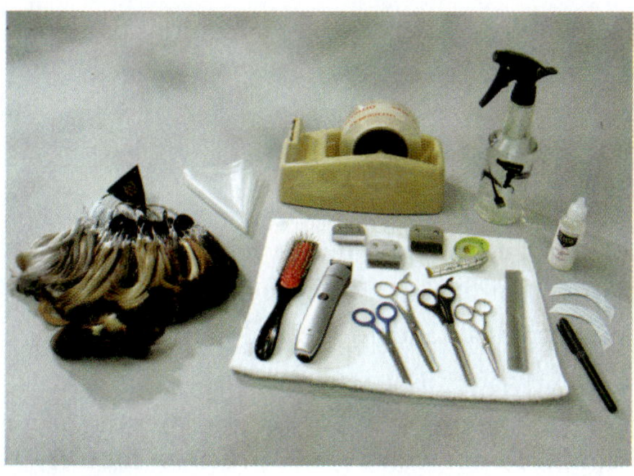

Figure 16–2 Supplies for hairpiece services.

- ☐ Acetone or remover solvent
- ☐ Alcohol
- ☐ Blow-dryer
- ☐ Client record cards
- ☐ Clippers
- ☐ Comb
- ☐ Double-sided adhesive tape
- ☐ Envelopes
- ☐ Grease pencil
- ☐ Hair net
- ☐ Haircutting shears
- ☐ Measuring tape
- ☐ Plastic wrap
- ☐ Razor
- ☐ Scissors (for cutting pattern)
- ☐ Small brush
- ☐ Spirit gum
- ☐ Styling block
- ☐ Thinning shears
- ☐ T-pins
- ☐ Transparent tape
- ☐ Wig cleaner

MEASURING FOR THE HAIRPIECE

Once the client consultation has been performed and an understanding has been reached about the type of hairpiece to be purchased, a preliminary haircut should be performed.

To achieve a natural look, the client's hair should be allowed to grow fairly long to make it easier to blend it with that of the hairpiece. When performing the *preliminary cut*, the hair should be lightly trimmed, leaving a long neckline and length close to the ears at the sides. Make sure to trim the front section as well (Figure 16–3). After the preliminary cut is finished, the longest cuttings are gathered and put into an envelope for use as a texture and color guide for the manufacturer.

The sizes of men's hairpieces are commonly measured in inches. For example, a 6-by-4-inch piece would be 6 inches long from front to back, and 4 inches wide. In the manufacturer's code, the larger number refers to the length unless otherwise indicated. Tape measurements alone can be used

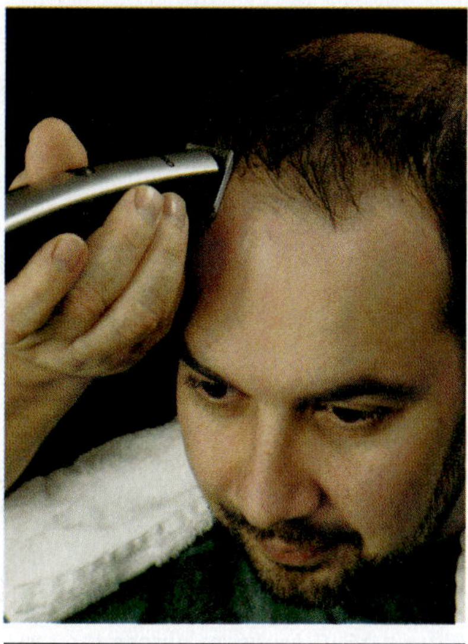

Figure 16–3 Trim the front section.

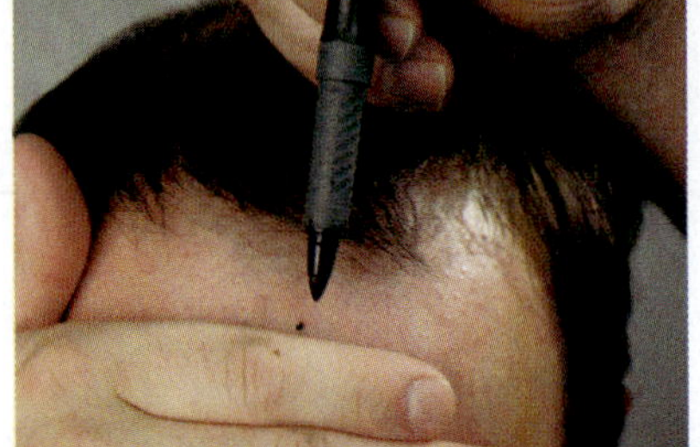

Figure 16-4 Mark the center where the hairpiece will begin.

for ordering stock hairpieces. Custom pieces, however, require a pattern of the client's head form in the area of hair loss.

Procedure for Hairpiece Pattern Making

Tape Measurement

For a front hairline to look natural, it should not be too low on the forehead. The original and natural hairline should be followed as closely as possible. The following procedure is a standard method of measuring for a hairpiece.

1. Place four fingers above the eyebrow with the last finger resting on the bridge of the nose. Make a dot with a grease pencil on the forehead directly in line with the center of the nose to indicate where the hairpiece is to begin (Figure 16–4).
2. Place the tape measure on the dot. Measure the length to where the back hair begins and mark the tape measure. Be sure to measure back to where substantial growth begins and disregard sparse hair between the forehead and bald crown areas (Figure 16–5).
3. The next measurement is across the top, directly over the sideburn. This is the place where the front hairline of the hairpiece blends in with the client's own hair at the sides of the head. Measure across the crown area if it is noticeably different from the front width (Figure 16–6). These measurements can be used to order a stock hairpiece.

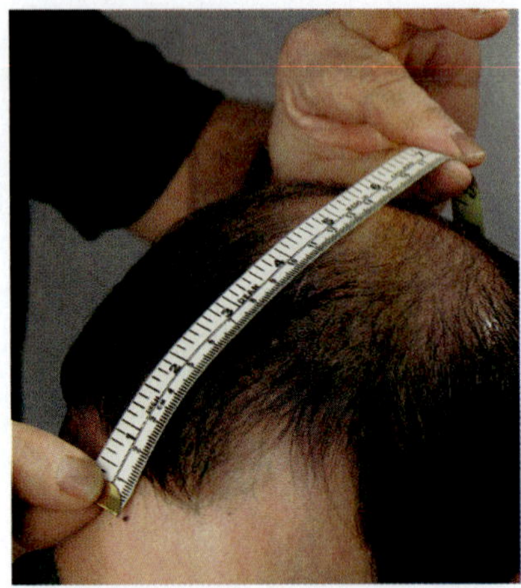

Figure 16-5 Measure from the dot to the back section.

Pattern Measurements

To create a pattern for a custom hairpiece, assemble the measuring tape, plastic wrap, 12 strips of ¾-inch transparent tape (preferably the dull-finish type for easy writing), and a grease pencil.

1. Place approximately 2 feet of plastic wrap on top of the client's head and twist the sides until they conform to the contour of the head.
2. Place three fingers above the eyebrows and make a dot on the pattern to indicate the new hairline. Place additional dots as follows:
   a) two dots on each side where the front hairline is to meet the client's own hairline

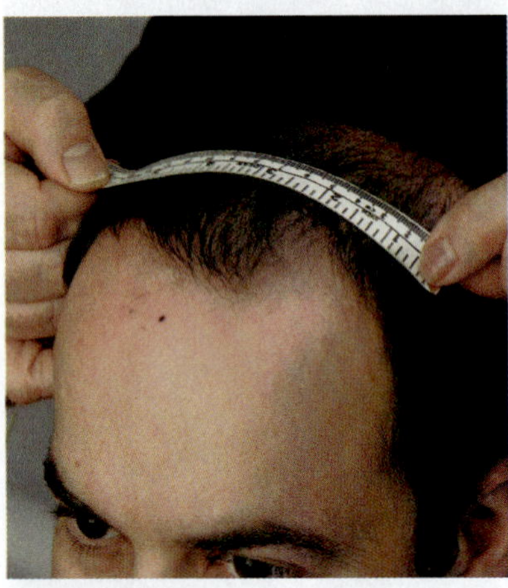

Figure 16-6 Measure across the top.

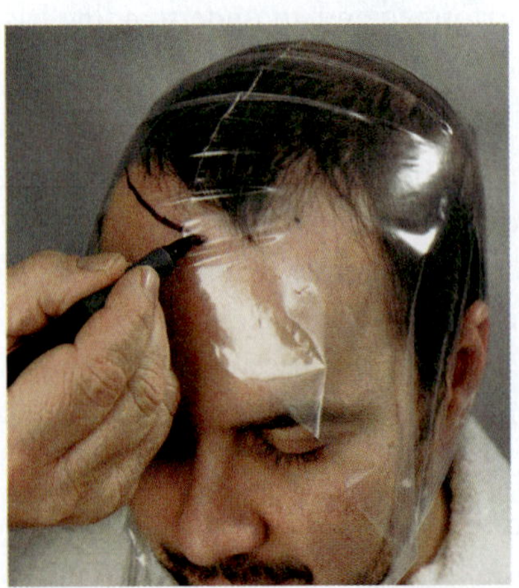

Figure 16-7 Apply plastic wrap.

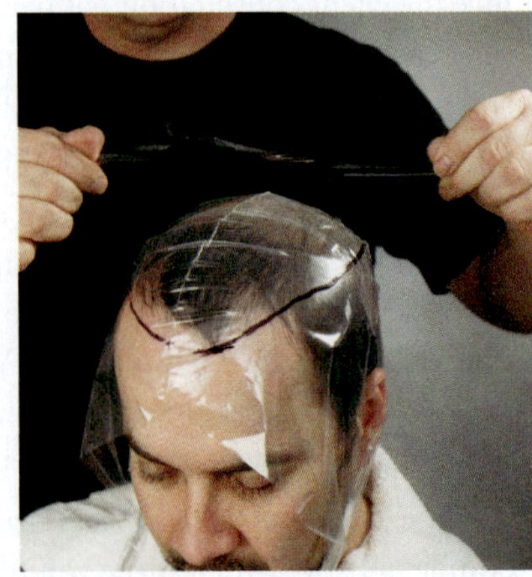

Figure 16-8 Place tape across the bald area to stiffen the pattern.

b) two dots in back of the head on each side of the balding spot

c) one dot at the center back edge of the bald spot to determine the length of the area to be covered

3. Connect the dots with a pencil to outline the balding area (Figure 16–7). Ignore minor irregularities and sparse areas.
4. While the client holds the plastic wrap, place each precut strip of tape across the bald area to stiffen the pattern and hold its shape (Figure 16–8).
5. Mark the front part of the pattern F and the back B as in Figure 16–9. Then remove and cut around the edge with scissors. After cutting the outline, replace the pattern over the balding area (Figure 16–10). Make sure the bald area is covered exactly. Although it is better to have a foundation that is slightly smaller than one that is too large, accuracy is very important.
6. Attach samples of the client's hair to the pattern or client card for color matching by the manufacturer.
7. Create a client record card (Figure 16–13), which can also serve as an information sheet when ordering stock and custom hairpieces. Send the measurements and/or pattern to the manufacturer with instructions covering the information in Figure 16-13. 3

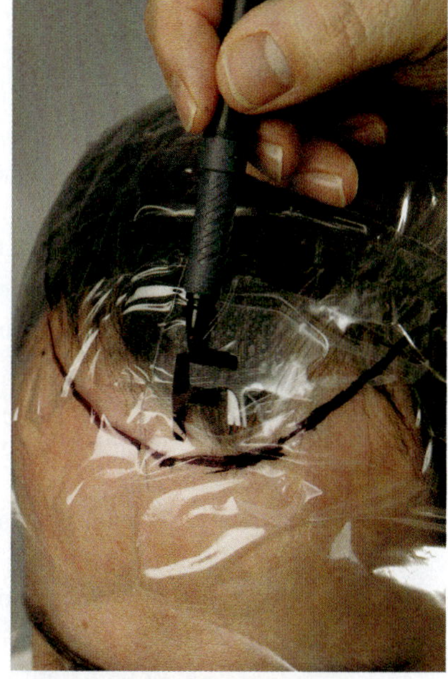

Figure 16-9 Mark the front (F) and back (B) on the pattern.

Applying a Non-Lace, Front Hairpiece

1. Before adjusting a hairpiece to the scalp, trim the front hairline and clean the entire bald area with a piece of cotton dampened with rubbing alcohol, or soap and water, then dry thoroughly.
2. Apply two-sided tape in a V-shape on the front reinforced area of the foundation (Figure 16–14). This tape holds the hairpiece close to the scalp. Place additional pieces of tape on the reinforced parts of the foundation at the sides and back of the hairpiece.
3. Place three fingers above the eyebrow to locate the hairline. Position the hairpiece at the hairline using the center of the nose as a guide. When the hairpiece is in the proper position, press down firmly on the various tape areas (Figure 16–15).

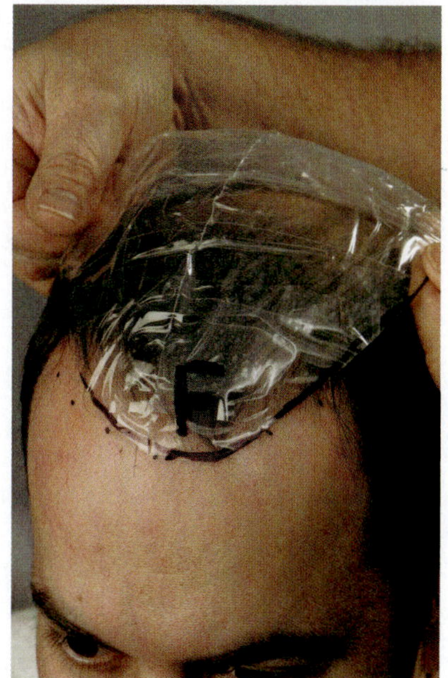

Figure 16-10 Check fit and size of pattern.

Cutting, Tapering, and Blending the Hairpiece

- *Back and sides.* When the hair is combed into the desired position, use a razor or shears to taper and blend the hair smoothly at the back of the head. Then taper and blend the sides. The tapering should be done gradually so that the blending with the client's natural hair will be undetectable.
- *Top section.* Depending on the density of the hairpiece, the fingers-and-shear method may be used to cut in the top section. Comb the hair up, bring it slightly forward, and cut. Repeat this operation as needed to blend using shears or thinning shears.
- *Blend crest with front.* Use the razor to blend the hairpiece with the natural side hair in the crest area. Cut a small amount of front hair short to soften the joining of the hairpiece with the client's hair (Figure 16–16).

1. Hairpiece without lace front (Figure 16-11)

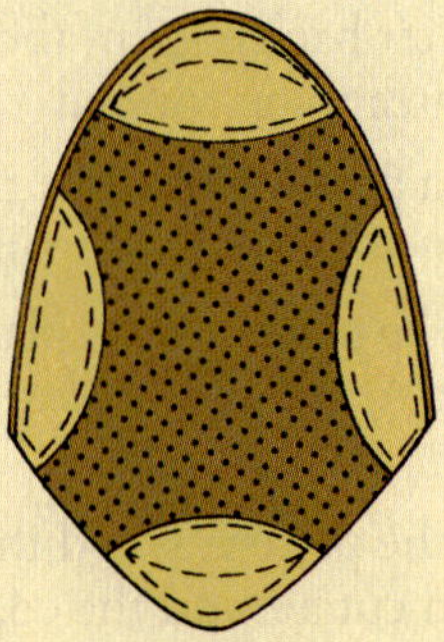

   a) Without side part ☐

   b) With left side part ☐

   c) With right side part ☐

2. Hairpiece with lace front (Figure 16-12)

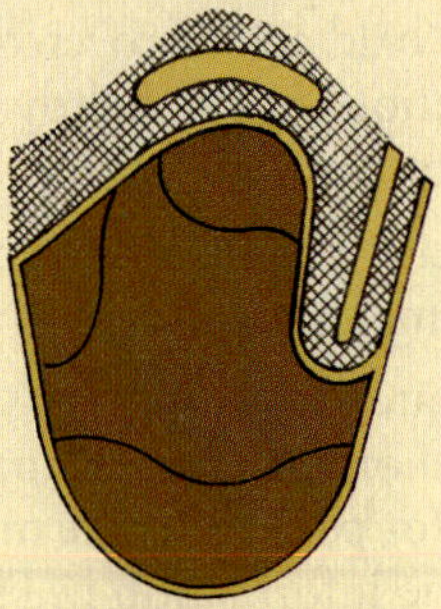

   a) With side part ☐

   b) With left side part ☐

   c) With right side part ☐

3. Hair color variations:

a) Front:	Natural	☐	Percentage of gray	☐
	Streaked	☐	Front and top lighter	☐
b) Temples:	Natural	☐	Percentage of gray	☐
c) Back:	Natural	☐	Percentage of gray	☐

4. Complexion:

   a) Ruddy: ☐

   b) Dark: ☐

   c) Light: ☐

5. Details:

   a) Partials ☐ Patches ☐ Fill-ins ☐

6. Photograph (may or may not be required by manufacturer).

Figure 16-13 Client record card.

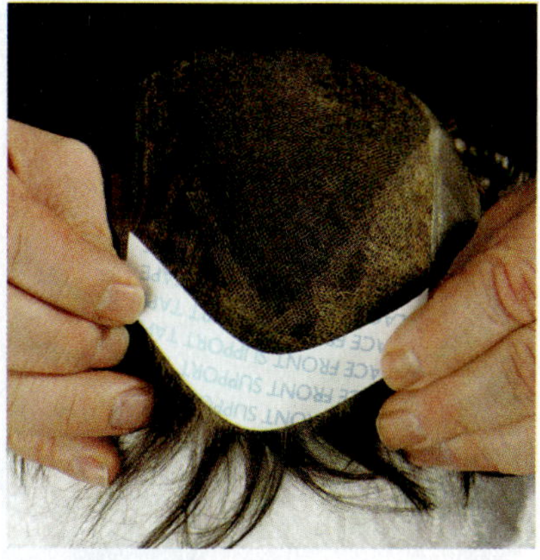

Figure 16–14 Apply two-sided tape in V-shape.

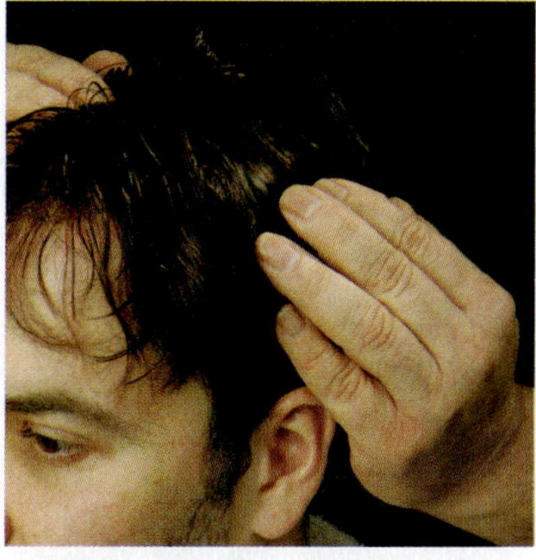

Figure 16–15 Attach the hairpiece, press down firmly on taped areas.

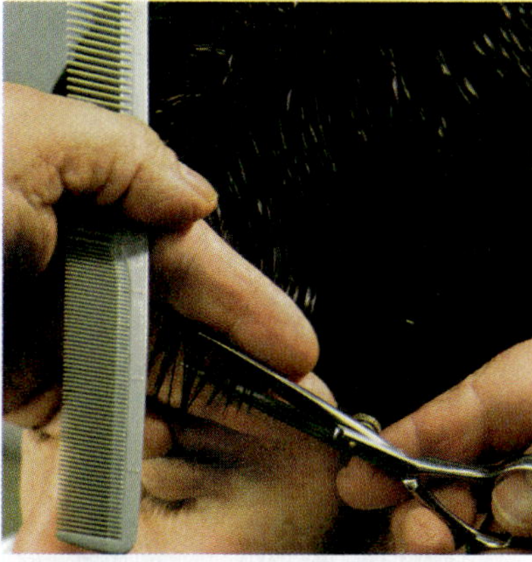

Figure 16–16 Trim front sections.

- *Thick front hairline.* If the front hairline appears heavy, use a razor for thinning. Be sure to make very narrow partings in order to form a natural-looking front hairline. To thin underneath hair, comb the hair forward and thin it with a razor. When combed back, the hair should lie flat.
- *Removing a hairpiece.* Reach up under the hairpiece with the fingertips at the front section and detach the tape from the scalp (Figure 16–17). Make sure the tape stays on the foundation so that it can be reactivated with spirit gum.

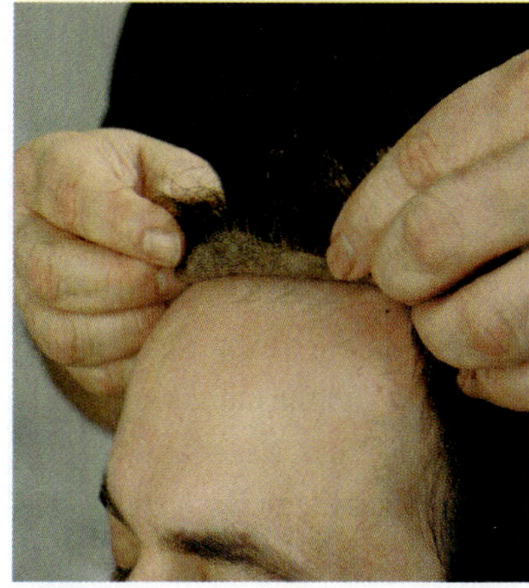

Figure 16–17 Removing a hairpiece.

Applying a Lace-Front Hairpiece

A hairpiece with a lace front is recommended when the hair is worn in an off-the-face style. It is scarcely visible from the front view and provides the required lightness for a natural-looking hairstyle.

1. Clean the bald area with rubbing alcohol or with soap and water.
2. Remove hair on the scalp where the tape or lace is to be attached (Figure 16–18).
3. Attach strips of tape (two-sided) to reinforced parts of the foundation, usually near the front, on the sides, and the back part of the hairpiece. Note that reinforced areas vary with the design of the foundation and the manufacturer's specifications. Never apply tape directly to the lace.
4. Adjust the hairpiece to the desired position using the three-finger method. Press it down into place (Figure 16–19).
5. Cut, taper, and blend the front lace hairpiece to match smoothly with the client's own hair (Figure 16–20).
6. Trim the lace to within ¼ of an inch of the hairline, or right down to the contour of the hairline, according to the client's preference.

   NOTE: The decision to trim or not to trim should be left until the hairpiece has been worn for a while. In the beginning, leave a small ¼ inch margin.

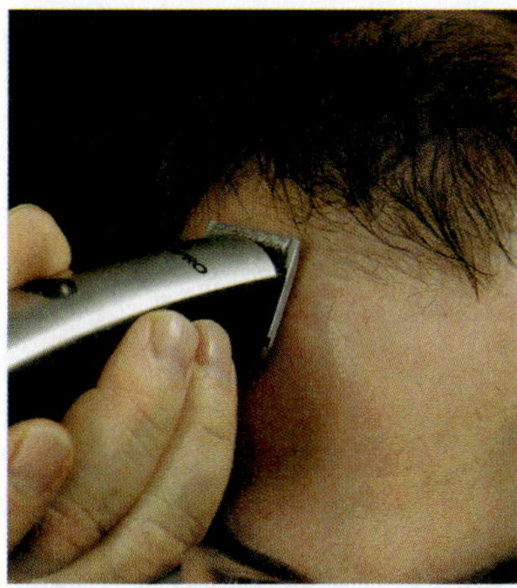

Figure 16–18 Remove hair on scalp where hairpiece will attach.

Removing a lace-front hairpiece: Before removing a lace-front hairpiece, dampen the lace with acetone or solvent in order to loosen it from the scalp

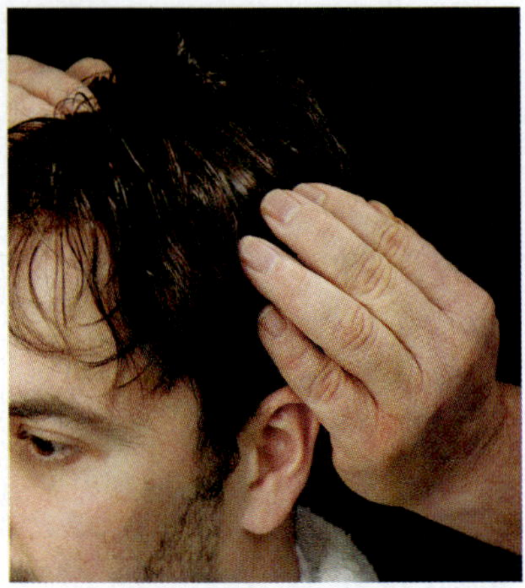

Figure 16–19 Adjust the hairpiece.

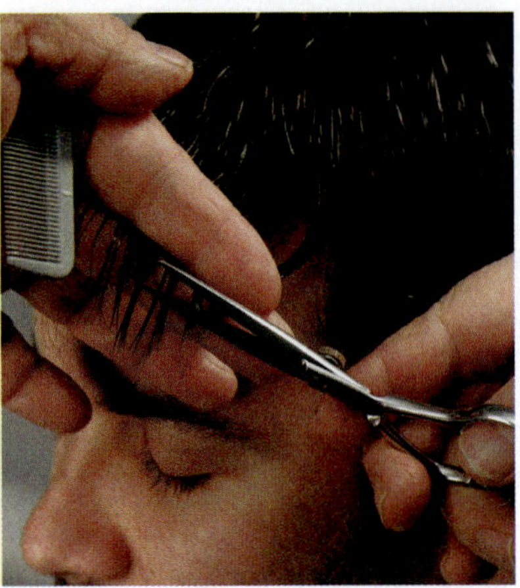

Figure 16–20 Cut, taper, and blend the hairpiece with the client's natural hair.

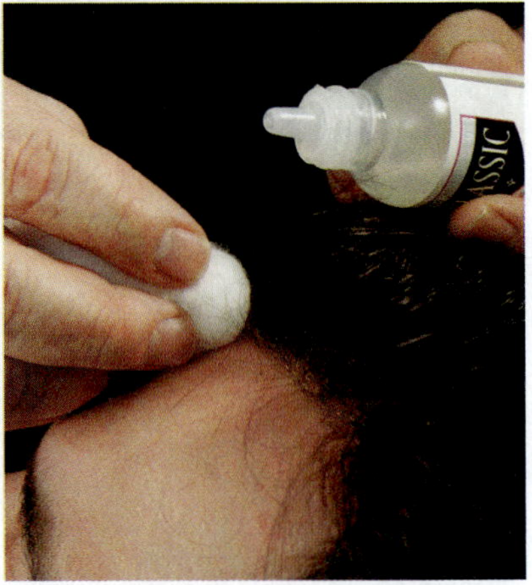

Figure 16–21 Dampen lace with solvent to remove hairpiece.

REMINDER

Reinforced areas of the hairpiece vary with the design of the foundation and the manufacturer's specifications. Never apply tape directly to the lace.

(Figure 16–21). Do not pull or stretch the lace. To apply solvent, use a piece of cotton or a brush. After the lace becomes loosened, use the fingertips to remove the tape from the scalp (Figure 16–22). Do not pull off the hairpiece by tugging on the hair. Clean the reinforced areas with a small brush dipped in acetone or other solvent.

Partial Hairpieces

For a small degree of hair loss, a partial lace fill-in may be all that is required. Partial hairpieces can be made for the front or crown areas of the head. The measuring, application, and cutting techniques are the same as those used for full-hairpiece styles. Be sure that the area to be covered is shaved to facilitate better adherence of the spirit gum and hairpiece.

Facial Hairpieces

Facial hairpieces are attached with spirit gum. Mustaches, sideburns, and beards may all be attached in the same manner. Clean the facial area and apply spirit gum to the appropriate section. Wait until the gum is tacky, position the piece, and gently press down with a lint-free cloth. Trim the piece to the desired style.

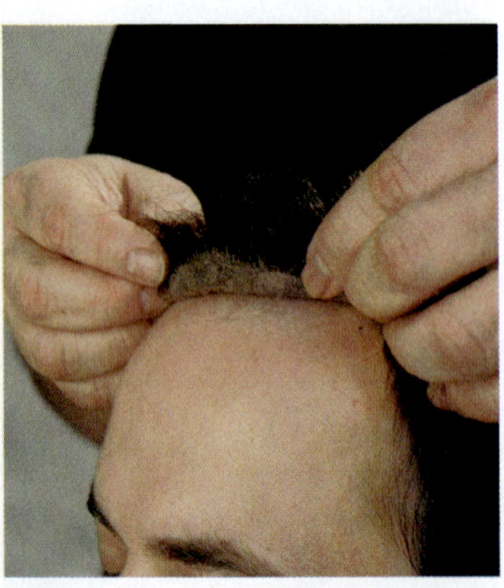

Figure 16–22 Remove hairpiece gently.

Full Wigs

While most men might not choose to wear a full wig, many women enjoy the coverage, convenience, and instant style changes they can achieve with wigs. Ready-to-wear wigs are usually made of modacrylic fibers such as Kanekalon, Dynel, and venicelon.

- *Construction and fit:* Full, ready-made wigs are constructed on a stretch cap made of lightweight elastic. The wig has permanent elastic bands at the sides designed to hold it in place. It should fit comfortably, but tightly enough to maintain its position without slipping, shifting, or lifting. Wigs come in a wide variety of colors and in many different styles.

- *Cleaning wigs:* Cleaning ready-made wigs is a fairly quick and easy process. Use the guidelines provided and the manufacturer's cleaning instructions to clean ready-made wigs.
  1. Brush the wig thoroughly to remove all surface dirt and residue.
  2. Mix a solution of warm water and mild shampoo in a bowl.
  3. Dip the entire wig into the solution; swish it around in the solution.
  4. Rinse the wig in clean, cold water.
  5. Blot it dry with a towel.
  6. Turn the wig inside out and dry it with a towel.
  7. Pin the wig to a head mold or **wig block** of the correct size.
  8. Carefully brush the hair into place.
  9. Permit the wig to dry naturally, pinned to the form.
  10. If necessary, use cool air to dry it quickly.
  11. When dry, brush it into the proper style.

CLEANING AND STYLING HAIRPIECES

With the proper care, a well-constructed hairpiece will last for years. Manufacturers furnish instructions on the care of their hairpieces that both the barber and client should follow carefully. Clients should have at least two hairpieces to ensure that one will always be in good condition while the other one is being serviced and maintained.

Cleaning Human Hair Hairpieces

Hairpieces must be kept clean just as natural hair must be kept clean. Cleaning should be performed carefully to help maintain the life of the hairpiece. Use the following guidelines and the manufacturer's recommendations to clean a hairpiece:

1. Remove all the old tape and clean any reinforced areas by dabbing them lightly with acetone or recommended solvent.
2. Put enough cleaner in a glass bowl so that the hairpiece can be submerged. Place the front of the hairpiece with the material side facing up into the solvent and allow to soak for three to five minutes. Swish the hairpiece back and forth (or dip it up and down) in the cleaner until all residue is removed from the hair and foundation.
3. With a small brush, gently tap the edge of the hairpiece until the adhesive has been removed. Do not rub or scrub.
4. If the solvent darkens, replace the cleaning agent until all residue is removed from the hair.
5. Place a towel on a flat surface and place the hairpiece with the material side facing upward on the towel.
6. Repeat the gum-removing procedure if any adhesive is left on the hairpiece.

7. If the adhesive forms a powder on the lace, place a little water on your fingertips and, in a sliding motion, allow the lace to absorb the water.
8. Gently press out the cleaner with the towel and allow to dry.
9. Fasten the dried hairpiece to the wig block with T-pins and comb out gently.
10. Set the piece in the desired style, cover with a hair net, and let it air-dry. Hairpieces may also be dried and styled with a blow-dryer while on the client's head. The scalp must be clean and dry and the hairpiece foundation thoroughly dried on a head mold before attaching it to the client's scalp. Moisten the hairpiece with a light water mist, being careful not to dampen the foundation. Style the hair as desired and cover with a styling hairnet. Use the blow-dryer on a low, warm setting to dry the hair in place.

Cleaning Synthetic Hairpieces

Synthetic hairpieces should never be cleaned in solvent. Attach the hairpiece to a plastic foam head mold with T-pins. Then immerse it in lukewarm water with a mild shampoo. Do not use hot water, which would cause the hairpiece to shrink or become matted and tangled. Swish the hairpiece around in the shampoo solution. Rinse with clean, lukewarm water. Permit the hairpiece to dry naturally, pinned on the mold overnight; if time does not permit, place it under a dryer with cool air. Some hairpieces may be dry-cleaned so always follow the manufacturer's instructions. 4

Basic Hairpiece Care

1. Use the manufacturer's tape, antiseptic, cleaner, and softeners.
2. When the hairpiece is not being worn, it should be placed on an appropriate block.
3. Some hairpieces should be removed for showering and swimming.
4. Clean the hairpiece after the first week of wear, and then every three to four weeks or as needed.
5. Never fold the hairpiece.
6. Always follow manufacturer's recommendations for removing the hairpiece.
7. Apply light hair dressings and sprays sparingly and with even distribution.
8. Set hairpieces with plain water.

Reconditioning Hairpieces

Reconditioning treatments should be given as often as necessary to prevent dryness or brittleness of the hair. Reconditioning treatments may also be used to liven up hairpieces that look dull and lifeless.

A small amount of reconditioner may be used, as directed by the manufacturer. If a slight color adjustment is necessary due to fading or yellowing, a suitable temporary color rinse is recommended. Select the rinse carefully so that the color matches that of the client's hair—be guided by your instructor.

Coloring Hairpieces

Permanent haircoloring products (aniline derivatives) can be used only on hairpieces made of 100 percent human hair. Use the following procedure and manufacturer's recommendations when coloring a hairpiece with permanent haircoloring products.

1. The hairpiece is first cleaned with a dry-cleaning solvent.
2. Cover the head form block with plastic material to prevent staining from the coloring product.
3. Secure the hairpiece firmly with T-pins or straight pins in the front, back, and sides.
4. Give a strand test on a small section of hair to determine the color desired. If using a tint with peroxide, apply it on a dry hair strand.
5. Mix the haircoloring of desired shade.
6. Apply with a haircoloring brush.
7. Comb the color product through lightly, being careful not to saturate the foundation.
8. Test every five minutes until the desired shade is obtained.
9. After processing, rinse thoroughly with warm water. Shampoo and condition according to manufacturer's directions.
10. Comb and set into the desired style.

Permanent Waving Hairpieces

Permanent waving a hairpiece requires time, creativity, and careful attention to detail. The objective is to create a natural look, so the hairpiece should be custom wrapped according to the contours of the head and the flow of the hair sewn into the hairpiece.

The rod placement does not rest on the scalp of the hairpiece as it would in a perm procedure on natural hair. Instead, the rods are *floated* to eliminate weight and rod marks on the base. Floating is accomplished by using T-pins to support the rod above the base of the hairpiece. The pins are inserted at both ends of the rod and are held in place by the rubber band of the perm rod. When the hairpiece has been rodded and secured with the T-pins, the procedure for completing the perming process is as follows:

1. Select a mild permanent wave solution appropriate for bleached or damaged hair types. Hold the wig block upside down and rotate while applying the solution. Allow the excess solution to drip into the sink before setting the block back on the stand.
2. Take a test curl every minute until processing is complete.
3. Rinse the hairpiece for 10 to 15 minutes. The hairpiece will be air neutralized and does not require the application of a neutralizing solution.
4. Thoroughly blot each rod with paper towels to absorb as much water as possible.
5. Remove the T-pins and hang the block upside down. Leave the rods in the hairpiece and cover with a plastic cap for 24 hours.
6. On day two, remove the cap and allow the piece to dry for another day. Remove the rods only when the hair is completely dry.

General Recommendations and Reminders

1. Comb hairpieces carefully to avoid matting, loss of hair, or damage.
2. Use a wide-tooth comb to avoid weakening or damaging the foundation.
3. Never rub or wring cleaning fluids from the hairpiece. Let it dry naturally.
4. Be careful not to cut too much hair when cutting, tapering, and blending a hairpiece.
5. Take accurate measurements to assure a comfortable and secure fit.
6. Recondition hairpieces as often as necessary to prevent dryness, brittleness, or dullness of the hair.
7. If required by the manufacturer, dry-clean hairpieces before styling.
8. Brush and comb hairpieces with a downward movement.
9. To avoid damage to the foundation never lighten or cold-wave a hairpiece.
10. If coloring is necessary, it must be done with care.

Selling Hairpieces

In order to sell men's hairpieces, it is important to know why men buy them. In the first part of this chapter, the results of a study concerning the perceptions of bald and balding men were discussed. When a man expresses an interest in wearing a hairpiece to his barber, he won't appreciate a hard-sell approach. His interest has already been made evident and he is simply looking for guidance and purchasing information at this stage. It is the barber's responsibility to educate the client about the possibilities and options available to him.

Just as a hard-sell approach should be avoided, the barber should never promise what cannot be delivered nor raise the client's expectations to an unreasonable level. For example, it is not professionally ethical to convince an elderly man that he can recapture the appearance of his 40s with a hairpiece. It simply cannot be done. The color of the hairpiece is also an important consideration. Dark opaque colors are not recommended for any age group, especially older persons. It is better to recommend a salt-and-pepper blend or medium-brown shade. The more natural looking the color, the less obvious the hairpiece will appear.

Marketing Techniques

- *Hairpiece display:* One or two correctly styled hairpieces displayed in the shop will alert clients to the fact that hairpiece services are performed there. Make certain that the sample is clean and nicely styled. It should be large enough to cover the average balding area of a man, since most clients will be men with an average amount of hair loss, and many may want to try it on.

  NOTE: Be sure to sanitize the hairpiece after each client.

- *Referrals and word-of-mouth:* These two methods may be a slower approach, and not to be relied on exclusively for new business, but they are still very effective forms of advertising. Personal referrals are the best evidence of pleased and satisfied clients.

- *Window displays:* Window displays can add to increased hairpiece sales. Before-and-after illustrations in the shop window let the walk-by and drive-by traffic know that hairpieces can be obtained through the barbershop. It can also offer encouragement to those clients whom you feel cannot be approached directly with the idea of wearing a hairpiece. As they become more comfortable with the idea of a hairpiece, or see other men in the shop receiving hairpiece services, they may feel more inclined to explore their own options.
- *Personal approach:* The personal approach may certainly be used to suggest a hairpiece to a client; however, it must be tactful approach. Wait for an opening during the consultation or haircut service when the client brings up his hair loss condition in the conversation and offer him the opportunity to try on a hairpiece. A quick demonstration may convince him of his improved appearance and lead to a sale.
- *Print ads:* Print ads include all printed advertising, from coupons to billboards. It is important to advertise hairpiece services because not all barbershops pursue this market. In many areas an extra line in the telephone book that mentions hairpieces will pay for itself. Your phone book also may contain a special listing for hair goods. This is another good classification in the phone directory to place an advertisement.

  In some communities, newspaper advertising is inexpensive and profitable. If a model is used, be sure to secure a model release for any photos that might be used in the ads. Even if the model is your best friend, do not assume that a release is unnecessary.
- *Personal experience:* If you wear a hairpiece yourself, you can develop an excellent promotional approach. Often, nothing is more convincing than your own before-and-after demonstration. The fact that you wear a hairpiece with assurance and complete ease can make a very strong impression on prospective hairpiece clients. 5✓

16

ALTERNATIVE HAIR RESTORATION TECHNIQUES

In addition to hairpieces, there are three other approaches to hair replacement available for men. The first are medicinal drugs known as *minoxidil* and *finasteride*, which are known by different brand names depending on the manufacturer. The second is surgery, which includes procedures such as hair transplantation, scalp reduction, and flap surgery. A third option is the hair weave.

A 2 percent solution of minoxidil applied twice daily has been shown to be moderately effective for about 50 percent of the men using it. Clinical studies conducted by Pharmacia and Upjohn (the maker, recently acquired by Pfizer, of the Rogaine brand minoxidil) revealed that 26 percent of the men reported average to dense hair growth and 33 percent minimal hair growth after four months of treatment with Rogaine. Minoxidil is available for both men and women and in two different strengths: 2 percent regular and 5 percent extra-strength formula.

FYI

As mentioned in Chapter 11, finasteride is an oral prescription medication for men only that provides men with an additional hair replacement option. Although it is considered more effective and convenient than minoxidil, its possible side effects include weight gain and loss of sexual function.

The three types of surgical hair restoration available are hair transplants, scalp reduction, and flap surgery.

- **Hair transplantation** is strictly a medical procedure that should be performed only by licensed medical professionals. The process consists of removing hair from normal areas of the scalp, such as the back and sides, and transplanting it into the bald areas under a local anesthetic. Small sections of hair from single strands to larger plugs of 7 to 10 hairs are surgically removed, including the hair follicle, papilla, and hair bulb, and reset in the bald area. With today's technological advances in hair restoration, micrographs have replaced the larger "plug" sections of the past few decades. The transplanted hair usually grows normally in its new environment while the area from which the hair was removed heals and shrinks in size to a very tiny scar.

  The surgeon must select the hair to be transplanted with care, taking into consideration color, texture, and type. Placement of the hair in the direction of natural growth to permit proper care and complimentary styling is also an important factor. Transplanted hair can last a lifetime if the service is performed properly. If the doctor is skilled and the individual cares for the hair as directed, hair transplants can be very successful as a method of permanently eliminating baldness.
- **Scalp reduction** is a process by which the bald area is removed from the scalp and surrounding scalp areas with hair growth are pulled together to fill in the spot.
- **Flap surgery**, like scalp reduction surgery, removes the bald scalp area. A flap of hair-bearing skin is then attached to what was the bald area.

The use of hair **weaves**, a form of nonsurgical hair replacement, has been practiced in barbershops for many years. While there are numerous claims of new techniques and exclusive methods in hair weaving, the usual procedure consists of sewing or weaving a foundation onto the remaining hair at the scalp, and then weaving wefts of human hair to the foundation.

Since the foundation is attached to the remaining hair on the head, the foundation tends to move out from the scalp as the natural hair grows. Continual adjustments are required to maintain the desired appearance. The foundation must be tightened and brought close to the scalp every four to eight weeks depending on the rate of natural hair growth. The hair must be shampooed carefully in sections to avoid pulling and causing damage to the foundation or pain to the client. And, as with natural hair, it should receive periodic conditioning treatments to add luster and to avoid dryness and damage. 6

chapter glossary

flap surgery	a surgical technique that involves the removal of a bald scalp area and the attachment of a flap of hair-bearing skin
hair transplantation	any form of hair restoration that involves the surgical removal and relocation of hair plugs, including scalp reduction and flap surgery
hairpiece	any small wig used to cover the top or crown of the head and integrated with the natural hair
hand-tied	handmade hairpieces in which each hair strand is sewn in individually
hard-base	a hairpiece base made of plastics or resins
lace-front	popular hairpiece style used for off-the-face styles
minoxidil	topical medication used to promote hair growth or reduce hair loss
root-turning	sewing hair into a hairpiece in the direction of natural growth, with the cuticle scales flowing in the same direction
scalp reduction	the surgical removal of a bald area, followed by the pulling together of the scalp ends
soft-base	hairpiece foundation made from silk gauze, nylon mesh, or plastic mesh
toupee	small hairpiece used to cover the top or crown of the head
weaves	a variety of methods by which strands of hair are sewn or tied into natural hair
wefted	strips of human or artificial hair woven by hand or machine onto a thread
wig block	head-shaped form of canvas-covered cork or plastic foam, to which a hairpiece is secured for cleaning and styling

chapter review questions

1. Explain why some men might choose to wear a hairpiece.
2. List three types of hair that are used to make men's hairpieces.
3. List the steps to measuring for a hairpiece.
4. List and describe five types of hairpiece bases.
5. List the steps to cleaning a human hair hairpiece.
6. List eight basic procedures associated with hairpiece care.
7. List three methods of surgical hair restoration.

part 4

ADVANCED BARBERING SERVICES

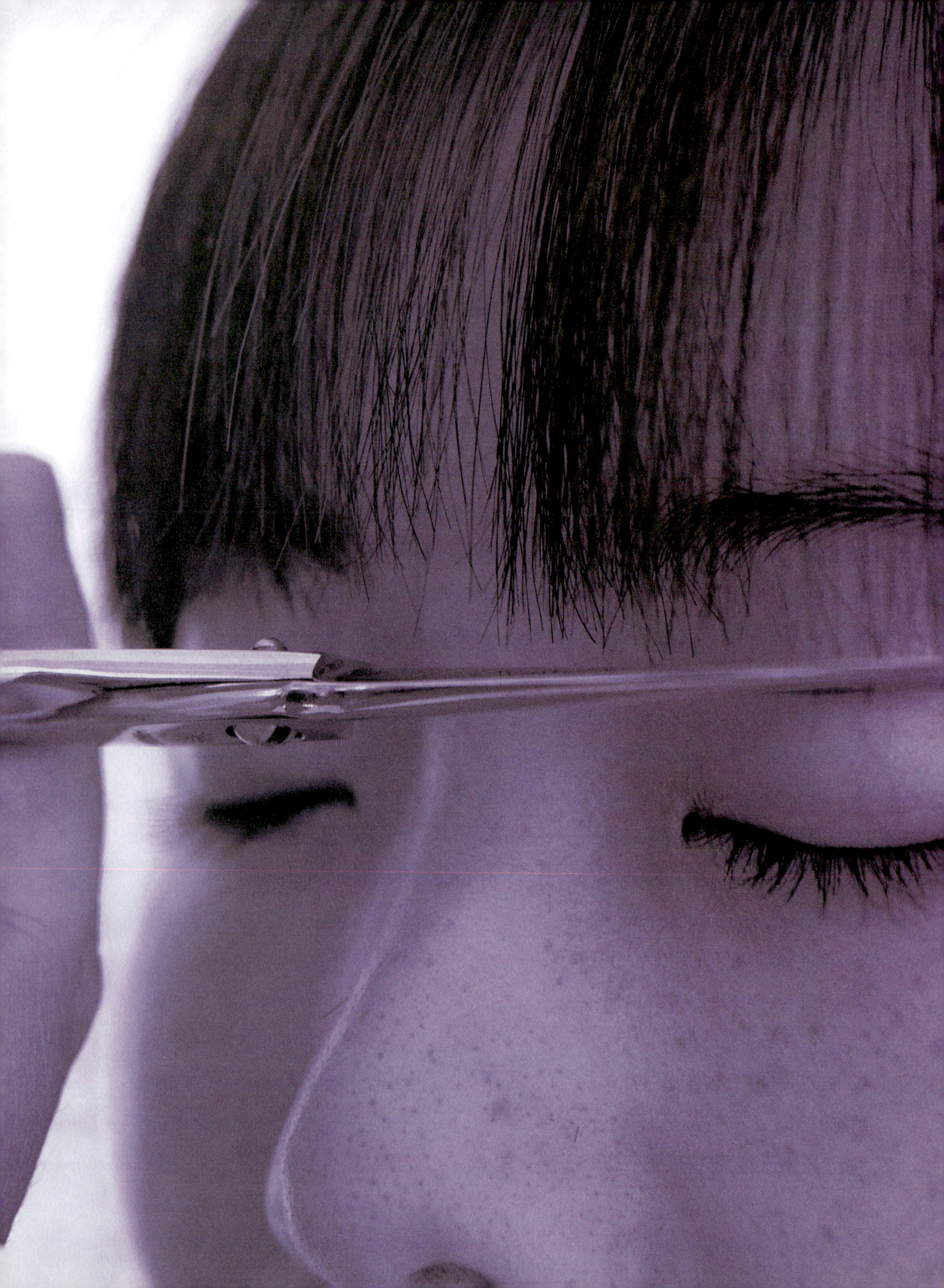

WOMEN'S HAIRCUTTING AND STYLING

Chapter Outline

Learning Objectives

After the completion of this chapter, you should be able to:

1. Perform four basic women's haircuts.
2. Demonstrate mastery of texturizing techniques.
3. Perform basic wet styling techniques.
4. Perform blow-dry styling techniques.
5. Perform thermal curling and straightening techniques.

Key Terms

base
pg. 476

blow-dry styling
pg. 470

blunt cut
pg. 447

circle
pg. 476

curl
pg. 476

graduated cut
pg. 452

hair pressing
pg. 479

half off-base
pg. 476

long layered cut
pg. 459

off-base
pg. 476

on-base
pg. 476

stem
pg. 476

thermal styling
pg. 476

uniform layered cut
pg. 452

In general, the concept of a barbershop infers a male domain. However, many women have been known to seek the haircutting services of a barber rather than visit the local beauty salon. It seems that no matter how traditional the atmosphere or the clientele of the barbershop, invariably a woman will walk in and request a service. Maybe she likes the way her husband's or son's hair has been cut, or perhaps she wants a precisely blended short, tapered cut. In either scenario, the professional barber should be willing and able to accommodate the request.

Other types of shops, such as unisex salons, maintain a fairly equal ratio of male to female clientele. In this environment, barbers must be proficient in cutting and styling women's hair as well as men's. Should you choose to work in a shop or salon that provides services to both men and women, embrace it for the learning experience it is and the enhanced effect it can have on your professional future.

In Chapter 14, you learned the basic foundations of haircutting and styling men's hair. This chapter will assist you in transferring that knowledge and application to the performance of women's cuts and styles. For the most part, the same terminology will be used to accomplish the four basic haircuts in this chapter. These include the blunt cut, graduated cut, uniform layered cut, and the long layered cut.

Since women's hairstyles do not usually end with the haircut, this chapter will also introduce some basic styling techniques for women's hair. Styling women's hair tends to be a more involved process than styling men's hair and includes techniques such as wet setting, finger waving, pin curls, hair wrapping, and thermal styling. This chapter addresses only those techniques that can be accomplished using a blow-dryer, thermal iron, or hair-wrapping method. For information and procedures regarding wet setting, finger waving, and pin curls refer to Chapter 12, Hairstyling, in *Milady's Standard Cosmetology* textbook.

BASIC HAIRCUTTING

Most men's haircuts are completed with very little styling or arranging beyond combing the hair into place. Conversely, most women's styles require styling and more finish work for optimum results. While some women prefer a "wash-and-wear" kind of style, the majority still choose a style that requires some form of daily arranging with a blow-dryer, curling irons, or other tools.

One of the main differences between cutting women's hair and cutting men's hair is that men's cuts usually appear more angular whereas women's cuts may be more rounded and soft-looking. This is important to keep in mind, especially when sculpting short hairstyles for women. Just because the hair is short doesn't mean that it has to look masculine. Points and curves along the design line versus straight horizontal lines will soften the look of a woman's short cut. Styling also plays an important role in the final look of a short haircut. A little wave, some soft feathering directed toward the face, height in the crown, or wisps at the neckline all help to soften the look of a short haircut design. Remember to visualize the finished cut and style before beginning the service.

General Haircutting Reminders

- Start with clean and conditioned hair.
- Pay attention to the head position.
- Pay attention to your body position.
- Pay attention to your finger placement. Comb through and practice the finger placement you will use before actually cutting the hair.
- Take consistent and clean partings to produce more precise results.
- Keep the hair moist when cutting.
- Work with natural growth patterns.
- Use consistent tension.
- Always work with a guide or guideline. If you cannot see the guide, don't cut! Take a thinner parting or reverse the procedure until reaching a visible guide.
- Use the mirror to check length and proportion. It is one of your most important tools.
- Plan for the shrinkage factor that results when the hair dries or when cutting wavy and curly hair textures.
- Always check and crosscheck your work.

The art of haircutting is made up of variations and combinations of four basic haircuts: blunt, graduated, uniform layers, and long layers. As with men's haircutting, a variety of elevations (Figure 17–1) and hand positions are used to create these effects. Review Chapter 15 if necessary.

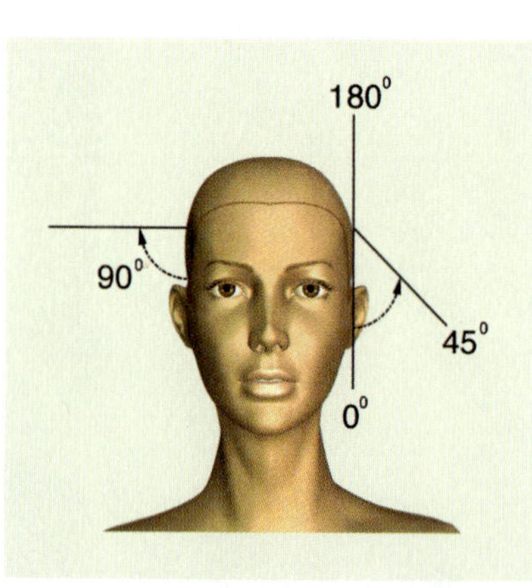

Figure 17-1 Cutting elevations.

THE BLUNT CUT (0 DEGREE)

The **blunt cut** is also known as a *one-length cut* because all the hair ends at one hanging level to form a weight line at the perimeter. Blunt cuts *look* like all the hair is the same length, but the hair is actually shorter underneath, with each subsequent parting being longer as it travels over the curves of the head to reach the weight line. The head should be held in an upright position to avoid shifting the hair out of its natural fall position. If the head is positioned forward, graduation will be created within the cut. The design line at the perimeter may be cut to reflect horizontal, convex, diagonal forward, or diagonal back lines (Figures 17–2 to 17–4). Figure 17–4 illustrates the *technical pattern* of a blunt cut with a diagonal forward design line.

Haircutting Tips for Blunt Cuts

- Shampoo and condition hair before cutting.
- Maintain uniform moisture while cutting.
- Work with the natural growth patterns of the hair.
- Keep the client's head upright and parallel to the floor.
- Take clean partings and subsections.
- Comb through the subsections twice from scalp to ends before cutting and cut parallel to the part.
- Follow the comb with the fingers to maintain control of the hair parting.
- Cut with uniform minimal to moderate tension, depending on hair texture and elasticity.

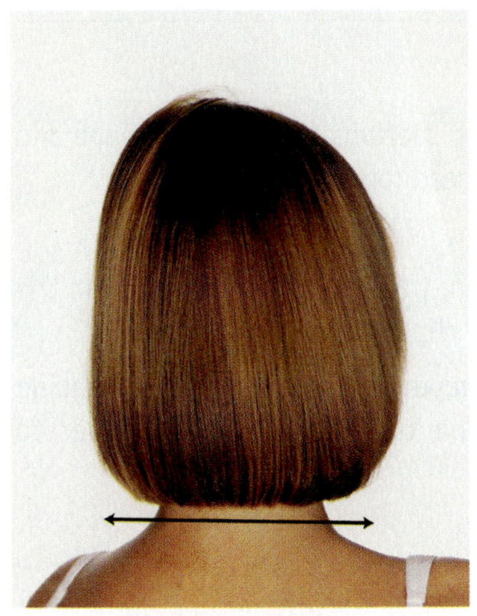

Figure 17-2 Horizontal blunt cut.

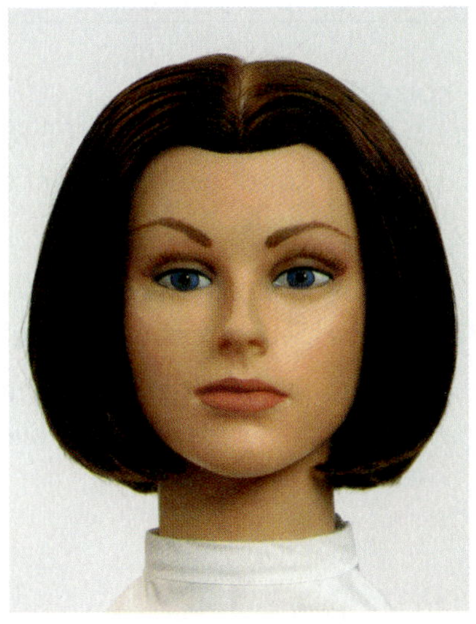

Figure 17-3 Finished blunt cut.

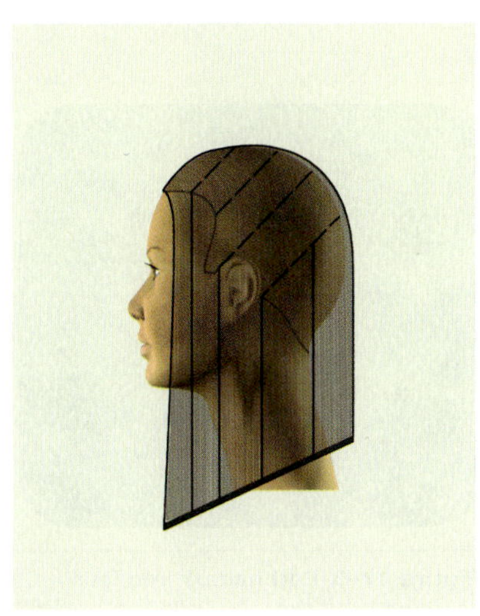

Figure 17-4 Blunt cut technical with diagonal forward design line.

PROCEDURE

BLUNT CUT

The method used to create the following blunt cut is somewhat different from other techniques you may be familiar with. Rather than working the four sections individually, this method provides a big-picture view of the haircutting areas and their relationship to each other throughout the entire haircut. Read through the procedure and discuss the steps before attempting the haircut. Remember to mist the hair as needed throughout the haircut. Be guided by your instructor for alternative methods of achieving a blunt cut.

Implements and Materials

- Towels
- Shampoo cape
- Shampoo and conditioner
- Chair cloth
- Neck strip
- Sectioning clips
- Brush
- Comb
- Shears
- Blow-dryer
- Spray bottle with water

Preparation

1. Conduct the client consultation and hair analysis.
2. Drape and perform shampoo service.
3. Towel dry hair and drape for haircut. Wash your hands.

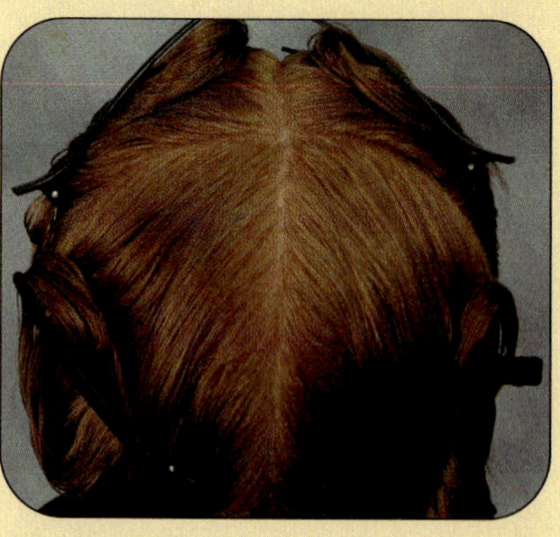

Figure 17-5 Part hair off into four sections.

Procedure

1. Comb the hair and part off into four sections from front to nape and from ear to ear over the top of the head form (Figure 17-5).
2. Secure sections with clips.
3. Beginning at the front right section, take a ½-inch parting from the hairline. Secure remainder of hair in clip (Figure 17-6).
4. Move to the back right section and repeat the parting process, making sure to connect the parting lines from the side, to behind the ear, to the nape (Figure 17-7).

5. Repeat this process on the left side of the head.
6. Comb through the ½-inch partings all around the head (Figure 17–8).
7. Move to the center back; comb through a section approximately 2 inches wide. Establish back guide at the desired length (Figure 17–9).
8. Move to the center front and establish a guide in the front section. Be sure that the length of the front guide will accommodate the intended line of the design line (Figures 17–10a and 17–10b). Example: for the horizontal design line, front guide length should be even with back guide length; for the diagonal forward design line, front guide length should be longer than back guide length; for the diagonal back design line, front guide length should be shorter than back guide length.

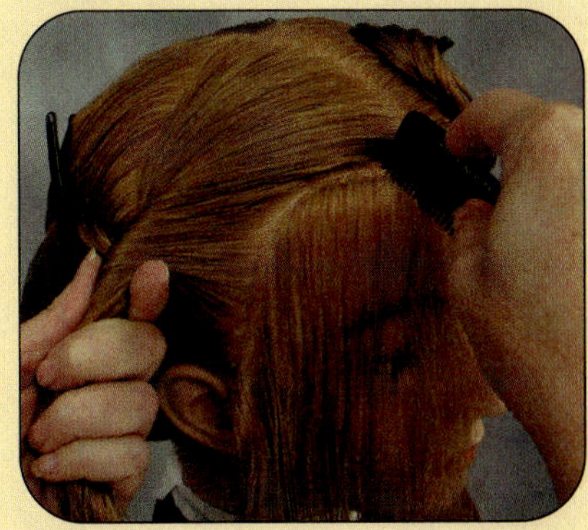

Figure 17–6 Take a ½-inch parting from the hairline.

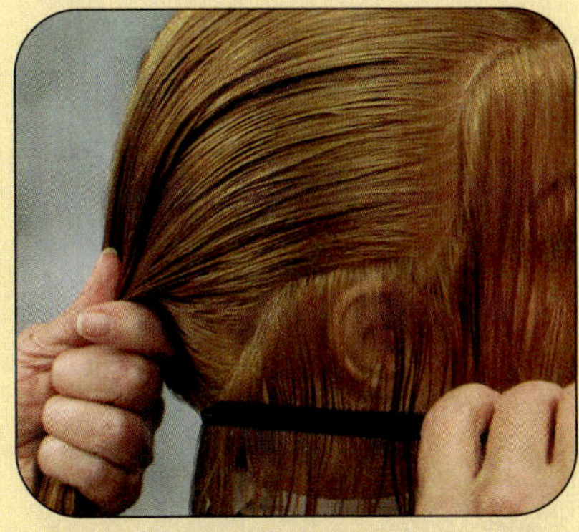

Figure 17–7 Connect the parting lines.

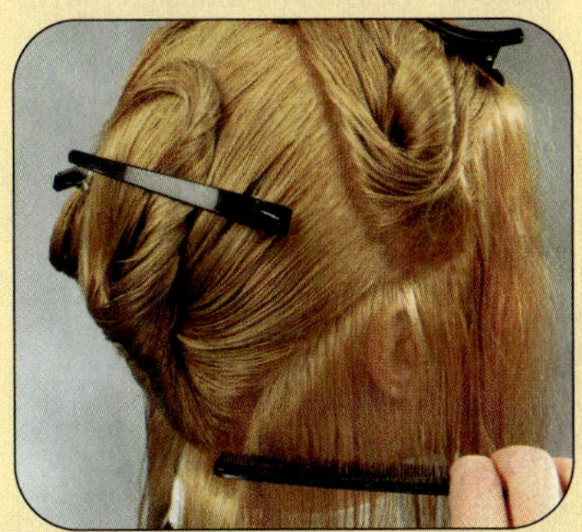

Figure 17–8 Comb through the ½-inch partings all around the head.

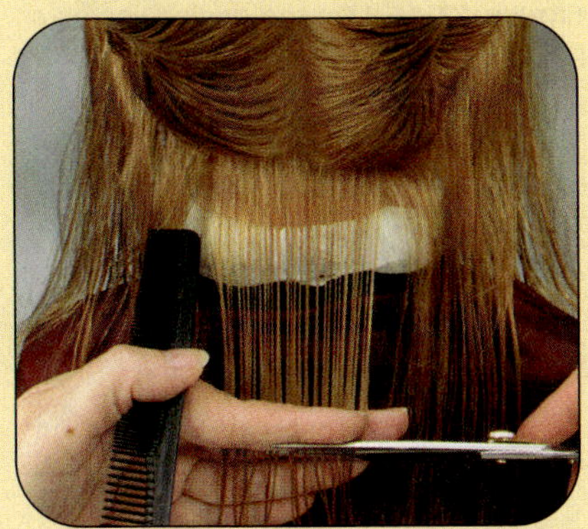

Figure 17–9 Establish back guide in center.

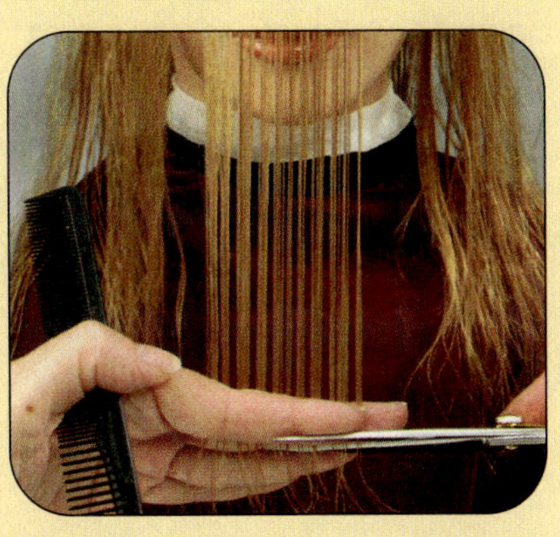

Figure 17–10a Cutting front guide.

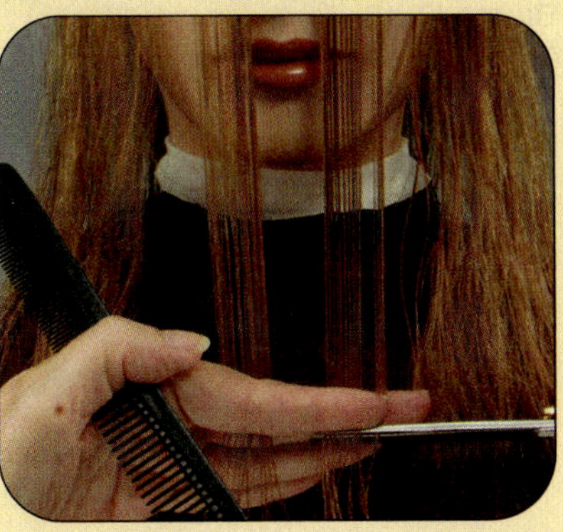

Figure 17–10b Cutting front guide allowing for protrusion of the nose.

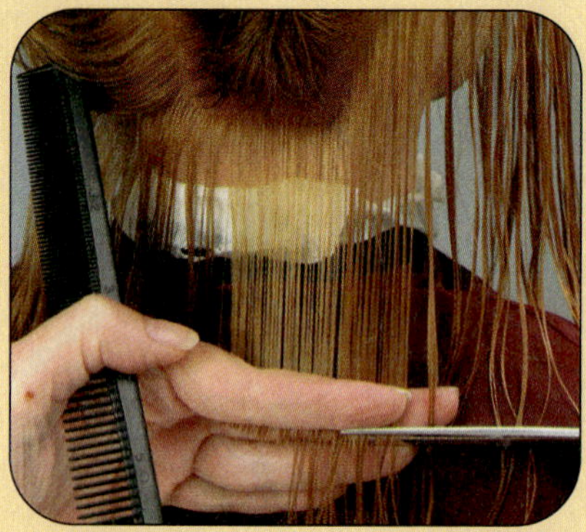

Figure 17-11 Use center guide to cut to back corners.

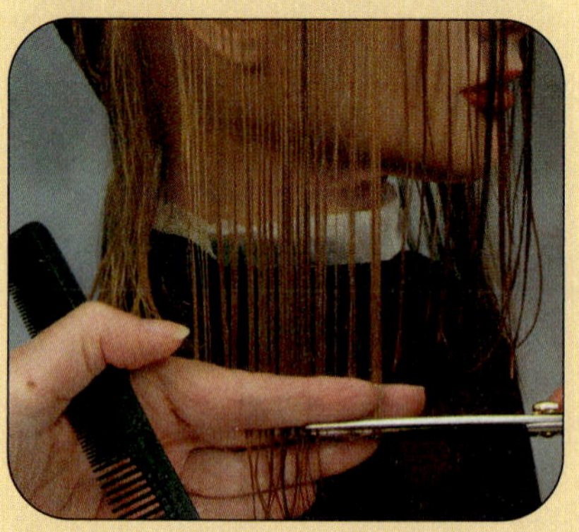

Figure 17-12 Cut in the design line until it meets the front guide length.

9. Move to the center back. Comb through the guide at a 0-degree elevation and, moving to the right, use the section as a guide to cut through to the corner of the back (Figure 17-11) and into the side area. Continue cutting the design line until it meets with the front guide (Figure 17-12).
10. Repeat the process working from the center back to cut in the left side design line until it meets the front guide.
11. Comb through and check the design line; fine-tune as necessary. Check the sides for even length (Figure 17-13). Do not proceed until the design line is as precise as possible.
12. Move to the back and release another ½-inch parting from both back sections (Figure 17-14). Comb through the first and second parting at 0 degrees and cut the second parting using the design line as a guide (Figure 17-15). Continue cutting the back section in this manner until the parting (usually around occipital height) meets the first side partings created in Step 9 (Figure 17-16).
13. All subsequent partings will be parted off from the four sections to create one parting all the way around the head (Figure 17-17).

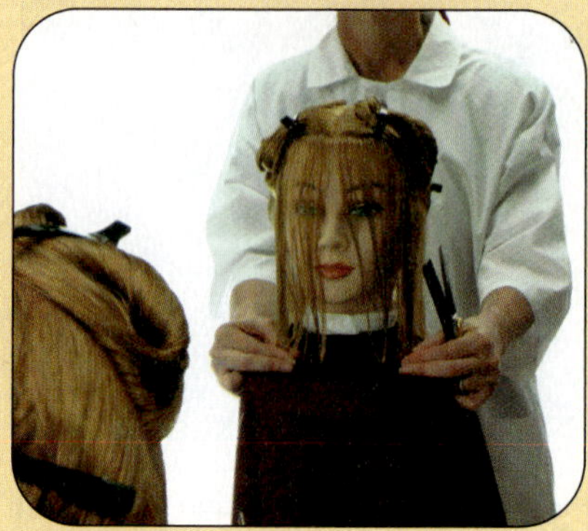

Figure 17-13 Check the sides for evenness.

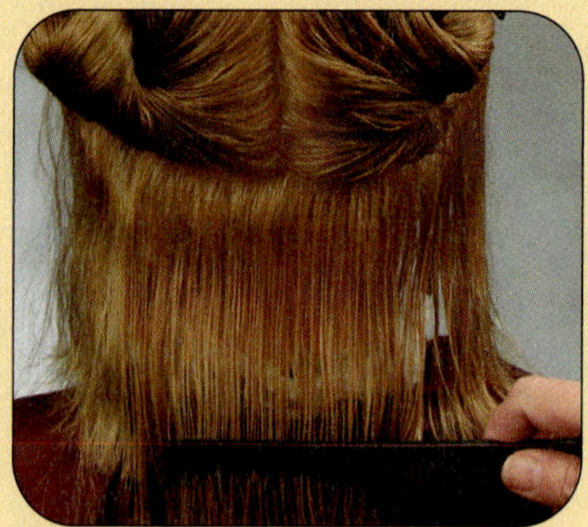

Figure 17-14 Release second parting in back section.

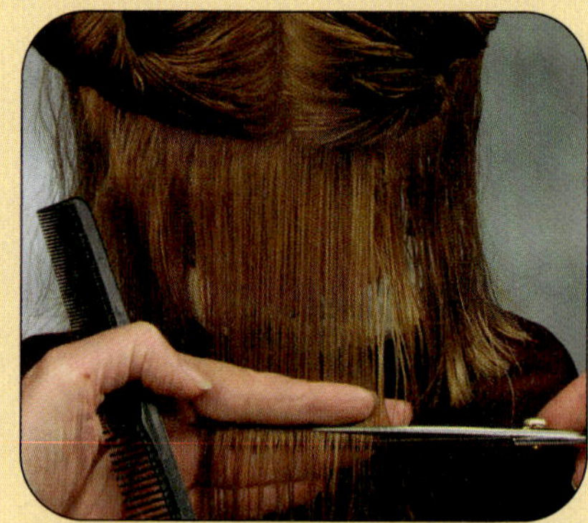

Figure 17-15 Use the design line as a guide for cutting the second parting.

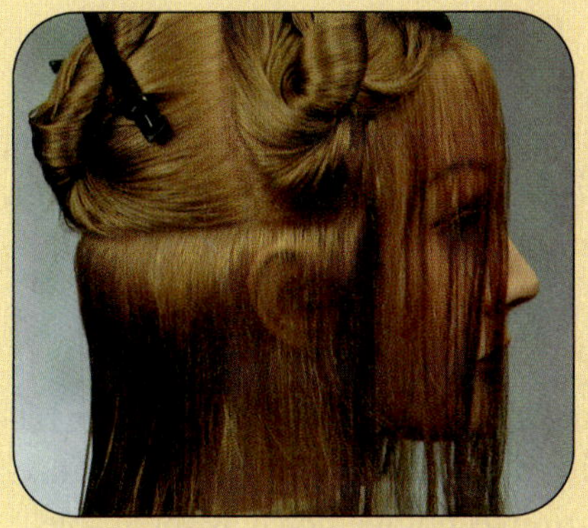

Figure 17-16 Cut back section until the parting meets the first side parting.

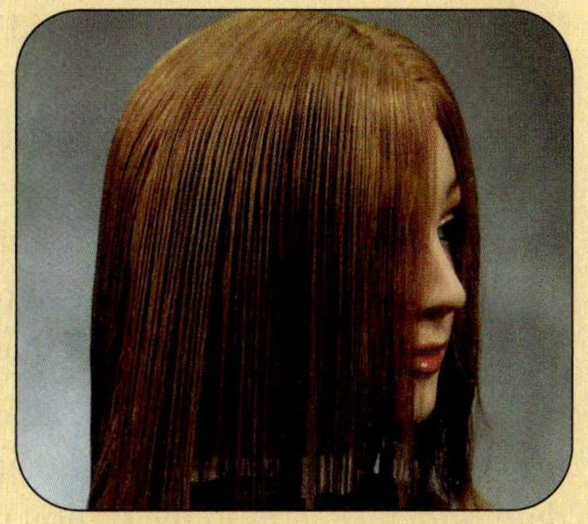

Figure 17-17 Subsequent partings are parted off from the four sections all around the head.

14. With the design line clearly established, cutting the subsequent partings can be performed from the back to sides to front or from the front to sides to back. Cut subsequent partings to the design line until all the hair is cut (Figure 17-18).
15. Check your work, fine-tune as necessary, style the hair, and check again (Figure 17-19).

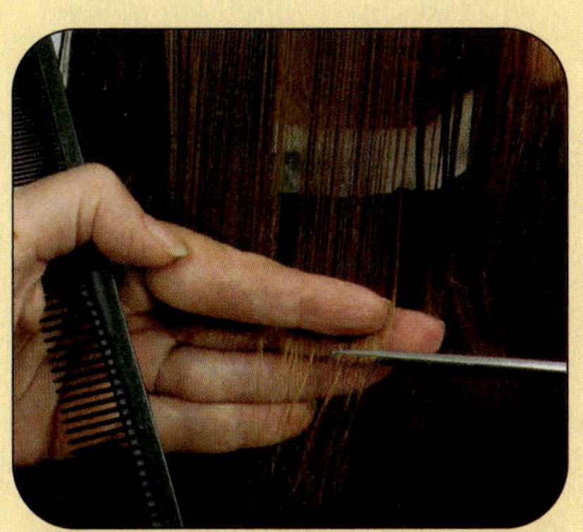

Figure 17-18 Cut subsequent partings at the design line.

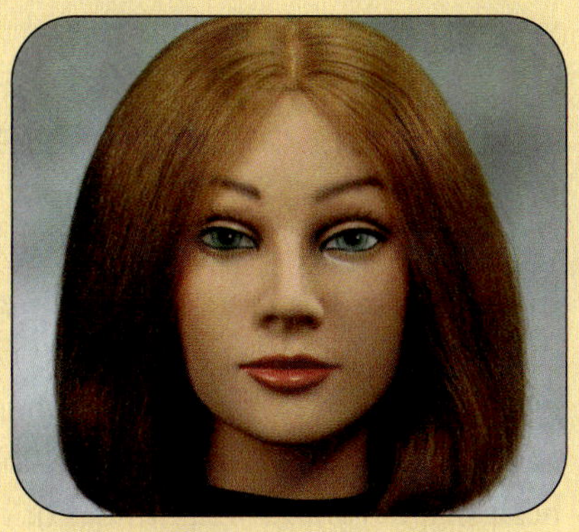

Figure 17-19 Finished blunt cut.

Cleanup and Sanitation

1. Disinfect tools, implements, and workstation.
2. Wash your hands.

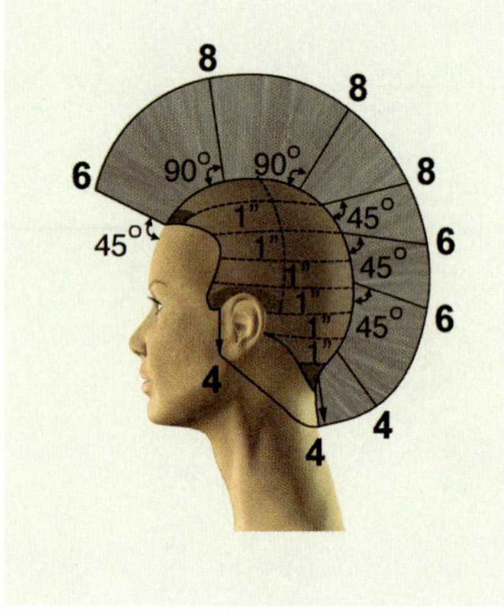

Figure 17-20 Graduated cut technical.

GRADUATED CUT (45 DEGREES)

A **graduated cut** has a wedge or stacked shape that is created by cutting with tension at low to medium elevations. The most common elevation is 45 degrees, which creates layers within the hair between 0 and 45 degrees. These layers build weight and volume along the perimeter of the hairstyle. See Figure 17–20 for the technical illustration of a graduated cut.

The graduated haircut can be accomplished with either horizontal or vertical partings. The horizontal method is described in the following procedure, with references to the vertical parting technique noted as applicable.

Haircutting Tips for Graduated Cuts

- Coarse, curly, and thick hair appears to graduate more than straight hair textures.
- Graduation makes fine hair of average density appear thicker and fuller.
- Avoid weight lines and graduation on fine, thin-density hair types.
- Maintain the same elevation around the perimeter when cutting in design lines.
- Maintain even/uniform tension and moisture throughout the haircut.
- Blend from one parting or subsection to another.

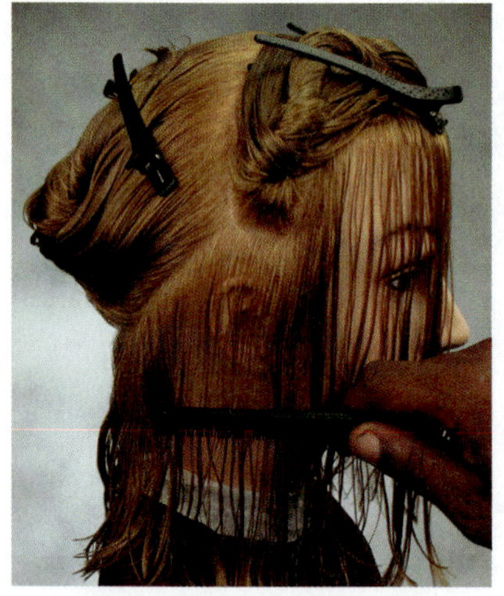

Figure 17-21 Uniform layered cut technical.

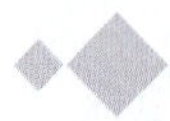

UNIFORM LAYERED CUT (90 DEGREES)

In a **uniform layered cut**, all of the hair strands are cut to the same length at a 90-degree projection, straight out from the growth source. A *traveling guide* is used on the interior sections to create layers within the entire haircut. When finished, the cut will look soft and textured and conform to the head shape without weight lines or corners at the perimeter.

A uniform layered cut can be used to cut short or long layered styles. The main points to remember are: hold the hair that is being cut at a 90-degree projection from *where it grows* and always use a guide from one section to the other. See Figure 17–21 for the technical illustration of a uniform layered cut.

Haircutting Tips for Uniform Layered Cuts

- Establish an interior guide first, then set a guide at the perimeter to avoid cutting off too much hanging length in the style.
- The thinner the parting, the more volume will be created within the cut.
- Work with the natural growth pattern, wave formation, and density of the hair.
- Always make sure the hair is blending from one section to another.
- Always check design lines for blending on the perimeter of the cut.

PROCEDURE

GRADUATED CUT

Implements and Materials

- Towels
- Shampoo cape
- Shampoo and conditioner
- Chair cloth
- Neck strip
- Sectioning clips
- Brush
- Comb
- Shears
- Blow-dryer
- Spray bottle with water

Preparation

1. Conduct the client consultation and hair analysis.
2. Drape and perform shampoo service.
3. Towel dry hair and drape for haircut. Wash your hands.

Procedure

1. Comb the hair and part off into four sections from front to nape and from ear to ear as in Figure 17–5 on page 448.
2. Secure sections with clips.
3. Beginning at the front right section, take a ½-inch parting from the hairline as in Figure 17–6 on page 449. Secure remainder of hair in a clip.
4. Move to the back right section and repeat the parting process, making sure to connect the parting lines from the side, to behind the ear, to the nape as performed in the blunt cut.
5. Repeat this process on the left side of the head.
6. Comb through the 1/2-inch partings all around the head (Figure 17–22).
7. Move to the center back; comb through a section approximately 2 inches wide. Establish the back guide at a 45-degree elevation (Figure 17–23).
8. Move to the center front and establish a guide at a 0 or low elevation in the front section. Be sure that the length of the front guide will accommodate the intended line of the design line.

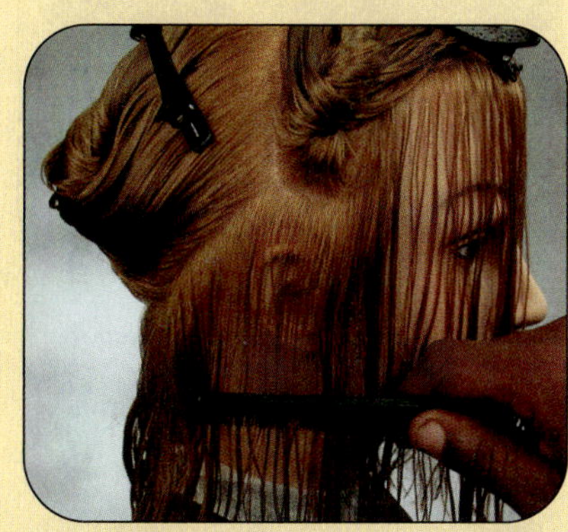

Figure 17–22 Comb through 1/2-inch partings.

17

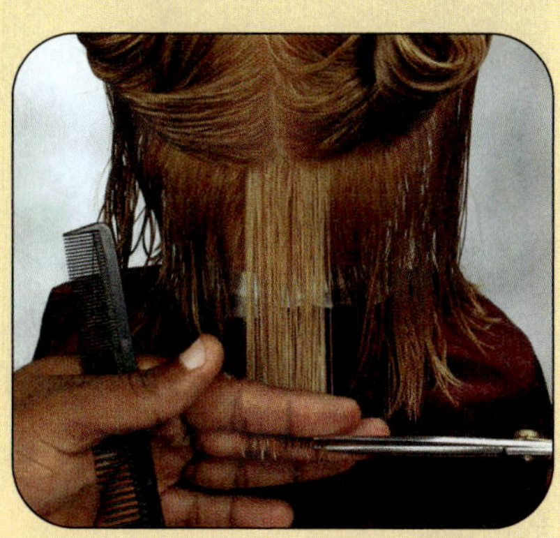

Figure 17–23 Establish guide at a 45-degree elevation.

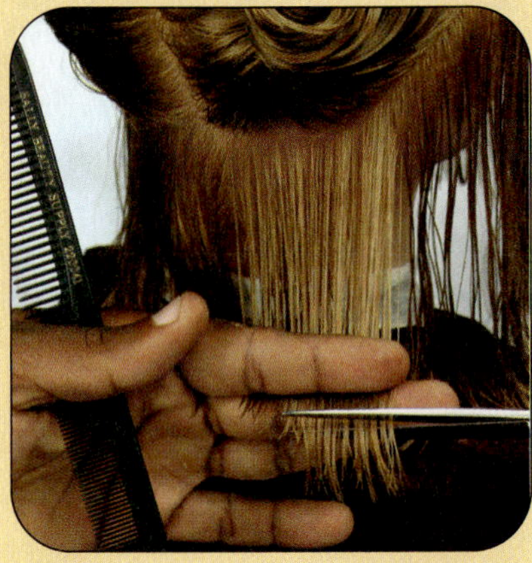

Figure 17-24 Cut to the right side using the guide at a 45-degree elevation.

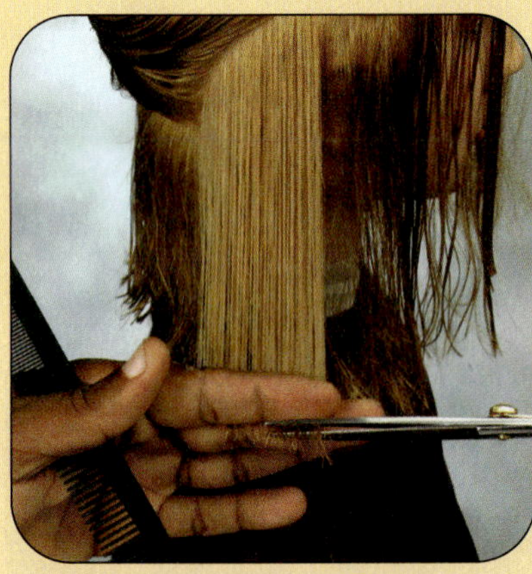

Figure 17-25 Cut into side section.

9. Move to the center back; comb through the guide horizontally at a 45-degree elevation. Cut to the right, using the guide to cut to the corner (Figure 17-24). Utilize a portion of the back guide to begin the side guide/design line, using a horizontal traveling guide at the perimeter (Figure 17-25). Continue cutting the design line until it meets with the front guide (Figure 17-26).
10. Repeat the process working from the center back to cut in the left side design line until it meets the front guide.
11. Comb through and check the design line; fine-tune as necessary. Check the sides for even length (Figure 17-27). Do not proceed until the design line is as precise as possible.
12. Move to the back and release another 1/2-inch parting from both back sections. Comb through the first and second horizontal partings, projecting to 45 degrees, and cut the second parting using the design line as a guide (Figure 17-28). Continue cutting the back section in this manner until the partings meet the side and front partings created in Step 9 (Figure 17-29).

    Vertical Cutting Option: Using the design line as a guide, take a vertical parting and position the fingers at a 45-degree angle as shown in Figure 17-30. Use this as a guide for cutting subsequent vertical partings around the head. Be careful to cut each section at the same elevation with the same angle of finger position. Also be sure that each section of hair blends from one vertical parting to another (Figure 17-31).
13. All subsequent partings will be parted off from the four sections to create one parting all the way around the head (Figure 17-32).
14. With the design line clearly established, cutting the subsequent partings can be performed from the back to sides to front or from the front

17

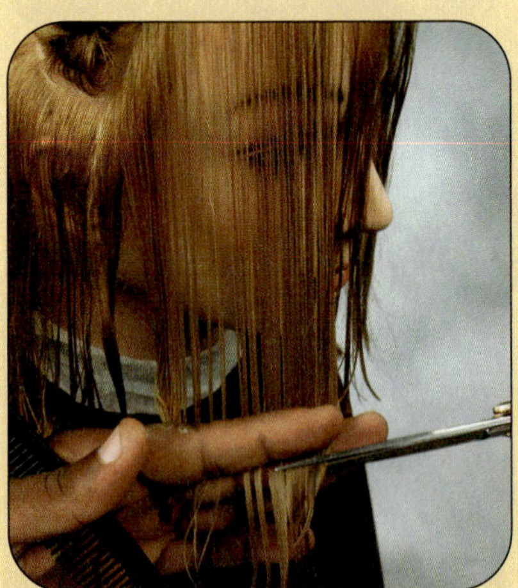

Figure 17-26 Cut until sides meet front guide.

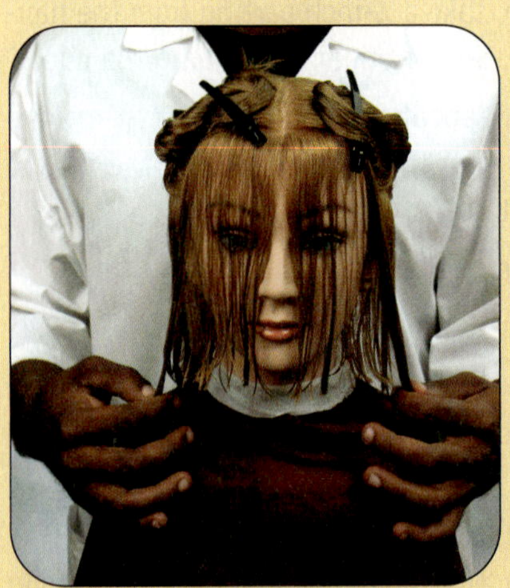

Figure 17-27 Check the sides for evenness.

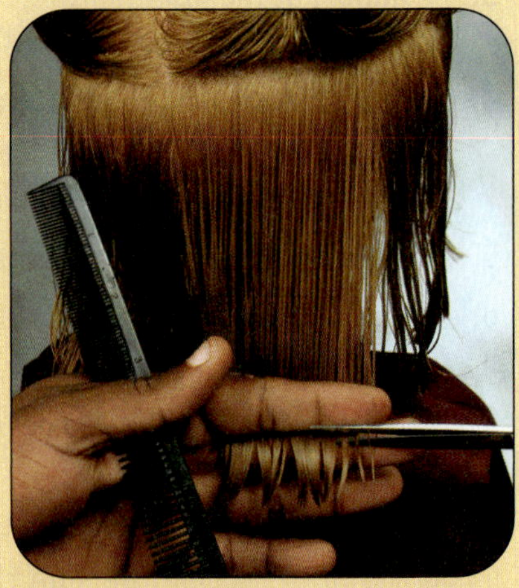

Figure 17-28 Hold first and second partings at 45 degrees and cut at the design line.

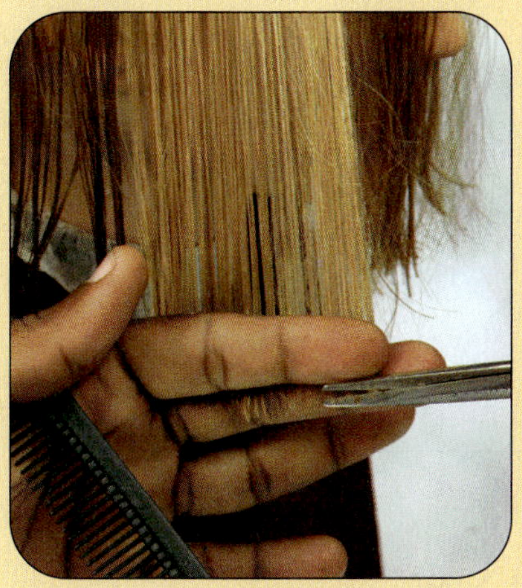

Figure 17-29 Continue cutting around the perimeter.

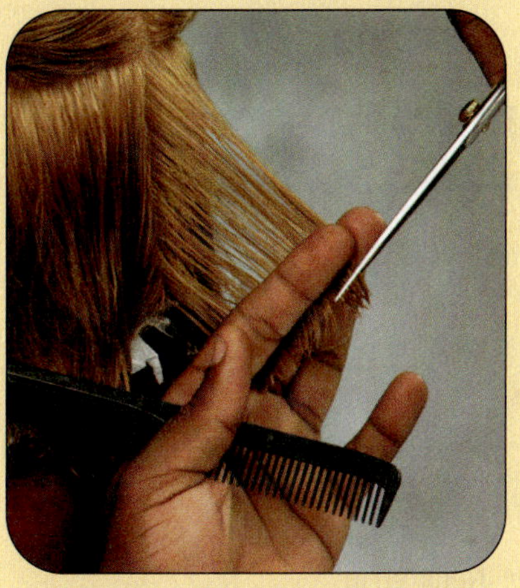

Figure 17-30 Use a vertical parting, position the fingers at a 45-degree angle, and cut to the design line guide.

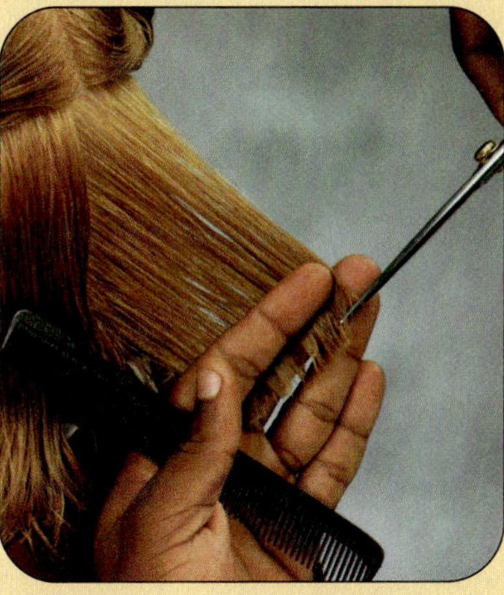

Figure 17-31 Check for blending from one vertical parting to another.

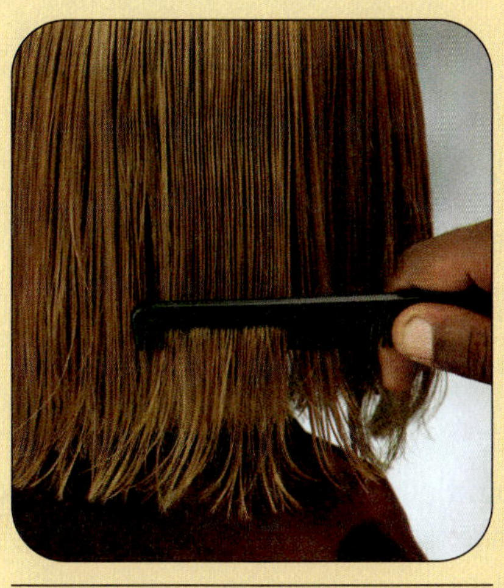

Figure 17-32 Subsequent parting from four sections creates one parting all around the head.

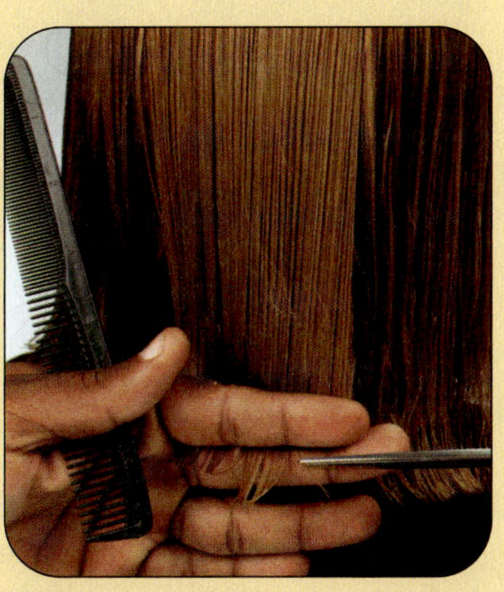

Figure 17-33 Cut subsequent partings at a 45-degree elevation.

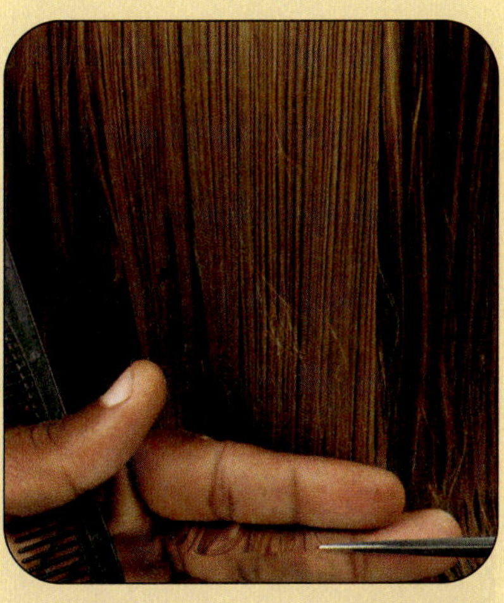

Figure 17-34 Check and fine-tune your work.

to sides to back. Cut subsequent partings at the design line with a 45-degree elevation until the haircut is completed (Figure 17–33).

15. Check your work, fine-tune as necessary (Figure 17–34), style the hair, and check again (Figure 17–35).

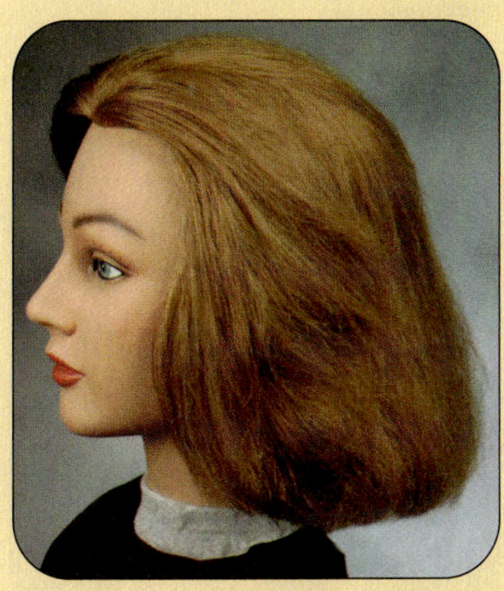

Figure 17-35 Finished graduated cut.

Cleanup and Sanitation

1. Disinfect tools, implements, and workstation.
2. Wash your hands.

PROCEDURE

UNIFORM LAYERED CUT

Implements and Materials

- Towels
- Shampoo cape
- Shampoo and conditioner
- Chair cloth
- Neck strip
- Sectioning clips
- Brush
- Comb
- Shears
- Blow-dryer
- Spray bottle with water

Preparation

1. Conduct the client consultation and hair analysis.
2. Drape and perform shampoo service.
3. Towel dry hair and drape for haircut. Wash your hands.

Procedure

1. Comb the hair into a natural fall position. If the hair is long, part off into five sections: top, two sides, and two back panels (Figure 17-36). Secure sections with clips if necessary.
2. Stand behind the client and comb a horizontal parting from the high point of the head form into a 90-degree elevation. Establish guide (Figure 17-37).
3. Use the first guide as a traveling guide to cut the top section toward the front area (Figure 17-38).
4. Comb the top section back. Move to the side. Starting at the forehead, part off the top section of hair, front to back, with the thumb and middle finger. Hold the original guide line and a ½-inch parting at the crown at 90 degrees, and cut (Figure 17-39). This establishes the guide for the crown and back sections.

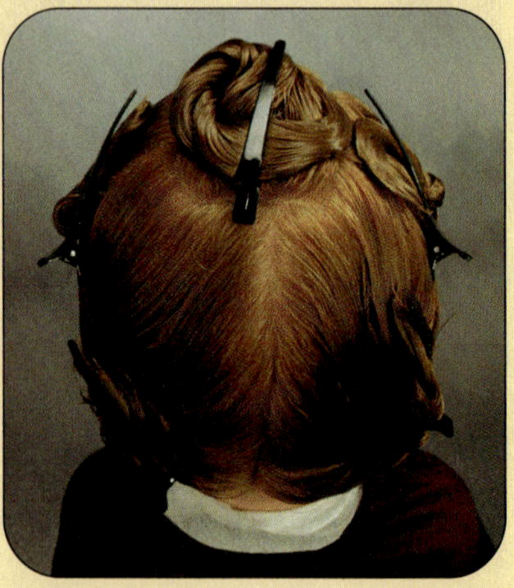

Figure 17-36 Part off hair into five sections.

17

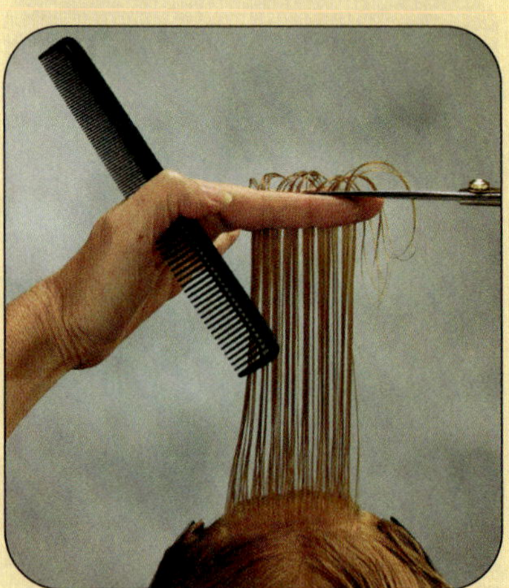

Figure 17-37 Establish top guide length.

5. Work forward, still maintaining a side-standing position. Following the arc and contour of the head, even off any length that does not blend with the traveling guide (Figure 17–40). If the horizontal partings were cut correctly, no more than ¼ inch of hair should need to be evened.
6. Comb the hair into natural fall. Pick up the crown area guide and hold at a 90-degree elevation. Use a vertical parting to cut the hair from the crown to the nape.
7. Once a vertical panel of hair has been cut to the appropriate length, use it as guide to cut the remainder of the back section. Vertical partings may be cut from the crown to the nape or from the nape to the crown (establish perimeter design line first), depending on preference (Figure 17–41).
8. Comb the back section into natural fall and establish a perimeter design line at 0 degrees.
9. Continue the design line into the sides and front areas. Check length on sides for evenness.
10. Move behind the client. Part off a vertical subsection from the hair on the right side. Hold the parting straight out to the side at 90 degrees. The design/guide line should be visible at the tips of the fingers when working on the right side of the client's head (Figure 17–42).

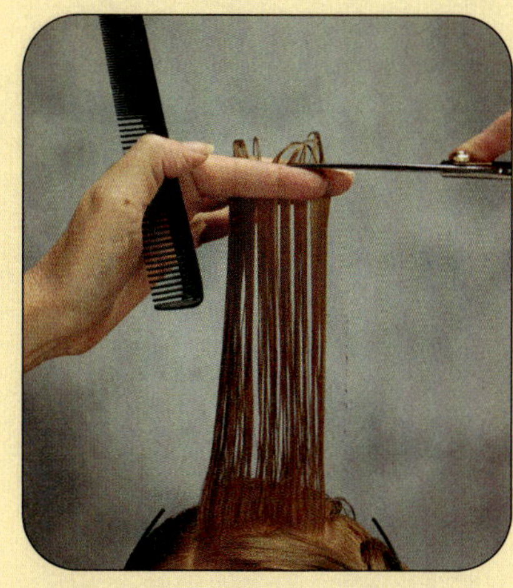

Figure 17–38 Cut toward front area using a traveling guide.

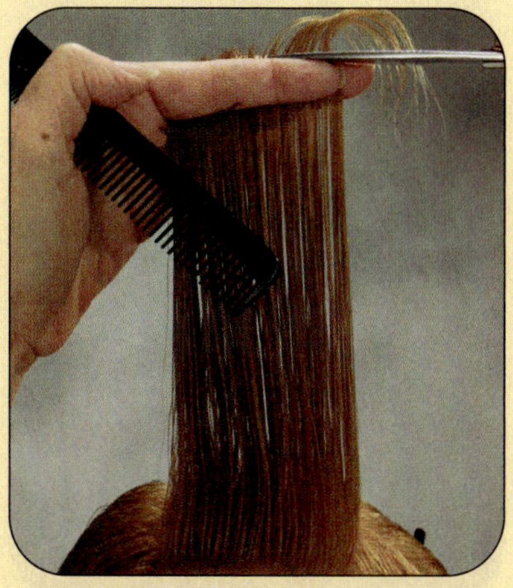

Figure 17–39 Stand at side and establish guide in crown area to meet top guide.

17

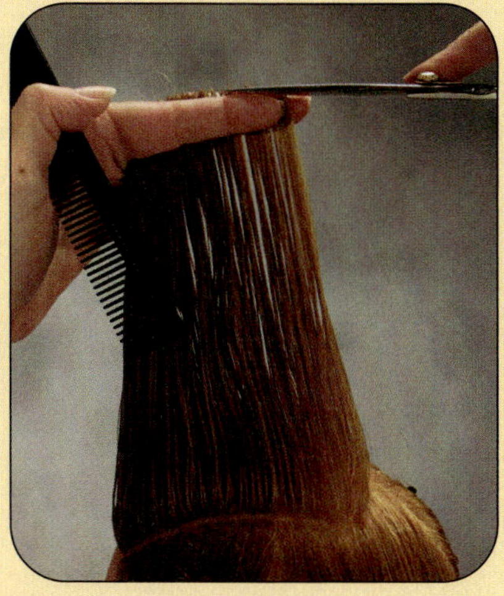

Figure 17–40 Follow the area of the form to the front area. Check blending.

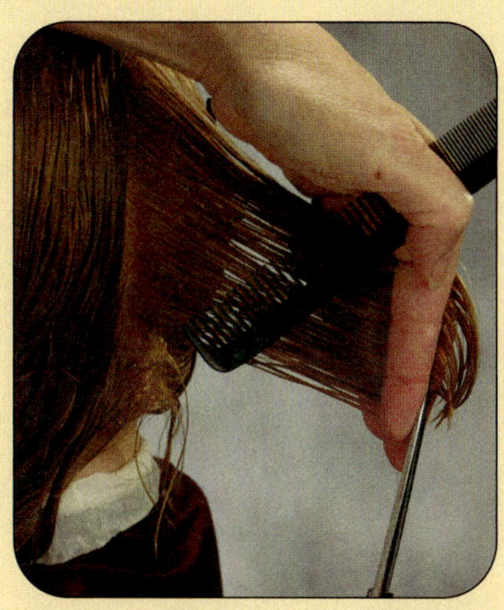

Figure 17–41 Use vertical partings to blend nape and back areas to the crest.

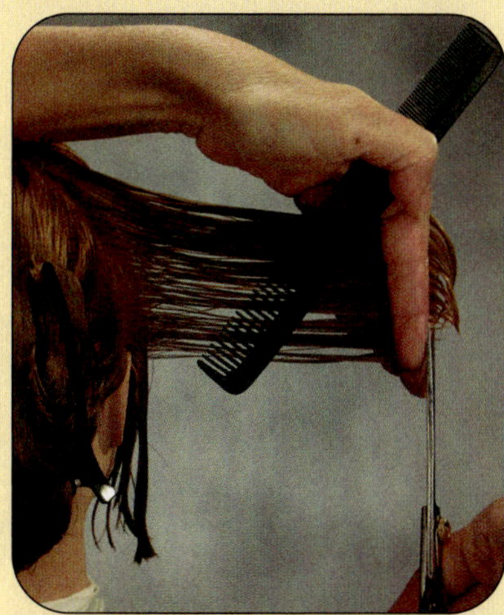

Figure 17–42 Use vertical partings at 90 degrees to cut the sides.

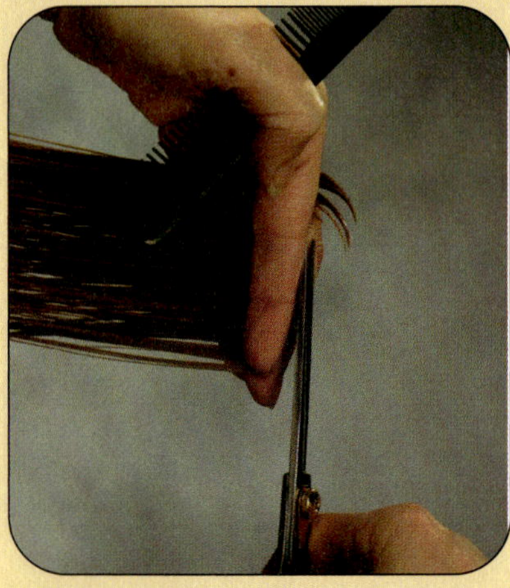

Figure 17-43 Cut off any hair that extends beyond the guide.

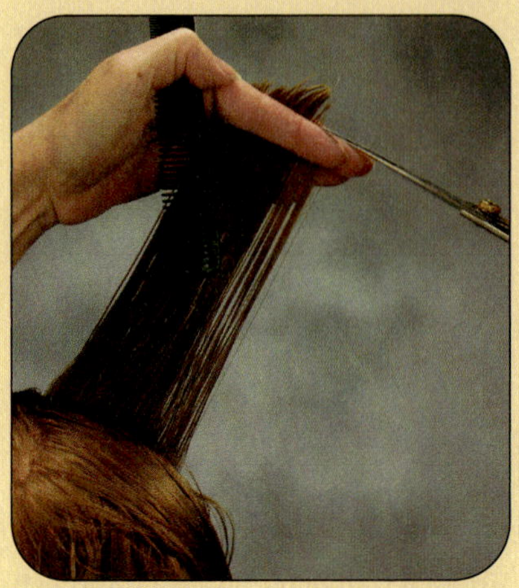

Figure 17-44 Blend the hair through the crest until it meets the top guide.

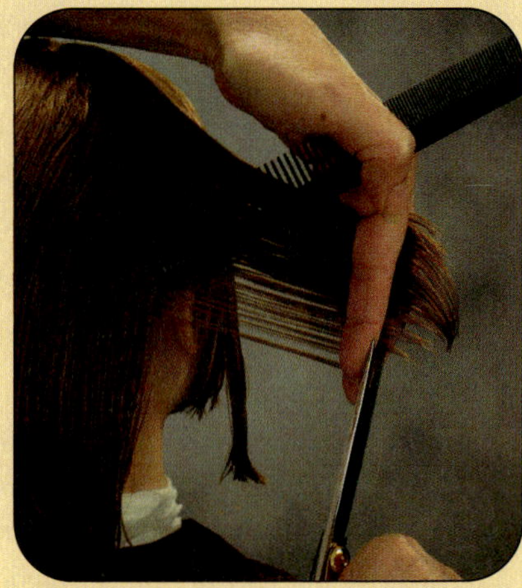

Figure 17-45 Blend the sides to the back section.

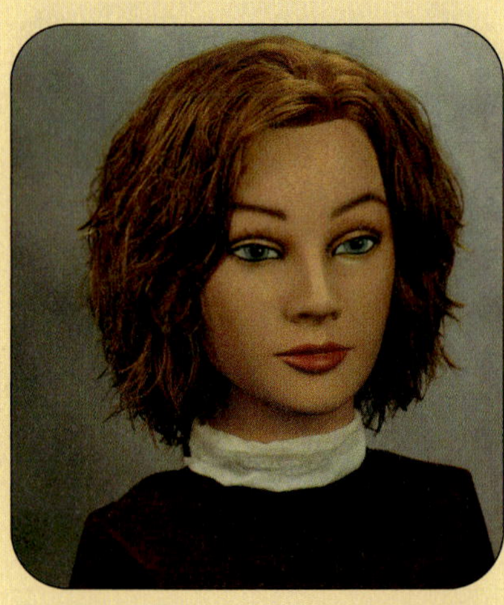

Figure 17-46 Uniform layered cut with scrunched styling.

17

11. Make a straight, vertical cut from the design/guide line, cutting off any hair that extends past the guide (Figure 17-43). Maintain uniform moisture.
12. Continue cutting partings of hair while following the contour of the head until reaching the guide in the top section (Figure 17-44). The hair should meet. Check the procedure by checking the blend of hair from the side design/guide line to the top section guide.
13. Proceed until all the side hair is cut. Use vertical partings to blend the side hair to the back hair (Figure 17-45). Repeat procedure on the left side. Option: Stand facing the client to facilitate working from the design/guide line up when blending the hair on the left side of the head.
14. Comb and check the cut. Style as desired. Figure 17-46 shows the uniform layered cut in a scrunched style.

Cleanup and Sanitation

1. Disinfect tools, implements, and workstation.
2. Wash your hands.

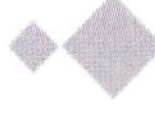

LONG LAYERED CUT (180 DEGREES)

A **long layered cut** consists of increased layering that is achieved by cutting the hair at a 180-degree elevation. This produces progressively longer layers from the top to the perimeter and begins with a stationary guide in the top section. Figure 17–47 depicts the technical pattern of a long layered cut.

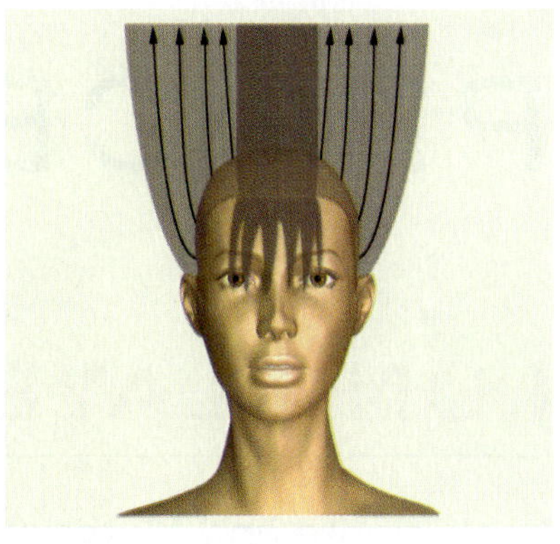

Figure 17–47 180-degree long layered technical.

Haircutting Tips for Long Layered Cuts

- Comb through parting or subsections from scalp to ends with even tension.
- Work with only as much hair as is comfortable and controllable. Create thinner working panels of hair if the combination of length and density becomes unmanageable.
- If in doubt about what the remaining hanging length of the hair will be when it is cut to the top guide, cut in the design line at the perimeter first.
- Avoid steps and gaps between the layers. Blend sections from long to short or short to long.

GALLERY OF CUTS: TECHNICALS AND FINISHED STYLES (FIGURES 17–48 THROUGH 17–53 AND 17–60 THROUGH 17–77)

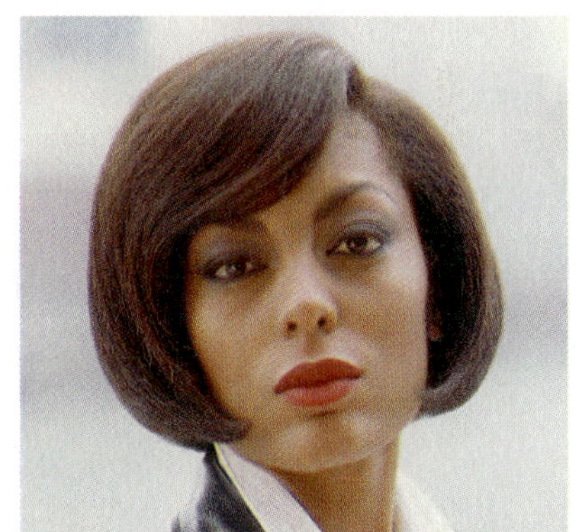

Figure 17–48 Blunt cut.

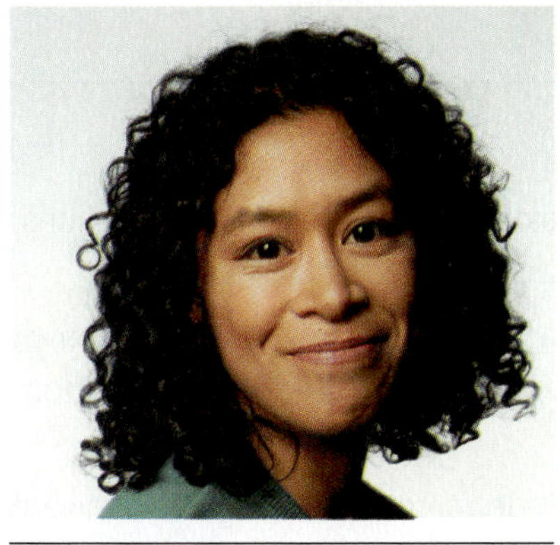

Figure 17–49 Blunt cut on curly hair.

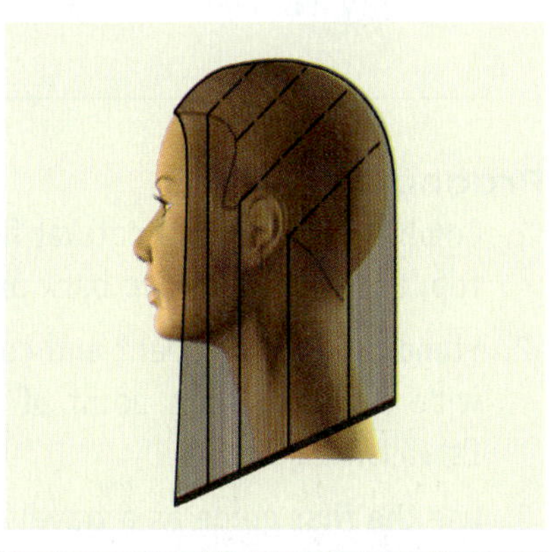

Figure 17–50 Blunt cut technical with diagonal forward design.

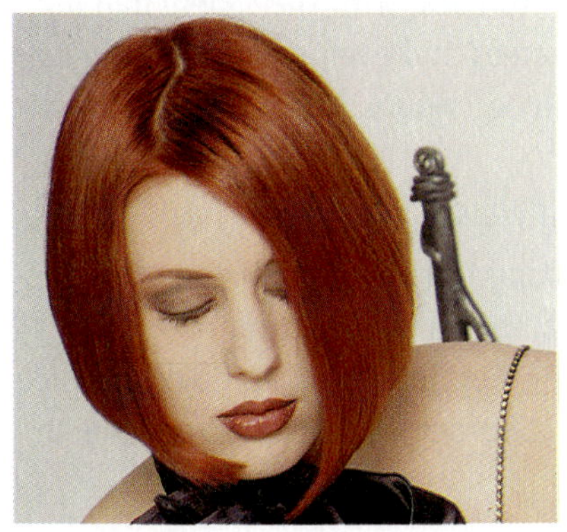

Figure 17–51 Diagonal forward bob.

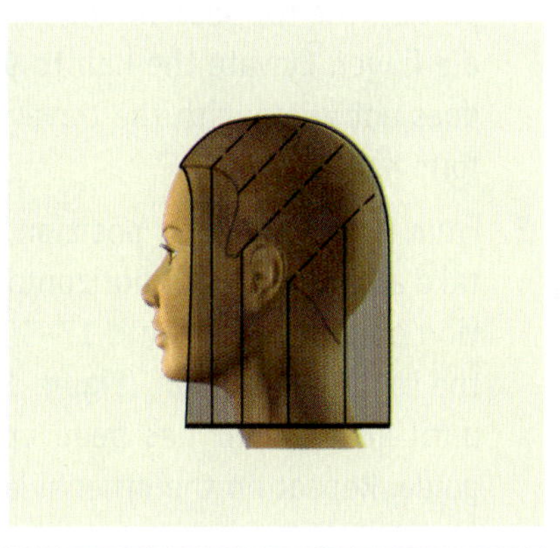

Figure 17–52 Blunt cut technical.

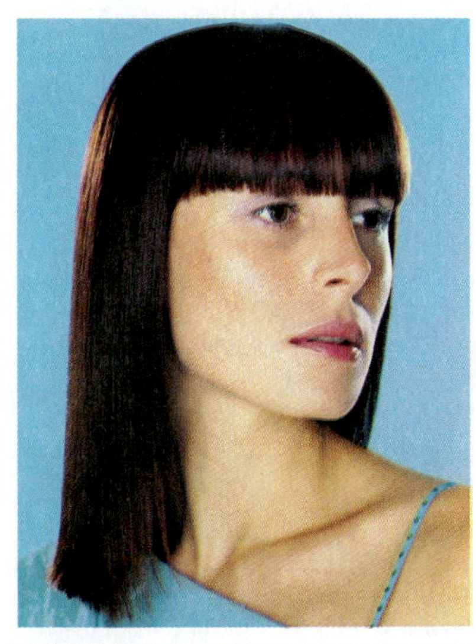

Figure 17–53 Longer blunt cut with one-length bangs.

PROCEDURE

LONG LAYERED CUT

Implements and Materials

- Towels
- Shampoo cape
- Shampoo and conditioner
- Chair cloth
- Neck strip
- Sectioning clips
- Brush
- Comb
- Shears
- Blow-dryer
- Spray bottle with water

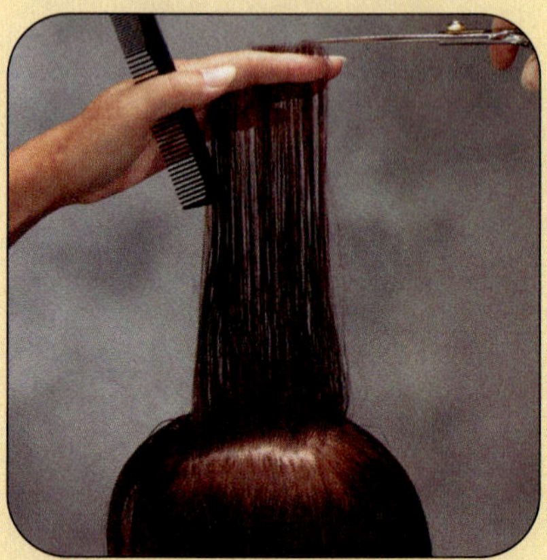

Figure 17-54 Check and blend top guide from a side position.

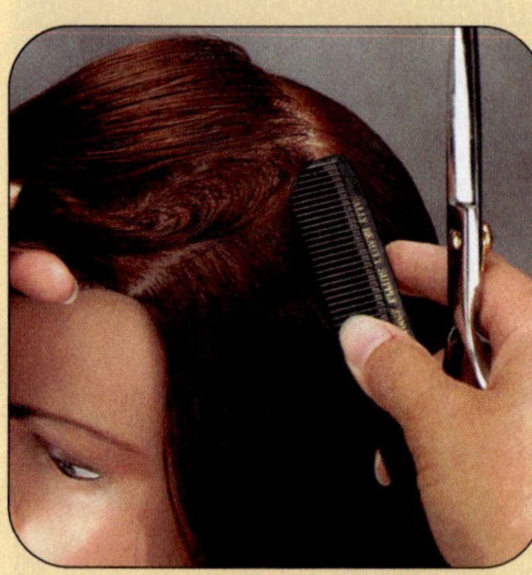

Figure 17-55 Hold the top guide and take a ¼- to ½-inch parting from the top of the crest area.

Preparation

1. Conduct the client consultation and hair analysis.
2. Drape and perform shampoo service.
3. Towel dry hair and drape for haircut. Wash your hands.

Procedure

1. Comb the hair into a natural fall position. Part off into five sections: top, two sides, and two back panels. Secure sections with clips.
2. Stand behind the client and comb a horizontal parting about an inch wide from the high point of the head into a 90-degree elevation. Establish a guide.
3. Use the first guide as a traveling guide to cut the top section toward the front area.
4. Comb the top section back. Move to the side. Starting at the forehead, part off the top section of hair, front to back, with the thumb and middle finger. Elevate the hair to 90 degrees and even off any length that does not blend with the traveling guide (Figure 17-54). Maintain uniform moisture.
5. From a side standing position, hold the top guide at 90 degrees and take a ¼- to ½-inch horizontal parting from the top of the crest section on the side (Figure 17-55). Comb the side parting of hair up to the top guide and cut (Figure 17-56). Continue working down the side until all the hair has been cut at 180-degree elevation to the top guide. Repeat on the other side.

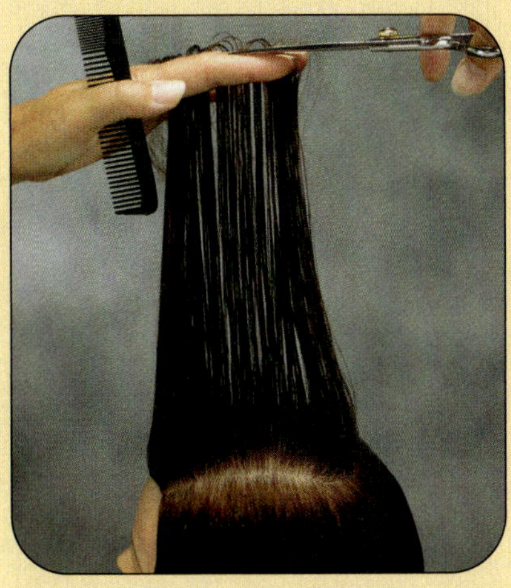

Figure 17-56 Comb crest side section to top guide and cut.

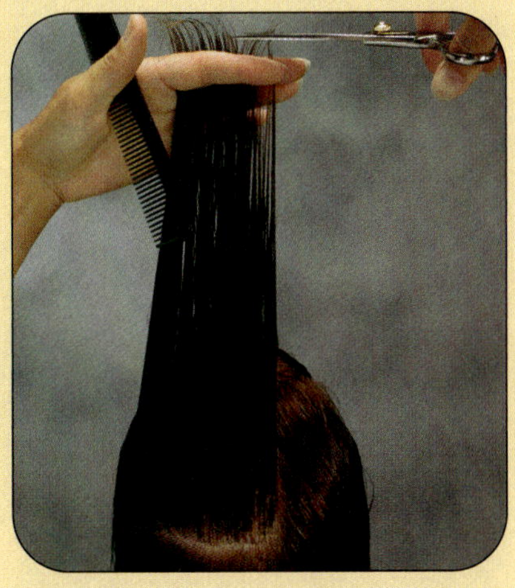

Figure 17-57 Cut back section in same manner as sides.

6. The back sections are cut in the same manner as the sides. Continue until both back panels are cut (Figure 17-57).
7. Comb the hair down into natural fall. Beginning at the center back, trim and fine-tune the perimeter design line (Figure 17-58). Check the sides for evenness. Check the layers for blending.
8. Style the hair as desired (Figure 17-59).

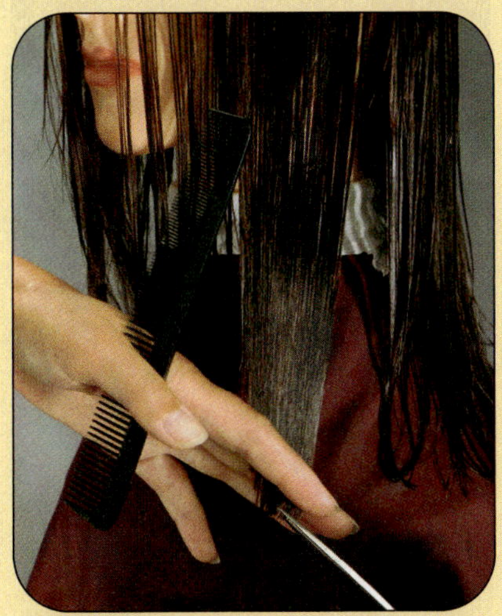

Figure 17-58 Trim the perimeter design line.

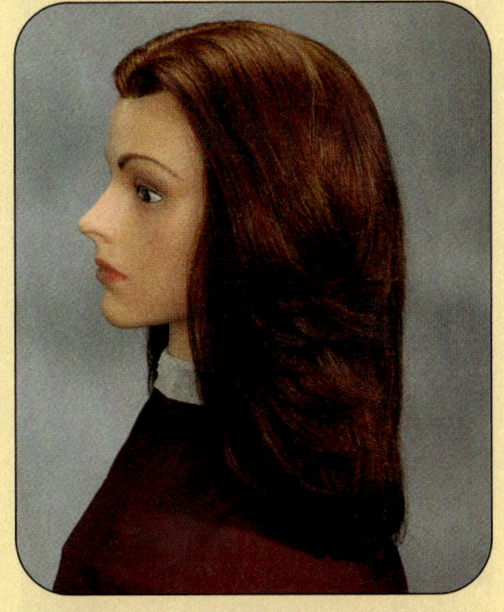

Figure 17-59 Finished 180-degree long layered cut.

Cleanup and Sanitation

1. Disinfect tools, implements, and workstation.
2. Wash your hands.

Figure 17-60 Graduated cut technical.

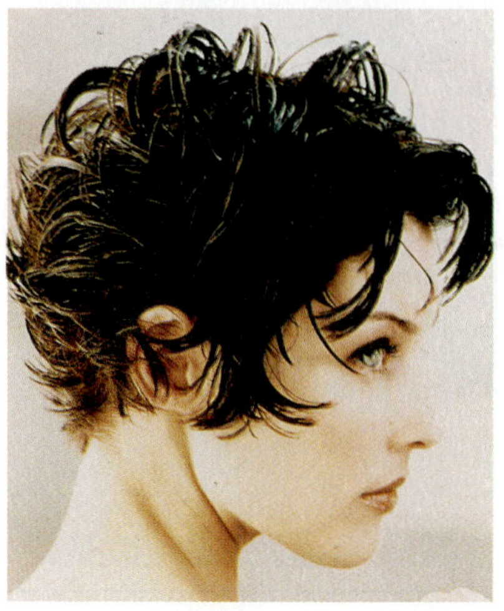

Figure 17-61 Graduated cut on curly hair.

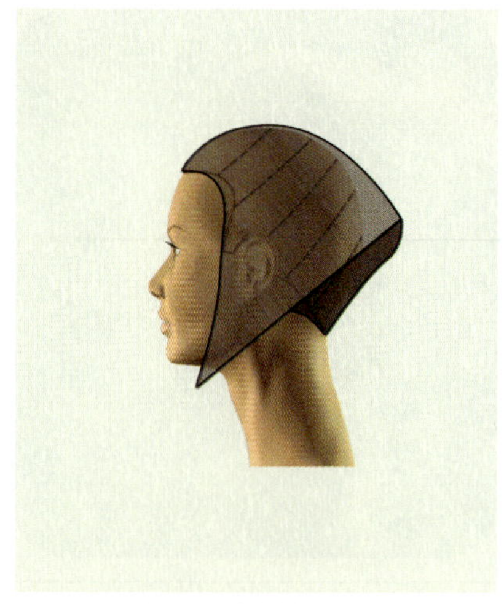

Figure 17-62 Graduated bob technical.

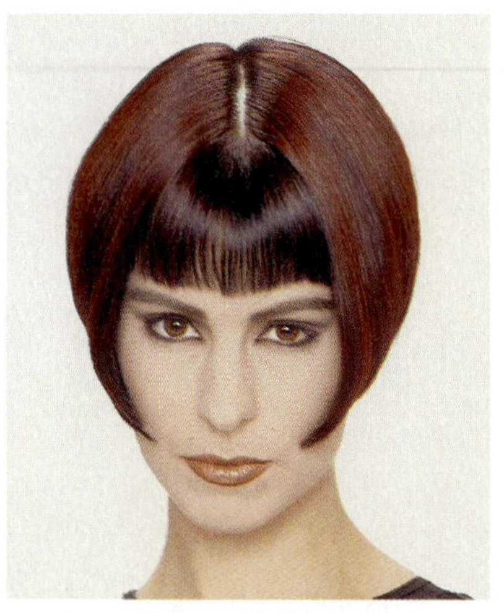

Figure 17-63 Finished graduated bob.

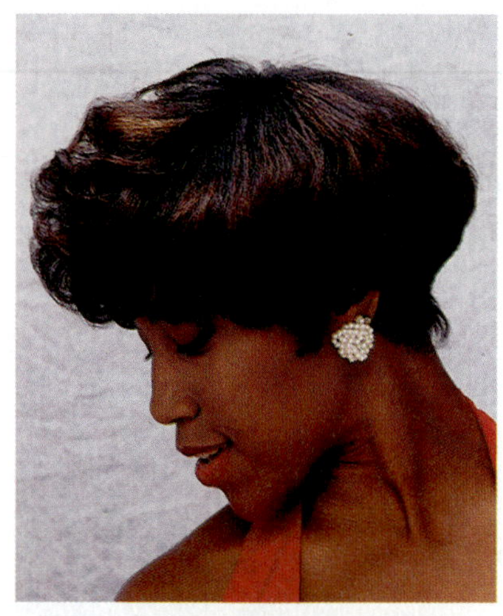

Figure 17-64 Bob variation.

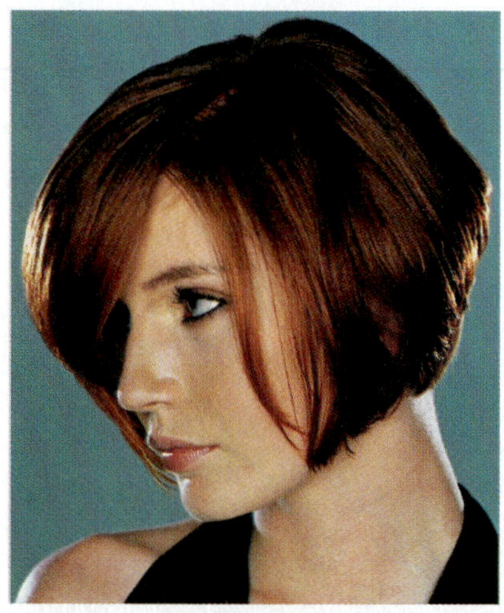

Figure 17-65 Bob variation.

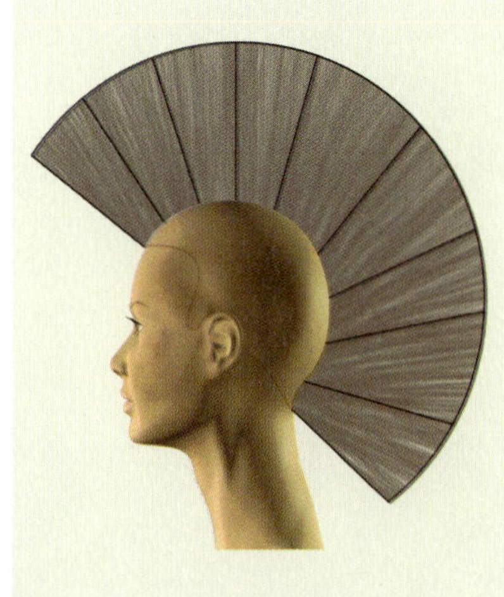

Figure 17-66 Uniform layered cut technical.

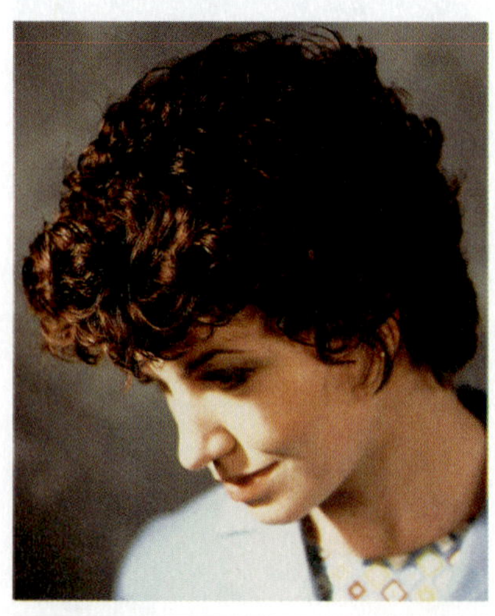

Figure 17-67 Uniform layered cut on curly hair.

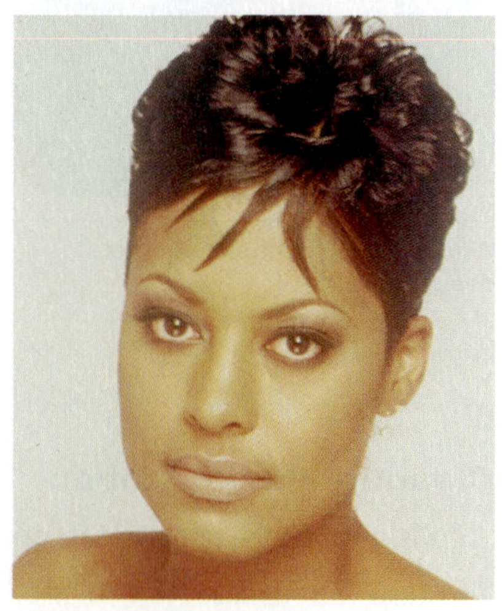

Figure 17-68 Uniform layer with taper variation.

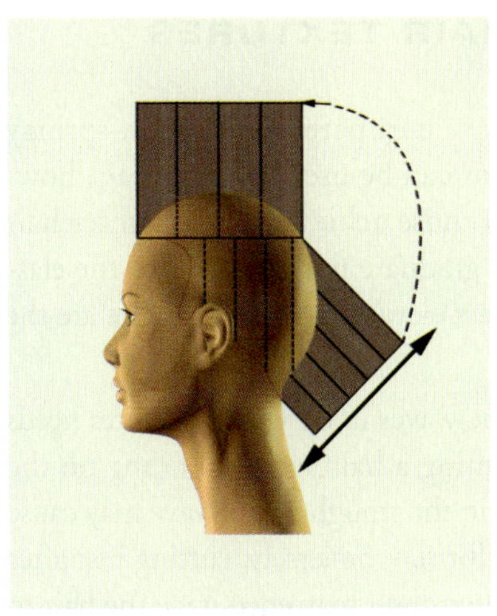

Figure 17-69 Uniform layer with taper variation technical.

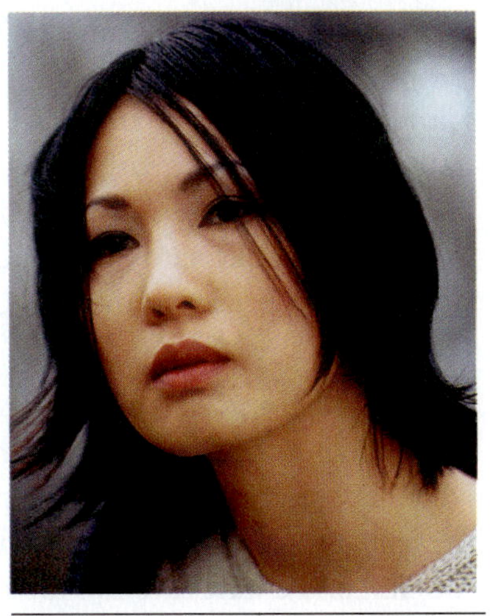

Figure 17-70 Uniform layer variation.

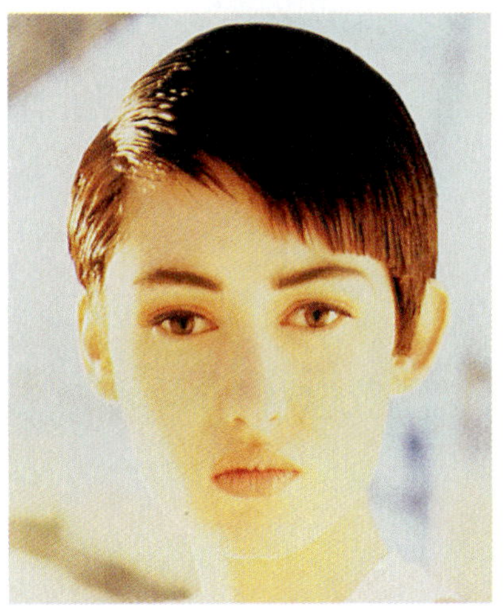

Figure 17-71 Uniform layer with taper variation.

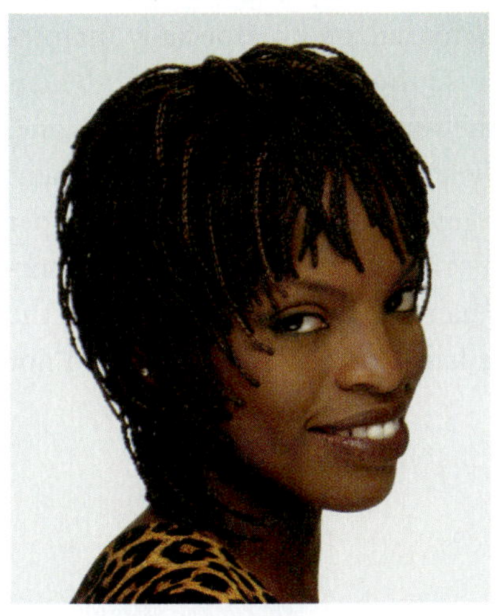

Figure 17-72 Uniform layer braided style.

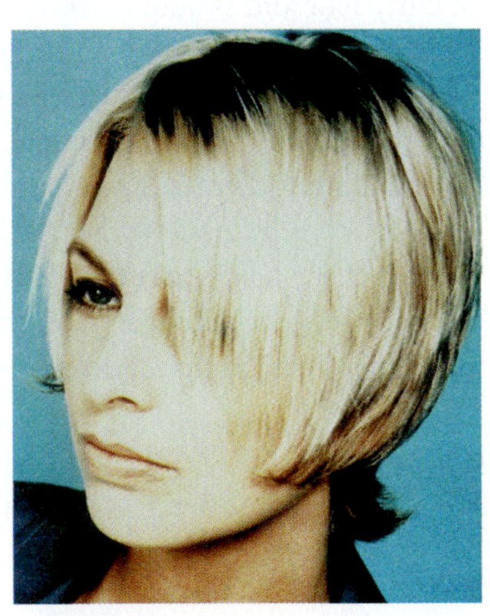

Figure 17-73 Uniform layered cut variation.

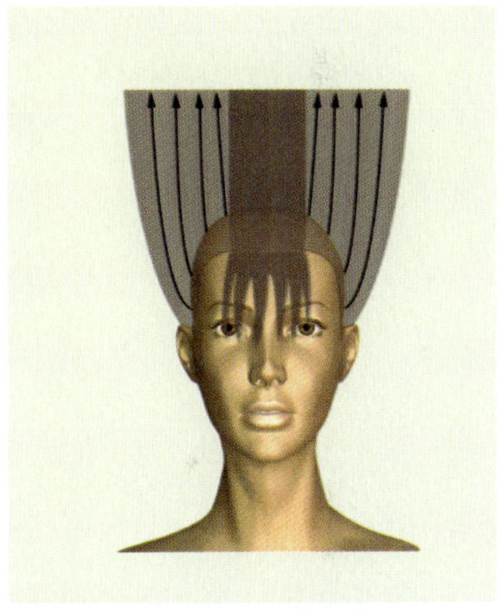

Figure 17-74 180-degree long layered technical.

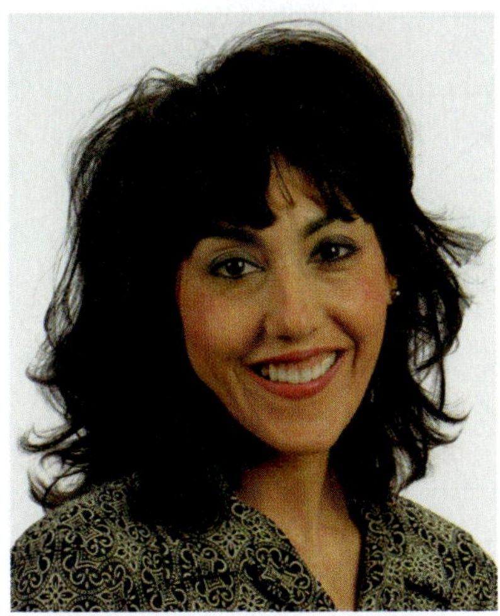

Figure 17-75 Long layered cut.

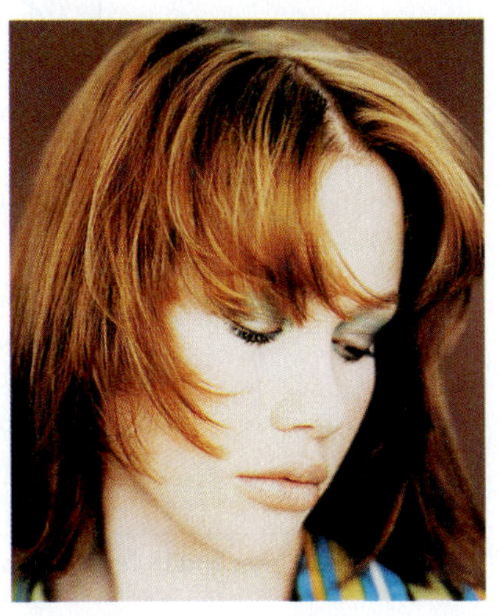

Figure 17-76 Long layered cut.

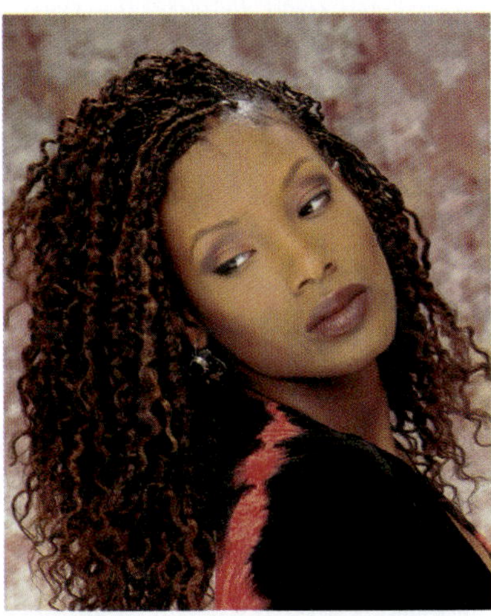

Figure 17-77 Long layered braided style.

CUTTING CURLY HAIR TEXTURES

Curly hair types range from large, loose curl patterns to tight, springy curls. Any of the four cutting elevations can be used on curly hair; however, the results will be different from those achieved on straighter hair types. For example, curly hair tends to graduate naturally due to the elasticity and *curl* pattern of the hair. Use less elevation if strong angles are the objective.

The trough and crest formation of the waves in curly hair textures needs to be taken into account when performing a haircut. Depending on the amount of curl, cutting the hair parting in the trough of the wave may cause the hair ends to flip out from the head form. Conversely, cutting just after the crest of the wave as it dips toward the trough may encourage the hair to fall inward toward the head form (Figure 17–78).

Knowing where to cut on the wave is helpful when cutting all lengths of curly hair and should be considered when analyzing the hair texture. It is most important when cutting shorter hairstyles, especially maintenance cuts on regular customers, because the amount of hair to be cut may have to be adjusted according to the wave pattern at any given time. For example, a client with wavy to curly hair has a standing appointment every four weeks. Assume that the hair grows at an average of ½ inch per month. If the hair was cut at a point just after the crest of the wave during the previous haircut service, those hair ends may now be part of the subsequent trough that develops as the hair curls naturally. It would not

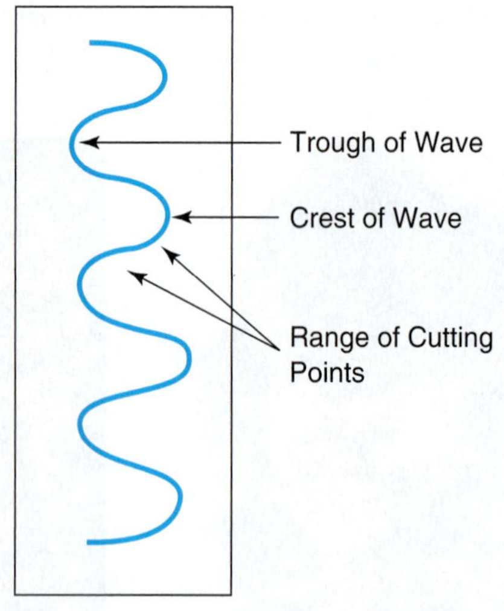

Figure 17-78 Crest and trough formation of waves.

be correct to automatically cut off ½ inch of hair during the next visit because it may encourage the curl to wave out from the head form. Cutting a little less or a little more will place the cut line at the crest of the wave again and encourage the hair to curl toward the head form instead of away from it.

Clipper Cutting Natural Curly Styles

Depending on the overall length of the hair, short natural cuts on extremely curly hair can be created by using the freehand clipper or fingers-and-shear cutting technique. The hair is tapered at the perimeter and may be tapered, rounded, or wedged from the sides to the top section. When using clippers, the hair should be clean and dry. Fingers-and-shear cutting is usually performed on clean damp hair.

The decision to use clippers or shears will depend on the density and texture of the hair. Thick, coarse hair types are easier to cut with the clippers. Curly hair of medium density and a softer curl may lend itself to shear cutting. The rule for fingers-and-shear cutting on extremely curly hair is that if a parting can be made and held between the index and second finger, fingers-and-shear cutting can be performed.

Haircutting Tips for Clipper Cutting Curly Hair

- Observe the density and curl pattern closely. Sometimes extremely curly hair gives the illusion that the scalp won't be seen if the hair is cut close, but in reality, it may continue to curl in upon itself in small tufts, leaving partings throughout the hair and scalp exposed.
- Use your comb as a guard around the hairline to avoid cutting the hair too close to the head.
- After each cut with the clipper, comb or pick the hair to check the effect.
- Create flattering and proportionate design forms throughout the crest and top sections.

OTHER CUTTING TECHNIQUES

In addition to the basic haircuts, there are other techniques that can be used to create different effects in the appearance and behavior of the hair. These techniques include over-direction, razor cutting, and texturizing.

Over-Direction

Over-direction occurs when the hair is combed away from its natural fall position. This technique of shifting the hair into a different position facilitates length increase in a design and the ability to blend short and long lengths along a perimeter design line (Figure 17–79) or interior section.

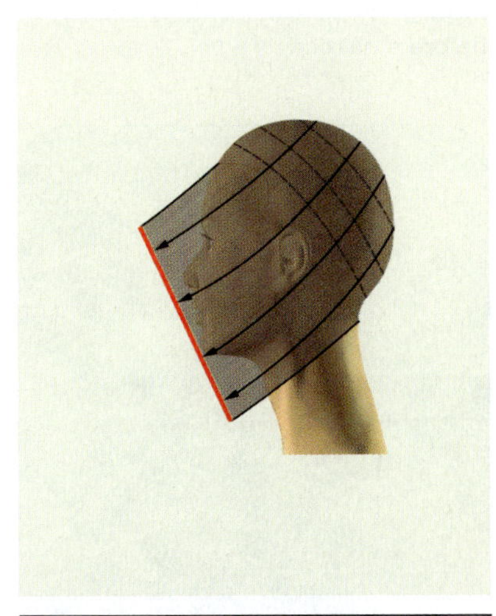

Figure 17-79 Over-direction in long layered cut: design.

17

PROCEDURE

CLIPPER CUT NATURAL STYLE

Implements and Materials

- Towels
- Shampoo cape
- Shampoo and conditioner
- Chair cloth
- Neck strip
- Clipper
- Comb and pick
- Shears
- Blow-dryer with diffuser attachment

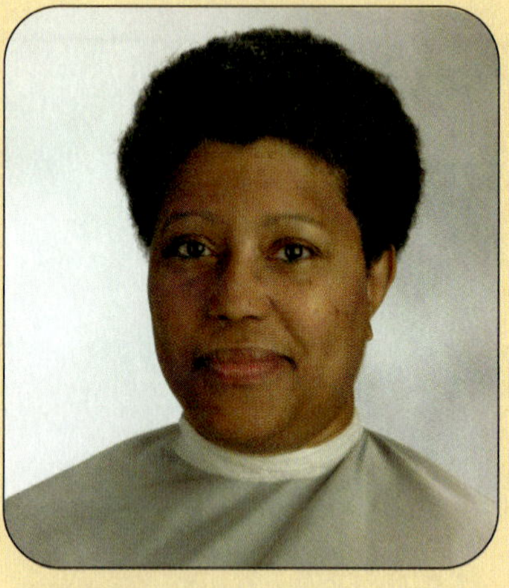

Figure 17-80 Consult with client before a haircut.

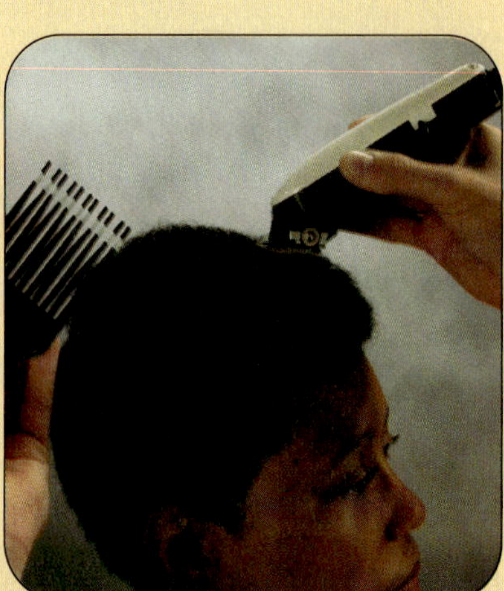

Figure 17-81 Establish a guide in the top center section.

Preparation

1. Conduct the client consultation and hair analysis (Figure 17-80).
2. Drape and perform shampoo service.
3. Dry hair with diffuser attachment and drape for haircut. Wash your hands.

Procedure

1. Pick the hair out, using a wide-toothed comb or pick.
2. Set a guide in the top center section (Figure 17-81).
3. Move to the back and have the client bow her head forward slightly. Begin the taper at the nape using a clipper-over-comb technique. Allow the hair to gradually increase in length as you move up toward the occipital area.
4. Move to the next working panel in the back section using the first cut as a guide. Cut to the occipital.
5. Continue cutting the back section in this manner, working one panel at a time while following the head shape.
6. Move to the right side and cut from the hairline over the ears to the crest area, creating a tapered, rounded, or wedged shape as desired (Figure 17-82). Blend the sides to the back section behind the ear (Figure 17-83). Repeat the procedure on the left side.
7. Blend the hair from the crest to top section. Remember to lift the hair out at 90 degrees with the pick or comb (Figure 17-84).

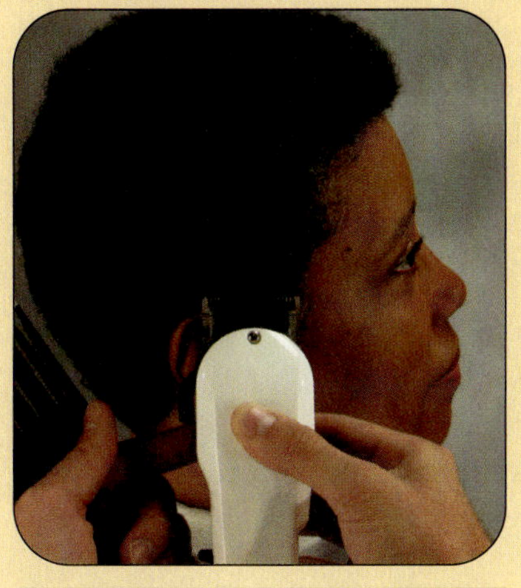

Figure 17-82 Cut from side hairline to crest in tapered, rounded, or wedged shape.

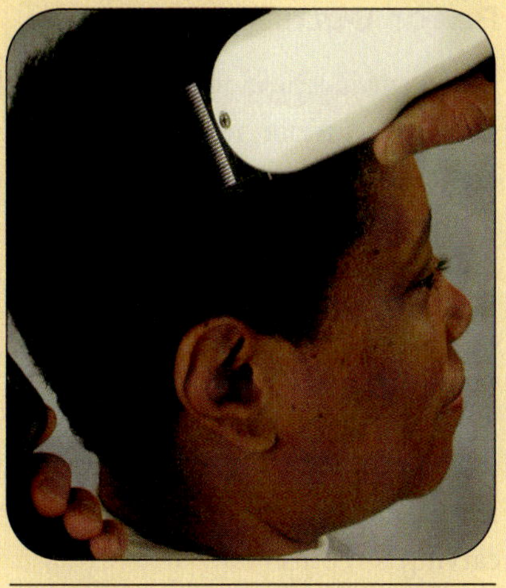

Figure 17-83 Blend sides to back.

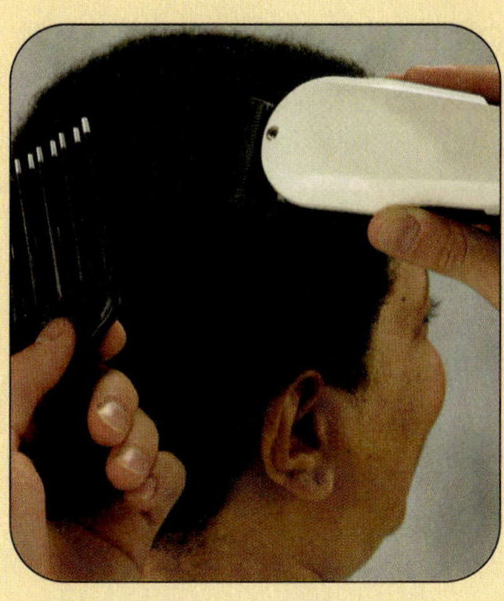

Figure 17-84 Blend crest to top.

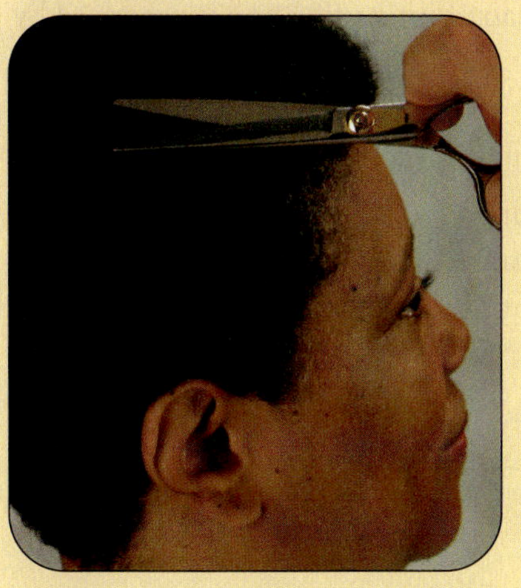

Figure 17-85 Check and finish with shear work.

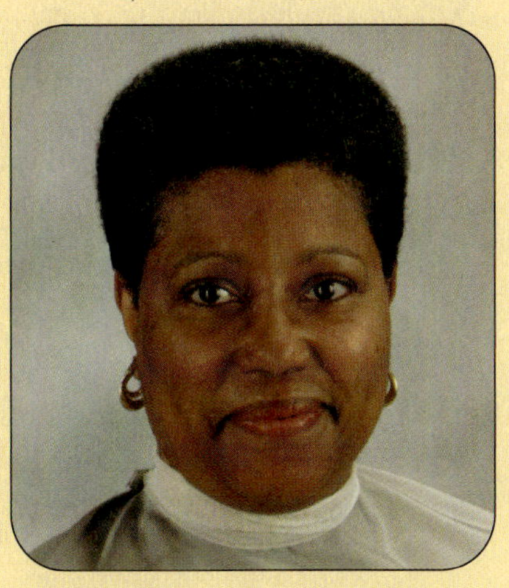

Figure 17-86 Finished haircut.

8. To complete the cut, comb through the hair in the direction that the client will be combing it. Check the cut and fine-tune with shears (Figure 17-85). Apply dressing to finished cut if desired (Figure 17-86).

Cleanup and Sanitation

1. Disinfect tools, implements, and workstation.
2. Wash your hands.

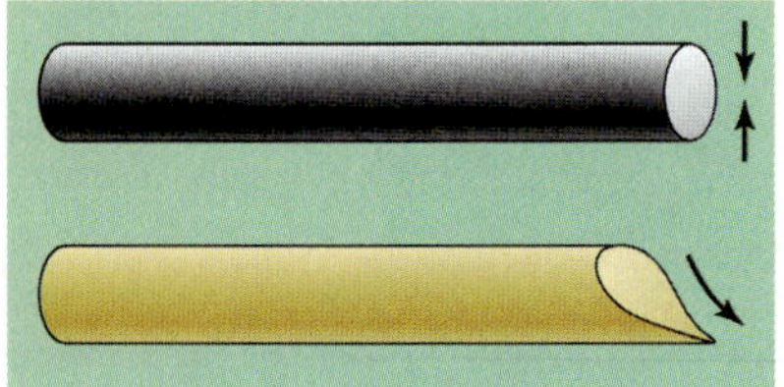

Figure 17-87 Shear cut and razor cut strands.

Razor Cutting

Razor cutting produces an angle at the ends of the hair that results in softer shapes with more movement and visual separation than shear cut hair ends. Generally, haircuts that can be accomplished with shears can also be performed with a razor. Review Figures 17–87 through 17–92 for razor applications on longer hair.

Texturizing

Texturizing techniques can be used to remove excess bulk, add volume, create movement, or create wispy and spiky effects. The most commonly used texturizing techniques are point cutting, notching, slithering, slicing, and carving.

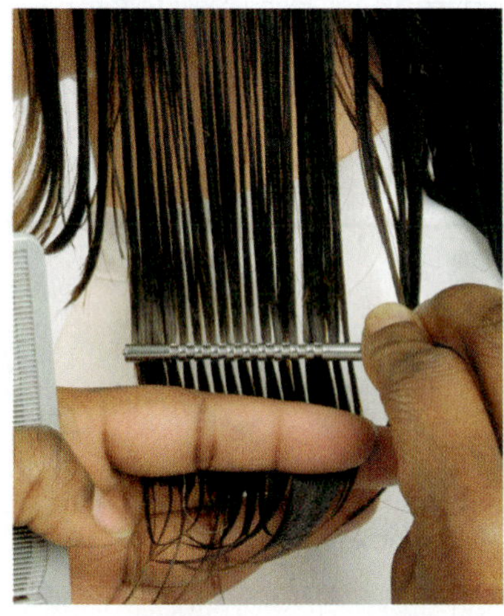

Figure 17-88 Incorrect razor angle.

- *Point cutting* is performed at the ends of the hair using the tips of the shears at a steep shear angle in relation to the hair parting (Figures 17–93a and 17–93b).
- *Notching* creates a chunkier effect than point cutting and is produced by positioning the shears at a flatter angle to the ends of the hair (Figure 17–94). Freehand notching is also accomplished with the tips of the shears, but is usually performed within the interior sections of the haircut.
- *Slithering* is the process of thinning the hair to graduated lengths with the shears, which produces volume and movement. The hair is cut using a sliding shears movement with the blades kept partially opened (Figure 17–95).
- *Slicing* also removes bulk and adds movement in the hair. The blades are kept open and only the portion of the blade near the pivot is used for cutting (Figure 17–96).

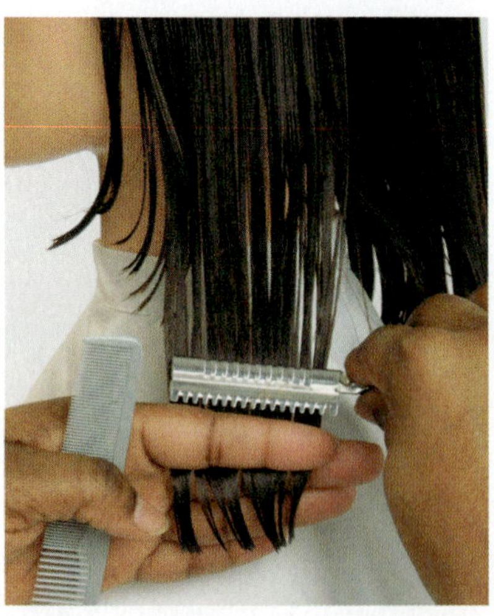

Figure 17-89 Razor cutting parallel to subsection.

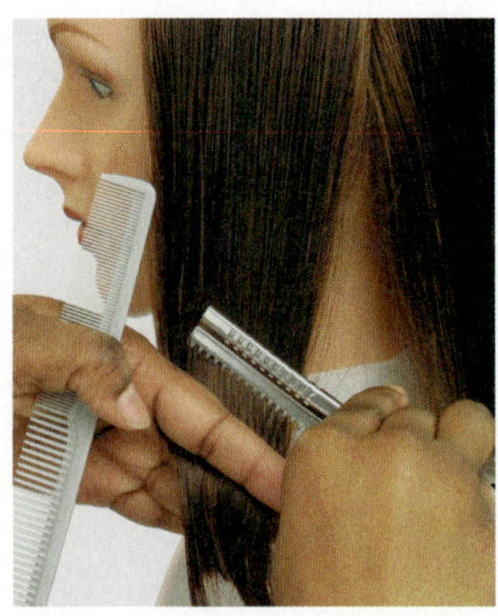

Figure 17-90 Razor cutting at a 45-degree angle.

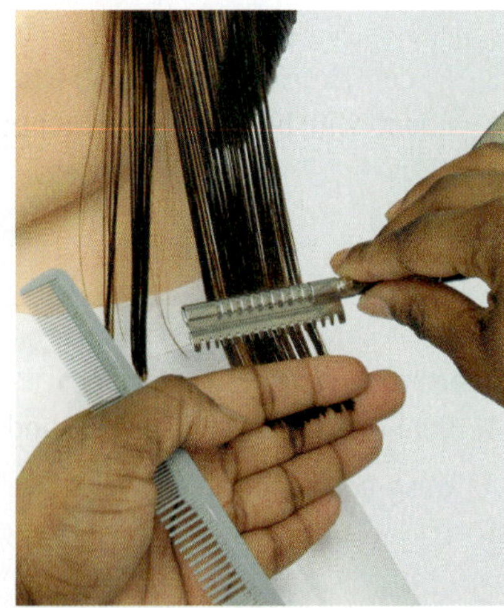

Figure 17-91 Hand position on horizontal section.

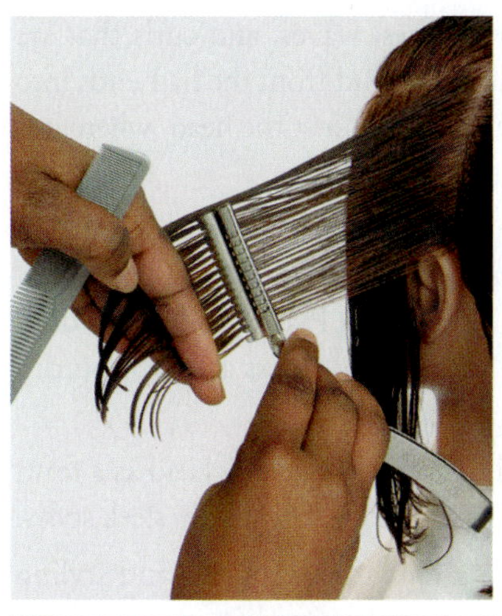

Figure 17-92 Hand position on vertical section.

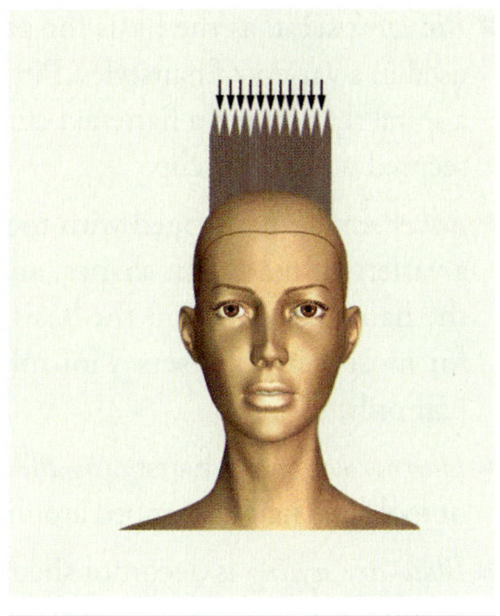

Figure 17-93a Point cutting with steeper shears angle.

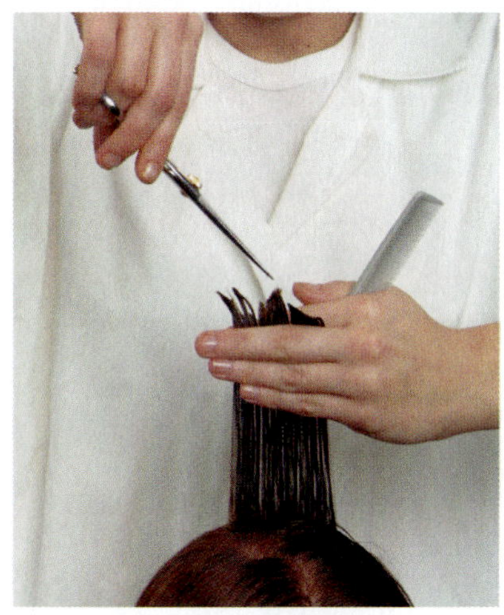

Figure 17-93b Point cutting.

- *Carving* is a version of slicing that creates separation in the hair. The shears are moved throughout the hair with an open and closing movement that carves out sections of hair (Figure 17–97). Carving the ends of the hair will create texture and separation at the perimeter. 2

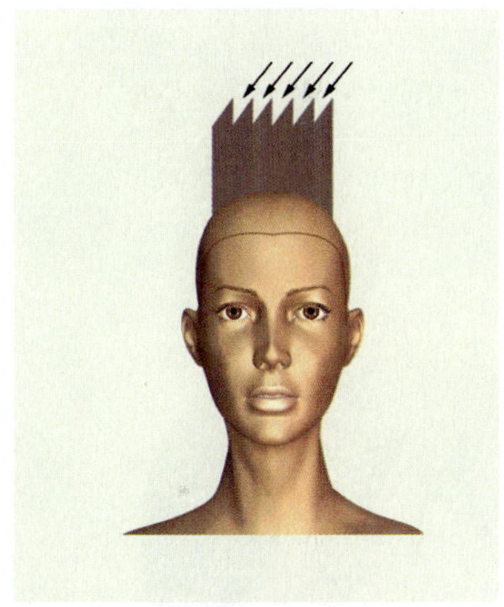

Figure 17-94 Notching.

HAIRSTYLING

As with haircutting, the first step in the hairstyling process is the client consultation. Guide the client toward the most suitable hairstyle design for her face shape, hair texture, and lifestyle. Keep styling magazines accessible for easy reference during the consultation. Hairstyling techniques include wet hairstyling, blow-dry styling, thermal styling, and natural dry styling.

Terminology and Techniques

This section provides a basic description of techniques and terminology used in women's hairstyling. The procedures for hair wrapping, blow-dry styling, and curling iron work are also included. For wet setting, finger waving, and pin-curling procedures see Chapter 12, Hairstyling, in *Milady's Standard Cosmetology* textbook.

- *Wet hairstyling* is accomplished through the processes of finger waving, pin curls, hair wrapping, and roller sets. The tools needed for these processes include rollers, pin curl clips, sectioning clips, all-purpose combs, brushes, and setting lotion.
- *Finger waving* is the process of shaping and directing the hair into an S-shaped pattern through the use of the fingers, comb, and setting lotion.

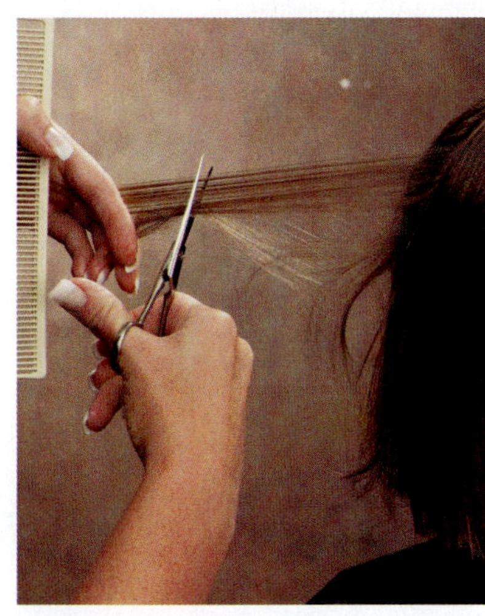

Figure 17-95 Slithering.

17

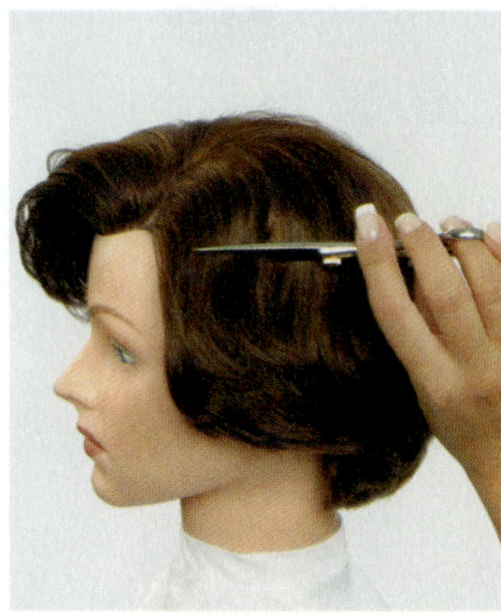

Figure 17-96 Slicing.

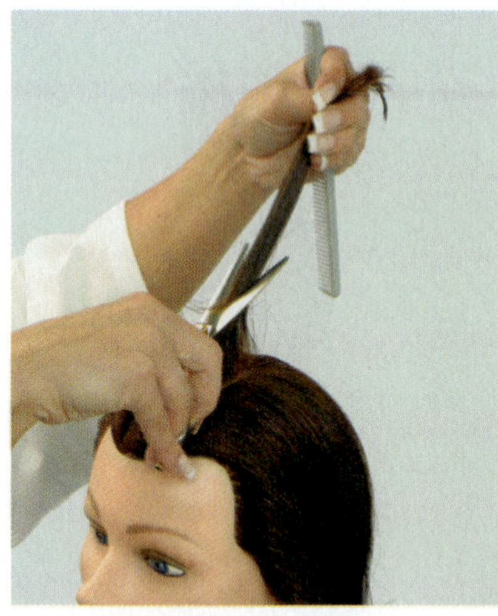

Figure 17-97 Carving.

- *Pin curls* serve as the basis for patterns, lines, waves, and curls that are used in a variety of hairstyles. Pin curls are wound from the hair ends into a spiral that creates a flattened curl formation against the head, where it is secured with a hair clip.
- *Roller sets* are performed with tools called rollers. Rollers are available in a variety of materials, shapes, and sizes that are used to set a pattern in the hair that will form the basis for a hairstyle. Plastic rollers are used for most wet roller sets. Hot rollers and Velcro rollers are used on dry hair only.
- *Hair wrapping* is a hairstyling method that uses the client's head as a form or tool. The hair is wrapped around the head to create smooth, sleek styles.
- *Blow-dry styling* is accomplished with a blow-dryer, brush, and styling products (optional) in a similar manner to that used in men's styling. Blow-dry styling also serves to prepare the hair for thermal iron curling techniques.
- *Natural dry styling* usually requires minimal manipulation of the hair. Once the hair is towel dried, it may be combed into place or arranged in a freeform style with the hands and fingers. It is then allowed to dry naturally.
- *Thermal styling* includes the procedures of thermal waving and thermal hair straightening. Heated tools are used to wave, curl, or straighten the hair.

These techniques are described and illustrated in the following sections.

Hair Wrapping

The technique of hair wrapping uses the client's head as a form or tool that the hair is wrapped around. This technique helps to temporarily straighten wavy and curly hair into smooth, sleek styles. Hair wrapping may be used on wet or dry straight and relaxed hair textures to create a natural-looking curvature to the hairstyle.

When the hair-wrapping technique is applied to the entire head of hair, minimal volume results at the scalp. If height or volume is desired at the crown area, two or three large rollers should be placed in this section for additional lift.

Blow-Dry Styling

Blow-dry styling is the technique of drying and styling damp hair in one operation. Combined with the foundation of a good haircut, blow-dry styling is a quick and relatively simple option for the client's self-styling or shop-styling procedures. Review Chapter 6 to become reacquainted with various blow-dryer attachments and brush designs that can be used in the performance of blow-dry styling.

PROCEDURE

HAIR WRAPPING

Implements and Materials

- Towels
- Shampoo cape
- Shampoo and conditioner
- Chair cloth
- Neck strip or hair-wrapping strip
- Duckbill clips
- Setting or wrapping lotion or gel
- Comb
- Firm-bristled brush
- Spray bottle with water

Preparation

1. Wash your hands.
2. Conduct the client consultation and hair analysis.
3. Drape and perform shampoo service. Towel blot hair.

Procedure

1. Apply lotion or gel product. Comb or brush the hair clockwise around the head in the desired direction (Figure 17–98).
2. Use duckbill clips to keep the hair in place while wrapping (Figure 17–99).

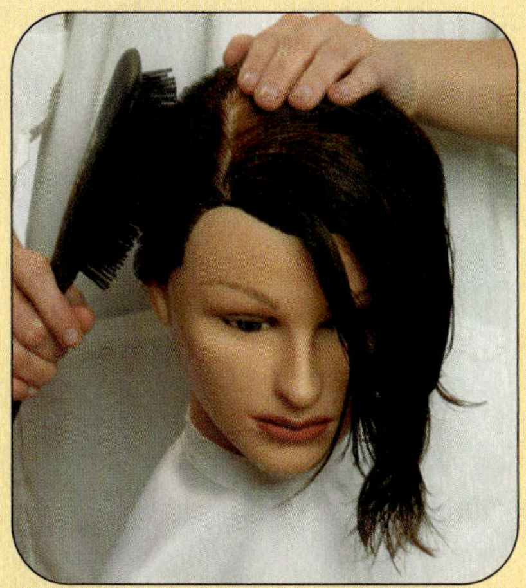

Figure 17–98 Wrap the first section.

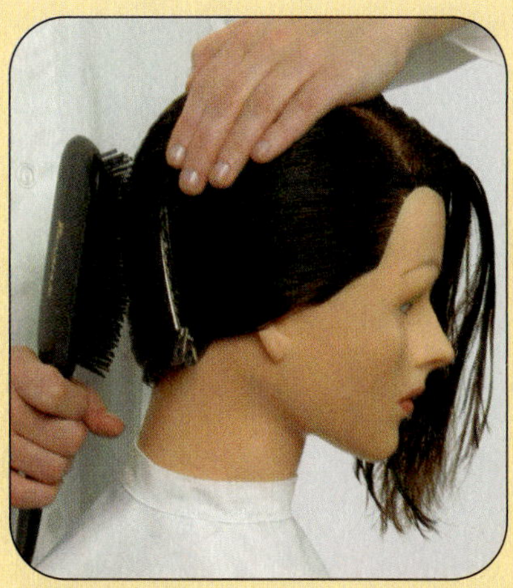

Figure 17–99 Hold wrapped hair with duckbill clips.

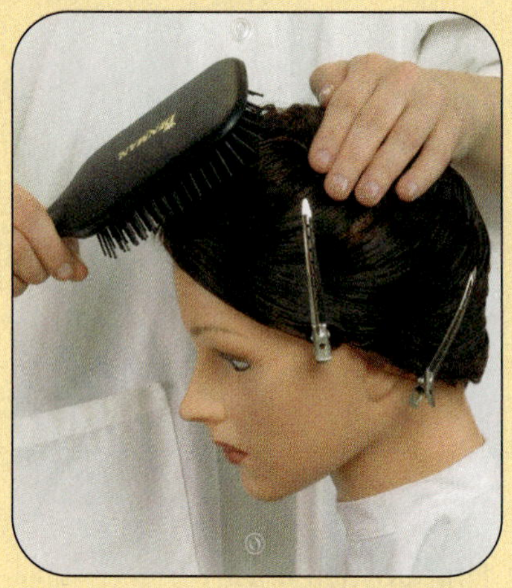

Figure 17-100 Continue wrapping hair.

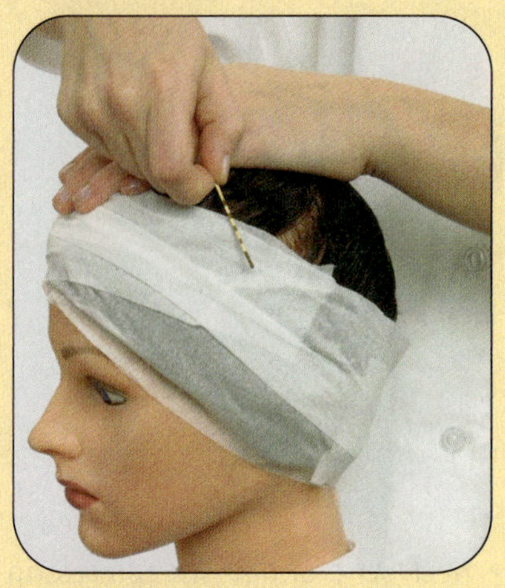

Figure 17-101 Wrap neck strip around hair.

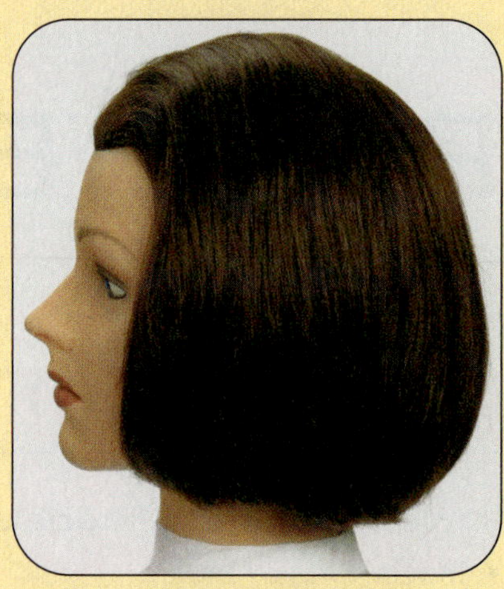

Figure 17-102 Finished style.

3. Continue wrapping the hair around the head. Follow the comb or brush with your hand to smooth and keep the hair tight against the head (Figure 17-100).
4. When the hair is wrapped, stretch a neckstrip or hair-wrapping strip around the head to keep the hair in place. Secure with a bobby pin and remove the duckbill clips (Figure 17-101).
5. Place client under hood dryer. When hair is thoroughly dried, allow it to cool before combing into the finished style (Figure 17-102). Apply holding spray or oil sheen as desired.

Cleanup and Sanitation

1. Disinfect tools, implements, and workstation.
2. Wash your hands.

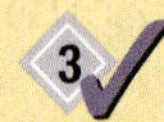

PROCEDURE

BLOW-DRY STYLING

Implements and Materials

- Towels
- Shampoo cape
- Shampoo and conditioner
- Chair cloth
- Neck strip or hair-wrapping strip
- Duckbill clips
- Styling lotion, mousse, or gel
- Comb
- Brush of choice
- Blow-dryer with attachments
- Spray bottle with water

Preparation

1. Wash your hands.
2. Conduct the client consultation and hair analysis.
3. Drape and perform shampoo service. Towel blot hair.

Procedure A

1. Distribute the styling product through the hair and comb through to the ends.
2. Use the comb to mold the hair into the desired shape (Figure 17–103).
3. Section the hair for blow-drying (Figure 17–104).

17

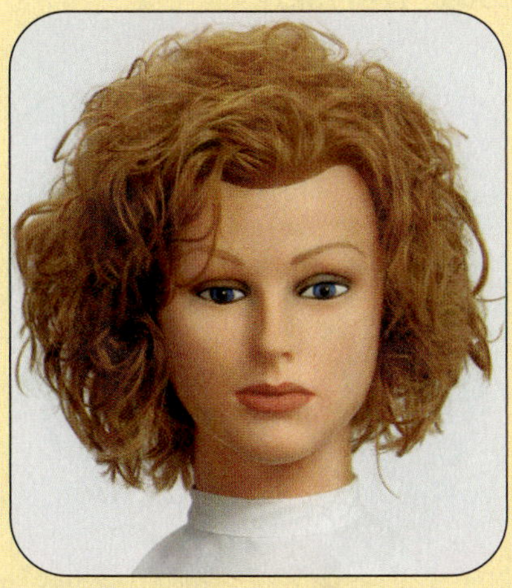

Figure 17–103 Mold the hair into the shape it will take when dry.

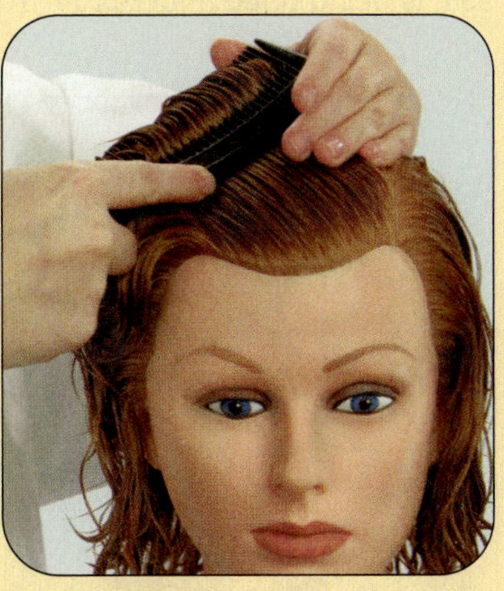

Figure 17–104 Section the hair for blow-drying.

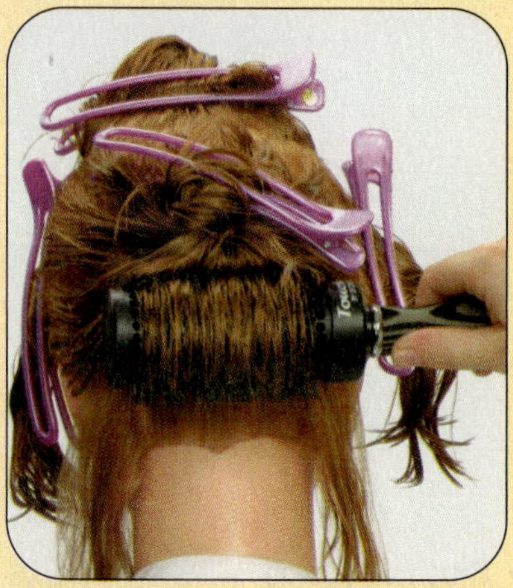

Figure 17-105 Blow-dry hair on brush.

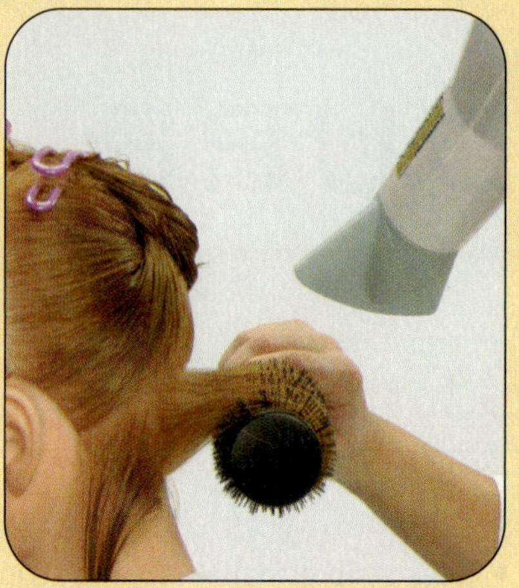

Figure 17-106 Direct the air stream to follow the brush.

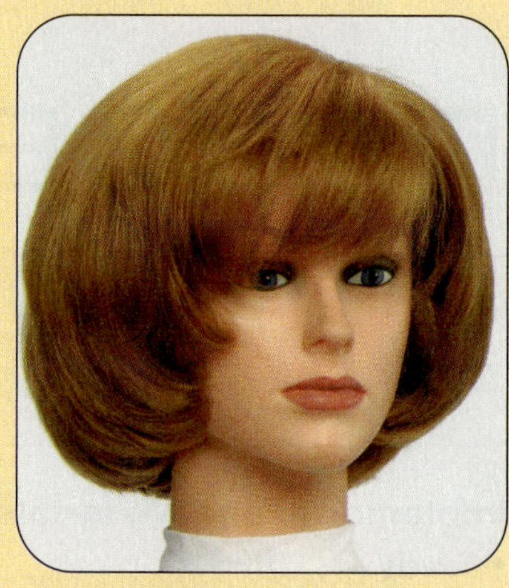

Figure 17-107 Finished style.

4. Beginning in the nape area, insert the brush at the base of the section. Roll the hair down to the base with medium tension at the projection appropriate for the desired volume (Figure 17-105).
5. Direct the stream of air from the blow-dryer over the hair in a back-and-forth motion in the same direction as the hair is wound (Figure 17-106).
6. Follow the same procedure throughout the sections of the head, using the appropriate projection of hair for a given area depending on the desired style.
7. Make sure the hair and scalp are completely dry before combing out the style. Finish with a holding spray or other appropriate product as the client desires (Figure 17-107).

Procedure B

Curly Style Option: To blow-dry short, curly hair into its natural wave pattern, use a diffuser and scrunch the hair as it is being dried (Figures 17-108 through 17-110).

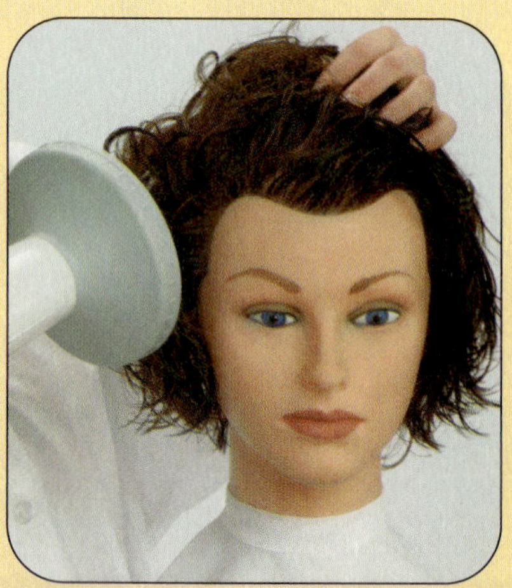

Figure 17-108 Hair being diffused.

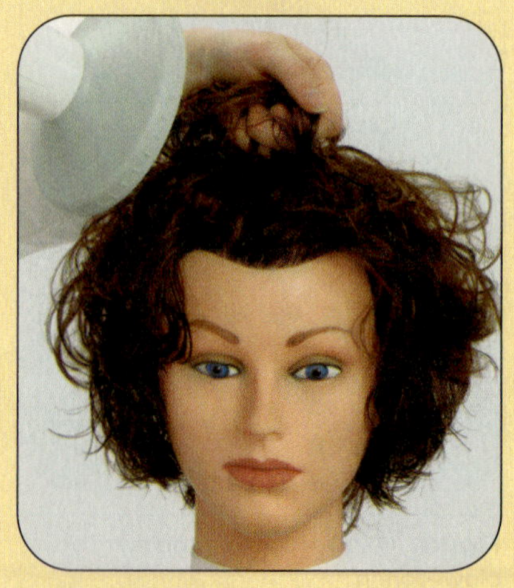

Figure 17-109 Scrunch the hair.

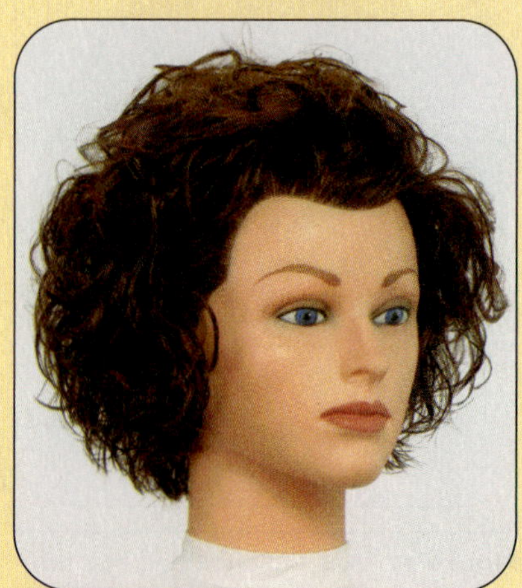

Figure 17-110 Finished hairstyle.

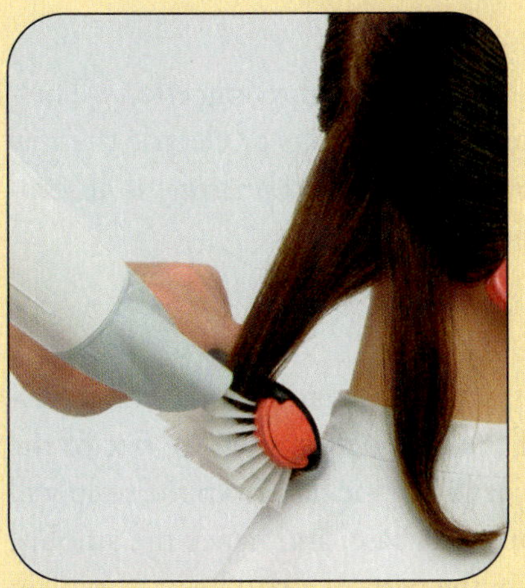

Figure 17-111 Hold the hair at low elevation.

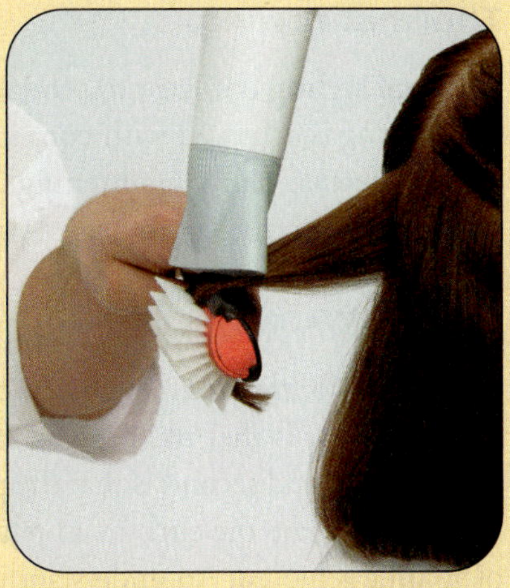

Figure 17-112 Hold the section straight out from the head.

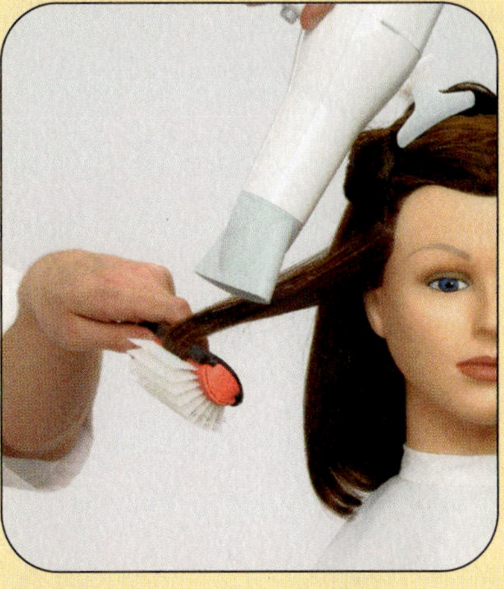

Figure 17-113 Side section turned under.

Procedure C

Long Layered Option: Use the following as a guide to blow-dry longer hairstyles.

1. Attach the nozzle for controlled styling. Part and section the hair to facilitate working on one section at a time.
2. Begin at a nape section. Draw the brush through the hair from scalp to ends at a low elevation and follow with the dryer heat (Figure 17-111).
3. For increased volume, elevate the section at 45 or 90 degrees (Figure 17-112).
4. When reaching the ends of the hair, turn the brush under or up depending on the desired style (Figures 17-113 and 17-114).
5. Continue the process until all the hair is dried. Comb or brush through the hair to finish. Apply holding spray as desired (Figure 17-115).

Figure 17-114 Side section flipped out.

Cleanup and Sanitation

1. Disinfect tools, implements, and workstation.
2. Wash your hands.

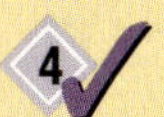

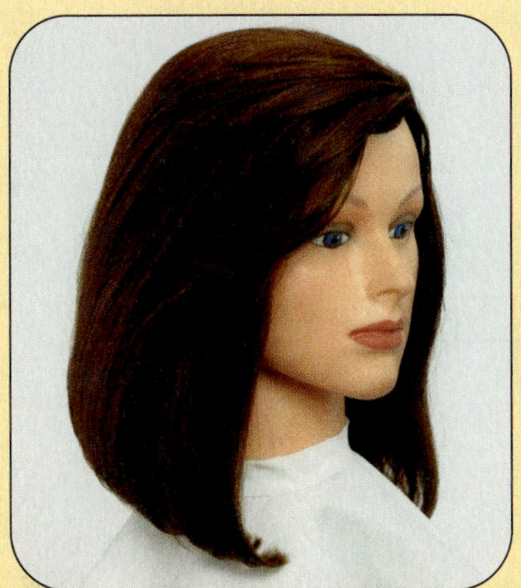

Figure 17-115 Finished style.

Thermal Styling

Thermal styling uses heat to produce waving or straightening effects. Thermal waving is achieved with conventional Marcel irons or electric thermal irons. Thermal hair straightening, also known as *hair pressing*, is accomplished through the use of heated pressing combs.

Thermal Waving

There are two important factors to consider when creating curls with a curling iron. First is that the barrel size of the iron determines the size of the wave or curl; and second is that the projection of the hair from the scalp will determine where the curl sits in relation to its base, and hence the amount of volume achieved. An understanding of the parts of a curl helps to explain the relationships between hair projection, bases, and volume.

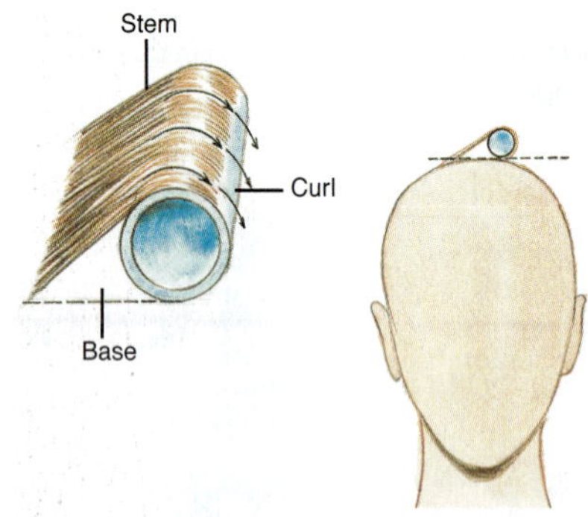

Figure 17-116 Parts of a roller curl.

The parts of a curl are the base, stem, and curl (**circle**) (Figure 17–116). The **base** is the foundation on which the barrel (or roller) is placed. The **stem** is the hair between the scalp and the first arc of the barrel; it gives the hair direction and mobility. The **curl** is the hair that is wrapped around the barrel. The ultimate size of the curl along the length of the hair shaft depends on how it is wrapped. A hair section that is wrapped in a spiral along the curling iron barrel will have a more uniform curl formation than a hair section that is repeatedly wrapped around itself over one section of the barrel.

There are three kinds of bases used in thermal (and roller) setting. They are on-base, half-base, and off-base.

- **On-base** roller placement sits directly on its base and produces a full-volume curl. On-base placement is achieved by slightly over-directing the hair in front of the base (Figure 17–117).
- **Half off-base**, or half-base, roller placement sits halfway on and halfway behind the base after rolling the hair parting at 90 degrees (Figure 17–118).
- **Off-base** roller placement produces the least amount of volume and sits completely off the base. The hair is held at 45 degrees from the base and rolled down to the scalp (Figure 17–119).

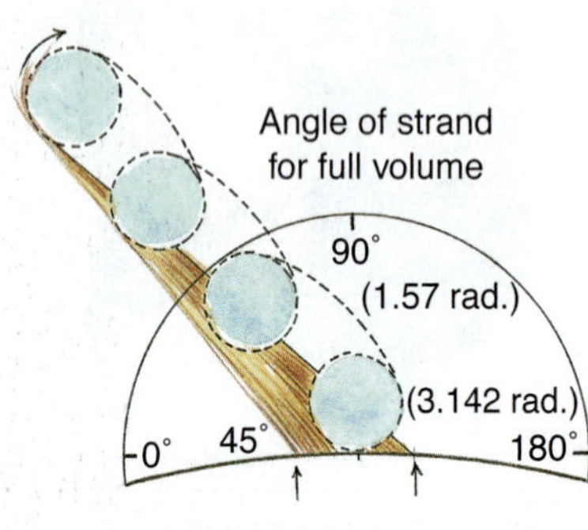

Figure 17-117 On-base: full volume.

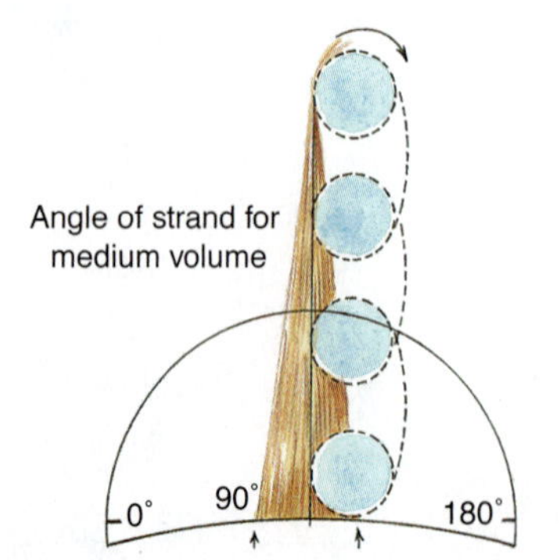

Figure 17-118 Half off-base: medium volume.

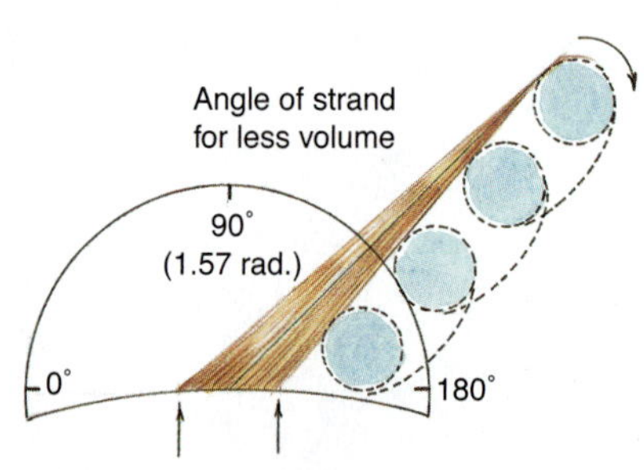

Figure 17-119 Off-base: less volume.

PROCEDURE

THERMAL IRON STYLING

Practice the following manipulative movements on a mannequin:

1. Practice turning the irons while opening and closing at regular intervals (Figures 17–120 through 17–122).
2. Rotate the irons downward, toward you, and upward, away from you (Figures 17–123 through 17–126).
3. Practice releasing the hair by opening and closing the irons with a quick, clicking movement.
4. Using a mannequin, practice rotating while opening and closing the iron on a hair section (Figure 17–127).
5. Guide the hair section toward the center of the curl while rotating the irons (Figure 17–128).

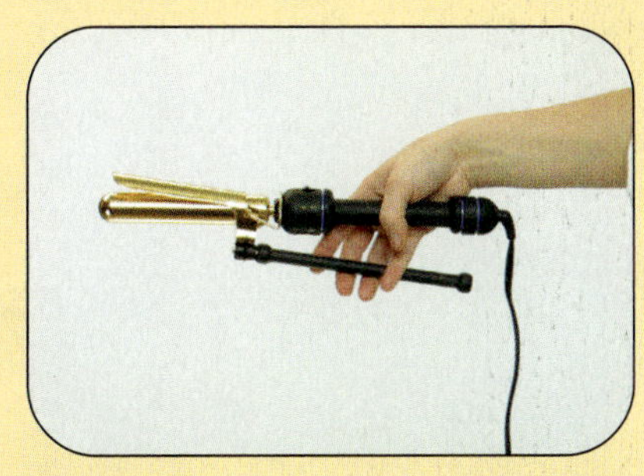

Figure 17–120 Use your little finger to open clamp.

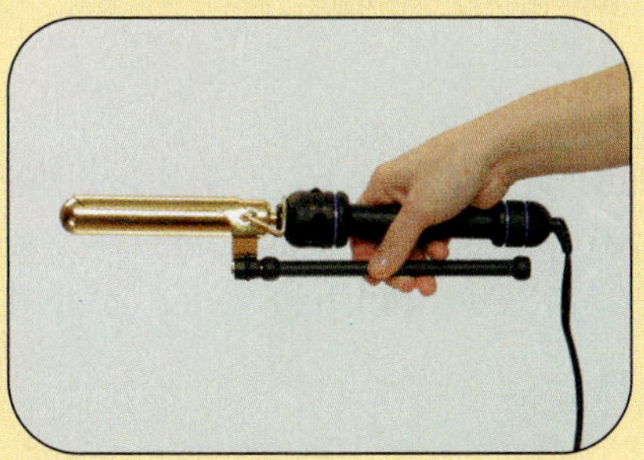

Figure 17–121 Use three middle fingers to close and manipulate irons.

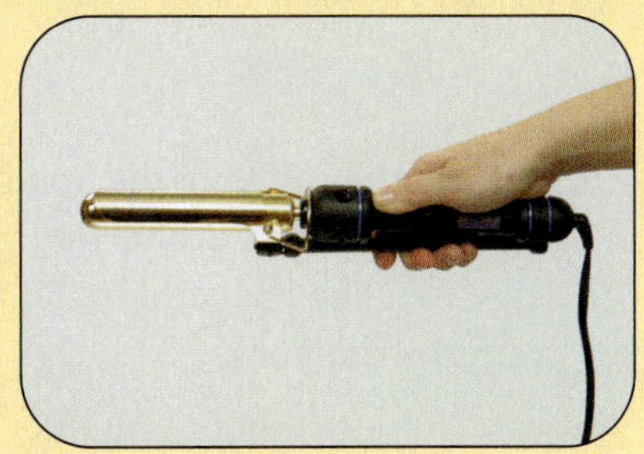

Figure 17–122 Shift thumb when manipulating irons.

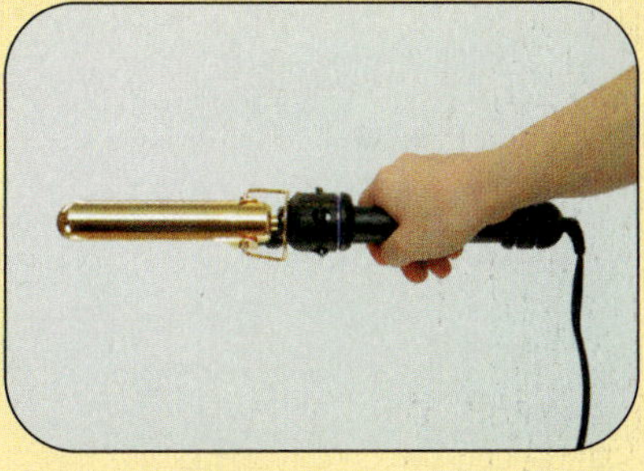

Figure 17–123 Close clamp and make a one-quarter turn downward.

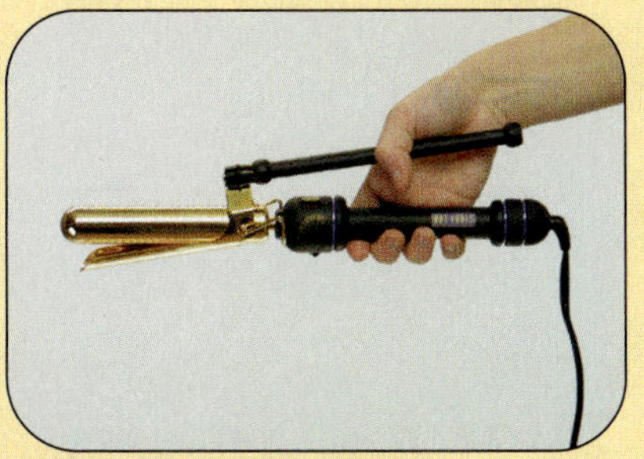

Figure 17–124 Irons have made a one-half turn. Use thumb to open clamp and relax hair tension.

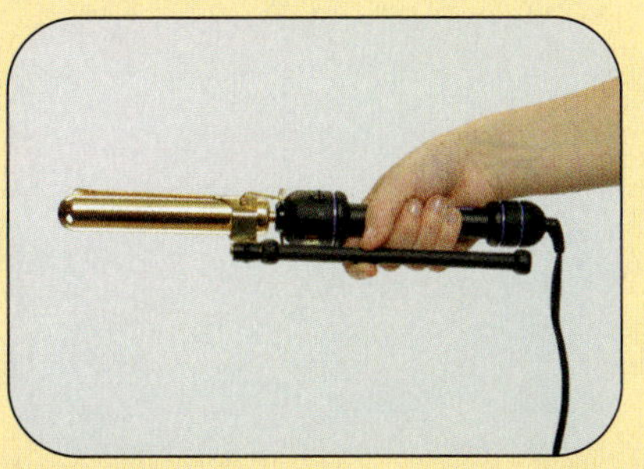

Figure 17–125 Rotate irons to three-quarters of a complete turn.

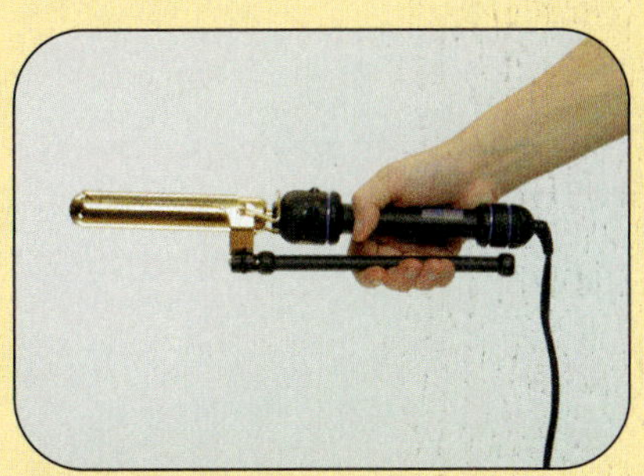

Figure 17–126 Full turn.

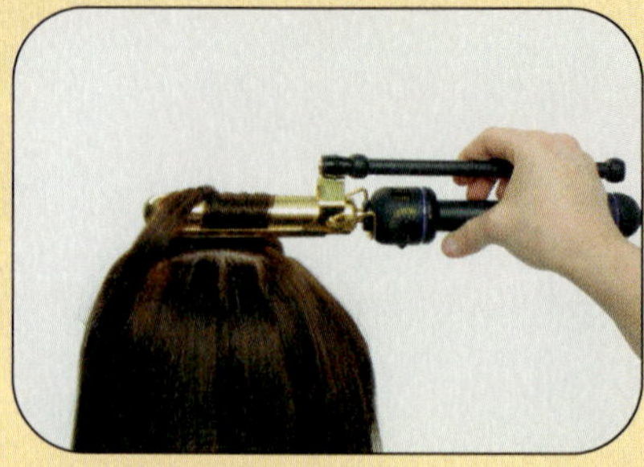

Figure 17-127 Rotate while opening and closing the irons.

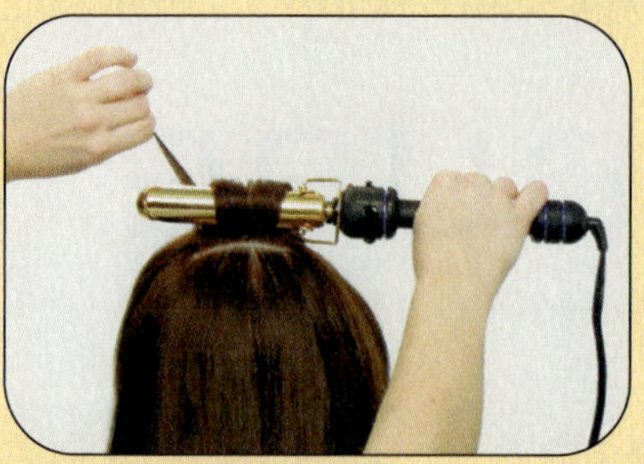

Figure 17-128 Guide hair strand into the center of the curl while rotating irons.

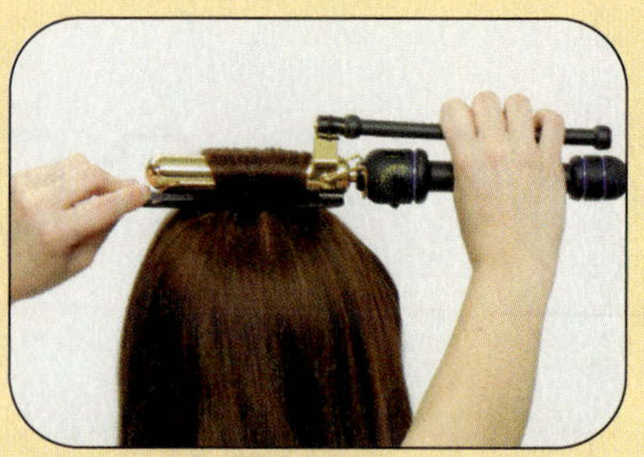

Figure 17-129 Remove curl using comb as guide.

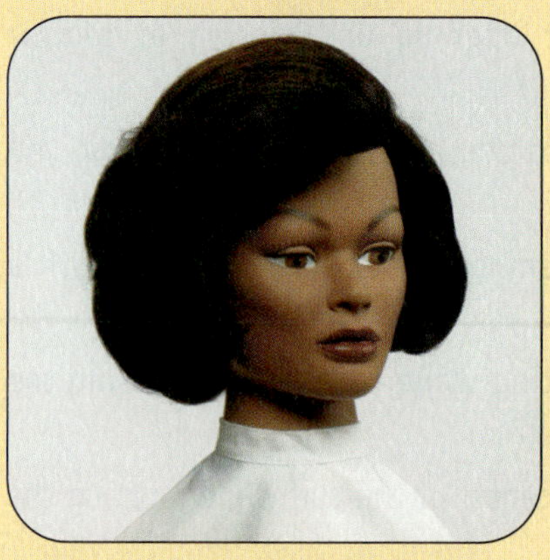

Figure 17-130 Finished thermal-curled medium-length hairstyle.

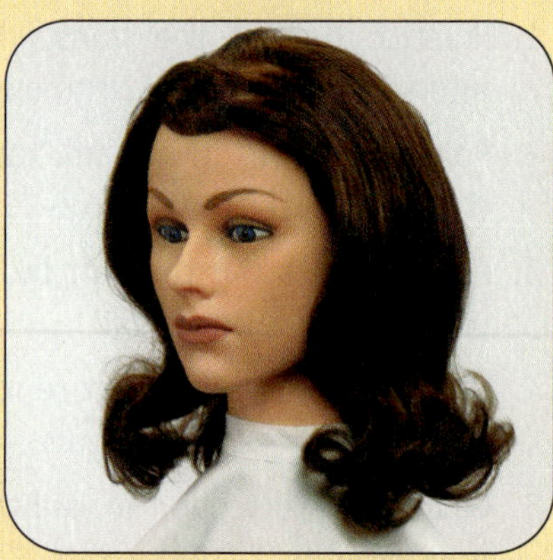

Figure 17-131 Finished thermal-curled long hairstyle.

6. Remove the curl from the iron by drawing the comb to the left and the curl to the right, using the comb to protect the scalp area (Figure 17-129). See Figures 17-130 and 17-131 for finished styles created with thermal irons.

Manipulating Thermal Irons

The manipulative techniques are basically the same for stove-heated irons and electric irons. Begin practicing by rolling the cold irons forward and then backward until comfortable with the tool (Figure 17–132).

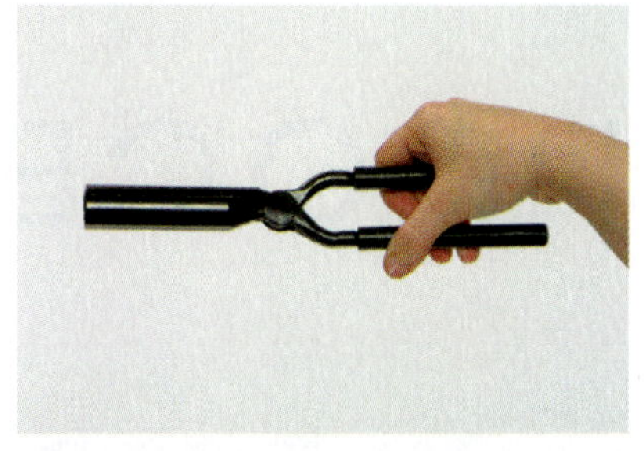

Figure 17-132 Rolling the iron.

Hair Pressing

Hair pressing temporarily straightens extremely curly or hard-to-manage hair by means of a heated pressing comb or iron. Pressings generally last until the next shampoo, although high humidity and other weather conditions can cause the hair to partially revert to its natural condition. In some cases, environmental conditions may determine whether a soft, medium, or hard press is used to straighten the hair.

- A *soft press* removes 50 to 60 percent of the curl and is accomplished by applying the pressing comb once to each side of the hair section.
- The *medium press* removes 60 to 75 percent of the curl and is performed in the same manner as the soft press, but with a little more pressure.
- A *hard press* removes 100 percent of the curl formation and involves two applications of the pressing comb on each side of the hair section.

Following a shampoo and blow-dry, the hair is prepared for the pressing service with an application of a pressing cream or oil. These products make the hair softer and help to prevent the hair from burning or scorching.

Safety Precautions

- Use thermal irons only after receiving instruction on their use.
- Keep irons clean and sanitized.
- Always test the temperature of the iron before using it on a client.
- Do not overheat irons.
- Handle and remove heated irons and stoves carefully.
- Do not place heated stoves near the station mirror as the heat can cause breakage.
- Place a hard rubber comb between the client's scalp and the iron. Never use a metal comb.
- Place heated stoves and irons in a safe place to cool.

PROCEDURE

HAIR PRESSING

Implements and Materials

- Towels
- Shampoo cape
- Shampoo
- Chair cloth
- Neck strip
- Clips
- Pressing cream or oil
- Styling pomade
- Comb
- Brush
- Blow-dryer with attachments
- Pressing comb
- Electric heater (stove)

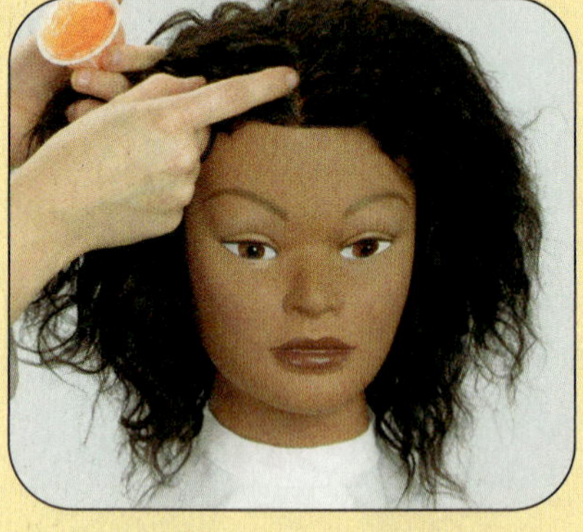

Figure 17-133 Apply pressing cream or oil to client's hair.

17

Preparation

1. Wash your hands.
2. Conduct the client consultation and hair analysis.
3. Drape and perform shampoo service. Towel blot hair.
4. Drape client with chair cloth and neck strip. Heat the pressing comb.

Procedure

1. Blow-dry the hair. Apply pressing cream or oil (Figure 17–133).
2. Comb and part off the hair into four sections (Figure 17–134).
3. Divide the first section into 1-inch subsections. Apply pressing cream or oil to the subsection as needed. Test the heated pressing comb (Figure 17–135).

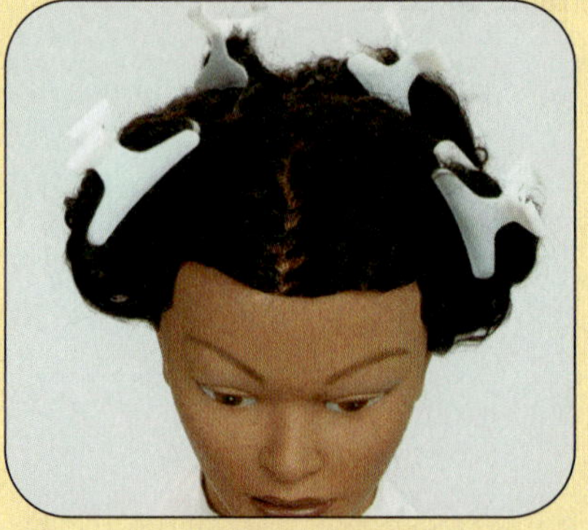

Figure 17-134 Divide hair into four sections.

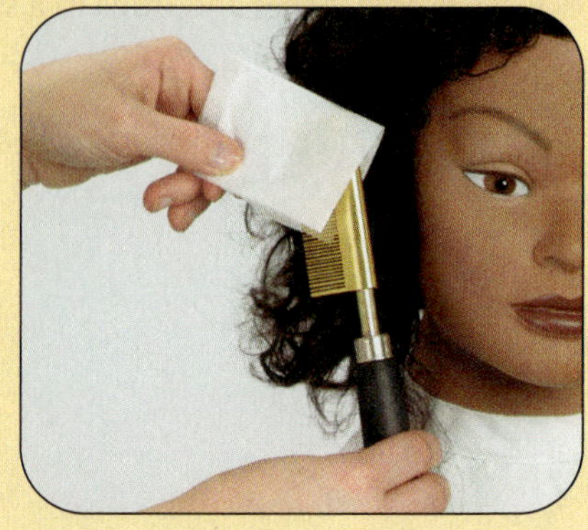

Figure 17-135 Test heated pressing comb.

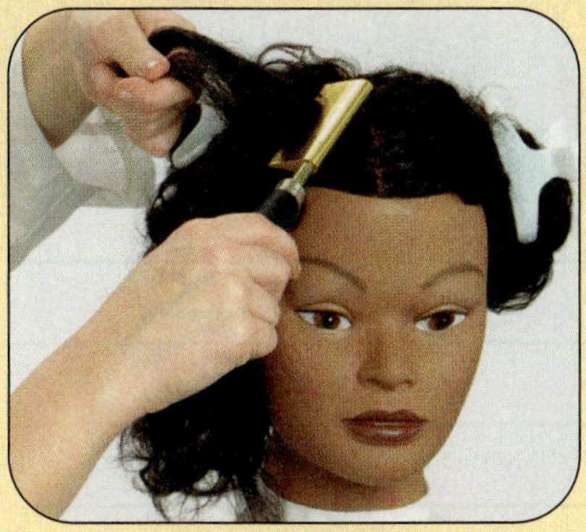

Figure 17-136 Insert comb into top side of hair section.

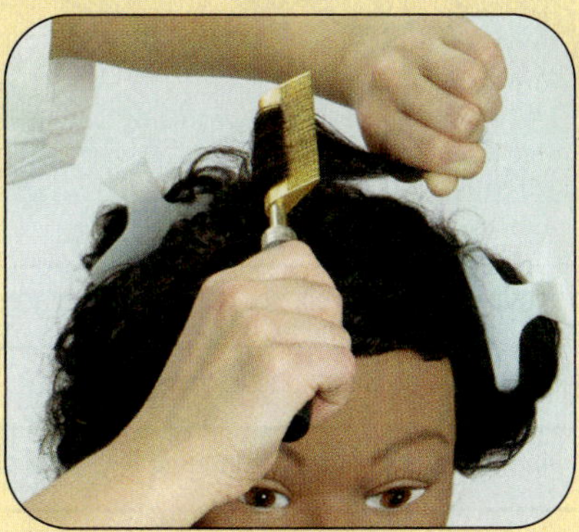

Figure 17-137 Press hair section with back of comb.

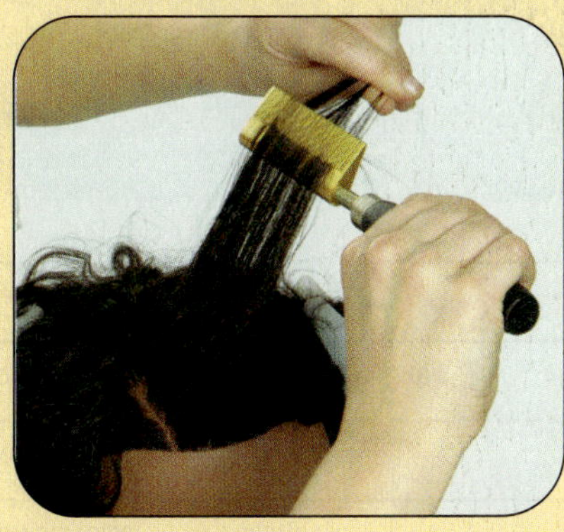

Figure 17-138 Bring pressing comb through ends of hair.

4. Hold the first subsection away from the scalp and insert the teeth of the comb into the top side of the hair section (Figure 17-136). Draw out the comb slightly, making a quick turn so that the back of the comb does the actual pressing (Figure 17-137).
5. Press the comb slowly through the hair until the ends pass through the teeth of the comb (Figure 17-138).
6. Reposition each completed section over to the opposite side of the head (Figure 17-139).
7. Continue this procedure until all the hair is pressed. Add pomade if desired.
8. Style and comb the hair or finish with curling iron according to client's wishes (Figure 17-140).

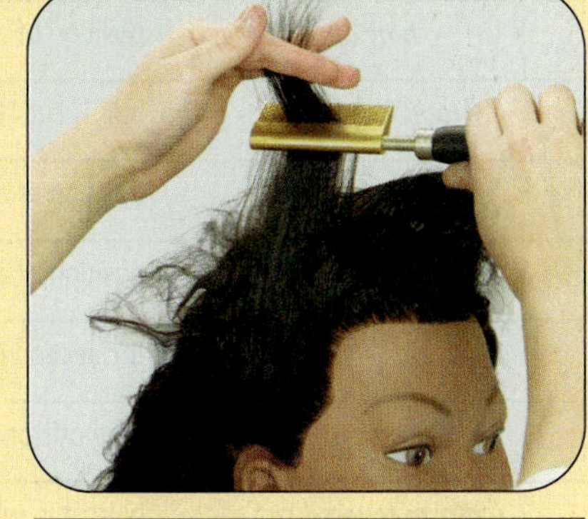

Figure 17-139 Bring finished section to one side.

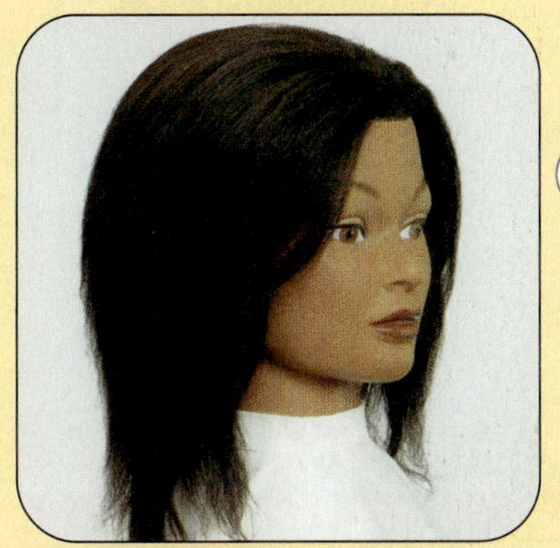

Figure 17-140 Finished pressed hairstyle.

chapter glossary

base	the area near the scalp at which a roller or iron barrel is placed
blow-dry styling	technique of drying and styling damp hair in one operation
blunt cut	haircut in which all the hair comes to one hanging level at 0 degrees to form a weight line
circle	also known as curl; part of a curl that forms a complete circle
curl	the hair that is wrapped around the barrel of an iron or a roller
graduated cut	graduated, wedge, or stacked shape at the perimeter of a haircut; usually cut at 45 degrees
hair pressing	method of temporarily straightening curly or unruly hair by means of a heated pressing comb
half off-base	position of a curl one-half off its base; provides medium volume and movement
long layered cut	hair is cut 180-degree elevation to create short layers at the top and increasingly longer layers at the perimeter
off-base	position of a curl off its base; provides maximum mobility and minimum volume
on-base	position of a curl directly on its base; provides maximum volume
stem	the section of a curl between the base and the first arc of the circle; gives the curl direction and movement
thermal styling	methods of curling or straightening on dry hair using thermal irons and pressing combs
uniform layered cut	haircut in which all the hair is cut at the same length with a 90-degree elevation

chapter review questions

1. List the four basic cuts and the elevations or projections used to achieve them.
2. Explain over-direction.
3. List the methods used in wet hairstyling.
4. Define on-base, half off-base, and off-base curl placement. Explain the effects of each.
5. Define thermal hairstyling.
6. Explain the hair-pressing procedure.

Learning Objectives

After completing this chapter, you should be able to:

1. Explain the effects of chemical texture services on the hair.
2. Identify the similarities and differences between chemical texture services.
3. List the factors of hair analysis for chemical texture services.
4. Perform a permanent wave service.
5. Perform a reformation curl service.
6. Perform a hair-relaxing service.

Key Terms

acid-balanced waves
pg. 502

alkaline or cold waves
pg. 501

ammonium thioglycolate (ATG)
pg. 501

base control
pg. 499

base cream
pg. 516

base direction
pg. 500

base relaxers
pg. 519

base sections
pg. 498

basic perm wrap
pg. 508

bookend wrap
pg. 497

chemical blow-out
pg. 520

chemical hair relaxing
pg. 487

chemical texture services
pg. 487

croquignole rodding
pg. 500

end wraps
pg. 497

endothermic waves
pg. 502

exothermic waves
pg. 503

glyceryl monothioglycolate (GMTG)
pg. 502

hydroxide relaxers
pg. 519

lanthionization
pg. 491

lotion wrap
pg. 501

neutralization
pg. 507

no-base relaxers
pg. 519

permanent waving
pg. 487

prewrap solution
pg. 504

reformation curl
pg. 487

texturize
pg. 519

thio relaxers
pg. 515

true acid waves
pg. 502

Chemical texture services such as permanent waving, reformation curls, and relaxers create chemical changes that permanently alter the natural wave pattern of the existing hair growth. These chemical services are used to curl straight hair, resize the curl in curly hair types, or straighten overly curly hair, respectively. When new hair growth occurs, retouch applications are required to maintain the altered texture and structure of the hair. Chemical texture services are practical, versatile, and lucrative services that provide clients with alternatives in haircut designs and styling.

CHEMICAL TEXTURE SERVICES DEFINED

Permanent waving is a process used to chemically restructure natural hair into a different wave pattern. Most permanent waving services are performed with the objective to create waves or curls in straighter hair types. Permanent waving requires the use of rods, end wraps, a waving lotion, and neutralizer. When performed properly, perms can increase the fullness of fine, soft hair, redirect resistant growth patterns until new growth occurs, and provide greater styling control.

A **reformation curl**, also known as a soft-curl perm, Jheri curl, or simply "a curl," is a process used to restructure very curly hair into a larger curl pattern. Reformation curls require a relaxing product to partially straighten the hair, rods, end wraps, waving lotion, and a neutralizer. This makes the procedure part chemical hair-relaxer service and part permanent waving service. The reformation curl procedure offers clients with tight curl textures an additional option to the natural look or total straightening with chemical relaxing products.

Chemical hair relaxing is the process used to rearrange the basic structure of over-curly hair into a straighter hair form. The relaxing process involves the use of a relaxing cream, neutralizer or neutralizing shampoo, and conditioning product. A properly performed chemical hair-relaxing service should leave the hair in a soft, straightened form that adapts well to wet setting, wrapping, or thermal styling techniques.

Chemical services require maintenance and periodic reapplications as new growth appears. The barber who develops the ability to perform chemical texture services has yet another skill by which to establish a loyal following of satisfied clients, repeat customers, and new referrals.

THE NATURE OF CHEMICAL TEXTURE SERVICES

The Chemistry

Chemical texture services create permanent changes in the structure and appearance of the hair. As you learned in Chapter 11, hair is composed of three layers: cuticle, cortex, and medulla. Because the medulla is considered to be "empty space" and may be present only in medium to thick, coarse hair types, the cuticle and cortex are the two layers most affected by chemical texture services.

The cuticle is the tough, outermost layer that protects the hair from damage. The degree to which hair is resistant to chemical changes depends on the strength of the cuticle. The alkaline solutions and substances used in chemical texture services soften and swell the cuticle, allowing for penetration into the cortex.

The cortex gives the hair its strength, flexibility, elasticity, and shape. These characteristics are derived from the millions of polypeptide chains found in keratin that make up the cortex of the hair. As you also learned in Chapter 11, as amino acids form proteins, chemical reactions produce peptide linkages. The amino acids are joined end-to-end by these peptide bonds creating parallel chains of peptide linkages. The parallel chains are then held together by sulfur (cystine), hydrogen, and salt cross-bonds to form a ladderlike structure. As the polypeptide chains twist together, they eventually form a fiber that becomes the cells of the cortex. As a result, the polypeptide chains in keratin are both physically and chemically bound together.

Hair develops and maintains its natural form by means of the physical and chemical cross-bonds in the cortical layer. The physical bonds are the weaker of the two types and are easily broken by the processes of shampooing and rinsing. Chemical bonds are broken or rearranged through chemical applications such as permanent waving, reformation curls, and chemical hair relaxers.

Alkaline substances used in chemical texture services create a chemical action that breaks the chemical bonds and allows for the softening and expansion of the hair. During this process, the cystine (disulfide or sulfur bonds) is altered slightly to become cysteine. Cysteine is an amino acid obtained by the *reduction* of cystine. This chemical action is important because it facilitates the chemical rearrangement of the inner structure of the hair as it assumes a new shape and form. After the hair has assumed the desired shape, it must be neutralized so that the hydrogen and sulfur cross-bonds in the cortical layer are permanently reformed. Cysteine is changed back to the cystine state during the process of oxidation and neutralization, which hardens the S bonds of the hair into the newly constructed form. Facilitated by both physical and chemical action, bonds within the cortex are rearranged and restructured when chemical texture services are performed. 1

Principal Actions of Chemical Texture Services

Chemical texture services involve two principal actions on the hair: physical and chemical. Compare the actions in Table 18–1.

The permanent wave process requires the *physical* actions of shampooing, rinsing, and wrapping the hair around rods. The *chemical* actions take place when a waving lotion and neutralizer produce permanent physical and chemical changes in the hair.

In permanent waving, the waving lotion (reducing agent) softens and swells the cuticle layer of the hair to allow penetration into the cortex, where the solution will break the disulfide bonds by a chemical process known as *reduction*. After processing and rinsing, the neutralizer neutralizes any

Action	Permanent Waving	Reformation Curl	Hair Relaxing
Physical	Shampooing and wrapping hair around rods	Shampooing and combing rearranger through the hair; Wrapping hair around rods	Smoothing or combing of the relaxing product; shampooing and rinsing
Chemical	Waving lotion: softens and breaks the internal hair structure Neutralizer: rehardens/ rebonds the internal structure of the hair	Rearranger: softens and breaks the internal hair structure Waving lotion (booster): softens and breaks the internal hair structure Neutralizer or neutralizing shampoo: rehardens/ rebonds the internal structure of the hair	Relaxer: softens and breaks the internal hair structure Thio relaxers may require an oxidizing neutralizer

Table 18–1 Physical and Chemical Actions of Chemical Texture Services

18

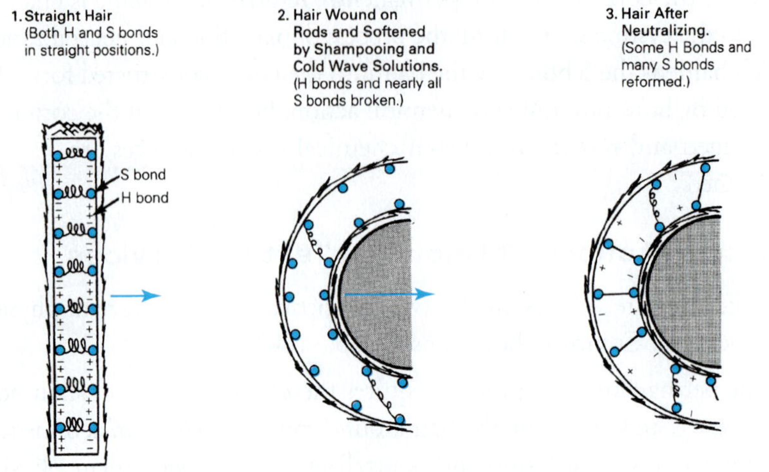

1. Straight Hair (Both H and S bonds in straight positions.)
2. Hair Wound on Rods and Softened by Shampooing and Cold Wave Solutions. (H bonds and nearly all S bonds broken.)
3. Hair After Neutralizing. (Some H Bonds and many S bonds reformed.)
S bond
H bond

Figure 18–1 Changes in hair cortex during permanent waving.

remaining waving lotion in the hair and rebonds the newly arranged disulfide bonds through a process called *oxidation* (Figure 18–1).

The reformation curl process requires the *physical* actions of shampooing, combing a *chemical* rearranger through the hair for partial relaxation of the natural curl, rinsing, and wrapping the hair on rods. The *chemical* actions used to produce permanent changes in the hair are facilitated by the rearranger, waving lotion (booster), and neutralizer.

In the reformation curl process, the rearranger serves the same purpose as the waving lotion in that it softens and swells the cuticle, allowing for penetration into the cortex. The difference between the waving lotion and the rearranger is one of consistency. Both have the same active ingredient, ammonium thioglycolate, but the waving lotion is in lotion form and the rearranger is in a cream form. Because the rearranger will be combed through the hair, it needs to be thicker for better adhesion and control. Once the natural curl is partially relaxed and rinsed, the waving lotion is used with rods to form a new-sized curl. The neutralization process is the same as with permanent waving.

The hair-relaxing process can be achieved with *thio relaxers* or *hydroxide relaxers*. Both product types require the *physical* actions of combing or smoothing the relaxing product through the hair, shampooing, rinsing, and conditioning. The primary *chemical* action that occurs in hair relaxing is the result of the relaxer product used to straighten the hair. Thio relaxing products, however, also require the use of a neutralizer to *chemically* oxidize the hair. Hydroxide relaxing products are neutralized through the *physical* actions of the shampooing and rinsing process because the disulfide bonds that have been broken by this type of relaxer cannot be reformed through oxidation.

When using an *ammonium thioglycolate (thio) relaxer* to straighten the hair, the reducing agent is a stronger strength than that used in permanent waving. Most thio relaxers have a pH above 10 and are manufactured in cream form for better adhesion and control. The relaxer cream softens and

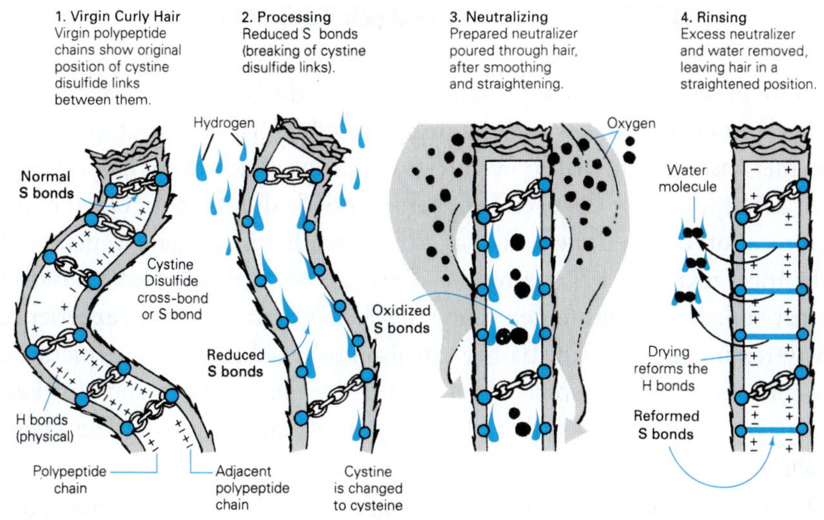

Figure 18-2 Chemical hair straightening—ammonium thioglycolate.

swells the hair and breaks apart the disulfide bonds. This action permits the removal of curl from the hair as the bonds are rearranged into a straighter position through the physical actions of combing and/or gentle pulling of the hair. The hair is then rinsed and neutralized with an oxidizing agent such as hydrogen peroxide that rebuilds the disulfide bonds broken by the relaxer (Figure 18–2).

Hydroxide relaxers are strong alkalis that can swell the hair up to twice its normal diameter. Hydroxide relaxers are not compatible with thio relaxers because they use a different chemistry and can have a pH as high as 13.0. At these high concentrations, the hydroxide product permanently breaks the disulfide bonds to the point where they can never be reformed. This process is known as **lanthionization** (lan-thee-oh-ny-ZAY-shun) and occurs as the disulfide bonds are converted to lanthionine bonds when the relaxer is rinsed and the hair is still at a high pH level (Figure 18–3).

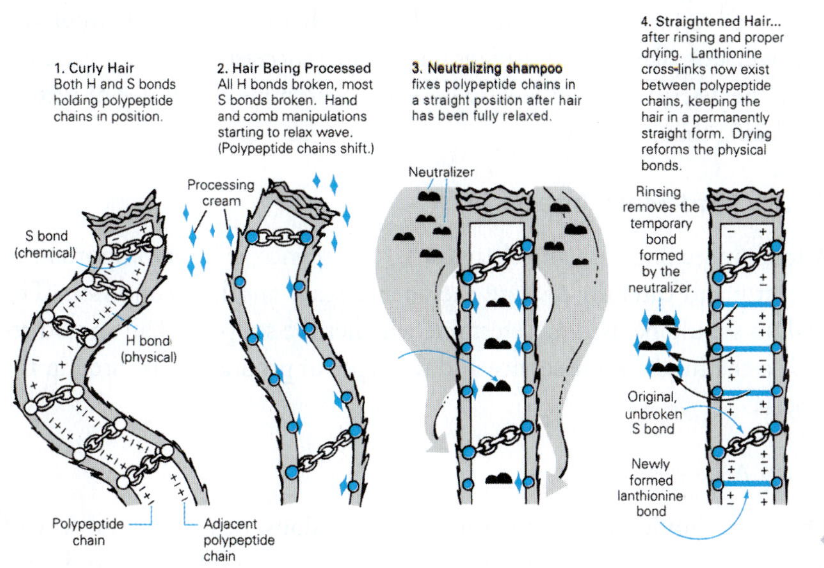

Figure 18-3 Chemical hair straightening—sodium hydroxide.

THE CLIENT CONSULTATION

Before proceeding with any chemical service, the barber must determine the client's expectations and the degree to which those expectations can be met based on the hair type and its condition. Each client has a different concept of how the chemical texture service should look. Open communication between the barber and the client helps to assure a successful chemical texture service outcome. This can be accomplished by asking open-ended questions to determine the client's desires and past experience with texture services. The barber can also use visual tools such as pictures, magazines, and stylebooks to ascertain the client's likes and dislikes. Review the following topics that may be discussed during the client consultation.

1. The desired hairstyle and amount of curl or straightening. Photos or magazine pictures help to make these specifications clear to both the client and the barber.
2. The client's lifestyle. Do they have leisure time or a demanding schedule that requires a low-maintenance style?
3. How the hairstyle relates to overall personal image. Is the client concerned about current fashion trends?
4. Previous experience. Was the last chemical texture service satisfactory? If not, what were the problems?

The consultation with the client takes only a few minutes, but it is time well spent. It helps to establish your credibility as a professional, inspires the client's confidence, and makes the entire chemical texture service experience more satisfactory for both the client and barber.

Keep the information learned during the consultation in the form of a written record that includes the client's address and home and business contact information. See Figure 18–4 for an example of an organized client record card.

In addition to determining the client's texture service desires, the barber also needs to have a clear understanding of what the finished haircut and style will look like. This information is key to a successful texture service because the desired finished look will help to determine the degree of texture or relaxing that is needed.

Scalp and Hair Analysis

Before proceeding with any chemical texture service, it is very important to correctly and carefully analyze the client's scalp and hair condition. The analysis should be used to determine whether the scalp and hair should receive a chemical texture service and the types of products to be used in the process.

Scalp Analysis

The scalp should be examined for cuts, abrasions, or open sores. Any of these conditions can make a chemical process uncomfortable and even

PERMANENT WAVE RECORD

Name .... Tel ....

Address ....

City .... State .... Zip ....

DESCRIPTION OF HAIR

Length	**Texture**	**Type**	**Porosity**	
☐ short	☐ coarse	☐ normal	☐ very porous	☐ slightly porous
☐ medium	☐ medium	☐ resistant	☐ moderately porous	☐ resistant
☐ long	☐ fine	☐ tinted	☐ normal	
		☐ highlighted		
		☐ bleached		

CONDITION

☐ very good ☐ good ☐ fair ☐ poor ☐ dry ☐ oily

Tinted with ....

Previouslt permed with ....

TYPE OF PERM

☐ alkaline ☐ acid ☐ body wave ☐ other ....

No. of rods .... Lotion .... Strength ....

RESULTS

☐ good ☐ poor ☐ too tight ☐ too loose

Date	Perm Used	Stylist	Date	Perm Used	Stylist

Figure 18–4 Client record card.

dangerous to a client's physical well-being. Do not proceed with the service if abrasions or signs of scalp disease are present. Refer the client to a physician as necessary.

Hair Analysis

The hair analysis includes the hair's porosity, texture, elasticity, density, length, and direction of hair growth.

Hair Porosity

The processing time for chemical services depends more on hair porosity than on any other factor. Generally, the more porous the hair, the less time processing will take. The porosity level of the hair determines the speed with which moisture will be absorbed into the hair, and it is directly related to the condition of the cuticle layer. Hair porosity is classified as resistant, normal, or porous. In the case of chemical texture services, these classifications help to determine the most appropriate strength of chemical product to use on different hair types. Do not proceed with the service if signs of breakage or overporosity are evident.

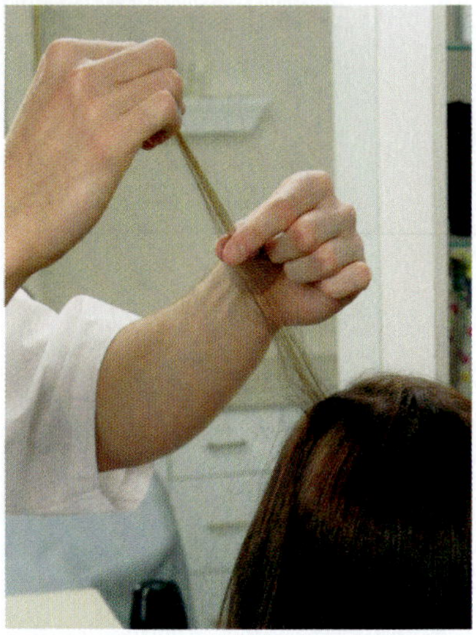

Figure 18–5 Porosity test.

- *Resistant* hair has a tight, compact cuticle layer that resists penetration of chemical solutions. This hair type requires a more alkaline solution to raise the cuticle and permit uniform saturation and processing.
- *Normal* porosity means that the hair is neither resistant nor overly porous. Chemical texture services performed on this hair type will usually process as expected.
- *Porous* hair has a raised cuticle layer that easily absorbs solutions. This hair type requires a less alkaline solution that will minimize swelling and help to prevent excessive damage to the hair.

To accurately test the porosity level, use three different areas: the front hairline, in front of the ears, and near the crown. Grasp some strands of dry hair. Hold the ends firmly with the thumb and index finger of one hand, and slide the fingers of the other hand from the ends toward the scalp. If the fingers do not slide easily, or if the hair ruffles up as your fingers slide down the strands, the hair is porous. The more ruffles that form, the more porous the hair; the fewer ruffles that form, the less porous it is. If the fingers slide easily and no ruffles are formed, the cuticle layers lie close to the hair shafts. This type of hair is the least porous and most resistant, and may require a longer processing time (Figure 18–5).

Hair Texture

Hair texture describes the diameter of a single strand of hair as being coarse, medium, or fine. While hair porosity is important in determining the processing time, hair texture also plays a part in the decision. For example, porous coarse hair will usually process faster than fine, resistant hair. If the resistant fine hair is of a wavy texture and the porous coarse hair is very straight, however, the fine hair will probably process faster because there is already a wave formation in the hair, which usually denotes greater elasticity of the hair. Hair texture should also be considered in deciding the size of the wave pattern and when planning a hairstyle.

18

- *Coarse* hair usually requires more processing than medium or fine hair and may also be more resistant to chemical processes.
- *Medium* hair is the most common hair texture. It is considered normal and does not usually pose any special processing problems.
- *Fine* hair is typically more fragile, easier to process, and more susceptible to damage from chemical services. Generally, fine hair will process faster and more easily than medium or coarse hair types.

Hair Elasticity

Hair elasticity is a very important factor to consider when performing chemical texture services because it is an indication of the strength of the cross-bonds in the hair. The greater the degree of elasticity, the longer the wave will remain in the hair because less relaxation of the hair occurs; thus the elasticity of the hair determines its ability to hold a curl. Hair elasticity is classified as normal or low.

- *Normal* elasticity is indicated by wet hair that can stretch up to 50 percent of its original length and then return to that length without breaking. Hair with normal elasticity usually holds the curl from wet sets and permanent waves.
- *Low* elasticity is indicated by wet hair that does not return to its original length when stretched and may not be able to hold curl patterns.

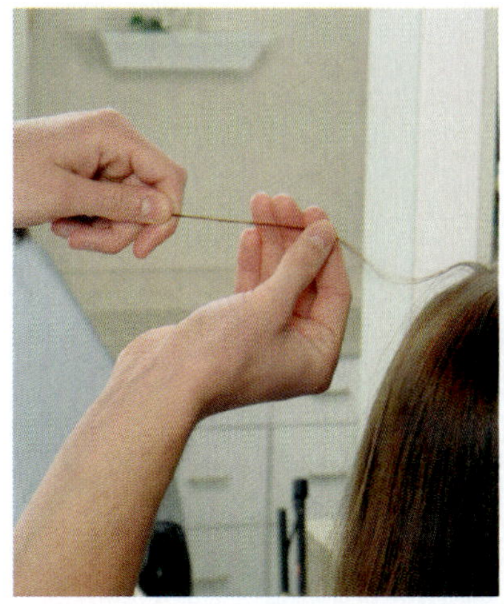

Figure 18–6 Elasticity test.

As a test of elasticity, start by taking some strands of damp hair and holding them between the thumb and forefinger of each hand. Slowly stretch the strands between your fingers (Figure 18–6). The farther they can be stretched without breaking, the more elastic is the hair. If the elasticity is good, the hair slowly contracts after stretching. Hair with poor elasticity will break quickly and easily when stretched.

Signs of poor elasticity include limpness, sponginess, and hair that tangles easily. Generally speaking, such hair will not develop a firm, strong wave. However, there are special waving solutions available that, if used in combination with smaller-diameter rods, may result in a satisfactory permanent wave or reformation curl process.

Hair Density

Hair density measures the number of hairs per square inch and indicates how thick or thin the hair is. Hair density is important to consider when performing chemical texture services because it helps to determine the number of blockings or subsections that will best facilitate the service. For example, when permanent waving, smaller blocks (subsections) and larger rods may be required for thickly growing hair. If the hair density is thin per square inch, however, smaller diameter rods are required to form a good wave pattern close to the head. Avoid large blockings on thin hair growth, as the strain may cause breakage. Hair density can also indicate the amount of product that will be needed.

Hair Length

Hair length is another factor to consider when performing chemical texture services. In permanent waving and reformation curl processes, hair length may determine the rodding technique to use. For example, waving hair of average length presents no real problem. If the client's hair length is 6 inches or more, however, the hair may not rod closely enough to the scalp to develop a good, strong wave pattern in that area. In addition, the weight of the hair may relax or stretch the curl to the extent that the majority of the wave pattern remains mid-shaft and on the hair ends with very little lift in the scalp area.

Like hair density, the length of the hair will also help to determine the amount of product that will be needed for the texture process.

Hair Growth Pattern

The growth direction of the hair causes hair streams, whorls, and cowlicks, which influence the finished hairstyle. These characteristics must be considered when selecting the wrapping pattern and rod placement for permanent waves or reformation curls and the direction of combing and smoothing when using chemical hair relaxers.

Now that the basics that apply to chemical texture services have been explored, it is time to focus on the products, methods, and procedures associated with each individual service. 3

PERMANENT WAVING

Permanent waving is a process that involves two principal actions on the hair: the physical action of wrapping the hair on perm rods and the chemical changes caused by the waving solution and neutralizer. Permanent waves are performed on hair that has been freshly shampooed and in a damp condition. A spray water bottle should be employed to maintain even moisture content throughout the hair while rodding the perm.

The Perm Wrap

In permanent waving, the size, shape, and type of curl are determined by the type, size, and shape of the tool and the method used to wrap the hair. These tools are called *rods* and the size of the rod determines the size of the curl (Figure 18–7).

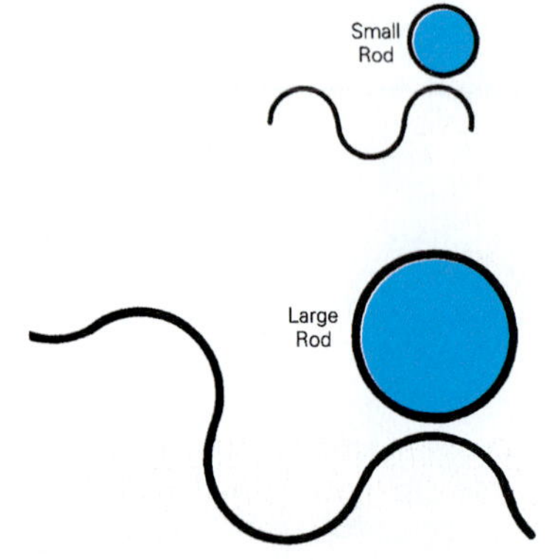

Figure 18-7 The size of the rod determines the size of the curl.

The proper selection of perm rods is essential for successful permanent waving. The most commonly used rods, concave and straight (Figures 18–8 and 18–9), are made of plastic and vary in diameter and length. The diameter of the rod controls the size of the curl. These diameters usually vary from ⅛ to ¾ inches (Figure 18–10). Rods are also available in short, medium, and long lengths that typically measure from 1¾ inches to 3½ inches. An elastic band is used to secure the hair and the rod into the desired position to prevent the curl from unwinding.

18

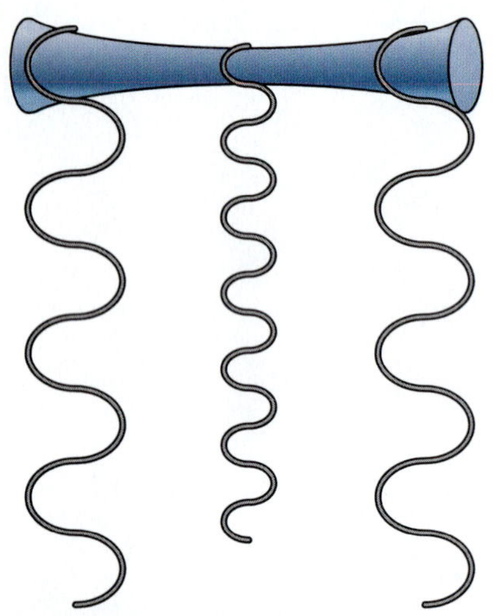

Figure 18-8 Concave rod and resulting curl.

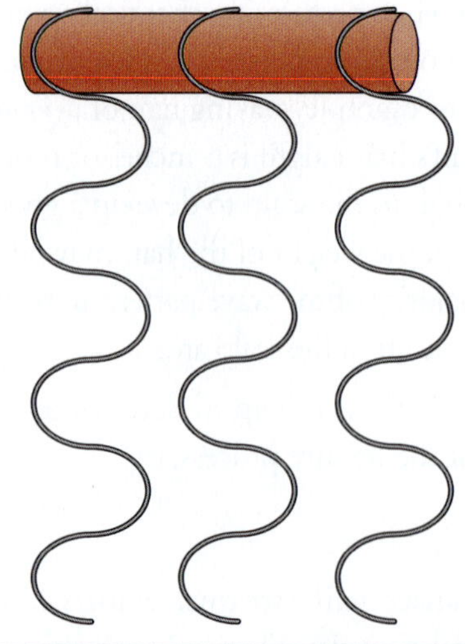

Figure 18-9 Straight rod and resulting curl.

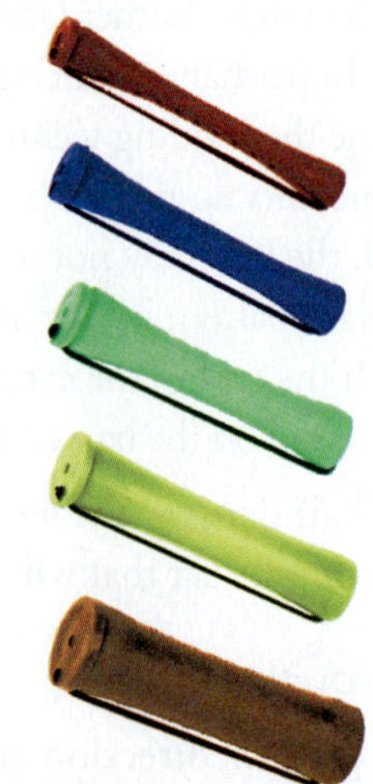

Figure 18-10 Rod sizes, top to bottom: extra small, small, medium, large, extra large.

Concave rods are the most commonly used perm rod. Concave rods have a smaller diameter in the center, which gradually increases to a larger diameter at both ends. This produces a tighter curl in the center and a larger curl on the sides of the hair parting (Figure 18–8). Concave rods are used when a definite wave pattern, close to the head, is desired.

Straight rods have a uniform circumference and diameter along the rod's length. This type of rod creates a consistently sized wave from one side of the hair parting to the other (Figure 18–9). Large, straight rods are usually used for a body wave that serves as a foundation for further styling .

Other perm tools include *bender rods* and *circle tools.* Bender rods are made of stiff wires covered by soft foam that permits bending in a variety of shapes. These rods measure about 12 inches long and have a uniform diameter (Figure 18–11).

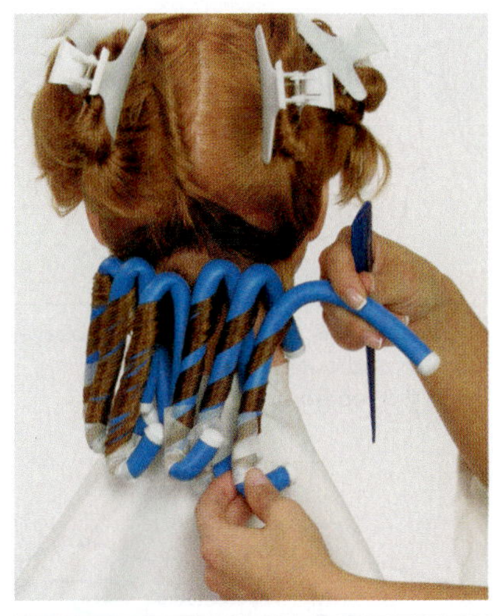

Figure 18–11 Spiral wrapping with soft bender rods.

The circle tool or loop rod is a plastic-coated tool that also measures about 12 inches with a uniform diameter along the length of the rod. These rods are secured by fastening the ends together to form a circle (Figure 18–12).

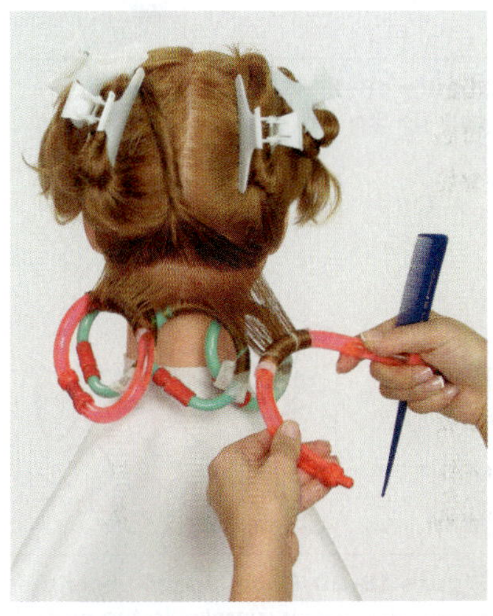

Figure 18–12 Circle tools.

End papers or **end wraps** are absorbent papers used to control the ends of the hair when wrapping and winding the hair on perm rods. End papers should extend beyond the ends of the hair to keep them smooth and straight, and to prevent "fishhooks." A fishhook is a flaw in the wrapping of the hair parting that results in the tip of the hair bending in a direction opposite to that of the rest of the curl. End papers are especially effective in helping to smooth out the wrapping of uneven hair lengths.

The most common end paper–wrapping techniques are the bookend wrap, the single flat wrap, and the double flat wrap.

- The **bookend wrap** uses one paper folded in half over the hair ends and eliminates excess paper (Figure 18–13). It can be used with short rods or short lengths of hair. Be careful to distribute the hair evenly over the entire length of the rod and avoid bunching the ends together toward the center of the rod. See Figures 18–16 through 18–22 for the step-by-step procedure for a bookend wrap.

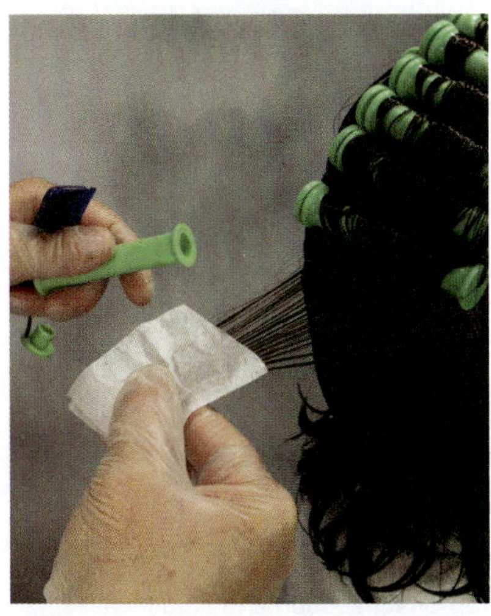

Figure 18–13 Bookend wrap rodding a reformation curl.

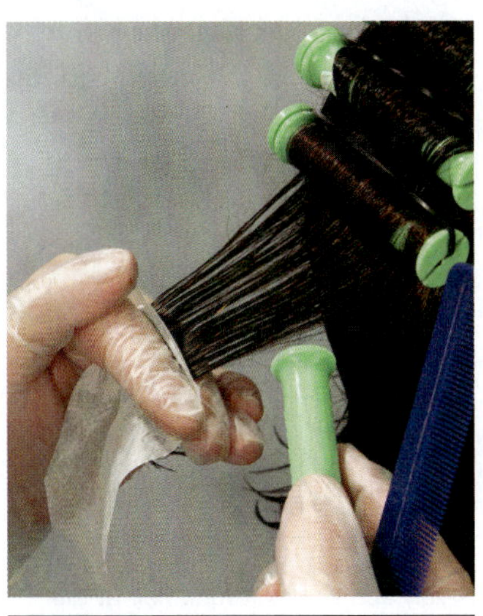

Figure 18–14 Single flat wrap rodding a reformation curl.

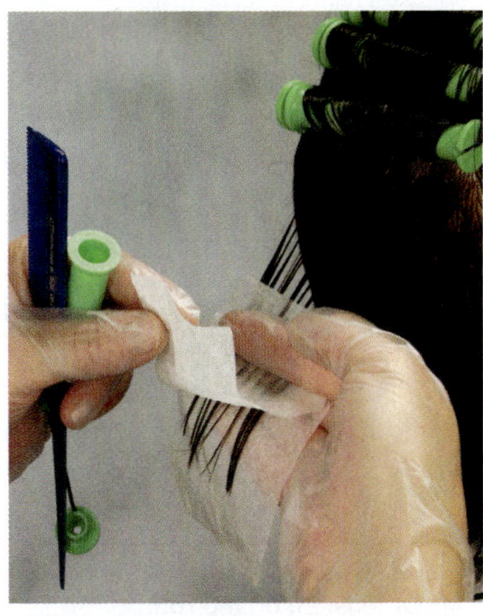

Figure 18–15 Double end wrap rodding a reformation curl.

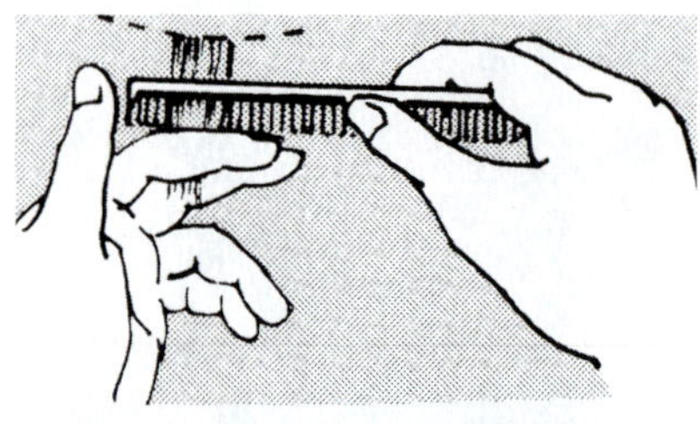

Figure 18-16 Part and comb subsection up and out until all the hair is evenly directed and distributed.

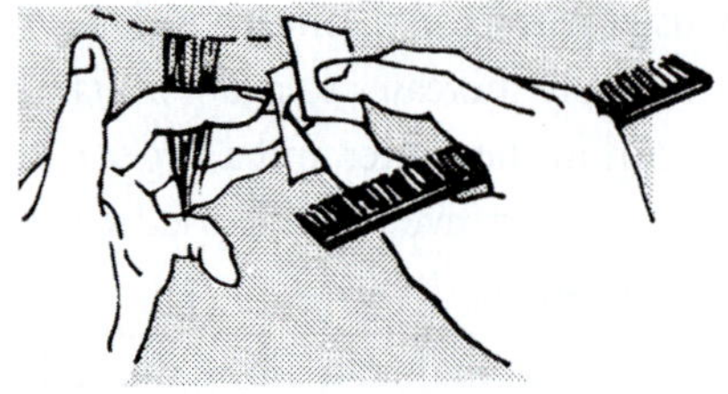

Figure 18-17 Hold subsection between the index and middle fingers. Fold and place the end paper over the subsection, forming an envelope.

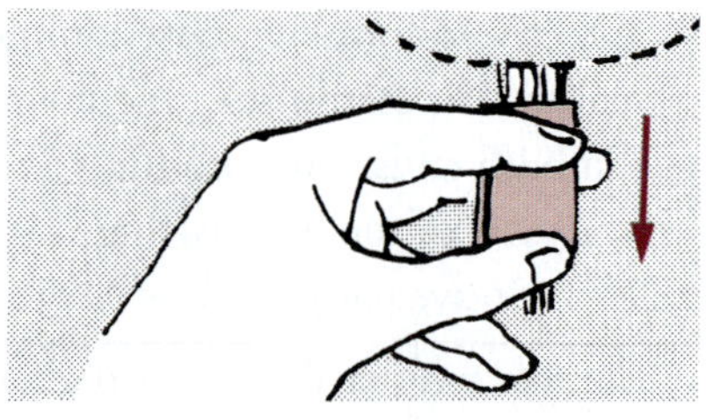

Figure 18-18 Hold the subsection smoothly and evenly. Slide the paper envelope a small fraction beyond the hair ends.

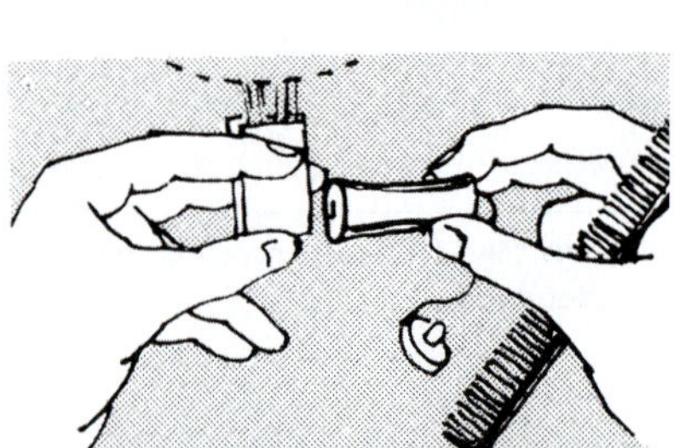

Figure 18-19 With the right hand, pick up the rod.

- The *single flat* or *single end wrap* uses one paper placed over the top of the hair parting being wrapped (Figure 18–14). See Figures 18–23 through 18–25 for the step-by-step procedure for a single flat wrap.
- The *double flat* or *double end wrap* uses two end papers, one placed under and one over the parting of hair being wrapped. Both papers should extend beyond the hair ends (Figure 18–15). See Figures 18–26 through 18–28 for the step-by-step procedure for the double flat wrap.

The preparation of the hair to receive the end wrap is the same for book-end, single, and double wrapping techniques (Figure 18–16).

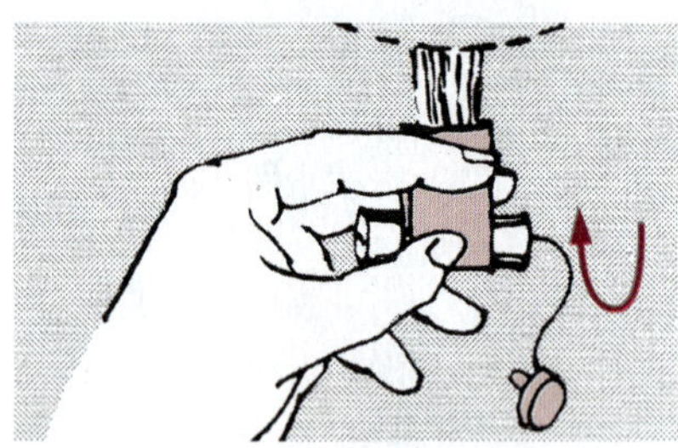

Figure 18-20 Place the rod under the folded end paper, parallel to the parting. Draw end paper and rod toward hair ends until they are visible above the rod, and start winding end paper and hair under, toward the scalp.

Sectioning

Perm wraps begin with sectioning the hair into panels. The size, shape, and direction of these panels will vary depending on the wrapping pattern and the type of tool being used. Each panel is further divided into subsections called **base sections**. The base sections are actually partings taken from the subsection that measure *almost* the same length and width of the rod or perming tool (Figures 18–29 and 18–30).

The number of base sections and rod sizes will vary with each client depending on the sectioning pattern used and the texture, density, and elasticity of the hair (Table 18–2). The average base section, or parting, should be slightly shorter than the length of the rod. If the rod is shorter than the length of the blocking, the hair will slip off the ends of the rod during winding and result in an uneven curl formation.

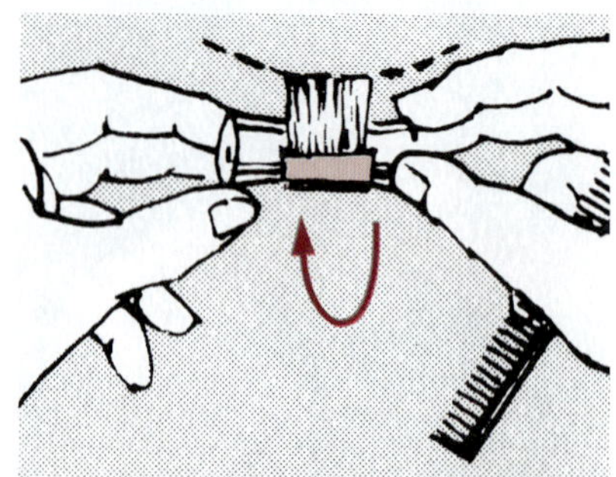

Figure 18-21 Wind the hair smoothly, without tension, on the rod.

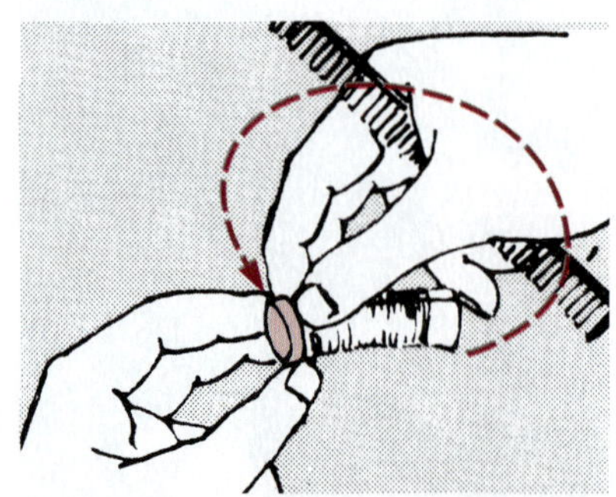

Figure 18-22 Fasten the rod band evenly across the wound hair at the top of the rod.

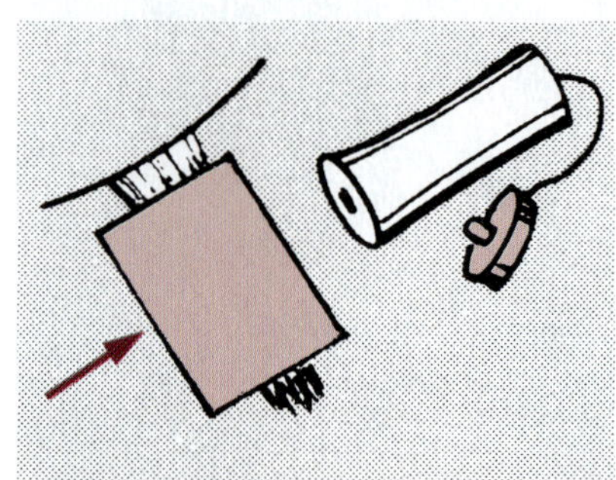

Figure 18-23 Place the end paper on top of subsection and hold it flat to prevent bunching.

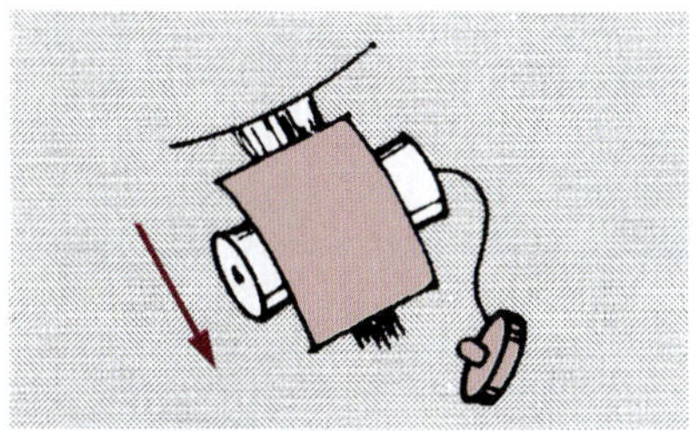

Figure 18-24 Place rod under the subsection, holding it parallel with the parting; then draw the end paper and rod downward until hair ends are covered.

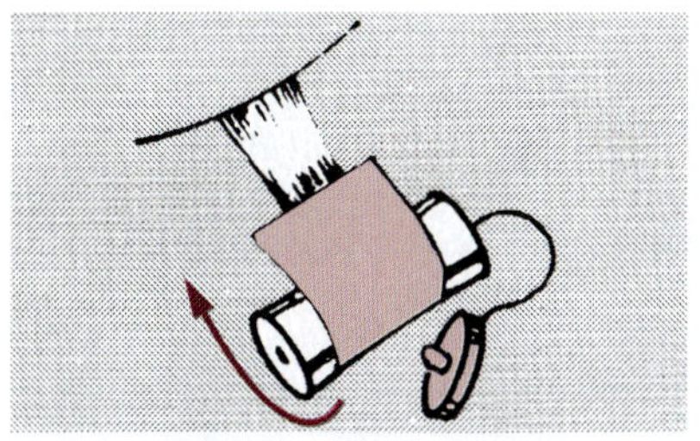

Figure 18-25 Roll the end paper and subsection under, using the thumb of each hand to keep the strands smooth. Wind subsection on the rod to the scalp without tension. Fasten band across top of rod in the same manner as for bookend paper wrap.

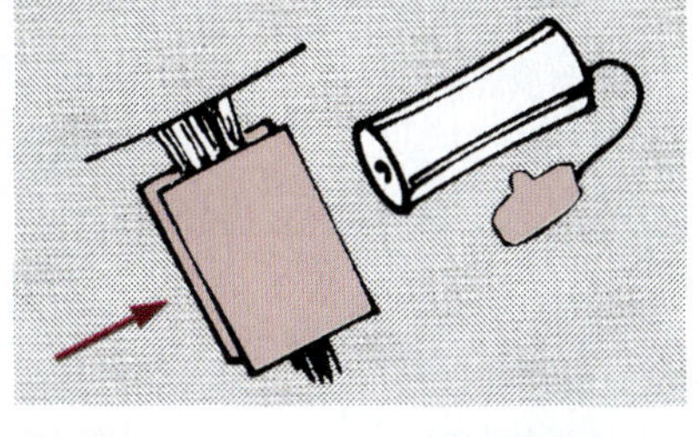

Figure 18-26 Place one end paper beneath the hair subsection and the other on top.

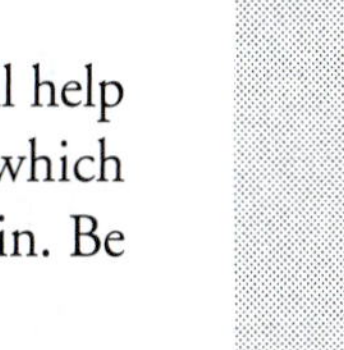

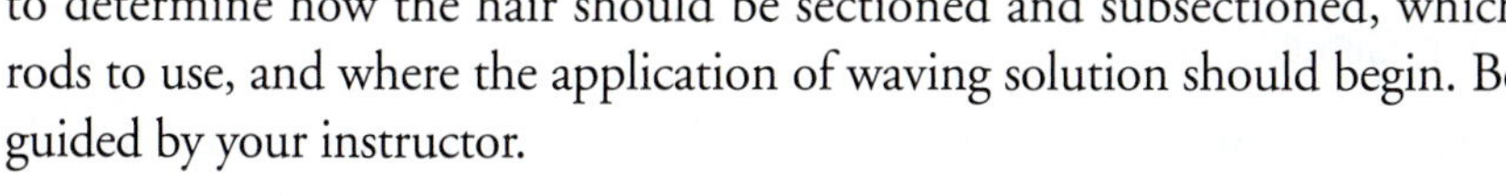

The texture, elasticity, porosity, and condition of the client's hair all help to determine how the hair should be sectioned and subsectioned, which rods to use, and where the application of waving solution should begin. Be guided by your instructor.

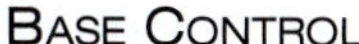

Base Control

Base control refers to the position of the perm rod or tool in relation to its base section and is determined by the angle at which the hair wrapped. Rods can be wound *on-base, half-base (half off-base),* or *off-base.*

In on-base placement, the hair is projected about 45 degrees beyond perpendicular (90 degrees) to its base section and the rod is placed on the base section (Figure 18–31). On-base placement results in greater volume at the scalp area.

Half off-base placement refers to wrapping the hair at an angle of 90 degrees to its base section (Figure 18–32). At this elevation of the hair, the rod is positioned half-off its base section.

Off-base placement is achieved by wrapping the hair at a 45-degree angle below perpendicular to its base section (Figure 18–33). The rod is positioned completely off its base section and creates the least amount of volume in the style.

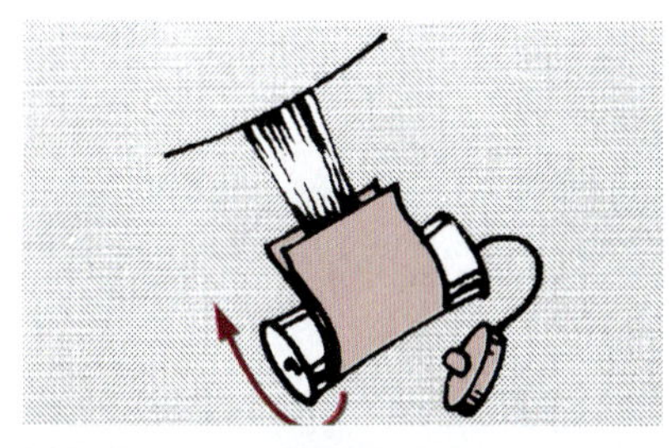

Figure 18-27 Place rod under double end papers, parallel with the parting. Draw both papers toward hair ends.

Figure 18-28 Wind the subsection smoothly on the rod to the scalp without tension. Then fasten the band across the top of rod as for bookend paper wrap.

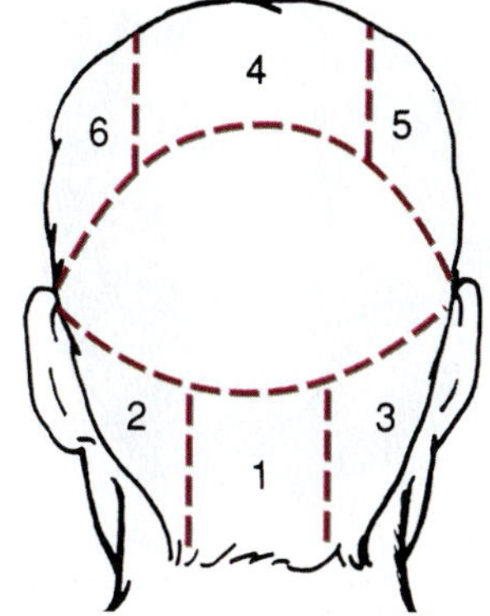

Figure 18-29 Sectioning.

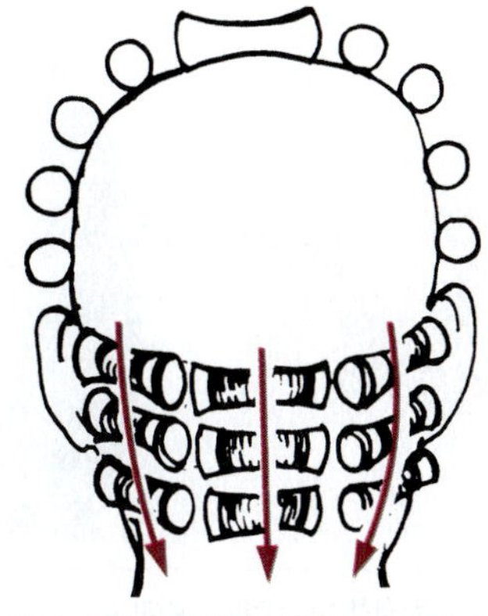

Figure 18-30 Blocking (subsections).

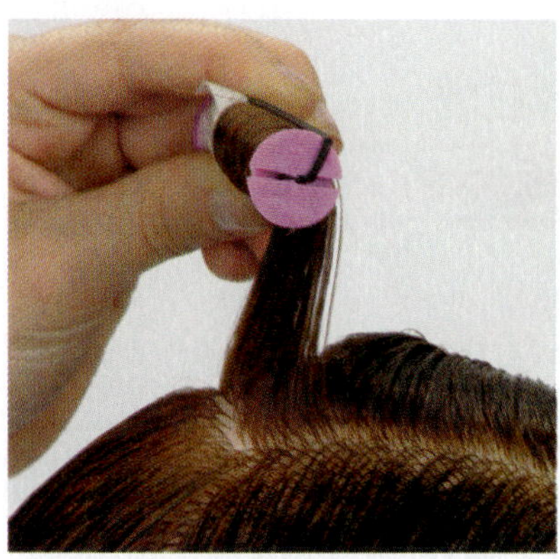

Figure 18-31 On-base placement.

Texture	Density	Elasticity	Base Section	Diameter of Rod
Coarse	Thick	Good	Narrow	Large
Medium	Average	Normal	Smaller	Medium
Fine	Thin	Poor	Smaller	Small
Damaged	Average	Very Poor	Smaller	Large

Table 18-2 Suggested Base Sections and Rod Sizes

Base Direction

Base direction refers to the directional pattern in which the hair is wrapped. Although wrapping with the natural direction of hair growth causes the least amount of stress on the hair, wrapping forward, backward, or to the side can create special effects in the final hairstyle.

Base direction also refers to the horizontal, vertical, or diagonal partings and positioning of the rod on the head, as pictured in Figure 18–34.

Rodding Techniques

The two basic methods used to wrap the hair around the perm rod are the croquignole and spiral rodding techniques.

When using the **croquignole rodding** technique, the hair is wound from the ends to the scalp. This overlapping of the hair layers with each revolution of the rod increases the size of the curl as it nears the scalp area, with a tighter curl at the ends (Figure 18–35).

Spiral rodding can be accomplished in two ways: from the ends to the scalp, or from the scalp to the ends. In both cases, the rod or perming tool

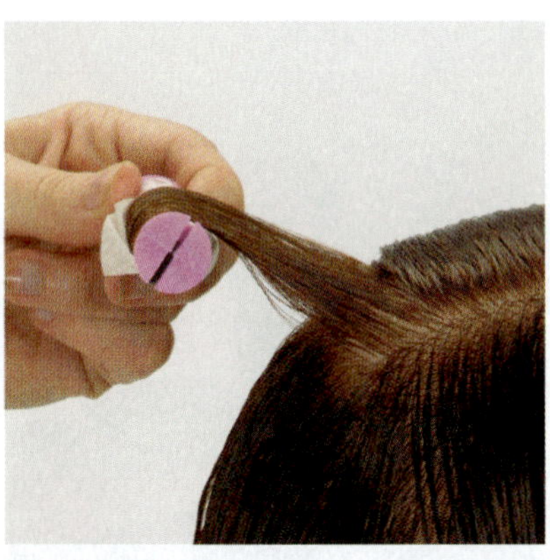

Figure 18-32 Half off-base placement.

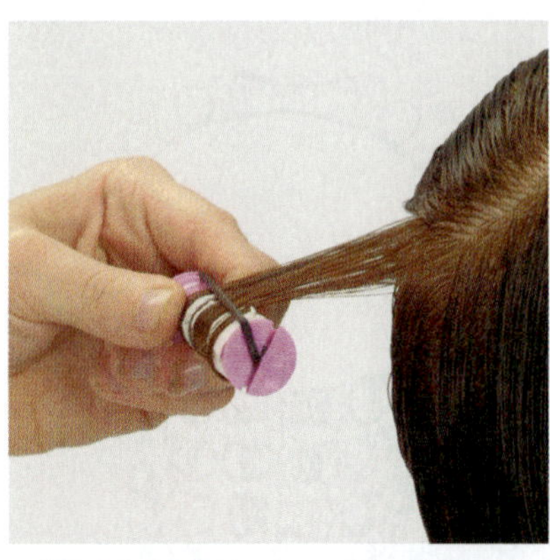

Figure 18-33 Off-base placement.

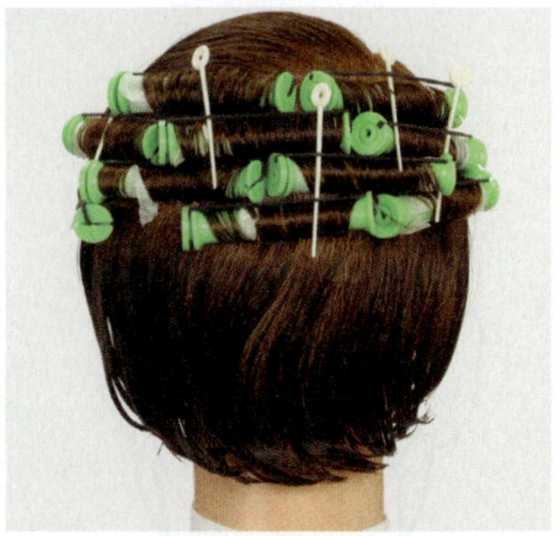

Figure 18-34 Horizontal base direction.

is positioned vertically as the hair parting is "rocked" or spiraled along the length of the rod. Straight rods are usually used for a spiral wrap and tend to produce a more uniform curl when the hair is spiraled properly along the rod (Figure 18–36).

To form a uniform wave the hair must be wrapped smoothly and neatly on each rod, without stretching. The hair should not be stretched or wrapped too tightly because that could interfere with the penetration and expansion process of the waving solution and the contraction process of the neutralizer. Tight wrapping can also result in hair breakage due to the amount of tension put on the hair.

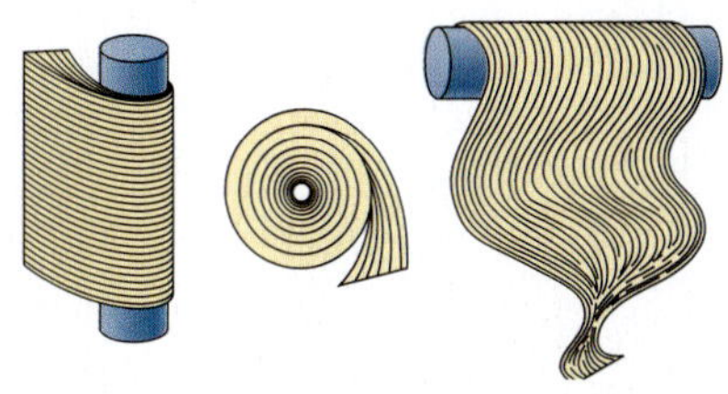

Figure 18-35 Croquignole perm wrap.

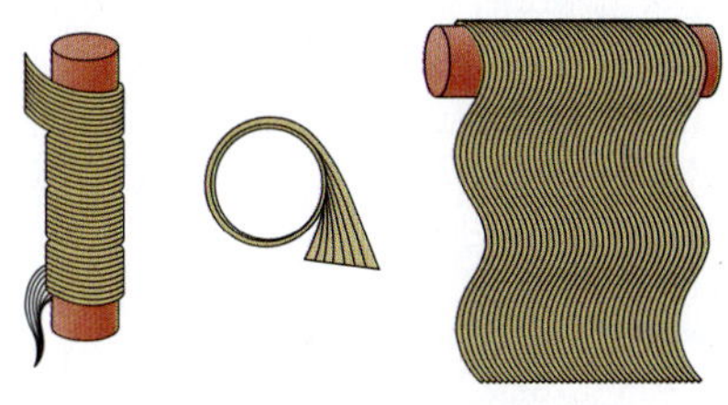

Figure 18-36 Spiral perm wrap.

Wrapping Methods

There are two types of wrapping methods used in permanent waving: the water wrap and the lotion wrap. Some permanent wave solutions allow only a water wrap while others may be lotion wrapped. Always be guided by the manufacturer's directions.

- A *water wrap* is simply the action of rodding the hair in a water-damp condition. Most perms are wrapped in this manner.
- A **lotion wrap** is the application of permanent wave solution to a working panel or section of hair just prior to rodding, for the purpose of "presoftening" resistant hair. This technique is usually used with alkaline (cold) waves to facilitate easier rodding of resistant, straight hair types—it "jump starts" the processing action. Once the hair is rodded, the remaining solution is applied to the entire head.

Types of Permanent Waves

Perm chemistry is constantly being refined and improved. Different formulas designed for a wide variety of hair types are available from today's manufacturers. Waving lotions and neutralizers for both acid-balanced and alkaline perms are available with new conditioners, proteins, and natural ingredients that help to protect and condition the hair during and after perming.

Stop-action processing is incorporated into many waving lotions to ensure optimum curl development. The curling takes place within a fixed time, without the risk of overprocessing or damaging the hair. Special prewrapping lotions have also been developed to compensate for hair with varying degrees of porosity.

Alkaline Perms or Cold Waves

The first **alkaline or cold waves** were developed in 1941.The main active ingredient or reducing agent in alkaline perms is **ammonium thioglycolate (ATG)**. This chemical compound is made up of ammonia and thioglycolic acid. The pH of alkaline waving lotions generally falls within the range of 9.0 to 9.6, depending on the amount of ammonia. These high pH levels cause the hair shaft to swell and the cuticle layer to lift, allowing penetration into the cortex. Some alkaline perms are wrapped with waving lotion, others with water. Either type may require a plastic cap for processing. Always read the manufacturer's directions carefully before proceeding with the service.

The benefits associated with alkaline perms are strong curl patterns, faster processing time (5 to 20 minutes), and room temperature processing. Alkaline perms are generally used when perming resistant hair types, when a strong or tight curl is desired, or when the client has a history of early curl relaxation.

True Acid Waves

The first **true acid waves** were introduced in the early 1970s. These perms have a pH range between 4.5 and 7.0 and use **glyceryl monothioglycolate (GMTG)** as the primary reducing agent. This lower pH is gentler on the hair and typically produces a softer curl and less damage than alkaline cold waves. Most true acid waves require the addition of heat from a hair dryer to accelerate the processing and are considered to be *endothermic* perm products. **Endothermic waves** require the use of an outside heat source to activate chemical reactions and processing.

It should be noted that although a pH of 7.0 is neutral on the pH scale, a pH of 5.0 is neutral for hair. Since every step in the pH scale represents a tenfold change in pH, a pH of 7.0 is 100 times more alkaline than the pH of hair. Even pure water will cause the hair to swell and expand.

The benefits of true acid waves are softer curl patterns, slower but more controllable processing time (usually 15 to 25 minutes), and gentler treatment for delicate hair types. Generally, true acid perms should be used when perming delicate/fragile or color-treated hair; when a soft, natural curl or wave pattern is desired; or when style support, rather than strong curl, is desired.

Acid-Balanced Waves

Most of today's acid waves have a pH between 7.8 and 8.2, which puts them into the category of **acid-balanced waves**. Acid-balanced waves process at room temperature and do not require the heat of a hair dryer for processing.

Although glyceryl monothioglycolate is the primary reducing agent in acid-balanced waves, these waving products usually contain some ammonium thioglycolate as well. All acid-balanced waves have three product components: permanent waving solution, activator, and neutralizer. The permanent waving solution usually contains ATG and the activator GMTG. These products must be added together immediately prior to use.

Acid-balanced waves process more quickly and produce firmer curls than true acid waves.

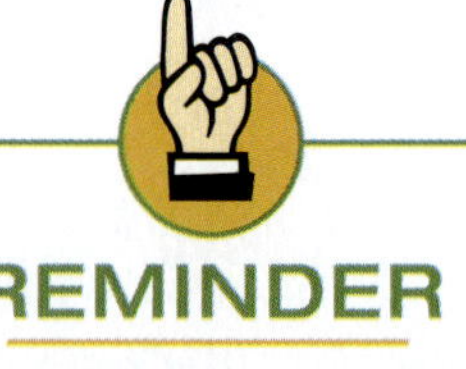

REMINDER

Repeated exposure to GMTG has been known to cause allergic sensitivity in practitioners and clients. Watch clients closely for signs of allergy or irritation. If problems develop, suggest they see a dermatologist.

Exothermic Waves

Like acid-balanced perms, all **exothermic waves** have three components: permanent waving solution, activator, and neutralizer. The activator in an exothermic wave, however, contains an oxidizing agent (usually hydrogen peroxide) that causes a rapid release of heat when mixed with the waving solution. The chemical reaction that releases heat and causes the waving solution to become warm can usually be felt when holding the bottle of solution. This rise in temperature increases the rate of the chemical reaction, which in turn shortens the processing time.

CAUTION

Accidentally mixing the contents of the activator tube with the neutralizer instead of the permanent waving solution will cause a violent chemical reaction that can cause injury, especially to the eyes.

Ammonia-Free Waves

Ammonia-free waves use alkanolamines (al-kan-all-AM-eenz) to replace ammonia and are gaining in popularity because of their low odor. Ammonia-free does not mean free of damage, so although these new products may not smell as strong as ammonia, they can still have a high alkaline pH. For example, an ammonia wave starts out at a pH of 9.6, but quickly drops to 8.2 during processing because ammonia evaporates quickly. Alkanolamines evaporate slowly, which is why they do not give off odors, and maintain the same pH level throughout the entire processing time. This constant pH level can ultimately be more damaging to the hair than waves containing ammonia.

Thio-Free Waves

Thio-free waves use cysteamine (SIS-tee-uh-meen) or mercaptamine (mer-KAPT-uh-meen) as the primary reducing agent. When used at high concentrations, these thio compounds can be just as damaging as regular thio formulations.

Low-pH Waves

Sulfates, sulfites, and bisulfites offer an alternative to ATG but are weak and do not produce a firm curl. Sulfite perms are usually marketed as *body waves.*

Strengths of Waving Solutions

Although the strength of a waving solution can be adjusted by increasing the amount of the active ingredient, today's wide range of perming products virtually eliminates the need to do so. Be cautioned that if the strength of a solution is adjusted through the addition of ammonia, the pH level should not exceed 9.6.

Most manufacturers market three or more strengths of permanent waving products:

- *Mild:* for damaged, porous, or tinted hair
- *Normal:* for normal hair with good porosity
- *Resistant:* for resistant hair with less porosity

Prewraps

Some permanent waving product packages contain a **prewrap solution** that is applied to the hair before rodding the perm. In most cases, the prewrap is simply a leave-in conditioner that helps to equalize the porosity of the hair to ensure even penetration of the waving lotion and to protect the hair from unnecessary damage. Always follow the manufacturer's directions.

Perm Selection

For a successful permanent waving service, it is essential to select the proper waving product for the client's hair type and desired result. After a thorough client consultation, the barber should be able to determine which type of permanent is best suited to the client's hair condition. Most resistant hair types require an alkaline wave; alkaline or acid-balanced perms can be used on most normal hair types; and acid-balanced or true acid perm formulas would be the best choice for most tinted, highlighted, or delicate hair types. Use Table 18–3 as a general guide to the selection of the most common types of permanent waves.

Perm Type	Active Ingredient	Wrapping Method	Process	Recommended Hair Type
alkaline/cold wave pH: 9.0 to 9.6	ammonium thioglycolate (ATG)	lotion wrap or water wrap	room temperature	coarse, thick, or resistant
exothermic wave pH: 9.0 to 9.6	ammonium thioglycolate (ATG)	water wrap	exothermic	coarse, thick, or resistant
true acid wave pH: 4.5 to 7.0	glyceryl monothioglycolate (GMTG)	water wrap	endothermic	extremely porous or very damaged hair
acid-balanced wave pH: 7.8 to 8.2	glyceryl monothioglycolate (GMTG)	water wrap	room temperature	normal, porous, or damaged hair
ammonia-free wave pH: 7.0 to 9.6	monoethanolamine (MEA)/ aminomethylpropanol (AMP)	water wrap	room temperature	porous to normal
thio-free wave pH: 8.0 to 9.6	mercaptamine/cysteamine	water wrap	room temperature	porous to normal
low-pH waves pH: 6.5 to 7.0	ammonium sulfite/ ammonium bisulfite	water wrap	endothermic	normal, fine, or damaged

Table 18–3 Permanent Wave Selection

Permanent Wave Processing and Wave Formation

The strength of any permanent wave is based on the concentration of its reducing agent. In turn, the amount of processing time is determined by the strength of the permanent waving solution and the porosity level of the hair. Most of the processing takes place within the first 5 to 10 minutes, so the amount of processing should be determined by the strength of the solution and not how long the perm processes. If the hair is not sufficiently processed after 10 minutes, it may require reapplication of the solution. The next time the client receives a perm service a stronger solution may be used. Conversely, if the client's hair has been overprocessed, a weaker solution should have been used.

As the hair is processing, the waves form a deep-ridged pattern. The wave has reached its peak when it forms a firm letter S shape (Figures 18–37). The S pattern reaches a desirable peak only once during the perm process. Shortly after the S is well formed, the hair may become frizzy unless processing is stopped. Frizziness indicates that the processing time has reached its absolute maximum. Beyond this point, the hair becomes overprocessed and damaged.

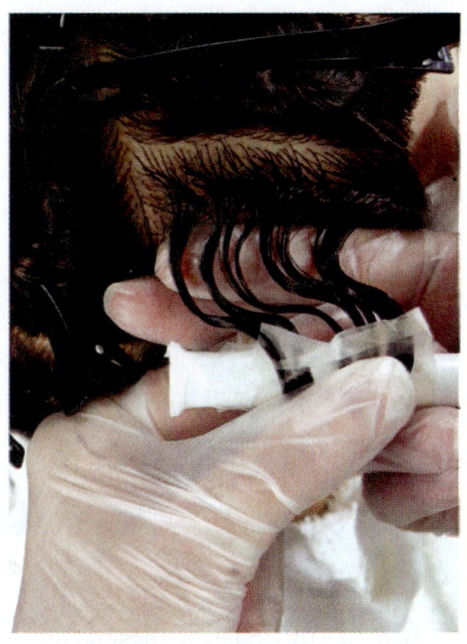

Figure 18–37 S pattern.

Results	Advantages	Disadvantages
firm, strong curls	processes quickly at room temperature	unpleasant ammonia odor; may damage delicate hair
firm, strong curls	faster processing time	unpleasant ammonia odor; may damage delicate hair
soft, weak curls	low pH produces minimal swelling	requires heat from hair dryer; will not produce firm, strong curls
soft curls	minimal swelling; processes at room temperature	repeated exposure may cause allergic sensitivity in clients and stylists
medium to fine curls	no unpleasant ammonia odor	overall strength varies with different manufacturers
medium to fine curls	may be gentler, depending on formula	overall strength varies with different manufacturers
weak curl or body wave	minimal swelling	requires heat from hair dryer; produces weak curls

Table 18–3 Permanent Wave Selection cont'd

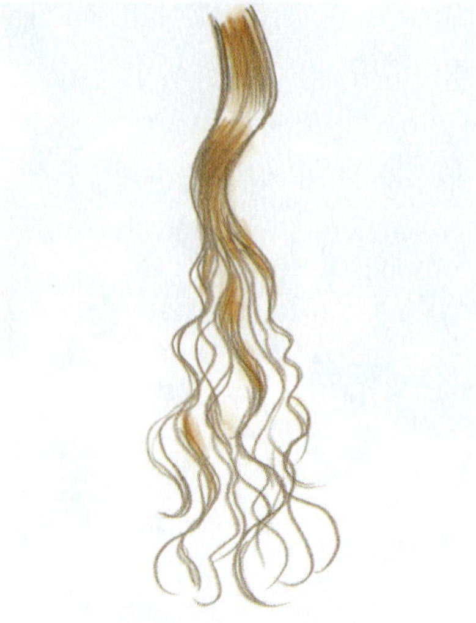

Figure 18-38 Underprocessed hair.

Different conditions and hair textures will cause the quality of wave patterns to vary. Hair of good texture will show a firm, strong pattern, whereas hair that is weak or fine will not produce a firm pattern.

Underprocessed hair has not been sufficiently softened to permit the breaking and rearrangement of the disulfide bonds. This results in a limp or weak wave formation with undefined ridges within the S pattern. The hair retains little or no wave formation and is unable to hold the desired curl (Figure 18–38). Reapplication of the permanent waving solution is necessary to complete the process.

Overprocessed hair can also appear to be too weak to hold a curl (Figure 18–39). Any solution that can process the hair properly can also overprocess it. Solution left on the hair too long results in overprocessing and if too many *disulfide bonds* are broken, the hair may not have enough strength to hold the desired curl.

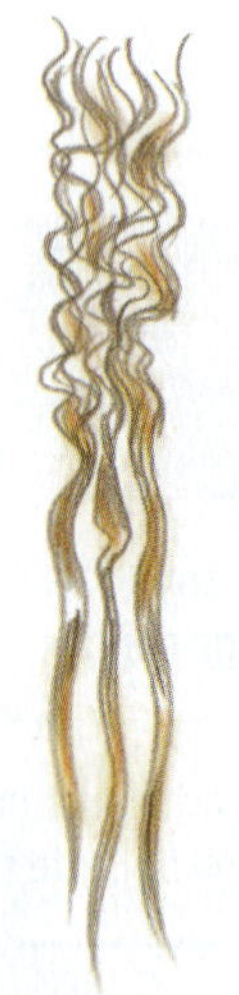

Figure 18-39 Overprocessed hair.

Signs that the hair has been overprocessed include weak curl formation, a very curly when wet appearance but completely frizzy when dry, and an inability to be combed into a suitable wave pattern. In hair that has been overprocessed, the elasticity of the hair has been damaged to the point where it is unable to contract into the wave formation. Overprocessed hair usually feels harsh after being dried and should be given reconditioning treatments.

Preliminary Test Curls

Test curls help to determine how the client's hair will react to the permanent waving process. A test curl provides information about how to obtain the best possible results out of the perm service. Test curls enable the barber to observe the following aspects of the hair:

- Speed of wave formation
- Degree of wave formation
- Exact time when peak of wave formation is reached
- Identification of resistant areas
- Appropriateness of product selection

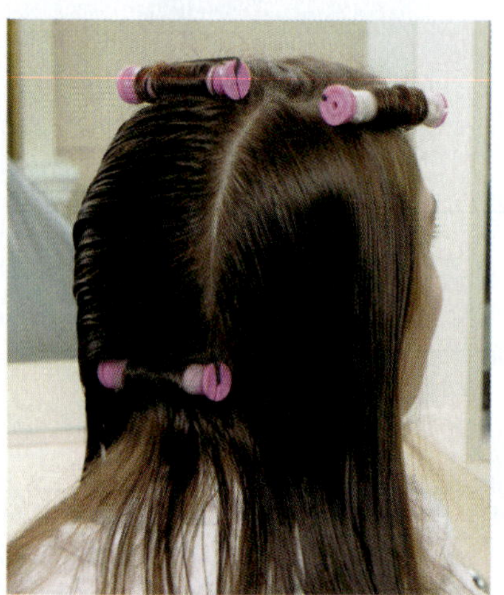

Figure 18-40 Wrap rods in three areas of the head.

Preliminary test curls are performed by rodding one parting of hair in three different areas of the head: the top, side, and nape. The procedure for performing preliminary test curls is as follows:

1. Wrap one tool in each different area of the head (top, side, nape) See Figure 18–40.
2. Wrap a cotton coil around each tool.
3. Apply waving lotion (Figure 18–41).
4. Set a timer and process according to manufacturer's directions.
5. Check each subsection frequently for proper curl development by unwinding the hair about 1½ turns of the rod (Figure 18–42).
6. Curl development is complete when a firm S is formed.

7. Rinse with warm water and neutralize. Do not proceed with the perm if the test curls are damaged or overprocessed. If the test curls are satisfactory, proceed with the perm, but avoid reperming the test curl partings.

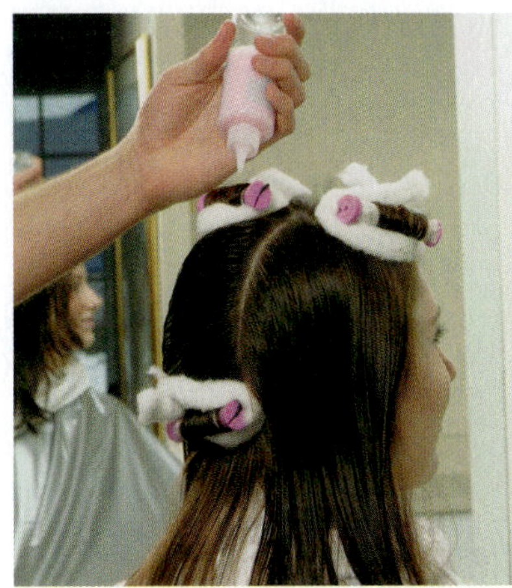

Figure 18-41 Apply waving lotion to test curls.

Neutralization

Neutralizers are actually *oxidizers* that stop the action of permanent wave solutions and harden the hair into its new form. This process is known as **neutralization**. The most common neutralizer is hydrogen peroxide with a concentration range between 5 volume (1.5 percent) and 10 volume (3 percent). Other types of neutralizers are sodium bromate and sodium perborate.

The two important functions of a neutralizer are to deactivate any waving solution that remains in the hair after rinsing and to rebuild the disulfide bonds that were broken by the waving solution. If the hair is not properly neutralized, the curl will relax or straighten within one to two shampoos. As with waving solutions, there may be slightly different procedures recommended for individual products. To achieve the best possible results, always read the directions carefully.

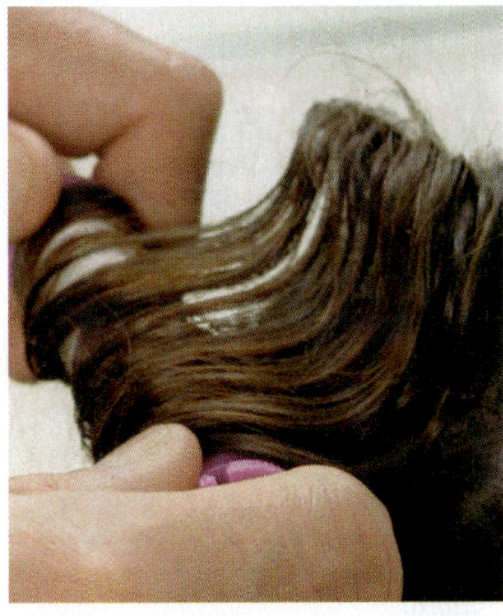

Figure 18-42 Check for S formation.

After thoroughly rinsing the permanent wave solution from the hair, it should be blotted until no excess water is absorbed into the towel. This is an important step to the neutralization process because excess water left in the hair prevents even saturation of the neutralizer and dilutes its properties.

The neutralizer should be applied to the top and bottom of each rod to assure saturation and even distribution of the product. Always give clients a towel to protect their eyes from excess or dripping neutralizer. A cotton coil should also be used for additional safety and client comfort.

Rinsing the Neutralizer

Depending on the permanent wave manufacturer's directions, neutralizers are rinsed from the hair in one of two ways: with the rods in place or after the rods have been removed from the hair.

The most commonly used method is to rinse the neutralizer from the hair with the rods in place. After a thorough rinsing with tepid water, followed by blotting, the rods are carefully removed in preparation for styling. Some directions may require a second rinse after the removal of the rods.

An alternative method is to carefully remove the rods without stretching after neutralization has taken place. Apply the balance of the neutralizing solution and allow it to remain on the hair for an additional minute. Then rinse with tepid water and proceed with setting and/or styling the hair.

Postperm Care

In the past, most practitioners have recommended a 48- to 72-hour waiting period before shampooing freshly permed hair. Since the bonds in the hair are reformed immediately, there is no scientific basis for this waiting period. When permanent waves are processed and neutralized properly, they should

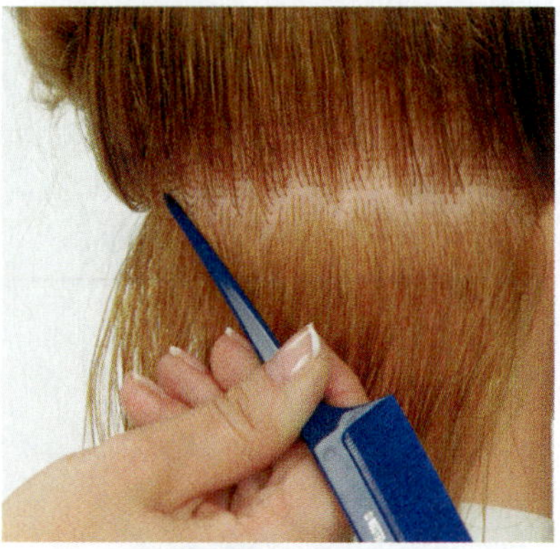

Figure 18-43 Weave technique.

stand up to shampooing with a mild *acid-balanced shampoo* product. Be sure to educate your clients about the most appropriate shampoos and conditioners to use after a perm service. Unless there are signs of scalp irritation, deposit-only haircolor can also be applied sooner than three days after a permanent wave.

Reconditioning treatments have a place in the after care of a permanent wave and between permanent waves. Effective postperm care helps to keep the hair in the best possible condition until the next chemical service. Suggest the following guidelines to permanent wave clients.

1. Shampoo the hair as needed with an acid-balanced shampoo.
2. Use a moisturizing hair conditioner.
3. Schedule regular shop visits for trims and/or conditioning treatments to maintain the hairstyle.

Permanent Waving Wrapping Patterns

Once the client consultation has been completed, the barber should have a definite plan of action designed to achieve the desired results. This plan should include the selection of a permanent waving product, rod size(s), and the wrapping pattern that will be used for the service.

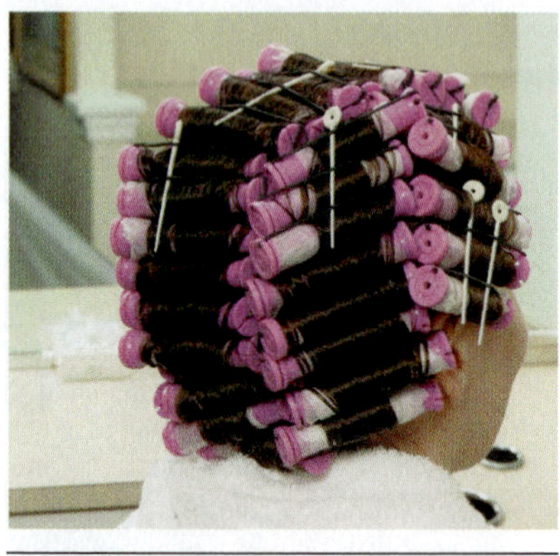

Figure 18-44 Basic perm wrapping pattern.

There are five common wrapping patterns that are used in permanent waving. They are the basic, curvature, bricklay, spiral, and piggyback wraps. The parting technique most often used is a straight part. Zigzag partings known as the *weave technique,* however, can be used for an entire perm or to create smooth transitions from rodded areas to nonrodded areas within a partial perm (Figure 18–43).

- **Basic perm wrap**: In this wrapping pattern, all the tools (rods) within a panel are positioned in the same direction on equal-size bases (Figure 18–44). All base sections are horizontal and approximately the same length and width of the rod. The base control is half off-base.
- *Curvature perm wrap*: This wrapping pattern is one of the best to use for men's styles as it produces a more natural-looking wave pattern. The movement curves within sectioned-out panels with partings and bases following the natural curvature and hair distribution of the head (Figure 18–45).
- *Bricklay perm wrap:* The base sections are offset from each other row by row to prevent noticeable splits in the hair (Figure 18–46). The bricklay pattern facilitates better blending of the hair from one area to another and may be preferred for men's styling over the basic perm wrap pattern.
- *Spiral perm wrap:* The spiral perm wrap is more a technique than a pattern. Unlike the preceding wrapping patterns, which are performed at an angle perpendicular to the rod, the spiral wrap is performed at an angle that positions the hair in a spiral pattern along the length of the rod or tool (Figure 18–47). This technique produces a uniform curl formation from the scalp to the ends and is especially appropriate for long hair designs .
- *Piggyback perm wrap:* The piggyback perm wrap uses two rods or tools for each parting of hair to facilitate even curl formation on long hair. The first

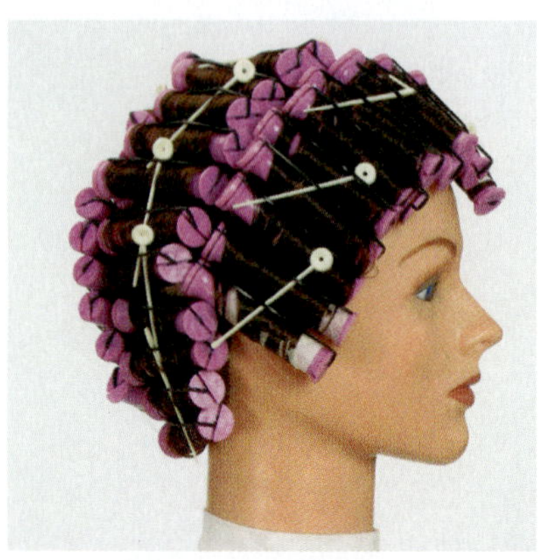

Figure 18-45 Curvature perm wrapping pattern.

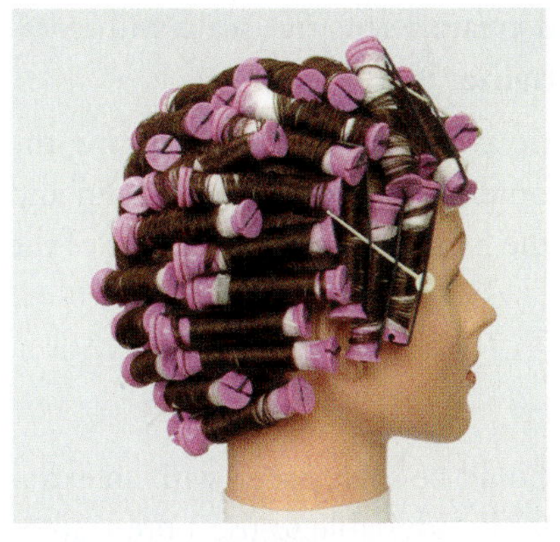

Figure 18–46 Bricklay perm wrapping pattern.

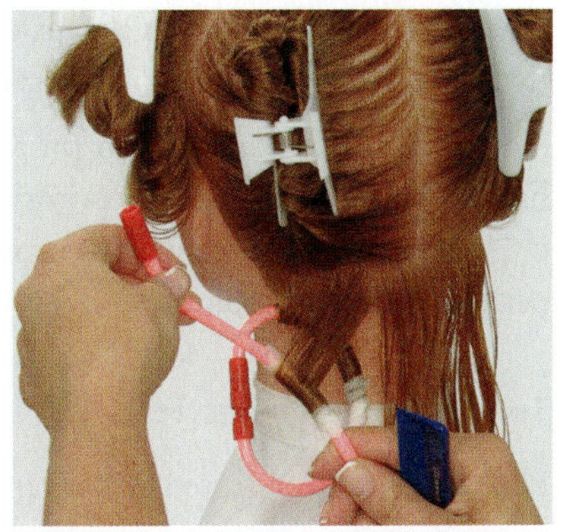

Figure 18–47 Spiral perm technique.

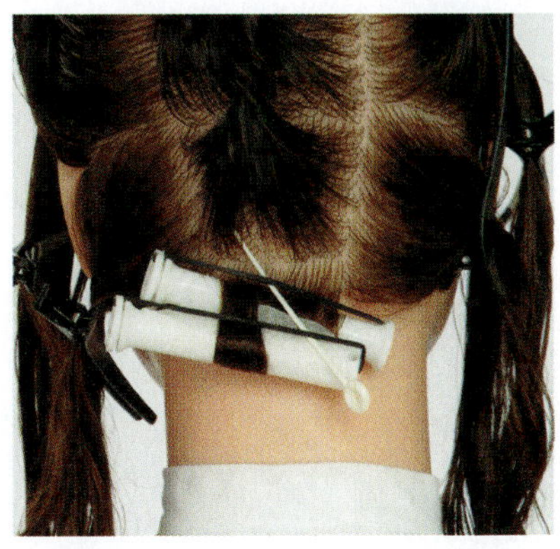

Figure 18–48 Double-tool piggyback perm technique.

rod is placed about midway between the scalp and hair ends. This section is rodded toward the scalp and leaves a tail of hair that extends from the midshaft point to the hair ends. The "tail" is then rodded from the ends to the midway point and secured and positioned across the first rod (Figure 18–48). In this way, the second rod is "piggybacking" the first the rod.

Partial perms

Partial-perming means that only a section of the hair is permed. In men's permanent waving, this is usually the top and crest area of the head (Figure 18–49). Partial perms can be used to create volume and lift in these areas or to reperm previously permed sections that have been trimmed due to normal hair growth and maintenance haircuts.

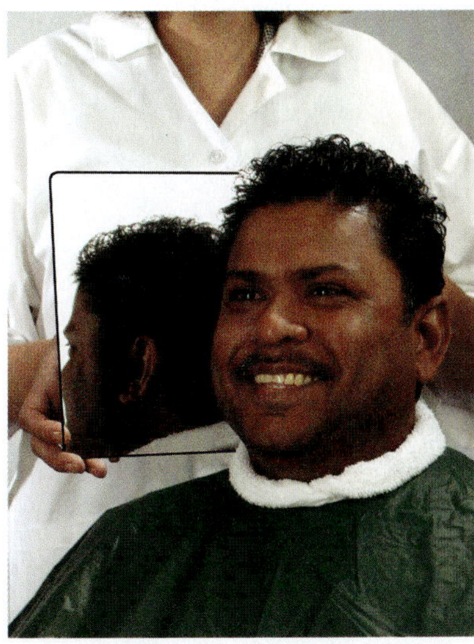

Figure 18–49 Partial perm style.

The same wrapping patterns and techniques used for a full perm can be used for a partial perm with the following considerations:

- To make a smooth transition from the rodded section to the nonrodded section, use the next larger rod size so that the curl pattern of the permed hair will blend into the nonpermed hair.
- After wrapping the area to be permed, place a coil of cotton around the wrapped rods as well as around the entire hairline.
- Before applying the waving lotion, apply a heavy, creamy conditioner to the sections that will not be permed to protect this hair from the effects of the waving lotion.

Many clients need the added texture and fullness that only a perm can give. A perm can help to temporarily overcome common hair problems such as redirecting a cowlick, making limp or unmanageable hair easier to style, or making sparse hair look fuller. Although men's and women's hairstyles may be different, the techniques for permanent waving are essentially the same.

Special Problems

Dry, Damaged Hair

Dry, brittle, damaged, or overporous hair should be given reconditioning treatments prior to a permanent wave service. Avoid any treatment requiring massage or heat as this could create a sensitive scalp and irritation when the waving solution or neutralizer is applied.

Special fillers that contain protein are available for reconditioning the hair and help to equalize its porosity. Some fillers also contain lanolin and cholesterol, which may help to protect the hair against the harshness of the permanent waving solution.

Tinted or Lightened Hair

Hair that has been tinted or lightened should be shampooed with an extra-mild shampoo before waving. It may also be advisable to use a prewrap or other leave-in conditioning product.

While prewraps and leave-in conditioners may be sufficient for stronger hair types that have been previously tinted or lightened, extremely porous hair will probably not benefit from these applications. Extremely porous hair may absorb too much conditioner, which, in turn, may interfere with waving solution penetration and curl formation.

Always select permanent waving solutions that are formulated for tinted and lightened hair conditions and always take the time to perform preliminary test curls.

Hair Tinted with Metallic Dye

Some over-the-counter haircoloring products still use metallic dyes in the formulations. Hair tinted with a metallic dye must first be treated with a dye remover to avoid hair discoloration or breakage. Do not wave the hair if the test curls break or discolor. This type of haircoloring product is difficult to remove so the best option is to cut the color-treated hair in a series of shop visits until all the color is removed. Then proceed with the perm service on virgin hair, followed by the application of professional haircoloring products.

Curl Reduction

Sometimes a client is displeased after a permanent wave because the hair seems too curly. If the hair is fine, do not suggest curl reduction before shampooing two or three times. This type of hair relaxes to a greater extent than does normal or coarse hair. Usually, after the second shampoo, the hair has relaxed to a satisfactory level.

If the hair has a normal or coarse texture, curl reduction may be done immediately following neutralization or after a few days.

Permanent waving solution may be used to relax the curl, where required. Carefully comb it through the hair to widen and loosen the wave. When sufficiently relaxed, the hair is rinsed, towel blotted, and neutralized. CAUTION: Do not attempt curl reduction on hair that has been overprocessed, as such treatment will only further damage the hair.

Air Conditioning/Heating Units

Because of its cooling effects, air conditioning will usually slow the action of permanent waving solutions and additional processing time may be required. Make sure that clients are seated in an area of the shop away from drafts, vents, and fans to avoid slowing the processing time. Conversely, sitting too close to a heating vent or hood hair dryers can speed up the processing time.

Safety Precautions for Permanent Waving

- Always protect clients clothing with the proper waterproof drape.
- Use two towels: one under the drape and one over the drape.
- Always examine the client's scalp before a perm service. Do not proceed if abrasions are present.
- Do not proceed with the perm if the client has ever experienced an allergic reaction to the products.
- Do not perm excessively damaged hair or hair that has been treated with hydroxide relaxers.
- Always apply a protective cream barrier around the client's hairline before applying the waving solution.
- Immediately replace cotton coils or towels that have become saturated with solution.
- Always protect the client's eyes when applying waving and neutralizing solutions by providing the client with a clean towel to hold over the eyes during the application. In case of accidental exposure, rinse thoroughly with cool water.
- Always follow the manufacturer's directions.
- Do not dilute or add anything to waving or neutralizing solutions unless specified in the manufacturer's directions.
- Wear gloves when applying solutions.
- Do not save opened or unused products, as the strength and effectiveness will change if not used promptly.
- Unless otherwise specified in the product instructions, apply waving and neutralizing solutions liberally to the top and underside of each rod.
- Start at the crown and progress systematically down each section. (Some barbers prefer to start at the top of head.) Be sure that the surface area of the wound hair is wet with lotion so penetration is even.
- Follow the same application pattern for the neutralizer as used with the waving solution to avoid missing any rods.
- Sometimes it is necessary to resaturate the rods during processing. This may be due to evaporation of the solution, dryness of the hair, hair that was poorly saturated the first time, improper selection of solution strength, or failure to follow manufacturer's directions. Reapplying the solution will hasten processing so watch the wave development closely, as negligence may result in hair damage.

prewrap solution	usually a type of leave-in conditioner that may be applied to the hair prior to permanent waving to equalize porosity
reformation curl	a soft-curl permanent; combination of a thio relaxer and thio permanent, whereby the hair is wrapped on perm rods; used to make existing curl larger and looser
texturize	a process used to semistraighten extremely curly hair into a more manageable texture and wave pattern
thio relaxers	relaxers that usually have a pH above 10 and a higher concentration of ammonium thioglycolate than is used in permanent waving
true acid waves	perms that have a pH between 4.5 and 7.0 and require heat to speed processing; process more slowly than alkaline waves and do not usually produce as firm a curl

chapter review questions

1. Explain the physical and chemical changes that occur in the hair as a result of chemical texture services.
2. List and define characteristics of the hair used in an analysis for chemical texture services.
3. List the similarities and differences between permanent wave, reformation curl, and hair-relaxing procedures.
4. List the steps involved in permanent waving.
5. List at least five safety precautions to use in permanent waving.
6. List the steps involved in the reformation curl service.
7. List the steps involved in relaxing with thio relaxers.
8. List the steps involved in relaxing with hydroxide relaxers.
9. Explain the difference between base and no-base relaxers.
10. Identify the chemical texture services that require a pre-service shampoo.
11. Explain the difference between a texturizer and a chemical blow-out.
12. List at least five safety precautions to use in chemical hair relaxing.

Pigment

Fine-textured hair

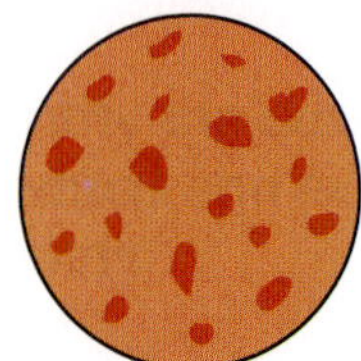

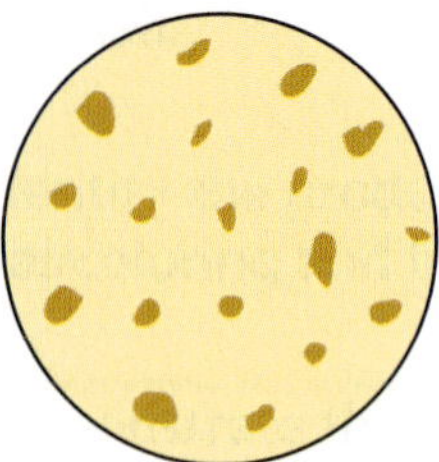

Figure 19–2 Melanin distribution according to hair texture.

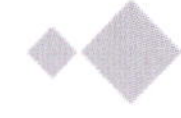

CHARACTERISTICS AND STRUCTURE OF HAIR

The client's hair structure will affect the quality and ultimate success of the haircolor service. The strength of the cuticle and the amount of elasticity and natural pigment in the cortex are important considerations in determining haircoloring options and product selection. Other hair structure factors relevant to a haircoloring or lightening service are texture, density, porosity, and natural color.

- *Texture:* The diameter of the individual hair strand determines whether the hair texture is classified as fine, medium, or coarse. Melanin is distributed differently within the different textures. Melanin granules in fine hair are grouped tightly, so the hair takes color faster and may appear darker. Medium-textured hair has an average response time to haircolor products and coarse hair may take longer to process (Figure 19–2).
- *Density:* To assure proper coverage, the density of the hair should be taken into account when applying haircolor or lighteners.
- *Porosity:* The porosity level of the hair influences its ability to absorb liquids. Porous hair accepts haircolor products faster and permits a darker saturation than less porous hair. Hair with a low porosity level has a tight cuticle, which makes it resistant to moisture and chemical penetration with the result that it can require a longer processing time. In hair that has an average porosity level, the cuticle is slightly raised and the hair tends to process in an average amount of time. High porosity is indicated by a lifted cuticle. Such hair may take color quickly but it may also fade sooner than other porosity levels, due to an inability to hold the color for the normal amount of time.
- *Natural color:* Natural hair color ranges from black to dark brown to red, and from dark blond to lightest blond. *Eumelanin* gives black and brown color to hair and *pheomelanin* is the melanin found in yellowish-blond, ginger, and red tones. The three factors that determine all natural colors, from jet black to light blond, are the thickness of the hair, the total number and size of pigment granules, and the ratio of eumelanin to pheomelanin. White hair is actually the color of keratin without the influence of melanin and therefore does not contain either type.
- **Contributing pigment** is the pigment that lies under the natural hair color. The foundation of haircoloring is based on modifying this pigment with haircoloring products to create new pigments or colors.

Gray hair is normally associated with aging, although heredity is also a contributing factor. In most cases, the loss of pigment increases as a person ages, resulting in a range of gray tones from blended to solid. The amount of gray in an individual's hair is measured in percentages, as presented in Table 19–1, and requires special care when formulating haircolor applications. (The challenges and solutions associated with coloring gray hair are discussed later in the chapter.)

Percentage of Gray Hair	Characteristics
30%	More pigmented than gray hair
50%	Even mixture of gray and pigmented hair
70 to 90%	More gray than pigmented; most of remaining pigment is located at the back of the head
100%	Virtually no pigmented hair; tends to look white

Table 19-1 Determining the Percentage of Gray Hair

COLOR THEORY

Color is a form of visible light energy. Although the human eye sees only six basic colors, the brain is capable of visualizing the combinations of different wavelengths relevant to the three primary and three secondary colors (see Chapter 9).. The movement of light rays that are absorbed or reflected by natural hair pigment or artificial pigment added to the hair creates the colors we see.

The Laws of Color

The **laws of color** regulate the mixing of dyes and pigment to make other colors. They are based in science and adapted to art. The laws of color serve as guidelines for harmonious color mixing. For example, equal parts of red and blue mixed together always make violet.

Primary Colors

Primary colors are basic or true colors that cannot be created by combining other colors. The three primary colors are yellow, red, and blue (Figure 19–3). All other colors are created by some combination of red, yellow, or blue. Colors with a predominance of blue are cool-toned colors and colors that are predominantly red are warm-toned colors.

Blue is the darkest and only cool primary color. Blue creates depth or darkness to any color to which it is added.

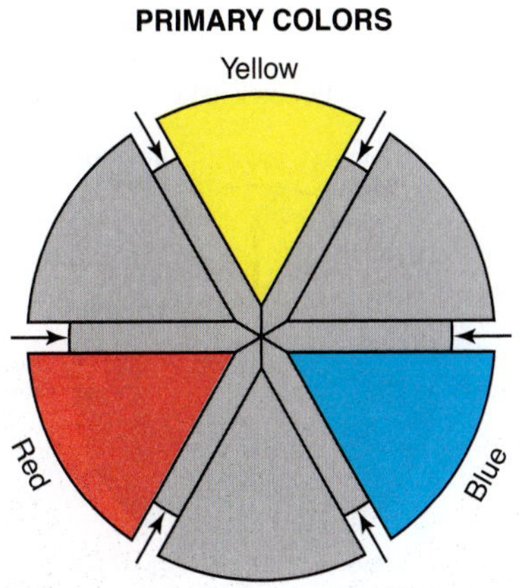

Figure 19-3 Primary colors.

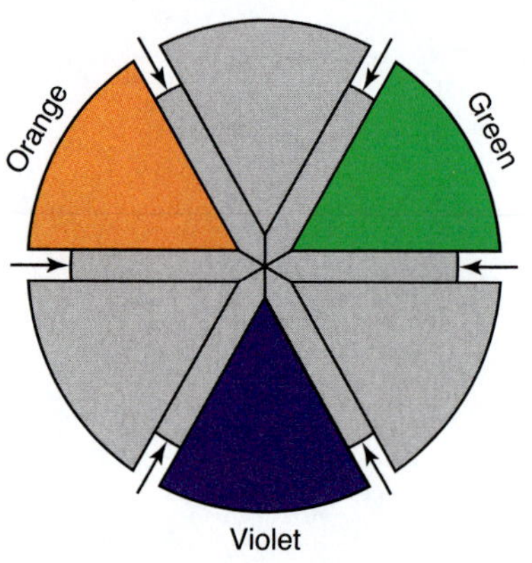

Figure 19-4 Secondary colors.

Red is the medium primary color. When added to blue-based colors, red makes them appear lighter. Conversely, red added to a yellow color will cause it to become darker.

Yellow is the lightest of the primary colors and will lighten and brighten other colors.

Secondary Colors

Secondary colors are created by mixing equal amounts of two primary colors. Mixed in equal parts, yellow and blue create green, blue and red create violet, and red and yellow create orange (Figure 19–4). Natural hair color is made up of a combination of primary and secondary colors.

Tertiary Colors

Tertiary colors are created by mixing equal amounts of one primary color with one of its adjacent secondary colors. Presented in their order on the color wheel, tertiary colors are yellow-green, blue-green, blue-violet, red-violet, red-orange, and yellow-orange (Figure 19–5).

NOTE: Quaternary colors are all other combinations of all three primary colors.

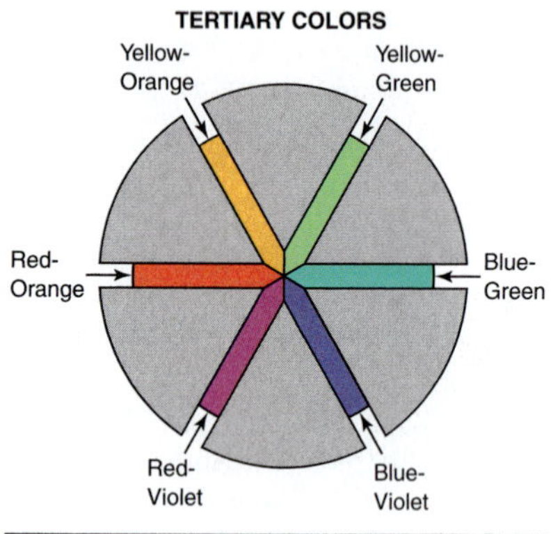

Figure 19-5 Tertiary colors.

Complementary Colors

Complementary colors are any two colors situated directly across from each other on the color wheel (Figure 19–6). When mixed together their action is to neutralize each other. For example, when mixed in equal amounts, red and green neutralize each other, creating brown. Orange and blue neutralize each other, and yellow and violet neutralize each other.

Complementary colors are always composed of a primary and a secondary color, and complementary pairs always consist of all three primary colors. For example, the color wheel shows that the complement of red (a primary color) is green (a secondary color). Green is made up of blue and yellow (both primary colors). So, all three primary colors are represented to varying degrees in the complementary pair of red and green.

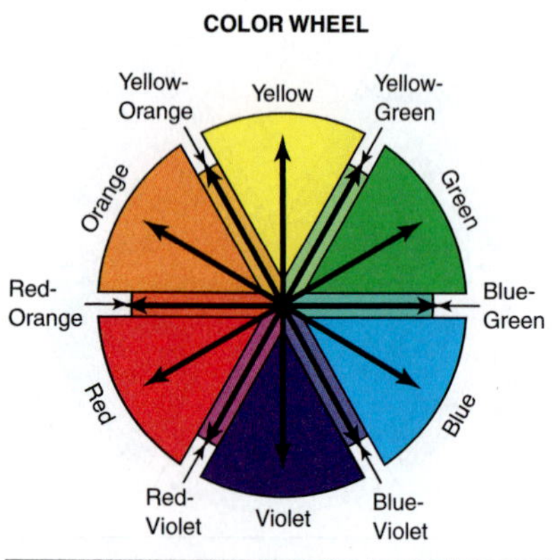

Figure 19-6 Complementary colors.

Tone or Hue of Color

The **tone** or hue is the basic name of a color, such as red, yellow, blue-green, etc. Tone is also used to describe the warmth or coolness of a color. The warm colors, also known as highlighting colors, are red, orange, and yellow. The cool colors, also known as ash or drab, are blue, green, and violet.

Level

The **level** of color is the density of a color and indicates the degree of lightness or darkness of a color. Colors lighten when mixed with white and darken when mixed with black. In haircoloring, the Level System is used to analyze the lightness or darkness of a hair color. Hair colors, both natural and color-treated, are arranged on a scale of 1 to 10, with 1 being black and

10. Lightest blond
9. Very light blond
8. Light blond
7. Medium blond
6. Dark blond
5. Light brown
4. Medium brown
3. Dark brown
2. Very dark brown
1. Black

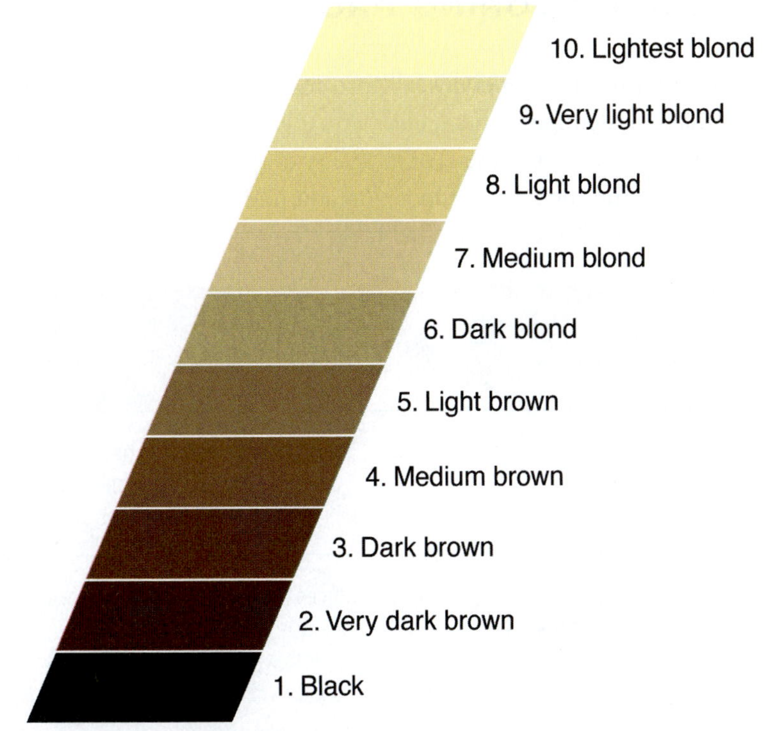

Figure 19–7 The Level System.

10 indicating lightest blond (Figure 19–7). The Level System is crucial to formulating, matching, and correcting colors.

Saturation

Saturation, or intensity, refers to the degree of concentration or amount of pigment in the color. It is the strength of a color. For example, a saturated red is very vivid. Any color can be more or less saturated. The more saturated the product the more dramatic the change in hair color.

Base Color

Artificial haircolors are developed from primary and secondary colors to form base colors. A **base color** is the predominant tone of a color, which greatly influences the final color result. For example, a violet base color will produce cool results and help to minimize yellow tones. Blue base colors minimize orange tones, and a red-orange base creates warm, bright tones in the hair.

Identifying Natural Level and Tone

The first step in performing a haircolor service is to identify the natural level of the hair. This is accomplished by holding the manufacturer's swatches or a color ring up to the client's hair for matching. It is important to identify the natural level of the hair so that an accurate determination can be made as to what the final hair color results will look like. These results will be based on the combination of the natural hair color and the artificial color that is added to it. 1

HAIRCOLORING PRODUCTS

Haircoloring products generally fall into four classifications: temporary, semipermanent, demipermanent, and permanent (Table 19–2). These classifications indicate color fastness, or its ability to remain on the hair, and are determined by the chemical composition and molecular weight of the pigments and dyes within the products (Table 19–3).

Category	Uses
Temporary color	Creates subtle color change Shampoos from the hair Neutralizes yellow hair
Semipermanent color	Introduces a client to haircolor services Adds subtle color results Tones prelightened hair
Demipermanent color	Blends gray hair Enhances natural color Tones prelightened hair Refreshes faded color Filler in color correction
Permanent haircolor	Changes existing haircolor Covers gray Creates bright or natural-looking haircolor changes

Table 19-2 Review of Haircolor Categories and Their Uses

19

Characteristic	Temporary	Semipermanent	Demipermanent	Permanent
Molecular weight of dye molecule	Large	Medium	Medium-small	Small
pH	Acid	Slightly alkaline	Moderately alkaline	Alkaline
Reaction or change	Physical	Chemical & physical	Chemical & physical	Chemical & physical
Color fastness	Removed with shampooing	Fades gradually	Fades slower than semipermanent color	Permanent
Color changes	Deposits	Deposits	No-lift, Deposit only	Lifts and deposits

Table 19-3 Four Classifications of Color

Temporary Haircolor (Nonoxidation Color)

Temporary colors utilize pigment and dye molecules of the greatest molecular weight, making these molecules the largest in the four classifications of hair color. The large size of the color molecule prevents penetration into the cuticle layer, producing only a coating action on the outside of the strand. This coating action usually results in very subtle color changes, lasting only until the next shampoo (Figure 19–8).

The chemical composition of a temporary color is acidic in reaction, creating a physical change rather than a chemical change in the hair shaft. As a result, patch tests are not required when applying temporary color. Temporary rinses have a pH range of 2.0 to 4.5.

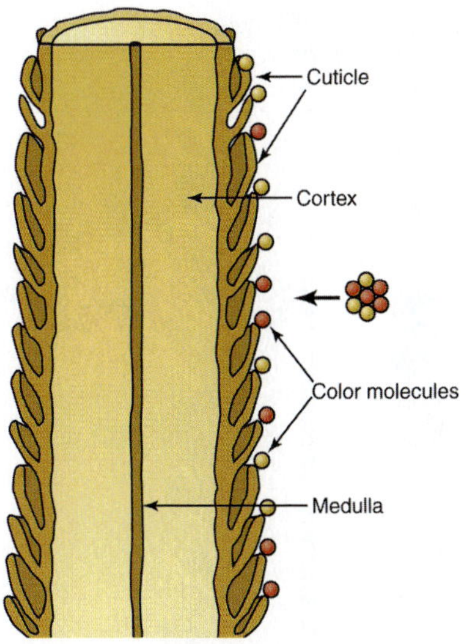

Figure 19-8 Action of temporary haircolor.

Types of Temporary Haircolor

- *Color rinses* are used to highlight the color or add color to the hair. These rinses contain certified colors and remain on the hair until the next shampoo. Two types of color rinses are available: instant and concentrated. Instant rinses are applied straight from the bottle and remain in the hair. Concentrated rinses are mixed with hot water before application, processed for 5 to 10 minutes, and then rinsed. Both types of rinses may leave traces of the darker shades on combs, brushes, and clothing.
- *Color-enhancing shampoos* combine the action of a color rinse with that of a shampoo. These shampoos generally contain certified colors, produce highlights, and impart slight color tones to the hair.
- *Crayons* are sticks of coloring compounded with soaps or synthetic waxes, that are sometimes used to color gray or white hair between hair tint retouches. Crayons are often used by men as a temporary coloring for mustaches. They are available in several standard colors: blond; light, medium, and dark brown; black; and auburn.
- *Haircolor sprays* are applied to dry hair from aerosol containers. Color sprays are usually available in vibrant colors and are generally used for special or party effects.
- *Haircolor mousses and gels* combine slight color and styling effects in one product.

Semipermanent Haircolor (Nonoxidation Color)

Traditional **semipermanent haircolor** products are also known as *direct dyes* because they do not develop color. Semipermanent pigment molecules are of a lesser molecular weight than those of temporary colors. This facilitates the physical capability to partially penetrate into the cortex. While some color does enter the cortex, most of the pigment molecules stain the cuticle layer through absorption. These molecules are also small enough to diffuse out of the hair during shampooing and tend to fade with each shampoo. Most semipermanent colors will last from six to eight shampoos (Figure 19–9).

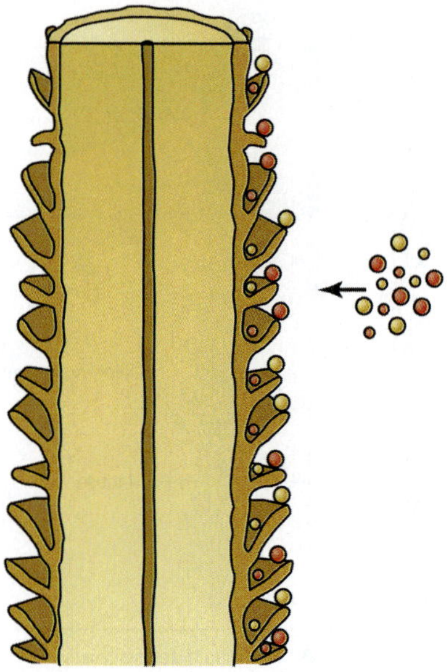

Figure 19–9 Action of semipermanent haircolor.

The chemical composition of semipermanent color is mildly alkaline in reaction, causes the cortex to swell, and raises the cuticle to allow some penetration. This chemical composition combines small color molecules, solvents, alkaline swelling agents, and surfactants to create a type of color that is known as self-penetrating. Self-penetrating colors tend to make a mild chemical change as well as a physical change.

Most semipermanent colors do not contain ammonia and may be used right out of the bottle. Although normally gentle on the hair, semipermanent colors require a patch test prior to application to prevent the occurrence of product sensitivity or allergic reaction.

Semipermanent haircolors typically fall within the 7.0 to 9.0 pH range; however, some formulations use salt bonds to improve colorfastness and may range between 7.0 and 8.0 on the pH scale. Due to the slight alkalinity of semipermanent color, these haircolor services should be followed with a mild, acid-balanced shampoo and conditioning. This will neutralize any residual alkalinity and help to restore the hair to normal pH levels.

Semipermanent haircolor may be used to:

- cover or blend partially gray hair without affecting its natural color (most semipermanent colors are designed to cover hair that is no more than 25 percent gray).
- highlight, enhance, or deepen color tones in the hair.
- serve as a nonperoxide toner for prelightened hair.

Demipermanent Haircolor (Oxidation Color)

Demipermanent haircolor, also known as *no-lift, deposit-only haircolor* (referred to as semipermanent by some manufacturers), is longer lasting than traditional semipermanent color. These products are designed to deposit color without lifting (lightening) natural or artificial color in the hair and are considered a type of oxidation color. As such, they are not used directly out of the bottle but must be mixed with a low-volume developer or activator immediately before use. The oxidizing agent in the developer causes an oxidation reaction, which develops the color (Figure 19–10).

Demipermanent and other deposit-only colors darken the natural hair color when applied. They are available in gel, cream, or liquid forms and require a patch test before application.

Demipermanent haircolor may be used to:

- impart vivid color results.
- cover nonpigmented hair.
- refresh faded permanent color.
- deposit tonal changes without lift.
- reverse highlight.
- perform corrective coloring.

Permanent Haircolor (Oxidation Color)

Permanent haircolor is mixed with a developer (hydrogen peroxide) and remains in the hair shaft. When the hair grows, a touch-up or retouch application is required to blend the color of the previously colored hair with the new hair growth. Permanent haircolor products usually contain ammonia, oxidative tints, and peroxide and require a patch test.

Permanent haircolor products can lighten and deposit color in one process. They can lighten natural hair color because they are more alkaline than demipermanent oxidation colors and are usually mixed with a higher-volume developer. The amount of lift is controlled by the pH of the color and the concentration of peroxide in the developer. As the pH of the color and concentration increase, the amount of lift increases as well. Permanent haircolor products are usually mixed with an equal amount of 20-volume peroxide and are capable of lifting one or two levels. When mixed with higher volumes of peroxide, permanent colors can lift up to four levels. Since some manufacturers recommend a 2:1 ratio of developer to haircolor, always read the manufacturer's directions.

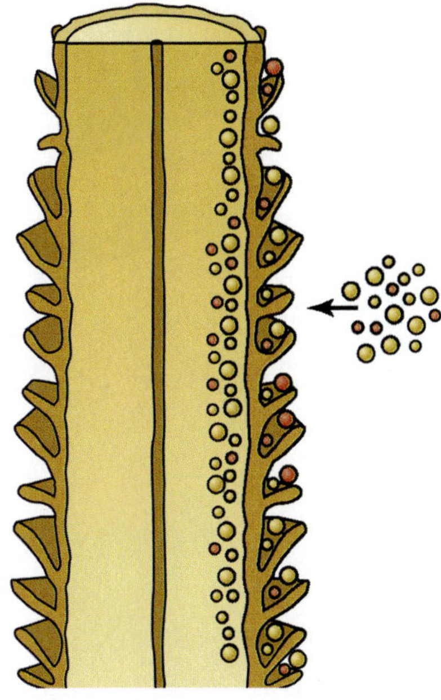

Figure 19–10 Action of demipermanent color.

Permanent haircolor is considered a penetrating tint because after the tint is mixed with an oxidizer it has the ability to penetrate through the cuticle into the cortex of the hair shaft. This action is facilitated by **aniline derivatives** that diffuse into the cortex and then form larger permanent tint molecules that become trapped within the cortex. In this way, the cortex undergoes permanent chemical and structural changes (Figure 19–11).

Permanent tints are alkaline in reaction and generally range between 9.0 and 10.5 on the pH scale. After processing, the hair is shampooed and as it dries it begins to return to its normal pH. This causes the cortex to shrink and the cuticle to close. Both actions tend to further trap the color molecules. Except for residual color product following the haircolor application,

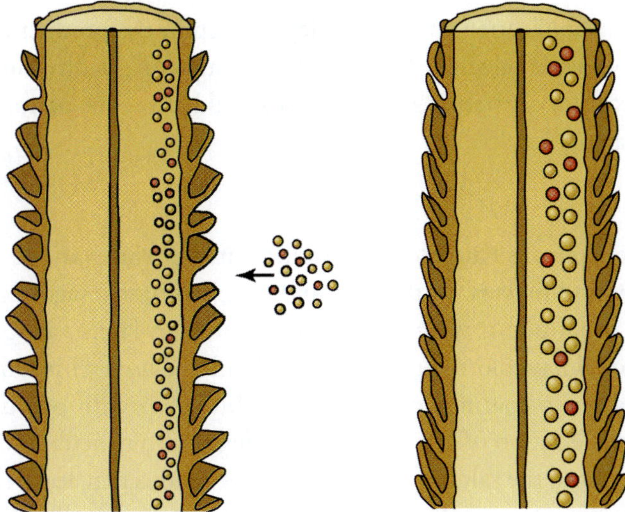

Figure 19–11 Action of permanent haircolor.

19

permanent haircolor does not wash out during the shampoo process. Eventually the color will fade and may require refreshing. When new growth occurs, **a line of demarcation** will develop between the old and new growth and will require a retouch.

Permanent haircoloring products are generally regarded as the best products for covering gray hair. This is because they simultaneously remove natural pigment through the action of lifting while adding artificial color to both the gray and pigmented hair.

Types of Permanent Haircolor

Permanent hair colors fall into four classifications: oxidation tints, vegetable tints, metallic or mineral dyes, and compound dyes.

Oxidation Tints

Oxidation tints are also known as aniline derivative tints, penetrating tints, synthetic-organic tints, and amino tints. Oxidation tints can lighten and deposit color in a single process and are available in a wide variety of colors. *Toners* also fall into the category of permanent color. Toners are aniline derivative products of pale, delicate shades designed for use on prelightened hair.

Most oxidation tints contain aniline derivatives and require a predisposition (patch) test before the service is performed. As long as the hair is of normal strength and kept in good condition, oxidation tints are compatible with other professional chemical services.

Oxidation tints are sold in bottles, canisters, and tubes, in either a semiliquid or cream form. These products must be mixed with hydrogen peroxide, which activates the chemical reaction known as oxidation. This reaction begins as soon as the two compounds are combined, so the mixed tint must be used immediately. Any leftover tint must be discarded since it deteriorates quickly.

Timing the application of the tint depends upon the product and the volume of peroxide selected. Consult the manufacturer's directions and your instructor for assistance. A strand test should always be performed to ensure satisfactory results.

Vegetable Tints

Vegetable tints are haircoloring products made from various plants, such as herbs and flowers. In the past, indigo, chamomile, sage, Egyptian henna, and other plants were used to color the hair. Henna is still used as a professional haircoloring product, but should be used with some caution. Henna has a coating action that can build up with overuse and prevent the penetration of other chemicals. Henna also penetrates the cortex and attaches to the salt bonds. Both of these actions may leave the hair unfit for other professional treatments. Even though vegetable tints are considered permanent, they are nonoxidation color products.

Metallic or Mineral Dyes

Metallic dyes are advertised as color restorers or **progressive colors**. The metallic ingredients, such as lead acetate or silver nitrate, react with the keratin in the hair, turning it brown. This reaction creates a colored film coating that produces a dull metallic appearance. Repeated treatments damage the hair and can react adversely with many professional chemical services. Metallic dyes are not professional coloring products.

Compound Dyes

Compound dyes are metallic or mineral dyes combined with a vegetable tint. The metallic salts are added to give the product more staying power and to create different colors. Like metallic dyes, compound dyes are not used professionally.

Hydrogen Peroxide Developers

A **developer** is an oxidizing agent that supplies oxygen gas for the development of color molecules when mixed with an oxidative haircolor product. This action creates a color change in the hair when the oxidizer combines with the melanin in the hair. Most developers range between 2.5 and 4.5 on the pH scale.

Hydrogen peroxide (H_2O_2) serves as the primary oxidizing agent used in haircoloring. As the oxygen and melanin combine, the peroxide solution begins to diffuse and lighten the melanin within the cortex. The smaller structure and spread-out distribution of the diffused melanin gives the hair a lighter appearance. This diffused melanin is called oxymelanin.

In its purest form, hydrogen peroxide has a pH level of about 7.0. When diluted with water and other substances for use in haircoloring, hydrogen peroxide has a mild acidic pH of 3.5 to 4.0.

Strengths of Hydrogen Peroxide

Hydrogen peroxide alone produces a relatively mild lightening of the hair color and causes little damage to the hair shaft. When very pale shades are desired, however, further lightening must occur and a longer processing time or the mixture of a stronger formula is required.

In the scientific world, different strengths of hydrogen peroxide are identified as percentages. In haircoloring, the term "volume" is used to denote the different strengths of hydrogen peroxide (Table 19–4).

Volume is the measure of the potential oxidation of varying strengths of hydrogen peroxide. The lower the volume, the less lift is achieved; the higher the volume, the greater the lifting action.

Permanent haircolor products use 10-, 20-, 30-, or 40-volume hydrogen peroxide for proper color development. A 10-volume solution is recommended when less lightening is desired for color enhancement. The majority of permanent coloring products use 20-volume hydrogen peroxide for

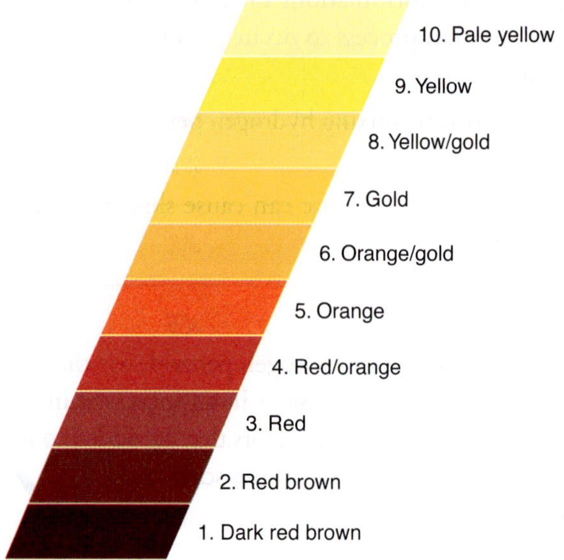

Figure 19-13 Ten degrees of decolorization.

Hair lighteners are used to create blond shades that are not possible with permanent haircolor and to achieve the following:

- Lighten the hair to the final shade
- **Prelightening** to prepare the hair for the application of a toner or tint (double-process application)
- Lighten hair to a particular shade
- Brighten and lighten an existing shade of color

Types of Lighteners

Lighteners are available in three forms: oil, cream, and powder. Oil and cream lighteners are considered **on-the-scalp lighteners** and powder lighteners are **off-the-scalp lighteners**. Each type has unique abilities, chemical compositions, and formulation procedures.

- *Oil lighteners* are usually mixtures of hydrogen peroxide with sulfonated oil. As on-the-scalp lighteners, they are the mildest form of lightener and may be used when only one or two levels of lift are desired.

Color oil lighteners add temporary color and highlight the hair as they lighten. They contain certified colors, may be used without a patch test, and remove pigment while adding color tones. Color oil lighteners are classified according to their action on the hair as follows:

1. Gold: lightens and adds golden to reddish tones depending on the base color of the hair
2. Silver: lightens and adds silvery highlights to gray or white hair and minimizes red and gold tones in other shades

3. Red: lightens and adds red highlights
4. Drab: lightens and adds ash highlights. Tones down or reduces red and gold tones

Neutral oil lighteners remove pigment without adding color tone. These oil lighteners may be used to presoften hair for a tint application.

- *Cream lighteners* are the most popular type of on-the-scalp lightener. They contain conditioning agents, bluing, and thickeners, which makes them easy to apply, and will not run, drip, or dry out. Cream lighteners provide the following benefits.
  1. The conditioning agents give some protection to the hair.
  2. The bluing agent helps to drab undesirable red and gold tones.
  3. The thickener provides control during application and prevents overlap.
- *Powder lighteners*, also called paste or quick lighteners, contain an oxygen-releasing booster and inert substances for quicker and stronger action. Paste lighteners will hold and not run, but will dry out quickly and do not contain conditioning agents.

  Note: If the scalp shows any sensitivity or abrasions, lighteners are not recommended.

Contribution of Underlying Pigment

The natural pigment that remains in the hair after lightening contributes to the artificial color that is added. It is essential to lighten the hair to the correct stage because the pigment that remains in the hair will impact the final result of the hair lightening and coloring process.

Use Figure 19–14 as a guide to determine the contributing pigment or undertones of color at various hair color levels.

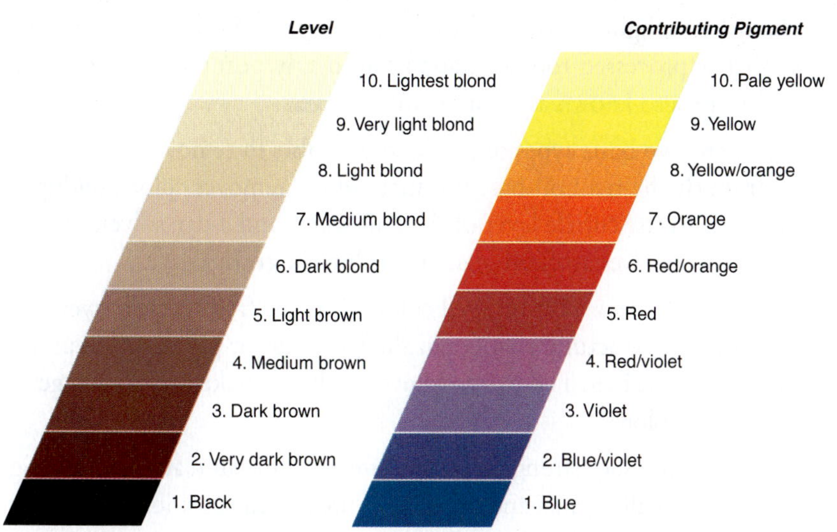

Figure 19-14 Contributing pigment (undertones).

19

Toners

A **toner** is a haircoloring product that is applied to prelightened hair for the purpose of achieving the desired color or tones in the hair. Traditional toners are permanent aniline derivative haircoloring products that have a smaller percentage of the formula that creates delicate shades of color. Toners differ from tints only in the degree of color saturation and require a patch test.

Toners are available in pale and delicate colors. They usually have a very different color than the final shade that they produce and may appear to be purple, blue, orange, or pink in the bottle. As toner color oxidizes it goes through several visual color changes; therefore, a strand test should be done to determine the processing time required for a desired shade.

After the hair goes through the desired stages of lightening, the color left in the hair is known as its foundation or contributing color. Achieving the correct foundation is necessary for proper toner development. This is usually the lightest degree of contributing pigment that remains after the lightening process.

Toner manufacturers provide literature that recommends the proper foundation to achieve a desired color. As a general rule, the more pale the desired color, the lighter the foundation must be. It is important to follow the guide closely. Overlightened hair will grab the base color of the toner, while underlightened hair will appear to have more red, yellow, or orange than the intended color.

Since toning is more of a technique than a particular product, semipermanent, demipermanent, and permanent haircolor can also be used as "toners" to achieve the desired hair color. CAUTION: Advise clients that lightening dark hair to a pale blond tone can be very damaging to the hair.

Dye Removers

The removal of haircoloring agents is sometimes desired if the client wants to change to a lighter shade, if a coloring mistake has been made, or if the hair has processed too dark due to an overly porous condition. **Dye removers** are also known as color or tint removers.

There are two basic types of products available to remove artificial pigment from the hair: an oil-base product, which removes color buildup or stain that is in the cuticle layer of the hair shaft; and a dye solvent, which diffuses and dissolves artificial pigment within the cortical layer.

- *Oil-base dye removers* lift trapped color pigments from cuticle layers and do not create structural changes in the hair shaft or pigment (natural or artificial) of the hair. These dye removers will not make drastic changes in the level of color.
- *Dye solvents* produce strong lightening effects on melanin and artificial pigment, are nonallergenic, and do not require a predisposition test. Follow manufacturer's directions carefully.

Fillers

Fillers are preparations designed to help equalize porosity and/or to create a color base in the hair and equalize excessive porosity. The two general classifications of conditioner fillers are protein and nonprotein, both of which are manufactured in gel, cream, and liquid forms. Color fillers are available in clear, neutral, and a variety of color bases.

Stain Removers

Generally, soap and water will remove most tint stains from the skin. Stain removers are commercially prepared solutions that are designed for this purpose. When soap and water is not capable of removing haircolor from the skin, use one of the following methods:

1. Dampen a piece of cotton with the leftover tint. Use a rotary movement to cover the stained areas and follow with a damp towel. Apply a small amount of face cream and wipe clean. 4
2. Use a prepared stain remover.

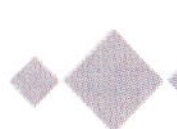

HAIRCOLORING PROCEDURES TERMINOLOGY

Successful haircoloring usually requires a series of steps to accomplish the desired end result. Due to the wide range of haircoloring products, application methods, and procedures, it is important to have a clear understanding of the terms used in haircoloring processes. Some common procedural terms are *patch test, strand test, soap cap, tint back, record keeping,* and the *client consultation.*

Patch Test

An individual's reaction to aniline derivative tints can be unpredictable. Some clients may show an immediate sensitivity while others may suddenly develop an allergy to the product after years of use. To identify a client who has a sensitivity to aniline derivatives, the U.S. Federal Food, Drug, and Cosmetic Act prescribes that a **patch test**, also known as a *predisposition test,* be given 24 to 48 hours prior to each application of an aniline derivative tint or toner.

Strand Test

A **strand test** is performed for color applications to determine how the hair will react to the haircolor product, how long it will take to process, and what the final outcome will look like. After the results of the patch test, the strand test is the next step in performing a haircolor service.

RELEASE FORM

I, the undersigned, ________________________________
(name)

residing at ________________________________
(street, address)

____
(city, state and zip)

about to receive services in the Clinical Department of
____

and having been advised that the services shall be performed by either students, graduate students, and/or instructors of the school, in consideration of the nominal charge for such services, hereby release the school, its students, graduate students, instructors, agents, representatives, and/or employees, from any and all claims arising out of and in any way connected with the performance of these services.

The Proprietor Is Not Responsible for Personal Property

Signed ________________________________

Date ________________________________

Witnessed ________________________________

THIS RELEASE FORM MUST BE SIGNED BY THE PARENT OR GUARDIAN IF THE CLIENT BEING SERVED IS UNDER 18 YEARS OF AGE.

Figure 19-22 Sample school release form.

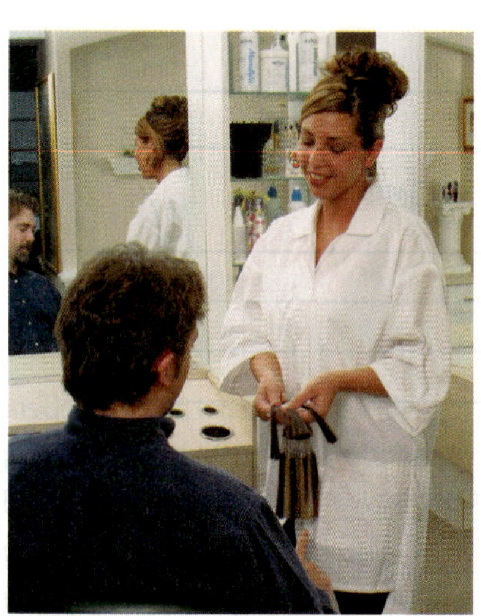

Figure 19-23 A client consultation should precede every haircolor service.

3. Perform a hair and scalp analysis and log the results on a record card. Use color swatches to determine client's natural level.
4. Ask the client leading questions about the desired end result, which tells you whether he or she wants temporary or permanent change, all-over color or highlights, etc.
5. Show examples of appropriate colors and make a determination with the client.
6. Review the procedure, application technique, maintenance, and cost with the client.
7. Gain approval and begin the service.
8. Record end results on the client record card.

HAIRCOLOR APPLICATION TERMS

There are a variety of different haircolor application methods. Review the following to become familiar with the terms used in haircoloring procedures.

Virgin Application

A **virgin application** refers to the application of haircolor to hair that has not been previously colored. Hair that is in a "virgin" state is usually healthy hair that has not suffered any chemical damage. A virgin application also indicates that the haircoloring product will be applied to the entire hair strand versus the new growth only.

Retouch Application

When permanent haircolor or lighteners are used, new hair growth will become obvious between haircolor applications. The new growth, or regrowth, is that section of the hair shaft between the scalp and the hair that has been previously treated. This creates a line of demarcation between the natural color of the hair and the previously colored or lightened hair that requires blending by way of another color or lightener application. The term **retouch application** is used to describe this blending process.

Single-Process Haircoloring

Single-process haircoloring is a process that lightens and colors the hair in a single application. Examples of single-process coloring are virgin tint applications and tint retouch applications. Single-process haircoloring is also known as single-application coloring, one-step coloring, one-step tinting, and single-application tinting.

Double-Process Haircoloring

Double-process coloring requires two separate and distinct applications to achieve the desired color. The hair is lightened before the depositing color is applied, allowing the practitioner to independently control the lightening and coloring actions. Double-process haircoloring is also known as double-application coloring, two-step coloring, two-step tinting, and double-application tinting. Double-process haircoloring may include the use of lighteners and toners, presofteners and tints, or fillers and color.

Presoftening

Presoftening is the process of treating gray or other extremely resistant hair types to facilitate better color penetration. Presoftening swells and opens the cuticle. It can be accomplished with a mixture of 1 ounce of 20-volume peroxide and 8 drops of 28 percent ammonia water, or with an oil or cream bleach product.

Highlighting

Highlighting is the process of coloring some of the hair strands lighter than the natural or artificial color to add the illusion of sheen and depth. Frosting, tipping, and streaking are forms of highlighting.

Lowlighting

Lowlighting or *reverse highlighting* is the process of coloring strands or sections of the hair darker than the natural or artificial color. Contrasting dark areas appear to recede and make detail less visible to the eye.

Cap Technique

The **cap technique** involves pulling strands of hair through the holes of a perforated cap with a plastic or metal hook. The number of strands pulled through the cap determines the degree of highlighting or lowlighting that is achieved.

Foil Technique

The **foil technique** involves slicing or weaving out sections of hair to be placed on a piece of foil. The color or lightening product is usually brushed onto the hair section, after which the foil is folded and sealed for processing.

Free-Form Technique

The **free-form technique**, also called *balayage*, is the process of painting a lightener or color directly onto clean, styled hair. The effects can be subtle or dramatic, depending on the type of product (color or lightener) and the amount of hair that it is applied to.

HAIRCOLORING PRODUCT APPLICATIONS

Given the many choices in haircoloring formulations and applications, it is crucial that the barber provides the client with the appropriate product and follows the correct application methods. Use the following as a guide for haircoloring product selection and application.

Temporary Color Rinses

Temporary color rinses may be used to give clients a preview of how a color change will look. They are also a satisfactory option for clients who want to highlight the color of their hair or add slight color to gray hair. These rinses wash out when shampooed and are available in a variety of color shades. Temporary rinses are easily and quickly applied at the shampoo bowl and can serve as an introduction to other longer-lasting color services.

Temporary color rinses can be used to bring out highlights, temporarily restore faded hair color to its natural shade, neutralize yellow tones in white

PROCEDURE

TEMPORARY COLOR RINSE

Implements and Materials

- Temporary color product
- Applicator bottle (optional)
- Shampoo cape
- Towels
- Protective gloves
- Shampoo
- Color chart
- Record card
- Timer
- Comb

Preparation

If the client is to receive a haircut, perform the cut prior to the color rinse application.

1. Assemble all necessary supplies.
2. Prepare the client. Protect the clothing with a plastic cape and a towel.
3. Examine the client's scalp and hair.
4. Select the desired shade of color rinse.
5. Perform a strand test.

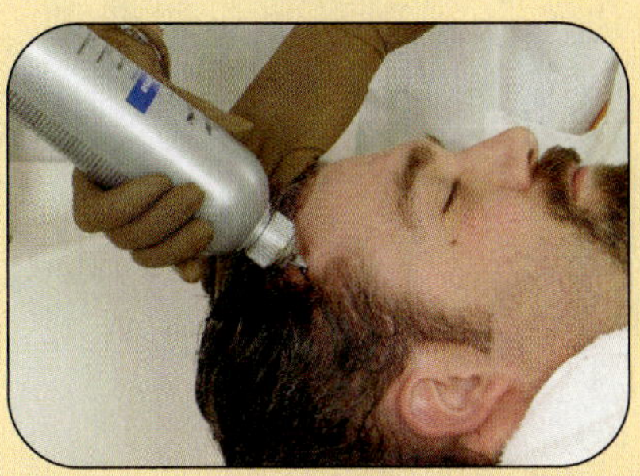

Figure 19-24 Apply color rinse at the shampoo bowl.

Procedure for Temporary Color Rinse Application

1. Shampoo, rinse, and towel blot hair. Excess moisture must be removed to prevent diluting the color. Put on gloves.
2. With the client reclined at the shampoo bowl, apply the color from the hairline through and around the entire head (Figure 19–24).
3. Use the comb to blend the color, applying more as necessary for even coverage (Figure 19–25).
4. Do not rinse product. Towel blot excess.
5. Proceed with styling (Figure 19–26).

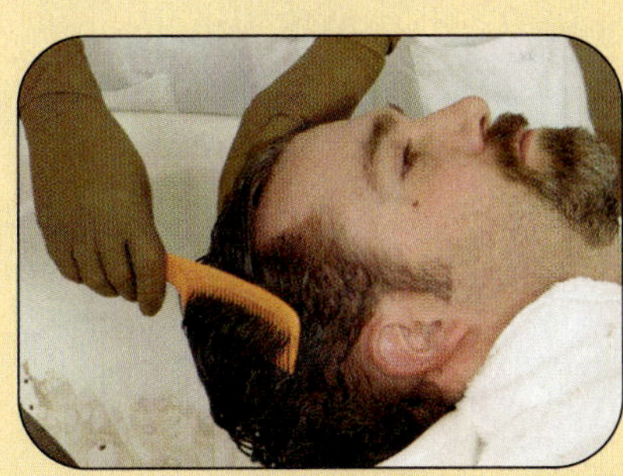

Figure 19-25 Blend color rinse through the hair.

Cleanup and Sanitation

1. Discard all disposable supplies.
2. Close and wipe off containers and store properly.
3. Sanitize implements, cape, and work area.
4. Wash hands.
5. Record results on client record card.

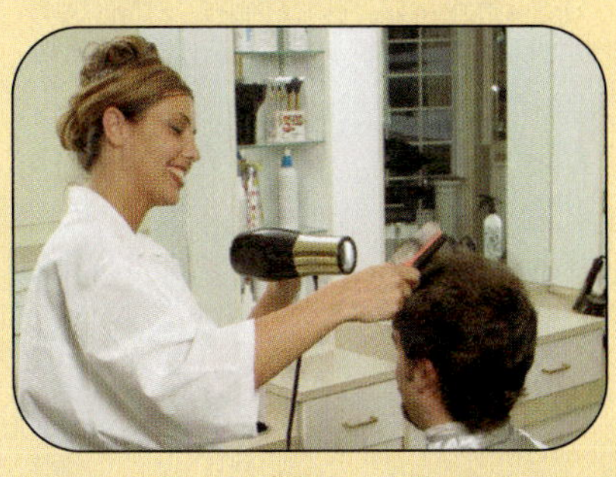

Figure 19-26 Style the hair.

or gray hair, or to tone down overlightened hair. Perform a preliminary strand test to determine proper color selection.

Semipermanent Haircolor

Semipermanent color products are appropriate for the client who may want more color change than is available with a temporary rinse, but who is hesitant about a permanent color change and its related maintenance. In this way, a semipermanent tint fills the gap between temporary color rinses and permanent haircolor without replacing either of them.

Since semipermanent products are deposit-only colors, the final outcome will depend on the hair's original color and texture, the color that is applied, and the length of development time. These haircoloring products are available in liquid and cream forms in a variety of colors. Some formulations are specifically designed in blue-gray or silver-gray hues to brighten or blend gray color tones.

Characteristics of Semipermanent Tints

The basic characteristics of semipermanent haircolor that influence the decision to choose this color product over another are as follows:

- Semipermanent tints do not require the addition of hydrogen peroxide.
- The color is self-penetrating.
- The color is applied the same way each time.
- Retouching is eliminated.
- The color does not rub off, because it has penetrated the hair shaft slightly.
- Hair will usually return to its natural color after four to eight shampoos, provided a mild, nonstripping shampoo is used.
- Semipermanent tints require a 24-hour patch test.
- Some semipermanent haircolors require preshampooing; others do not.

Selecting Semipermanent Color

The addition of artificial color to the natural pigment in the hair shafts creates a darker color. When using a color chart to determine the level and shade of semipermanent color to use, consider the natural color to represent half of the formula. Use the following guide to select the correct color to perform the strand test.

1. On hair with no gray (solid), select a color level that is two levels lighter than the desired shade. For example: A client with a natural level of 6 desires a level 7 shade. Therefore, a level 9 shade of color should be used.
2. The use of ash or cool shades will create a color that appears darker than if a warm shade is applied.
3. Warm colors appear shinier due to the reflection of light.
4. For clients with less than 50 percent gray, select a shade that matches the natural hair color
5. For clients with 50 percent or more gray hair, select a color one shade darker than the natural hair color.

PROCEDURE

SEMIPERMANENT COLOR APPLICATION

Implements and Materials

- Semipermanent color product
- Color chart
- Applicator bottle or brush
- Shampoo cape
- Towels
- Protective gloves
- Shampoo
- Conditioner
- Comb
- Plastic clips (optional, depending on length of hair)
- Plastic cap (optional, depending on manufacturer's directions)
- Cotton
- Protective cream
- Record card
- Timer

Preparation

1. Perform a preliminary patch test 24 hours before the service. Proceed only if the test is negative.
2. Perform client consultation and record results on client record card.
3. Drape client and apply protective cream.
4. Perform a strand test and record the results.

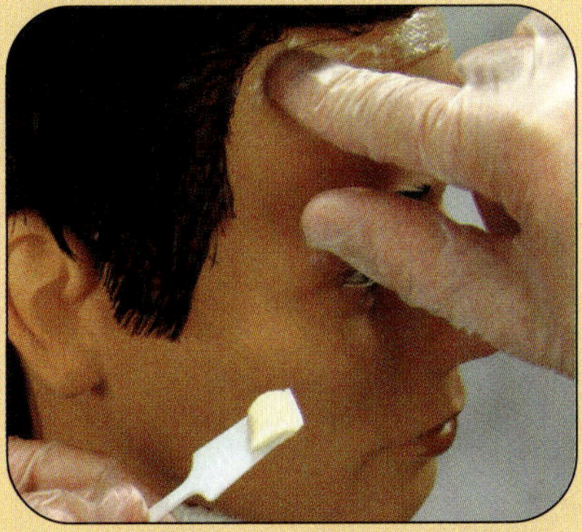

Figure 19-27 Apply protective cream around hairline.

Procedure for Semipermanent Color Application

1. Shampoo, rinse, and towel blot hair. Follow manufacturer's directions.
2. Part the hair into four sections. Put on gloves. Apply protective cream to hairline (Figure 19-27).
3. Working with $\frac{1}{4}$-inch to $\frac{1}{2}$-inch subsections, apply color to the entire hair shaft from scalp to ends (Figure 19-28). Use an applicator bottle or brush depending on the product's consistency. With the fingers, gently work the color through the hair until it is thoroughly saturated. Do not massage into the scalp. If the hair is long, pile it loosely on the top of the head.
4. Apply plastic cap if so instructed by the manufacturer's directions.
5. Process according to strand test results and manufacturer's directions. Check color.

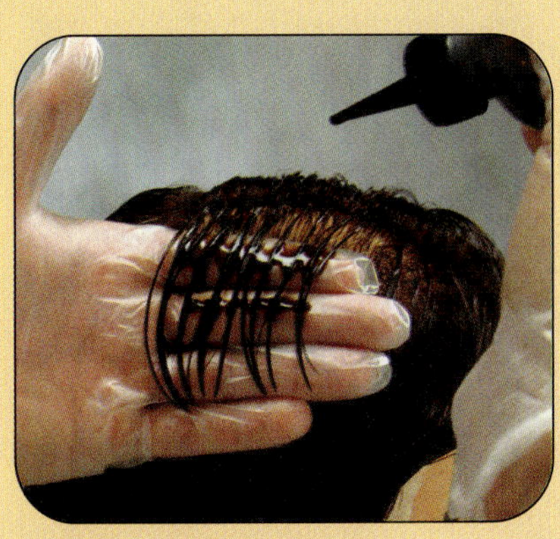

Figure 19-28 Apply semipermanent color from scalp to ends.

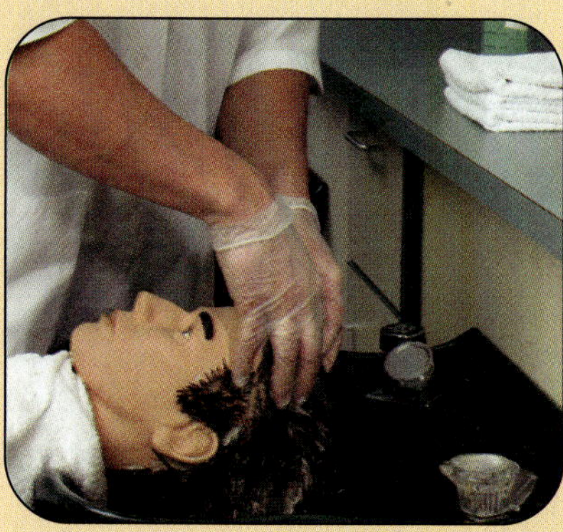

Figure 19–29 Work product into a rich lather.

6. Following color development, wet client's hair with warm water, lather, and work through hair (Figure 19–29).
7. Rinse thoroughly, shampoo, and condition. Remove stains as necessary.
8. Rinse, towel blot, and style.

Cleanup and Sanitation

1. Discard all disposable supplies.
2. Close and wipe off containers and store properly.
3. Sanitize implements and tools, cape, and work area.
4. Wash hands.
5. Record results on client record card.

Special Problems

Some semipermanent haircolor products have a tendency to build up on the hair shaft with repeated applications. If this should occur, apply the color to the new growth only, process until the desired color shade develops, then wet the hair with warm water and blend the color through the hair with a large-toothed comb.

Demipermanent Haircolor

Since demipermanent color is considered to be deposit-only color, the same procedures used for the application of a semipermanent haircolor product can be employed. Follow the manufacturer's guidelines for application, color selection, and processing time.

Permanent Haircolor

Practically all professional permanent haircoloring is done with the use of oxidizing penetrating tints that contain aniline derivatives. These penetrating tints are considered either single-process or double-process tints and are available in liquid, cream, and gel forms.

Single-Process Haircoloring

Single-process tints provide a simplified method of haircoloring. In one application, the hair can be colored permanently without requiring preshampooing, pre-softening, or pre-lightening. Single-process tints usually contain a lightening agent, shampoo, aniline derivative tint, and an alkalizing agent to activate the peroxide. Most color is formulated for use with 20-volume hydrogen peroxide. When other volumes of peroxide are used, the color results change. The choice of colors varies from deepest black to lightest blond.

Characteristics of Single-Process Tints

A single-application tint is applied on dry hair. If the hair is extremely oily or dirty and a shampoo is necessary, it must be dried thoroughly before applying the tint. Some characteristics of single-process tints are that they:

1. save time by eliminating preshampooing or prelightening.
2. color the hair lighter or darker than the client's natural color.
3. blend in gray or white hair to match the client's natural hair color.
4. tone down streaks, off-shades, discoloration, and faded hair ends.

Color Selection of Single-Process Tints

The porosity of the hair is one of the most important characteristics to consider when choosing hair color tint shades. Use the following guide for choosing the level of color when tinting darker.

- Normal porosity: half level lighter than desired color
- Slightly porous: one level lighter than desired color
- Very porous: one to two levels lighter than desired color

General rules for single-process color selection for gray hair are:

1. To match the natural color of hair and to cover gray, select the color closest to the natural shade.
2. To brighten or lighten hair color and to cover gray, select a shade lighter than the natural color. The selected tint must contain enough color to produce the desired shade on gray hair.
3. To darken the hair and cover gray, select a color darker than the natural hair color.
4. Study the manufacturer's color chart for correct color selections.

Use the following formula for color selection when tinting lighter than the natural color.

Formulation Step Example:

1. Identify the desired level. 6
2. Identify the natural level. -4
3. Subtract the natural level from the desired level. 2
4. Add the level difference to the desired level. +6
5. Total is the level of color needed. 8

SINGLE-PROCESS COLOR RETOUCH

To retouch new hair growth, use the same preparation steps as for coloring virgin hair. Then proceed as follows:

1. Refer to the client record card for correct color selection and other data.
2. Apply the tint first to new growth at sideburns, temples, and nape area.
3. Apply the tint to new growth in ¼-inch strands. Do not overlap. Check frequently for color development.
4. When color has almost developed, dilute the remaining tint by adding a mild shampoo or warm water. Apply and gently work the mixture through the hair with the fingertips. Comb and blend from the scalp to the hair ends for even distribution.
5. Process for the required time. Rinse with warm water to remove excess color.
6. Use an acid-balanced shampoo and rinse thoroughly.
7. Dry and comb, or style hair as desired.
8. Remove color stains, if necessary.
9. Fill out a record card.
10. Clean up in the usual manner.

Double-Process Haircoloring

Double-process haircoloring begins with hair lightening, followed by a tint or toner application. This double process requires two separate steps as presented in the following section.

Characteristics of Lighteners

Lightening creates a desired color foundation. This new color foundation may be the finished result or it may be the first step of a double-process

PROCEDURE

SINGLE-PROCESS COLOR APPLICATION FOR VIRGIN HAIR

Implements and Materials

- Single-process permanent color product
- Hydrogen peroxide
- Color chart
- Applicator bottle or brush and bowl
- Shampoo cape
- Towels
- Protective gloves
- Shampoo
- Conditioner
- Comb
- Plastic clips (optional, depending on length of hair)
- Plastic cap (optional, depending on manufacturer's directions)
- Cotton
- Protective cream
- Record card
- Timer

Preparation

1. Perform a preliminary patch test 24 hours before the service. Proceed only if the test is negative.
2. Perform client consultation and record results on client record card.
3. Drape client and apply protective cream.
4. Perform a strand test and record the results.

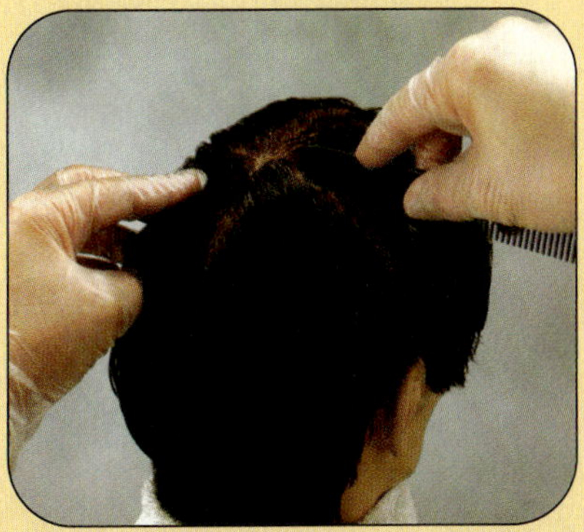

Figure 19-30 Part hair into four sections.

Procedure for Single-process Permanent Color Application

1. Follow manufacturer's directions.
2. Put on gloves and part dry hair into four sections (Figure 19-30).
3. Prepare color formula for either bottle or brush application method.
4. Begin in the section where the hair is most resistant or where there will be the most color change.
5. Part off 1/4-inch subsections and apply color to the mid shaft area (Figure 19-31). Stay at least 1/2 inch from the scalp and do not apply to the porous ends.
6. Process according to the strand test results and the manufacturer's directions.

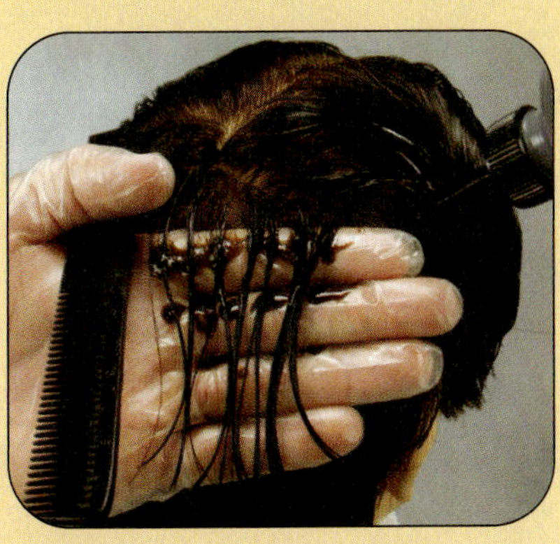

Figure 19-31 Apply color to midshaft.

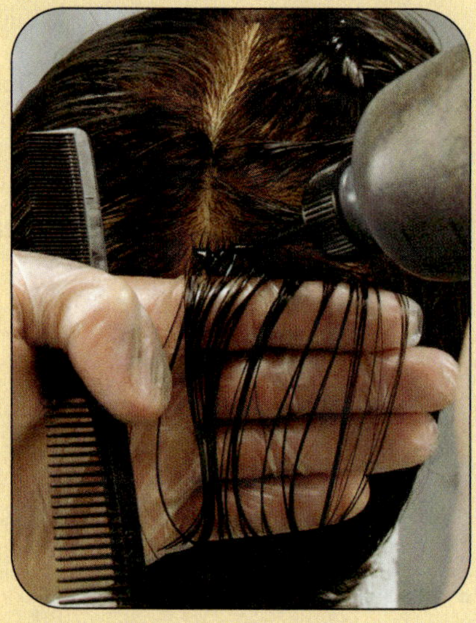
Figure 19-32 Apply product to scalp area.

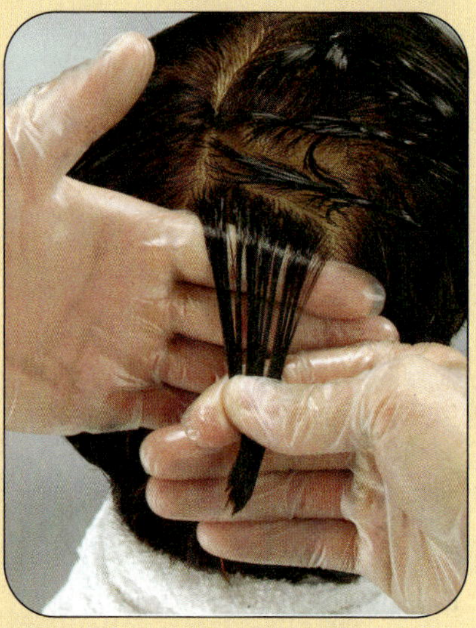
Figure 19-33 Pull color through to hair ends.

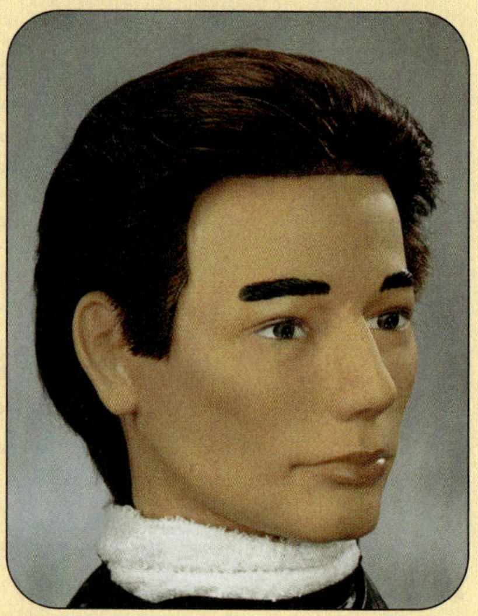
Figure 19-34 Style as desired by client.

7. Check color development. When desired color is reached, apply remaining product to hair at the scalp, then pull the color through to the hair ends (Figures 19-32 and 19-33).
8. Lightly wet client's hair with warm water and lather. Massage lather through the hair.
9. Rinse thoroughly, shampoo, and condition. Remove stains as necessary.
10. Rinse, towel blot, and style (Figure 19-34).

Cleanup and Sanitation

1. Discard all disposable supplies.
2. Close and wipe off containers and store properly.
3. Sanitize implements and tools, cape, and work area.
4. Wash hands.
5. Record results on client record card.

application. Consideration must be given to the existing hair color, processing and development time, resulting porosity, and color selection to achieve the desired shade.

Depending on the manufacturer's directions, hair lighteners can be used for the following processes.

- To lighten the entire head of hair
- To lighten the hair to a particular shade
- To brighten and lighten the existing shade
- To tip, streak, or frost certain sections of the hair
- To lighten hair that has already been tinted
- To remove undesirable casts and off-shades
- To correct dark streaks or spots in hair that has already been lightened or tinted

Selection of Lighteners

Remember to choose the appropriate lightener for the service. Cream and oil lighteners may be used on the scalp; powder lighteners are off-the-scalp products.

Together with the manufacturer's directions, be guided by the following general rules when choosing a lightening product.

1. Oil lighteners are the mildest form of lightener and may be used when only one or two levels of lift are desired.
2. Cream lighteners offer some protection to the hair, are controllable during application, and can be used to drab undesirable red and gold tones. For increased strength, up to three activators can be added for on-the-scalp applications and up to four activators for off-the-scalp processes.
3. Powder lighteners are strong enough to produce blonding effects, but should not be used for retouch applications.

Lightener Retouch

A *lightener retouch* is the term commonly used when a lightener is applied only to the new hair growth to match the rest of the lightened hair. The client's record card should be consulted as a guide to the lightener used previously and the time required for the shade to develop.

Cream lightener generally is used for a lightener retouch because it prevents the overlapping of the previously lightened hair. Black or dark brown hair usually requires more frequent retouch applications than lighter natural shades. When retouching, the lightener is applied to the new growth only. If a lighter or different level is desired overall, wait until the new growth is almost light enough or has developed fully. Then bring the remainder of the lightener through the hair shaft. One to five minutes should be ample time to create a lighter level effect.

PROCEDURE

STEP 1: LIGHTENING VIRGIN HAIR

Implements and Materials

- Lightener product
- Hydrogen peroxide
- Color chart
- Applicator bottle or brush and bowl
- Shampoo cape
- Towels
- Protective gloves
- Shampoo
- Conditioner
- Comb
- Plastic clips (optional, depending on length of hair)
- Cotton
- Protective cream
- Record card
- Timer

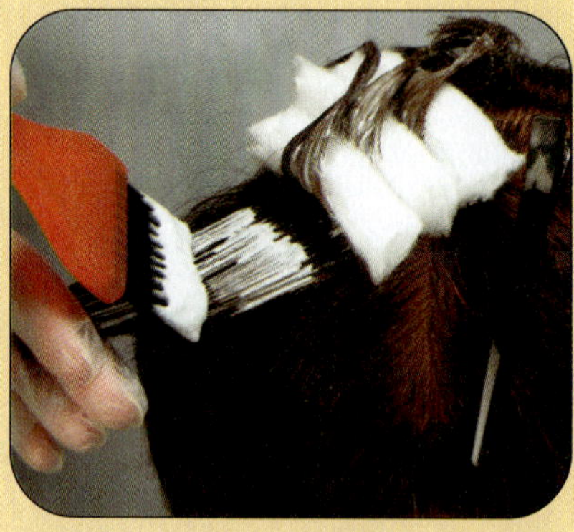

Figure 19-35 Apply lightener to top and underside of the subsection.

19

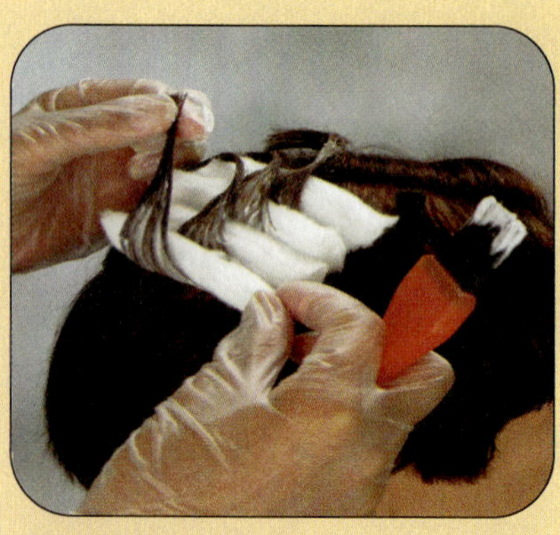

Figure 19-36 Place a strip of cotton along the part lines.

Preparation

1. Perform a preliminary patch test 24 hours before the service. Proceed only if the test is negative.
2. Perform client consultation and record results on client record card.
3. Drape client and apply protective cream.
4. Perform a strand test and record the results.

Procedure for Lightening Virgin Hair

1. Divide dry hair into four sections.
2. Apply protective cream around hairline. Put on gloves.
3. Prepare lightening formula. Use either bottle or brush application method.
4. Begin in the section where the hair is most resistant or where there will be the most color change.
5. Part off 1/8-inch subsections and apply lightener 1/2 inch from the scalp up to, but not through, the porous ends. Apply to top and underside of the subsection and place a strip of cotton along the part lines to prevent seepage to the scalp area (Figures 19–35 and 19–36).
6. Apply lightener to other sections in the same manner. Keep lightener moist with repeated applications if necessary. Do not comb the lightener through the hair.

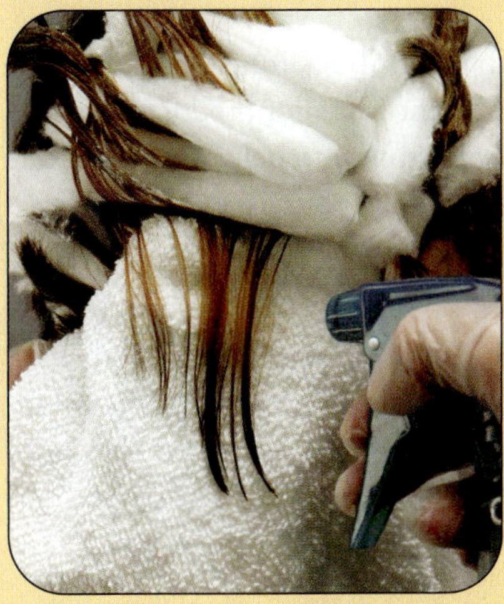

Figure 19-37 Test for lightening action.

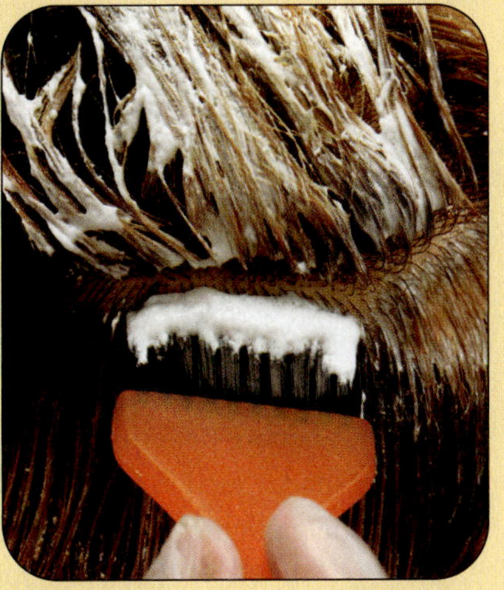

Figure 19-38 Remove cotton and apply lightener near the scalp.

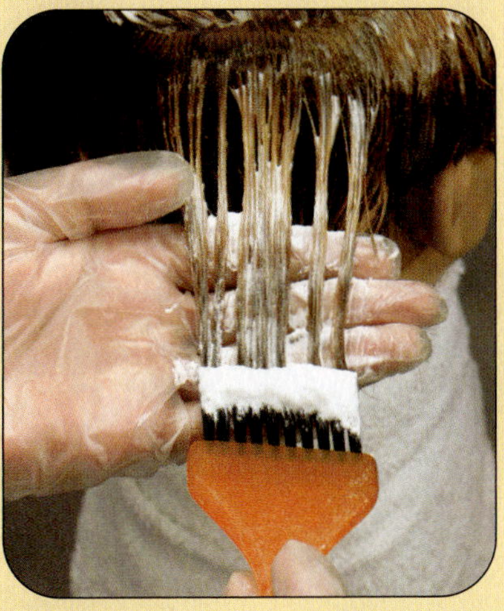

Figure 19-39 Apply lightening products to the ends.

7. Process according to the strand test results and manufacturer's directions. Check lightening action by misting as for a strand test about 15 minutes before the completion of the time required (Figure 19-37). If the level is not light enough, reapply the mixture and continue testing frequently until the desired shade is almost developed.
8. Remove cotton from scalp area and apply lightener near the scalp (Figure 19-38). Apply lightening product to the porous ends (Figure 19-39). Process until the entire hair shaft has reached the desired level.
9. Rinse thoroughly, shampoo, and condition. Dry the hair with a towel or under a cool dryer per the manufacturer's directions. Examine the scalp for abrasions.
10. Proceed with toner application if desired.

Cleanup and Sanitation

1. Discard all disposable supplies.
2. Close and wipe off containers and store properly.
3. Sanitize implements and tools, cape, and work area.
4. Wash hands.
5. Record results on client record card.

Toners

Other than a reduced ratio of dye load in the formula, toners have the same chemical ingredients and actions as permanent haircolor products. The difference in the formulation is what allows for toners to deliver pale, delicate shades of color to prelightened hair.

Color Selection of Toners

Pastel colors, such as silver, ash, platinum, and beige, are popular toners for lighter blond colors. Gray hair and skin tone changes that accompany advancing years may benefit from the lighter silver tones. When extremely pale toner shades such as very light silver, platinum, or beige are desired, the hair must be prelightened to pale yellow or almost white.

Toner Retouch

A toner retouch must be given the same careful consideration as you would give a two-color tint retouch application. The new growth must be prelightened to the same degree of lightness achieved in the previous toner application. The lightener is applied to the new growth only. To avoid damage to the hair, be careful not to overlap the lightener on previously lightened hair. After the lightening process has been completed, the toner is applied to the entire length of the hair in the usual manner.

Suggestions and Reminders

- Toners are completely dependent on the proper preliminary lightening treatment, which must leave the hair light and porous enough to receive the pale toner shades.
- Semipermanent and demipermanent color can also be used with lighteners to achieve specific tones and colors.
- Strand tests are vital to correct double-process applications.
- A complete explanation of the possible outcome should be discussed with the client. It is always possible that the hair cannot be decolorized sufficiently for the color choice without resulting in serious damage to the hair. Gold or red pigments remaining in the hair after lightening indicate under-lightening; ash tones indicate over-lightening. When this happens, the shade of toner should be chosen to neutralize the unwanted tones.

SPECIAL-EFFECTS HAIRCOLORING AND LIGHTENING

Special-effects haircoloring refers to any technique that involves the partial lightening or coloring of the hair. As previously defined in the Haircolor Application Terms section, highlighting is the process of lightening or coloring some of the hair strands lighter than the natural color. Frosting,

PROCEDURE

STEP 2: TONER APPLICATION

Implements and Materials

- Toner product
- Hydrogen peroxide
- Color chart
- Applicator bottle or brush and bowl
- Shampoo cape
- Towels
- Protective gloves
- Shampoo
- Conditioner
- Comb
- Plastic clips (optional, depending on length of hair)
- Cotton
- Protective cream
- Record card
- Timer

Preparation

1. Perform a preliminary patch test 24 hours before the service. Proceed only if the test is negative.
2. Perform client consultation and record results on client record card.
3. Drape client.
4. Prelighten the hair to the desired level.
5. Shampoo, rinse, condition, and towel dry the hair.
6. Perform a strand test and record the results.

Procedure for Toner Application

1. Divide dry hair into four sections.
2. Apply protective cream around hairline. Put on gloves.
3. If using an oxidative toner, mix the toner and developer. Use either bottle or brush application method.
4. Begin in the crown section and part off 1/4-inch subsections. Apply toner from the scalp up to, but not through, the porous ends. Apply to other sections.
5. Process according to the strand test results and the manufacturer's directions. Check toning action by misting as for a strand test. If proper color development has occurred, work the toner through the ends of the hair.

6. When the desired color has been reached, add water and massage toner into a lather.
7. Rinse thoroughly, shampoo, and condition. Remove any stains as necessary.
8. Style as desired.

Cleanup and Sanitation

1. Discard all disposable supplies.
2. Close and wipe off containers and store properly.
3. Sanitize implements and tools, cape, and work area.
4. Wash hands.
5. Record results on client record card.

tipping, and streaking are forms of highlighting application techniques. Lowlighting, or reverse highlighting, is the process of coloring strands or sections of the hair darker than the natural color. As an application process, tipping and streaking techniques can be used for lowlighting effects.

Frosting involves lightening strands of hair over various parts of the head. Either the cap technique or foils can be used for the process. The effect achieved will depend on where and how many strands of hair are treated.

Tipping is similar to frosting, except that only the ends of the hair strands are lightened or colored. Apply the product using either the cap technique or free-form technique for better placement and product control.

Streaking is also similar to frosting, but the strands of lightened or colored hair are usually thicker and more dramatic than those taken for a frosting effect. Streaking effects are best accomplished using the foil or free-form application techniques.

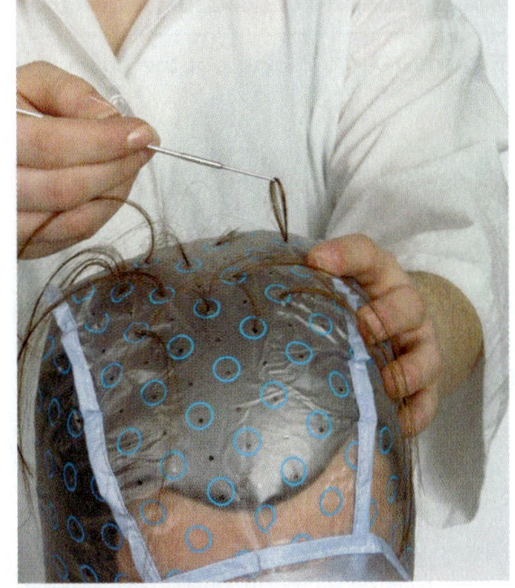

Figure 19-40 Draw strands through holes in the cap.

Cap Technique

As we have learned, the cap technique involves pulling strands of hair through the holes of a perforated cap with a plastic or metal hook (Figure 19–40). The number of strands pulled through the cap determines the degree of highlighting or lowlighting that is achieved throughout the hair.

Cap Technique Procedure

1. Perform a preliminary patch test 24 hours before the service. Proceed only if the test is negative.
2. Perform client consultation and record results on client record card.
3. Drape client.
4. Perform a strand test and record the results.
5. Shampoo and dry the hair.
6. Comb the hair gently.
7. Adjust a perforated cap over the head.
8. Draw the strands of hair through the holes with crochet hook. Prepare coloring or lightening product. Put on gloves.
9. Apply the color or lightener.
10. Cover loosely with a plastic cap if necessary for processing.
11. When the hair has processed remove the plastic cap if present.
12. Rinse and shampoo the color or lightener with the perforated cap in place. Towel dry.
13. Optional: Apply toner if necessary and process accordingly.
14. Style as desired.
15. Perform clean up and sanitation procedures.

Foil Technique

The *foil technique* involves weaving out alternating strands of hair from a subsection, or slicing out ⅛-inch partings from a straight part, to isolate the

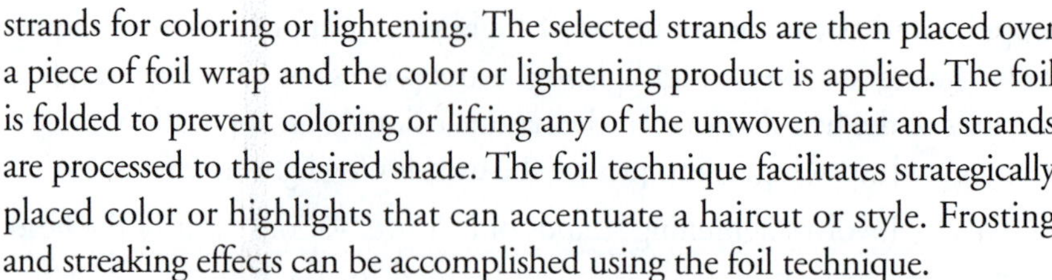

strands for coloring or lightening. The selected strands are then placed over a piece of foil wrap and the color or lightening product is applied. The foil is folded to prevent coloring or lifting any of the unwoven hair and strands are processed to the desired shade. The foil technique facilitates strategically placed color or highlights that can accentuate a haircut or style. Frosting and streaking effects can be accomplished using the foil technique.

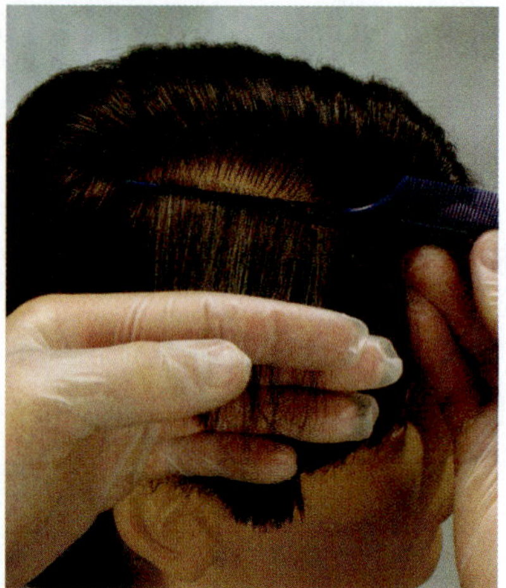

Figure 19-41 Slicing out the strands.

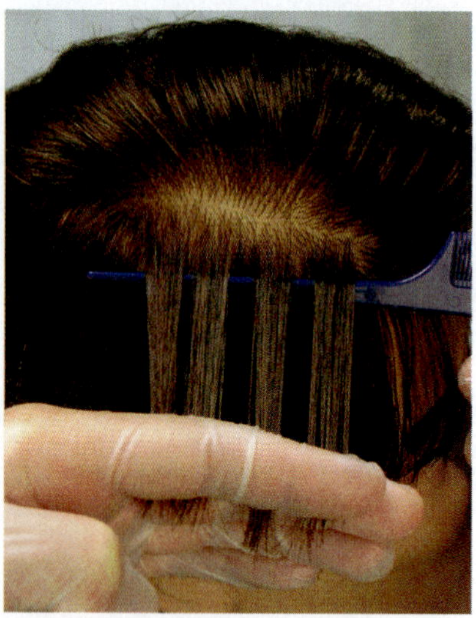

Figure 19-42 Weaving out the strands.

Foil Technique Procedure

1. Perform a preliminary patch test 24 hours before the service. Proceed only if the test is negative.
2. Perform client consultation and record results on client record card.
3. Drape client.
4. Perform a strand test and record the results.
5. Apply to dry hair if using permanent color or lighteners. Apply to damp hair if using traditional semipermanent colors.
6. Comb the hair gently. Prepare color or lightening product. Put on gloves.
7. Slice or weave out the strands from the first parting to be processed (Figures 19–41 and 19–42).
8. Place the foil under the hair and grasp it firmly at the scalp between the thumb and index finger (Figure 19–43).
9. Brush color or lightening product onto the hair (Figure 19–44).
10. Fold the foil in half from bottom to top until the ends meet at the scalp area (Figure 19–45).
11. Fold the left and right edges of the foil halfway and crimp lightly until secure (Figure 19–46). Clip the foil upward.
12. Continue the same process until all the areas to be foiled are completed (Figure 19–47).
13. Process according to strand test results. Check color or lightening level.

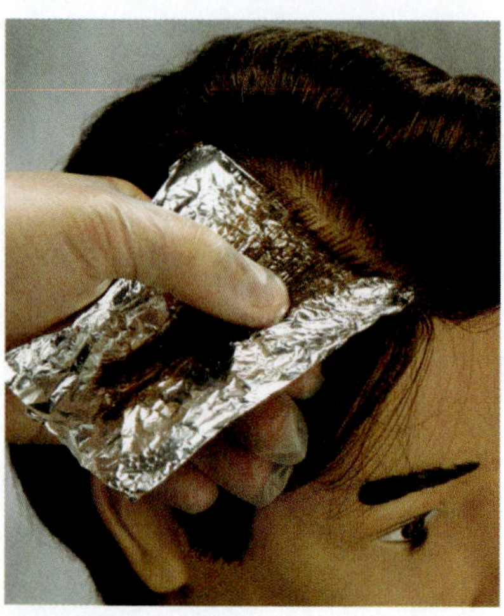

Figure 19-43 Place foil under hair section.

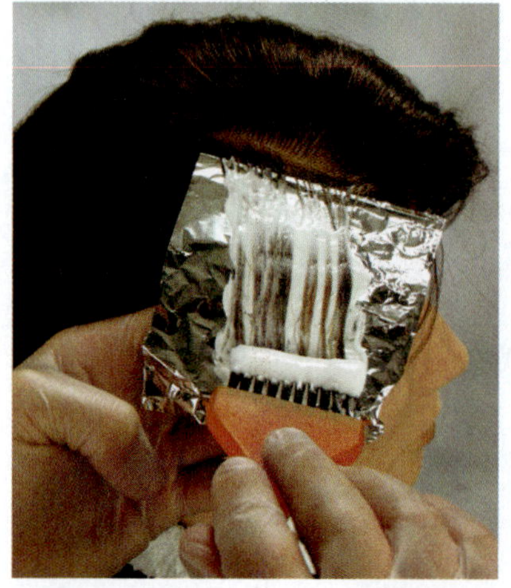

Figure 19-44 Brush product onto the hair.

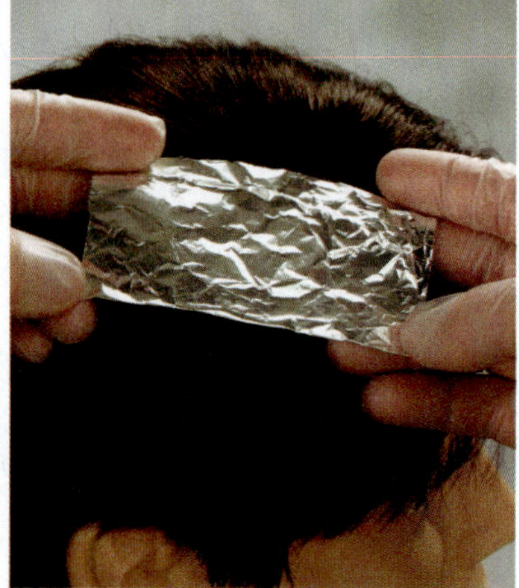

Figure 19-45 Fold foil from bottom to top.

14. When processing is complete, remove foils at the shampoo bowl.
15. Rinse, shampoo, and condition according to product directions.
16. Style hair as desired.
17. Perform clean up and sanitation procedures

    NOTE: When performing the foil technique over the entire head, the sequence of application should be: lower crown, back, sides, top, and front.

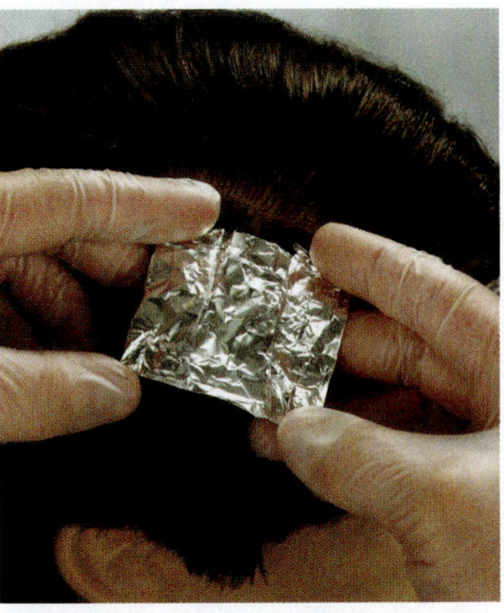

Figure 19-46 Fold left and right edges.

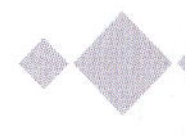

SPECIAL PROBLEMS AND CORRECTIVE HAIRCOLOR

Each haircoloring or lightening service has the potential to create unique problems. Some problems can be avoided by performing preliminary strand tests, but others can be the result of unique properties within the client's hair structure that are unforeseen. Most haircoloring and lightening problems can be resolved with a calm approach, an accurate assessment of the problem, and the knowledge to rectify the situation.

Gray Hair Challenges

Gray, white, or salt-and-pepper hair shades have characteristics that can present unique color challenges (Figure 19–48). Since both gray and white hair contain little melanin within the cortex, a large number of coloring services are performed with the intent to cover or enhance the color. Depending on the amount of gray, the hair may have a yellowish cast or process differently from one strand to another. Some gray hair also tends to be more resistant to chemical processes and may require presoftening before a service.

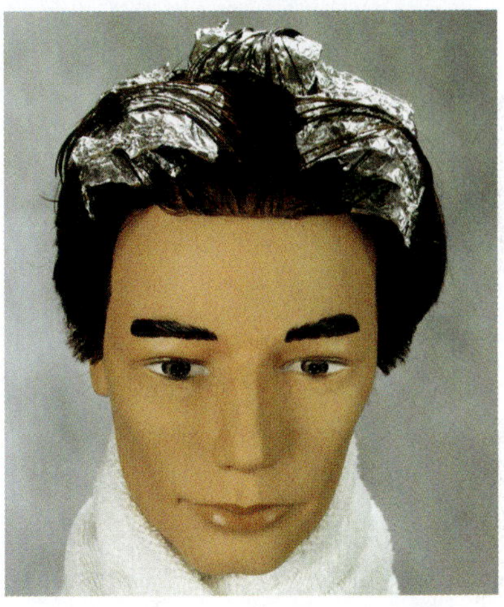

Figure 19-47 Completed foil wrap.

Yellowed Hair

Gray, white, and salt-and-pepper hair with a yellowish cast can be treated with violet-based colors that range from highlighting shampoos and temporary rinses to lightening agents. The longevity of the product used will depend on the client's desired result and the options offered by the barber. (If lightening and coloring services are not typically offered in the barbershop, it is highly recommended that, at a minimum, highlighting shampoos or temporary rinses with violet bases be available to shop clients.)

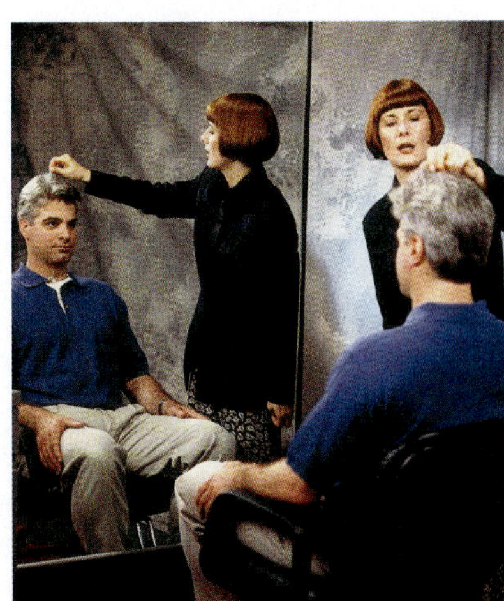

Figure 19-48 Gray hair presents certain challenges.

Determining the Percentage of Gray

Since most people retain some dark hair as they turn gray, the hair must be analyzed for level, hue, and the percentage of gray before the appropriate product selection can be made. Gray hair may be evenly distributed or isolated in various sections of the head, such as the temple areas. Use Table 19–5 as a guide for determining percentages of gray and recommended formulations.

Percentage of Gray	Characteristics	Semipermanent Color Formulation	Permanent Color Formulation
90–100%	Virtually no pigment; white	Desired level	Desired level
70–90%	Mostly nonpigmented	Equal parts: desired level & one level lighter	Two parts desired level & one part lighter level
50–70%	More gray than pigmented	One level lighter than desired level	Equal parts: desired level & lighter level
30–50%	More pigmented than gray	Equal parts: one level lighter & two levels lighter	Two parts lighter level & one part desired level
10–30%	Mostly pigmented	Two levels lighter than desired color	One level lighter

Table 19-5 Percentages of Gray and Recommended Formulations

Formulating for Gray Hair

Gray hair will usually accept the level of the color applied. Generally, lighter shades in the level 9 range may not provide complete coverage, whereas levels 6, 7, and 8 will often cover successfully. The difference in coverage ability is due to the smaller percentage of artificial pigments found in the lighter shades of a level 9 formulation.

When a client has 80–100 percent gray, lighter haircolors are usually more flattering than darker shades. The client's skin tone, eye color, and personal preference will determine whether warm or cool tones are used. Reminder: When a dark level of color is applied to hair with a low percentage of gray, the addition of artificial pigment to the natural pigment will create a color that may be darker than the intended result. In addition, the nonpigmented strands may process lighter. To avoid these outcomes, select a color that is one level lighter than the darkest natural color (Figure 19–49).

Occasionally, gray hair is so resistant that presoftening is necessary for better color penetration. Mix the product according to the manufacturer's directions and apply to the most resistant areas first. Process as directed and then perform a preliminary strand test with the desired color.

Fillers

Color fillers are dual-purpose haircoloring products that are able to create a color base and equalize excessive porosity in one application.

They are available in clear, neutral, and a variety of colors. A clear filler is designed to correct porosity without affecting color and does not deposit a color base. Neutral fillers (a balance of all three primary colors) have minimal saturation and color correction abilities but have full power to equalize porosity. Color fillers are preoxidized colors that remain true during application and that will be subdued by the tint.

If there is any doubt that the finished color will develop into an even shade, a color filler is recommended. The filler is applied after the hair has been prelightened and before the application of a toner or tint. Fillers are also used for clients who have tinted or lightened hair and desire to return it to the natural color. Color fillers have the ability to:

1. deposit color to faded hair shafts and ends.
2. help hair to hold color.
3. help to ensure a uniform color from the scalp to the hair ends.
4. prevent color streaking.
5. prevent off-color results.
6. prevent dullness.
7. facilitate more uniform color in a tint back to the natural shade.

Fillers use certified colors as pigments and are safe to use without a predisposition test. They may be used directly from the container and applied to the hair prior to tinting, or may be added to the remainder of the tint and applied to damaged hair ends. To obtain satisfactory results, select the color filler to match the same basic shade as the toner or tint to be used.

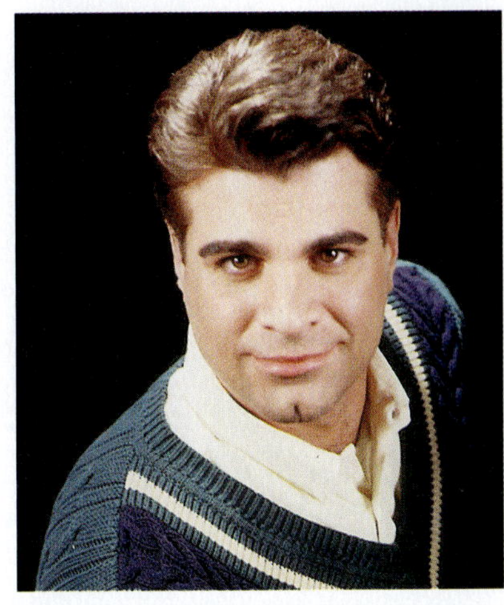

Figure 19-49 Many haircolor options cover gray successfully.

Reconditioning Damaged Hair

Hair that is damaged due to careless chemical applications, excessive heat, or misused styling products must be reconditioned before it can be tinted or lightened successfully.

Hair may need reconditioning for reasons other than damage resulting from the use of harmful products. Sometimes hair is naturally brittle, thin, and lifeless. Both neglect and the client's physical condition may contribute to these conditions.

Hair is considered damaged when it exhibits one or more of the following characteristics:

- Overporous condition
- Brittle and dry
- Breaks easily
- Little to no elasticity
- Rough and harsh to the touch
- Spongy and mats easily when wet
- Rejects color or absorbs too much color during a tinting process

Any of these conditions may create undesirable results during a tinting or lightening treatment. Therefore, damaged hair should receive reconditioning treatments prior to and after the application of these chemical agents.

Reconditioning Treatment

To restore damaged hair to a more normal condition, commercial products containing lanolin or protein substances should be used. The reconditioning agent is applied to the hair. If heat is applied, use a heating cap, a steamer, or a heating lamp according to the manufacturer's directions. Be guided by your instructor as to the frequency and length of time for each treatment.

Tint Back to Natural Color

Clients who have been tinting or lightening their hair may want to return to their natural shade. Each tint back to natural color must be handled as an individual situation. The determining factors in the selection of the tint shade are the present condition and color of the hair, the final result desired, and the original color. Check the natural shade of the hair next to the scalp.

Select an appropriate shade of filler to correspond with the tint to be used; otherwise it will be difficult to obtain a uniform color from the scalp to hair ends, due to uneven porosity levels. Perform strand tests as needed to determine the expected final outcome.

Coating Dyes

Many clients buy and use over-the-counter haircoloring products at home. Some such coloring agents are actually progressive dyes and must be removed prior to any other chemical service.

Hair treated with a compound, metallic, or other coating dye looks dry and dull and generally feels harsh and brittle to the touch. These colors usually fade to unnatural tones. Silver dyes have a greenish cast, lead dyes leave a purple color, and those containing copper turn red. If the barber is unsure as to whether the client has used a progressive dye, a test for metallic salts and dyes should be performed on the hair.

Test for Metallic Salts and Coating Dyes

1. In a glass container, mix 1 ounce (30 ml) of 20-volume (6 percent) peroxide and 20 drops of 28 percent ammonia water.
2. Cut a few strands of the client's hair, bind it with tape, and immerse it in the solution for 30 minutes.
3. Remove, towel dry, and observe the strand. Refer to the following for analysis of the hair:
   - Hair dyed with lead will lighten immediately.
   - Hair treated with silver will show no reaction at all. This indicates that other chemicals will not be successful because they will not be able to penetrate the coating.
   - Hair treated with copper will start to boil, and will pull apart easily. This hair would be severely damaged or destroyed if other chemicals such as those found in permanent colors or perm solutions were applied to it.
   - Hair treated with a coating dye either will not change color or will lighten in spots. Hair in this condition will not receive chemical

services easily and the length of time necessary for penetration may result in further damage to the hair.

Removing Coatings from the Hair

The removal of metallic dyes from the hair shaft may not always be effective the first time. Performing a strand test after the treatment will indicate whether the metallic deposits have been removed. If not, the entire application must be repeated until the hair shaft is sufficiently free of metal salts to perform other chemical services.

Materials Needed

70 percent alcohol

Concentrated shampoo for oily hair

Mineral, castor, vegetable, or commercially prepared color-removing oil

Procedure

1. Apply 70 percent alcohol to dry hair.
2. Allow alcohol to stand for five minutes.
3. Apply the oil to the hair thoroughly.
4. Cover the hair completely with a plastic cap.
5. Place under a hot dryer for 30 minutes.
6. To remove, saturate with concentrated shampoo.
7. Work the shampoo into the oil for three minutes, then rinse with warm water.
8. Repeat the shampoo steps until the oil is removed completely.

COLORING MUSTACHES AND BEARDS

An aniline derivative tint should never be used for coloring mustaches; to do so may cause serious irritation or damage to the lips or the delicate membranes of the nostrils. Harmless commercial products are available in a variety of formulations that are appropriate for coloring mustaches and beards.

Crayons are waxy sticks that are available in several colors: blond, medium and dark brown, black, and auburn. The end of the stick is used like a pencil to apply the product by rubbing it directly on the facial hair until the desired shade is reached.

Pomades usually consist of harmless ingredients and are formulated specifically for coloring mustaches and beards. These products are available in a variety of shades including black, brown, blond, chestnut, and white (neutral). The pomade is applied to the facial hair with a small brush and is stroked from the nostrils downward until full coverage is achieved.

Liquid pomades are also available and may be preferred for use on beards. Some pomades contain heavy waxing ingredients that can be used to style mustaches with rolled or twisted ends for dramatic looks. Liquid eyebrow and eyelash tint is also available in brown and black for coloring facial hair.

Procedure for Coloring Mustaches and Beards

Implements and Materials

Petroleum jelly

Coloring solutions (No. 1 and No. 2)

Stain remover

Towels

Applicator sticks

Procedure

1. Seat the client in a comfortable position and drape.
2. Place a clean towel across the chest.
3. Wash the facial hair with warm, soapy water.
4. Apply petroleum jelly around the hairline of the facial hair.
5. Apply solution No. 1. Remove the cap and moisten a cotton-tipped applicator in the solution. Touch the tip of the applicator to a towel to remove excess moisture. Apply the solution to the mustache/beard, moistening it completely. Replace the cap on bottle No. 1. Discard the applicator immediately. Moisten a fresh cotton-tipped applicator with stain remover and place it on the edge of a towel for future use. Replace the cap on the stain remover bottle.
6. Apply solution No. 2 to the mustache/beard in the same manner as solution No. 1. If the skin becomes stained, use stain remover immediately. Replace the cap on bottle No. 2.
7. Wash the mustache/beard with soap and cool water.
8. Remove any stains with stain remover. Replace the bottle cap.
9. Style the mustache/beard as desired.
10. Clean up in the usual manner.

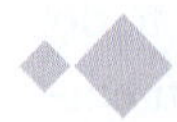

HAIRCOLORING AND LIGHTENING SAFETY PRECAUTIONS

Haircoloring

- Perform a 24-hour patch test before the application of a tint or toner.
- Examine the scalp before applying a tint.
- Do not apply tint if abrasions are present on the scalp.
- Use only sanitized swabs, brushes, applicator bottles, combs, and linens.
- Always wash your hands before and after serving a client.
- Do not brush the hair prior to a tint.
- Do not apply a tint without reading the manufacturer's directions.
- Perform a strand test for color and processing results.
- Choose a shade of tint that harmonizes with the general complexion.

- Use an applicator bottle or bowl (plastic or glass) for mixing the tint.
- Do not mix tint before ready for use; discard leftover tint.
- If required, use the correct shade of color filler.
- Make frequent strand tests until the desired shade is reached.
- Suggest a reconditioning treatment for tinted hair.
- Do not apply tint if metallic or compound dye is present.
- Do not apply tint if a patch test is positive.
- Give a strand test for the correct color shade before applying tint.
- Do not use an alkaline or harsh shampoo for tint removal.
- Do not use water that is too hot for removing tint.
- Protect the client's clothing by proper draping.
- Do not permit tint to come in contact with the client's eyes.
- Do not overlap during a tint retouch.
- Do not neglect to fill out a tint record card.
- Do not apply hydrogen peroxide or any material containing hydrogen peroxide directly over dyes known or believed to contain a metallic salt. Breakage or complete disintegration of the hair may result.
- Wear protective gloves.

Hair Lightening

- Analyze the condition of the hair and suggest reconditioning treatments, if required.
- When working with a cream or paste lightener, it must be the thickness of whipped cream to avoid dripping or running, causing overlapping.
- Apply lightener to resistant areas first. Pick up ⅛-inch sections when applying lightener. This will ensure complete coverage.
- Check strands frequently until the desired shade is reached.
- After completing the lightener application, check the skin and remove any lightener from these areas.
- Check the towel around the client's neck. Lightener on the towel that is allowed to come in contact with the skin will cause irritation.
- Lightened hair is fragile and requires special care. Use only a very mild shampoo, and cool water for rinsing.
- If a preliminary shampoo is necessary, comb the hair carefully. Avoid irritating the scalp during the shampoo or when combing the hair.
- Work as rapidly as possible when applying the lightener to produce a uniform shade without streaking.
- Never allow lightener to stand; use it immediately.
- Cap all bottles to avoid loss of strength.
- Keep a completed record card of all lightening treatments.

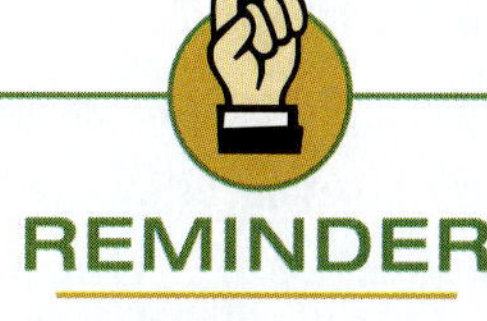
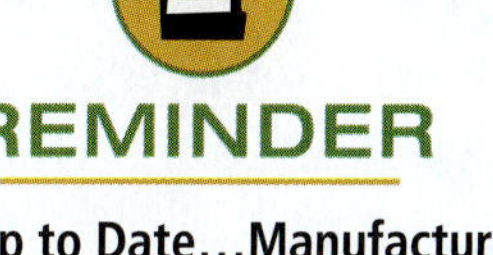

REMINDER

Keep Up to Date...Manufacturers are constantly improving and developing new haircoloring products. Be sure to attend seminars and trade shows as often as possible to stay current in your profession.

spotlight on

Robert Wagner

Robert Wagner had been a hair stylist/barber since 1986 when he realized his dream of opening a "rock 'n' roll barbershop" in E. Northport on New York's Long Island in 1998. A former marine, a tattooed biker, and a husband and father, Wagner has since expanded Rockabilly Barbers to two additional locations. The shops' unique combination of music, memorabilia, and cutting edge styles has attracted the attention of publications ranging from International Tattoo Art to The New York Times.

You must be a people person to be successful in the barbering and beauty industry, whether as a shop owner, operator, or both. You must also enjoy and be good at what you do. Be courteous, friendly, and always charitable and community-oriented. Be prepared to put in long hours. Be assertive and be willing to try new techniques. You must be innovative and persistent.

19

While in school, don't be afraid to experiment. You are there to learn and to hone the skills of your trade. Pay attention in school. Nothing is better than hands-on practice or application. Understanding barber and hair theory is a must to becoming a great barber, as opposed to being just an average barber. You must know how hair grows, including growth patterns, textures and densities, and why certain styles work better with certain textures.

Know your tools and use them all equally as well. Whatever you can do with one, be able to do with the other. Be familiar with all techniques of cutting and texturizing with clippers, scissors, and razors. Learn about products and what they do and how they work.

Remember, a great haircut isn't judged by the hair you cut off—it's judged by the hairstyle you leave behind. Be innovative. Know long hair styles and techniques as well as short hair styles and techniques, and keep up to date on fashion trends. Always know how to utilize and apply current hair products.

In any business, the customers always come first. They may not always be right. They may need you, as the professional, to educate them. For example, a client with very little hair on top of his head is not getting a spiked haircut or flat top.

Be tactful and polite when addressing matters like this. We are not magicians; suggest a style better suited for the person's hair type, texture, or lifestyle. Never let your customer leave your chair unsatisfied. Remember, your haircuts are your best advertisements.

Always try to establish a good rapport with customers as well as with your staff. Shake hands with your customers. Try to remember names or something about them so the next time you see them you can converse with them, making them feel welcome and comfortable.

If you establish a happy and positive atmosphere for your client and he or she is satisfied with the haircut, they will surely tell others. Word of mouth is truly the best form of advertising in this industry! Be a people person!

chapter glossary

activator	an additive used to quicken the action or progress of hydrogen peroxide
aniline derivatives	uncolored dye precursors that combine with hydrogen peroxide to form larger, permanent color molecules in the cortex
base color	the predominant tone of an existing color
cap technique	lightening technique that involves pulling strands of hair through a perforated cap with a plastic or metal hook
color fillers	tinted products used to even out color processing
complementary colors	a primary and secondary color positioned opposite each other on the color wheel
contributing pigment	pigment that lies under the natural hair color that is exposed when the natural color is lightened
demipermanent haircolor	deposit-only haircolor product similar to semipermanent but longer lasting
developer	an oxidizing agent, usually hydrogen peroxide, used to develop color
double-process haircoloring	a two-step combination of lightening and haircoloring
dye removers	products used to strip built-up color from the hair
fillers	preparations designed to equalize porosity and/or deposit a base color in one application
foil technique	highlighting technique using foil
free-form technique	also known as balayage; the painting of a lightener on clean, styled hair
haircolor	industry-coined term term referring to artificial haircolor products and services
hair lightening	the chemical process of diffusing natural or artificial pigment from the hair
highlighting	coloring or lightening some strands of hair lighter than the natural color
laws of color	a system for understanding color relationships
level	unit of measure used to identify the lightness or darkness of a color
lighteners	chemical compounds that lighten hair by dispersing and diffusing natural pigment
line of demarcation	a visible line separating colored hair from new growth
lowlighting	coloring some strands of hair darker than the natural hair color
off-the-scalp lighteners	lighteners that cannot be used directly on the scalp
on-the-scalp lighteners	lighteners that can be used directly on the scalp
patch test	test for identifying a possible allergy to haircolor products
permanent haircolor	haircolor that is mixed with a developer and remains in the shaft
prelightening	the first step of a double-process haircoloring; used to lighten natural pigment

presoftening	process of treating resistant hair for better color penetration
primary colors	red, blue, and yellow; colors that cannot be achieved from a mixture of other colors
progressive colors	haircolor products that contain compound or metallic dyes, which build up on the hair; not used professionally
retouch application	application of the product to the new growth only
secondary colors	colors obtained by mixing equal parts of two primary colors
semipermanent haircolor	deposit-only haircolor product formulated to last through several shampoos
single-process haircoloring	process that lightens and colors the hair in a single application
soap cap	equal parts of tint and a shampoo
strand test	the application of a coloring or lightening product to determine how the hair will react to the formula and the amount of time it will take to process
temporary colors	color products that last only from shampoo to shampoo
tone	the basic name of a color; also used to describe the warmth or coolness of a color.
toner	a semipermanent, demipermanent, or permanent haircolor product used primarily on prelightened hair to achieve pale and delicate colors
virgin application	the first time the hair is tinted
volume	the measure of the potential oxidation of varying strengths of hydrogen peroxide

chapter review questions

1. Define haircoloring and lightening.
2. List the colors of the color wheel. Identify primary, secondary, and complementary colors.
3. List four types of haircoloring products.
4. Identify types of nonoxidation and oxidation haircolor.
5. Explain the difference between semipermanent and demipermanent haircolor products.
6. List four types of permanent haircolor tints.
7. List the volumes of hydrogen peroxide used in haircoloring.
8. Explain how to test for an allergy to haircolor products.
9. Define strand test.
10. Define single-process and double-process haircoloring.
11. Explain the lightening process.
12. List the products used to color beards and mustaches.

Learning Objectives

After completing this chapter, you should be able to:

1. Identify the composition of the nail.
2. Identify and describe nail irregularities and diseases.
3. Demonstrate the proper use of manicuring implements, equipment, and products.
4. Recognize the five general shapes of nails.
5. Demonstrate male and female manicure and hand massage procedures.

Key Terms

cuticle
pg. 588

free edge
pg. 588

hangnails
pg. 592

leukonychia
pg. 592

lunula
pg. 588

melanonychia
pg. 592

nail
pg. 587

nail bed
pg. 588

nail folds
pg. 589

nail plate
pg. 588

nail root or matrix bed
pg. 588

onyx
pg. 587

onychatrophia
pg. 592

onychauxis
pg. 593

onychia
pg. 594

onychocryptosis
pg. 593

onychogryposis
pg. 594

onycholysis
pg. 594

onychomadesis
pg. 594

onychophagy
pg. 593

onychoptosis
pg. 594

onychorrhexis
pg. 593

onychosis
pg. 591

paronychia
pg. 594

pterygium
pg. 593

pyrogenic granuloma
pg. 595

tinea unguium
pg. 595

As with hair and skin services, nail care has been a part of human existence for thousands of years. This fact is evidenced through the recorded histories of Egypt and China dating back to 3000 BC. Egyptian men and women of high social rank painted their nails with henna, and by 600 BC the members of Chinese royalty were painting their nails with gold and silver paint. Later accounts of life in Rome and Babylon tell us that in addition to having their hair and beards dressed for battle, military men also colored their nails to match their lip color.

Barbershops of the first half of the twentieth century routinely provided manicures as part of the traditional shave, haircut, and shoeshine service. In fact, a newspaper article of 1912 noted that in addition to shampooing, applying facial cosmetics, facial hair tinting, removing comedones, and hair curling, "the modern barbershop has a manicure girl" (Owen, 1991).

It should not be surprising that many of today's barbershops offer manicures. As a result, it is advisable that you become acquainted with the manicuring procedure and become proficient in its execution. This knowledge will provide a foundation from which to either offer the service or oversee the procedure, as it may be performed by others in your employ. A basic understanding of nail composition and structure provides the first step in building this foundation of knowledge.

THE NAIL

The **nail** is a horny, translucent plate of hard keratin that serves to protect the tips of the fingers and toes. Nails are part of the integumentary system and are considered to be appendages of the skin. The technical term for nail is **onyx** (AHN-iks).

The condition of the nail, like that of the skin, reflects the general health of the body. The normal, healthy nail is translucent with the pinkish color

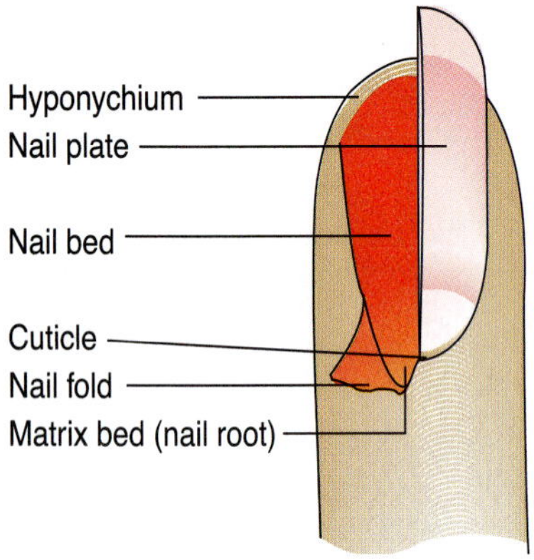

Hyponychium
Nail plate
Nail bed
Cuticle
Nail fold
Matrix bed (nail root)

Figure 20-1 The structure of the nail.

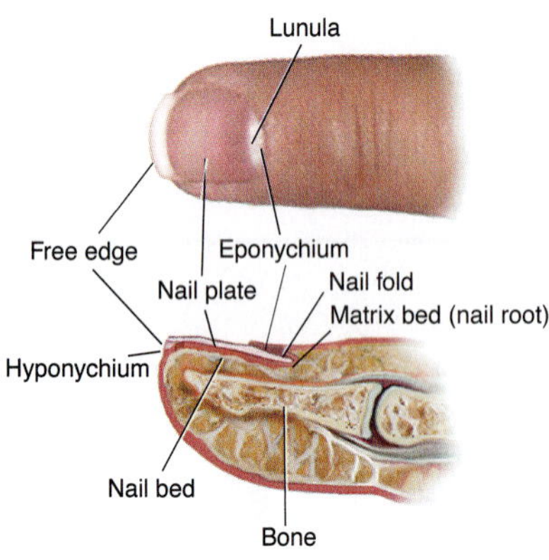

Figure 20-2 Cross section of the nail.

of the nail bed below showing through. Its surface should be smooth, curved, and unspotted, without any hollows or wavy ridges. No nerves or blood vessels are contained within the horny nail plate.

Nail Structure

The nail unit consists of six basic parts (Figures 20–1 and 20–2).

- Nail bed
- Nail root (matrix bed)
- Nail plate (nail body)
- Cuticular system (cuticle, eponychium, hyponychium)
- Specialized ligaments
- Nail folds

Nail Bed

The **nail bed** lies under the nail plate and is the portion of the skin upon which the nail body rests. It is supplied with blood vessels that provide the reddish tone from the lunula almost to the free edge and is abundantly rich in nerves that are attached to the nail plate.

Nail Root (Matrix Bed)

The **nail root**, or **matrix bed**, is imbedded under the skin and is where the nail is formed. Matrix cells produce the nail plate, which originates at the base of the nail. The matrix will continue to grow as long as it receives nutrition and remains healthy. The growth of nails may be retarded by poor health, a nail disorder, disease, or injury to the nail matrix. The visible portion of the matrix bed is called the **lunula** (LOO-nuh-luh) or half-moon. It is located at the base of the nail where the matrix and the connective tissue of the nail bed join.

Nail Plate

The **nail plate**, or nail body, is the visible portion of the nail, which rests upon and is attached to the nail bed. The nail body extends from the root to the **free edge**.

Although the nail plate seems to be made of one piece, it is actually constructed in layers. This structure can be seen in both length and thickness when a nail splits. The free edge is the end portion of the nail that reaches over the fingertips.

Cuticular System

The **cuticle** is the crescent of overlapping epidermis around the base of the nail. A normal cuticle around the nail should be loose and pliable. The *eponychium* (ep-oh-NIK-ee-um) is the extension of the cuticle that partly overlaps the lunula. The *hyponychium* (hy-poh-NIK-ee-um) is that portion of the epidermis under the free edge of the nail.

Specialized Ligaments

Specialized ligaments are bands of fibrous tissue that attach the nail bed and matrix bed to the underlying bone. These ligaments are located at the base of the matrix and around the edges of the nail bed.

Nail Folds (Nail Walls)

The **nail folds**, or nail walls, are folds of normal skin that surround the nail plate. These folds form the nail grooves on the sides of the nail that permit the nail to move as it grows. The mantle is the deep fold of skin in which the nail root is imbedded.

Nail Growth

Nail growth is influenced by nutrition, health, and disease. A normal healthy nail grows forward, starting at the matrix and extending over the fingertip. The average rate of growth in the normal adult is about ⅛ inch per month. Typically, nails grow faster in summer than they do in winter. Children's nails grow more rapidly, whereas those of elderly persons grow more slowly. The nail of the middle finger grows the fastest and the thumbnail the most slowly. Although toenails grow more slowly than fingernails, they are thicker and harder.

Nail Malformation

If the nail is separated from the nail bed through injury, it becomes distorted or discolored. Should the nail bed be injured after the loss of a nail, a badly formed new nail will result.

Nails are not shed in the same way that hair is shed. If a nail is torn off accidentally or lost through infection or disease, it will be replaced only if the matrix remains in good condition. The replacement nails frequently are shaped abnormally, due to interference at the base of the nail. Replacement of the nail takes about four to six months.

1 ✓

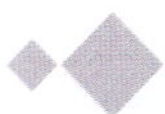

NAIL DISORDERS AND DISEASES

A *nail disorder* is a condition caused by injury to the nail, disease, or chemical or nutritional imbalance. Most, if not all, clients will have had some common nail disorder, and may have one when they are scheduled for a manicure. It is important to learn to recognize the symptoms of nail disorders so that a responsible decision can be made about whether or not to perform a service on the client (Table 20–1). In some cases, it may be necessary to recommend medical treatment. In others, the disorder may be improved cosmetically.

The rule is, if the nail or skin to be worked on is infected, inflamed, broken, or swollen, this may be a sign of disease and the service should not be performed. Instead, the client should be referred to a doctor (Table 20–2).

Disorder	Signs or Symptoms
Bruised nails	Dark purplish spots; usually due to injury
Corrugations/Furrows	Wavy ridges caused by uneven nail growth; usually result of illness or injury Depressions in the nail that run either lengthwise or across the nail; result from illness or injury, stress, or pregnancy
Discolored nails (blue nails)	Nails turn a variety of colors; may indicate systemic disorder
Eggshell nails	Noticeably thin white nail plate that is more flexible than normal; may be caused by diet, illness, or medication
Hangnail (Agnail)	The cuticle splits around the nail
Infected finger	Redness, pain, swelling, or pus; refer to physician
Leukonychia (white spots)	Whitish discoloration of the nails; usually caused by injury to the base of the nail
Melanonychia	Darkening of the fingernails or toenails
Onychatrophia	Atrophy or wasting away of the nail; caused by injury or disease
Onychauxis (hypertrophy)	Overgrowth in thickness of the nail; caused by local infection, internal imbalance, or may be hereditary
Onychophagy	Bitten nails
Onychorrhexis	Abnormal brittleness with striation (lines) of the nail plate
Plicated nails	Folded nails
Pterygium	Forward growth of the cuticle
Tile-shaped nails	Increased crosswise curvature throughout the nail plate
Trumpet nails (pincer nails)	Edges of the nail plate curl around to form the shape of a trumpet or cone around the free edge

Table 20-1 Overview of Nail Disorders

Disease	Signs or Symptoms
Onychia	Inflammation of the matrix with pus and shedding of the nail
Onychocryptosis	Ingrown nails
Onychogryposis	Thickening and increased curvature of the nail
Onycholysis	Loosening of the nail without shedding
Onychomadesis	Separation and falling off of a nail from the nail bed
Onychoptosis	Periodic shedding of one or more nails
Paronychia	Bacterial inflammation of the tissues around the nail; pus, thickening, and brownish discoloration of the nail plate
Pyrogenic granuloma	Severe inflammation of the nail in which a lump of red tissue grows up from the nail bed to the nail plate
Tinea (ringworm)	Reddened patches of small blisters; slight or severe itching
Tinea unguium (onychomycosis or ringworm of the nails)	Whitish patches on the nail that can be scraped off or long yellowish streaks within the nail substance

Table 20-2 Overview of Nail Diseases

Onychosis (ahn-ih-KOH-sis) is a technical term applied to any deformity or disease of the nail.

- *Bruised nails* occur when a blood clot forms under the nail plate. The clot is caused by injury to the nail bed. It can vary in color from maroon to black. In some cases, a bruised nail will fall off during the healing process. The application of artificial nail services to a bruised nail is not recommended.
- *Discolored nails* are a condition in which the nails turn a variety of colors including yellow, blue, blue-gray, green, red, and purple. Discoloration can be caused by poor blood circulation, a heart condition, or topical or oral medications. It may also indicate the presence of a systemic disorder. Artificial tips or wraps, or an application of colored nail polish, can hide this condition.
- *Eggshell nails* are thin, white, and curved at the free edge (Figure 20–3). The condition is caused by improper diet, internal disease, medication,

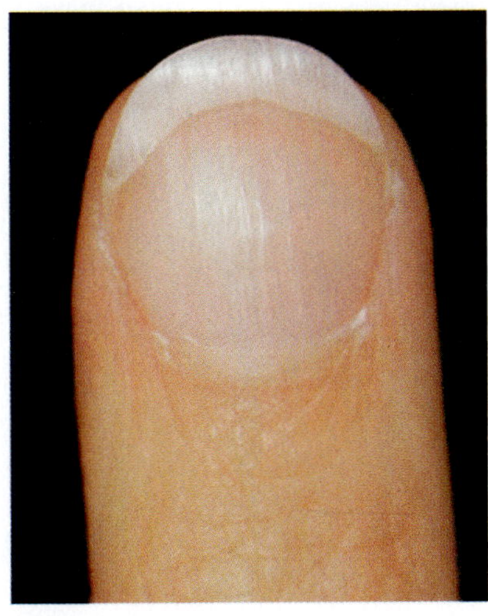

Figure 20-3 Eggshell nail.

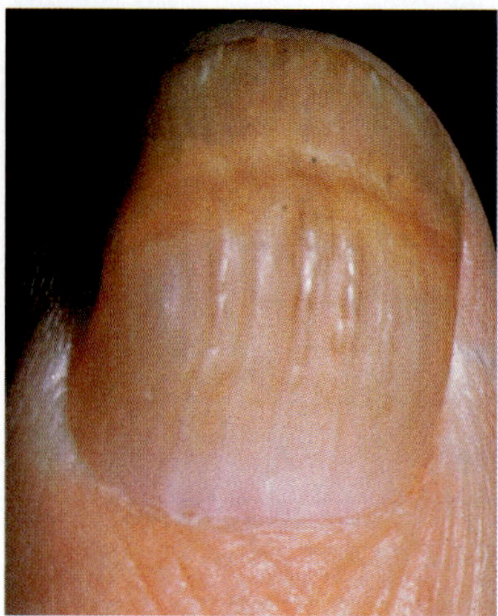

Figure 20-4 Furrows.

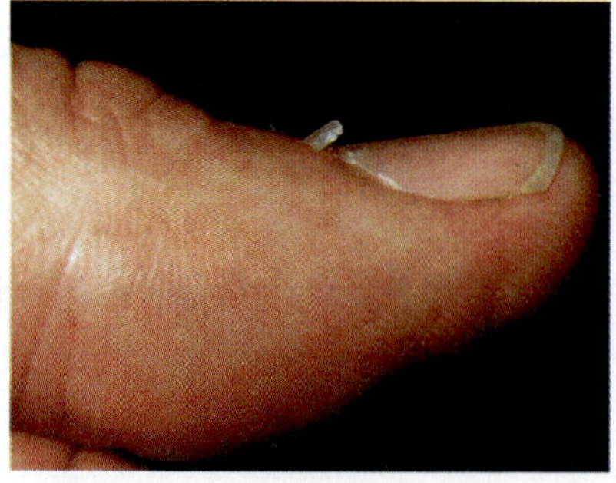

Figure 20-5 Hangnail.

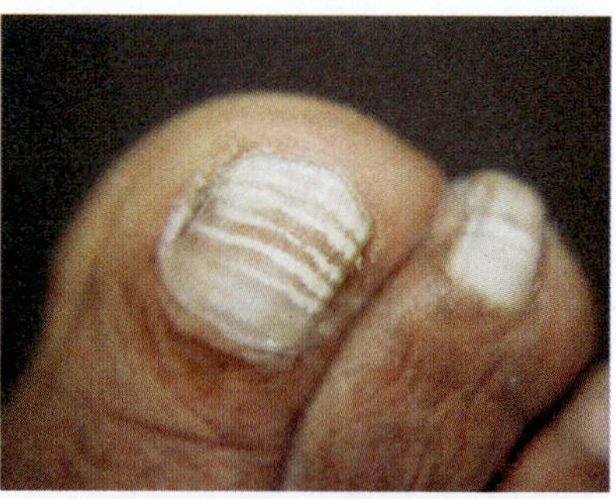

Figure 20-6 Leukonychia.

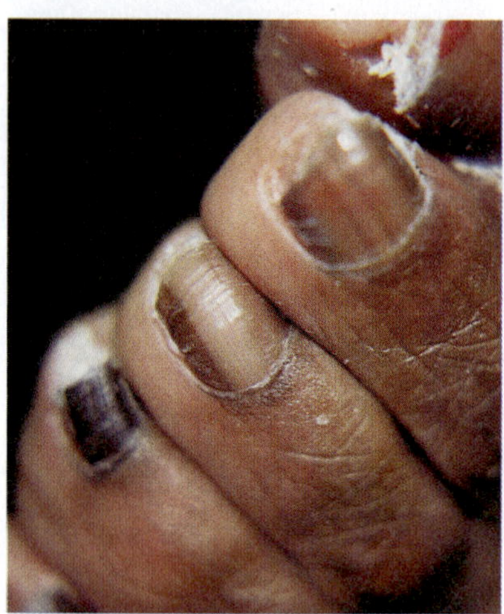

Figure 20-7 Melanonychia.

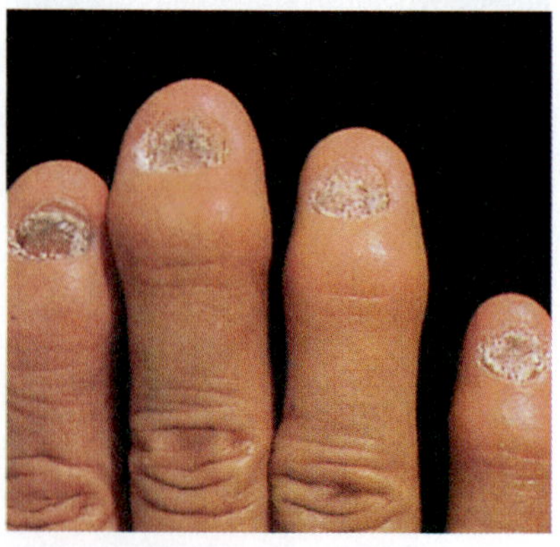

Figure 20-8 Onychatropia.

or nerve disorders. Be very careful when manicuring these nails. They are fragile and can break easily. Use the fine side of an emery board to file gently and do not use pressure with a metal pusher at the base of the nail.

- *Furrows*, also known as *corrugations*, are long ridges that run either lengthwise or across the nail (Figure 20–4). Some lengthwise ridges are normal in adult nails, and they increase with age. Lengthwise ridges can also be caused by conditions such as psoriasis, poor circulation, and frostbite. Ridges that run across the nail can be caused by conditions such as high fever, pregnancy, measles in childhood, or a zinc deficiency in the body. If ridges are not deep and the nail is not broken, the appearance of this disorder can be corrected. Carefully buff the nails with pumice powder to remove or shorten the ridges. The remaining ridges can be filled with ridge filler and covered with colored polish to give a smooth, healthy look.
- **Hangnails**, also known as *agnails* (AG-nayls), are a common condition in which the cuticle around the nail splits (Figure 20–5). Hangnails are caused by dry cuticles or cuticles that have been cut too closely to the nail. The disorder can be improved by softening the cuticles with oil. Although hangnails are a simple and common disorder, they can become infected if not serviced properly.
- **Leukonychia** (loo-koh-NIK-ee-ah) is a condition in which white spots appear on the nails as a result of air bubbles, a bruise, or other injury to the nail (Figure 20–6). Although the condition cannot be corrected, the nail will eventually grow out.
- **Melanonychia** (mel-uh-nuh-NIK-ee-uh) is a darkening of the nail as a result of increased and localized pigment cells within the matrix bed (Figure 20–7). Nail polish or an artificial nail service can hide this disorder.
- **Onychatrophia** (ahn-ih-kuh-TROH-fee-uh), also known as atrophy, describes the wasting away of the nail (Figure 20–8). The nail loses its shine, shrinks, and falls off. It can be caused by injury to the nail matrix or by internal disease. Handle this condition with extreme care. File the nail with the fine side of the emery board and do not use a metal pusher,

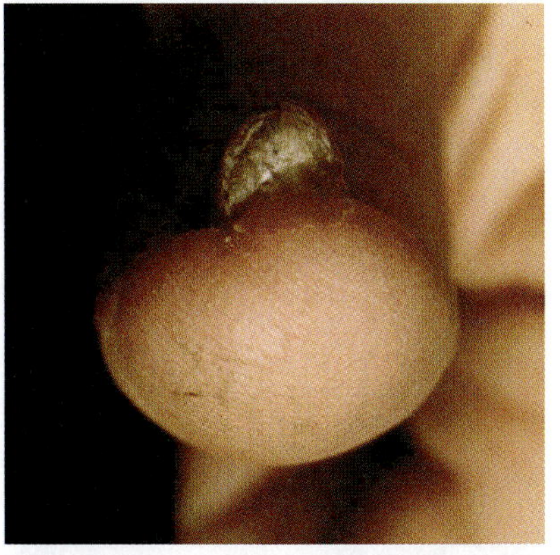
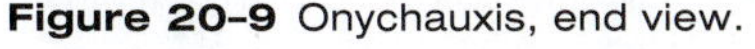

Figure 20-9 Onychauxis, end view.

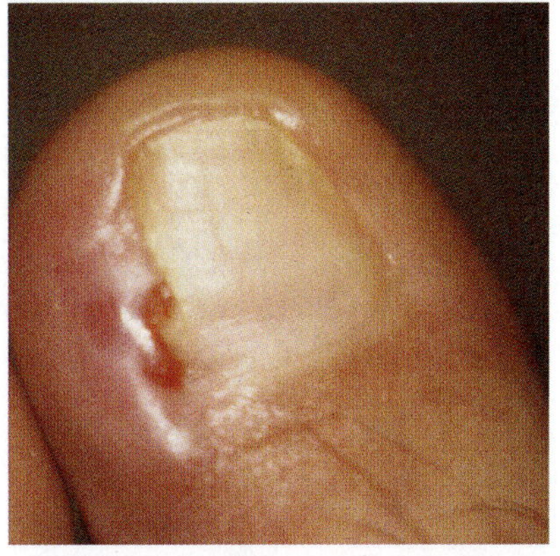

Figure 20-10 Onychocryptosis.

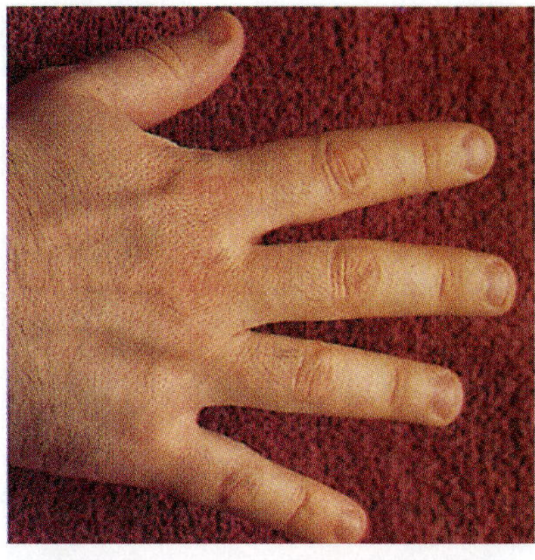

Figure 20-11 Onychophagy.

strong soaps, or washing powders. If the condition is caused by internal disease and the disease is cured, new nails may grow back.

- **Onychauxis** (ahn-ih-KAHK-sis), or hypertrophy, shows the opposite symptoms of onychatrophia. The condition is the overgrowth of nails in which the nails are abnormally thick (Figure 20–9). It is usually caused by an internal imbalance, local infection, or heredity. File the nail smooth and buff with pumice powder.
- **Onychocryptosis** (ahn-ih-koh-krip-TOH-sis), or ingrown nails, is a familiar condition in which the nail grows into the sides of the tissue around the nail (Figure 20–10). Improper filing of the nail and poor-fitting shoes are causes of this disorder. If the tissue around the nail is not infected and the nail is not imbedded too deeply in the flesh, trim the corner of the nail in a curved shape to relieve the pressure on the nail groove. This condition should be treated by a physician.
- **Onychophagy** (ahn-ih-koh-FAY-jee) is the medical term for nails that have been bitten enough to become deformed (Figure 20–11). This condition can be improved greatly by professional manicuring techniques. Give frequent manicures, using the techniques described in this chapter.
- **Onychorrhexis** (ahn-ih-koh-REK-sis) refers to split or brittle nails that also have a series of lengthwise ridges (Figure 20–12). It can be caused by injury to the fingers, excessive use of cuticle solvents, nail polish removers, and careless, rough filing. Nail services can be performed only if the nail is not split below the free edge. This condition may be corrected by softening the nails with a reconditioning treatment, proper filing, and discontinuing the use of harsh soaps or polish removers.
- **Pterygium** (teh-RIJ-ee-um) describes the common condition of the forward growth of the cuticle on the nail (Figure 20–13). The cuticle sticks to the nail and, if not treated, will grow over the nail to the free edge. The early stages of this condition can be treated by a reconditioning hot-oil manicure, which will soften the cuticle so it can be pushed back by the cuticle pusher and then removed.

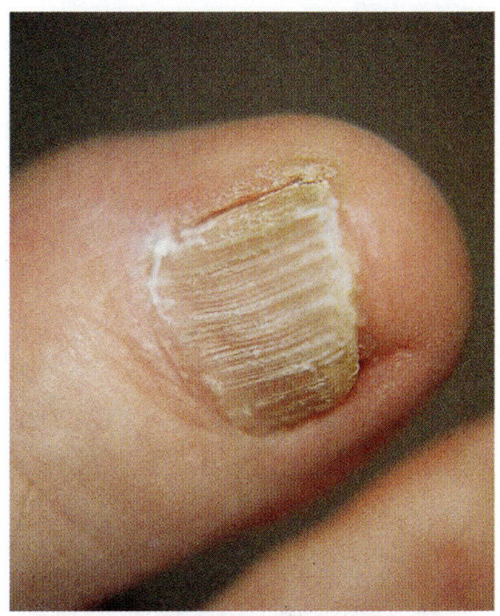

Figure 20-12 Onychorrhexis.

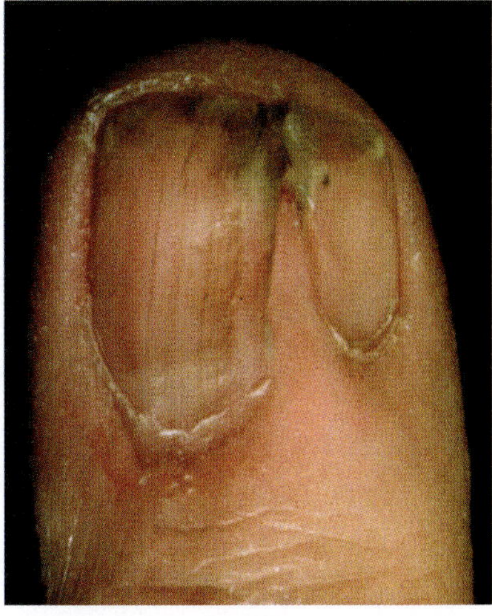

Figure 20-13 Pterygium.

Figure 20-14 *Pseudomonas aeruginosa*.

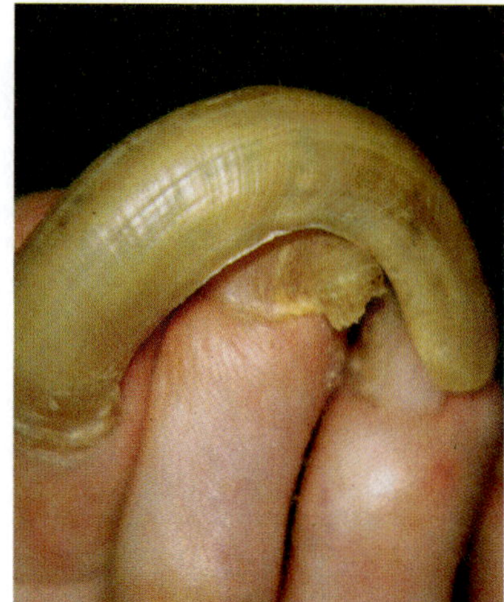

Figure 20-15 Onychogryposis.

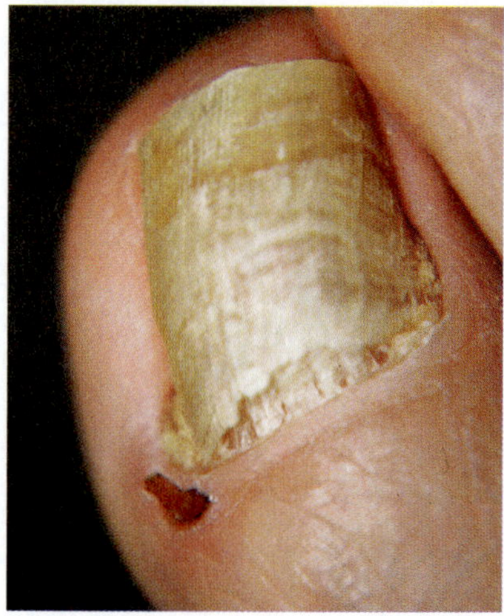

Figure 20-16 Onychomadesis of a toenail.

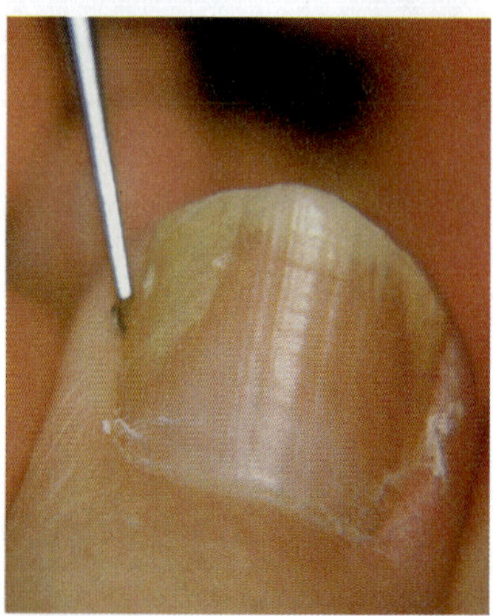

Figure 20-17 Onycholysis.

- *Nail mold* is not really a mold. It is a bacterial infection of the nail, caused by a bacteria called *Pseudomonas aeruginosa*, that can be caused by moisture that seeps between an artificial nail and the free edge of the nail (Figure 20–14). Mold starts with a yellow-green color and darkens to black if not properly treated. This condition should be treated by a physician.
- **Onychia** (uh-NIK-ee-uh) is an inflammation of the matrix with the formation of pus, redness, swelling, and shedding of the nail. Onychia is often caused by improperly sanitized implements and bacterial infection.
- **Onychogryposis** (ahn-ih-koh-gry-POH-sis) is a condition in which the nail curvature is increased and enlarged. The nail becomes thicker and curves, sometimes extending over the tip of the finger or toe (Figure 20–15). This condition results in inflammation and pain if the nail grows into the skin. The cause of this disorder is unknown.

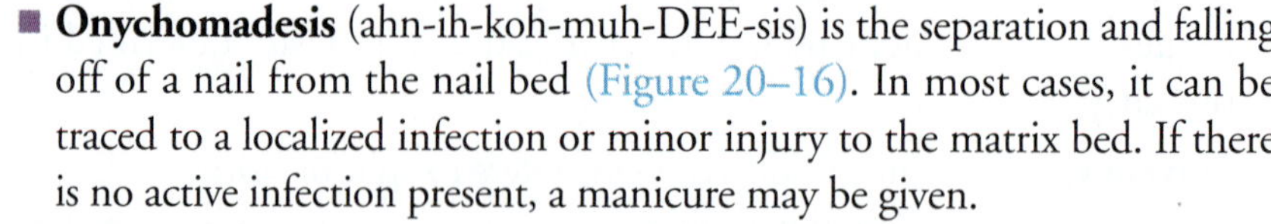

- **Onychomadesis** (ahn-ih-koh-muh-DEE-sis) is the separation and falling off of a nail from the nail bed (Figure 20–16). In most cases, it can be traced to a localized infection or minor injury to the matrix bed. If there is no active infection present, a manicure may be given.
- **Onycholysis** (ahn-ih-KAHL-ih-sis) is a condition in which the nail loosens from the nail bed, beginning usually at the free edge and continuing to the lunula, but does not come off (Figure 20–17). It is caused by an internal disorder, trauma, infection, or certain drugs.
- **Onychoptosis** (ahn-ih-kahf-TOH-sis) is a condition in which part or all of the nail sheds periodically and falls off. It can affect one or more nails. It occurs during or after certain diseases such as syphilis, as a result of fever, as a reaction to certain prescription drugs, or as a result of trauma.
- **Paronychia** (payr-uh-NIK-ee-uh) is a bacterial inflammation of the tissue around the nail (Figure 20–18). The symptoms are redness,

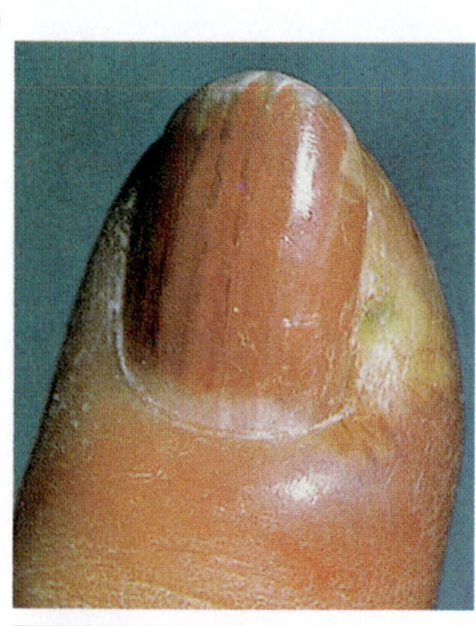

Figure 20-18 Paronychia.

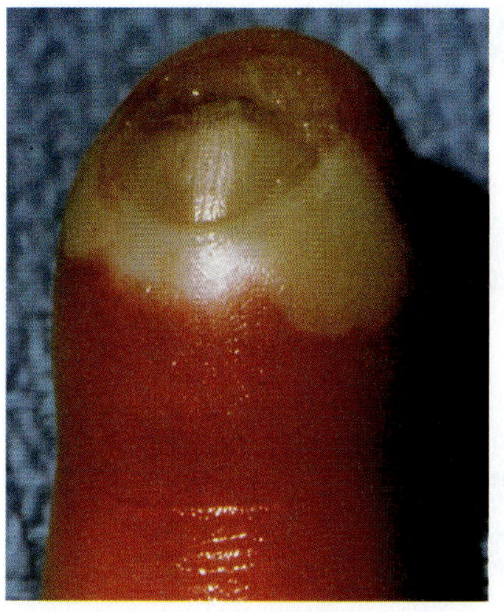
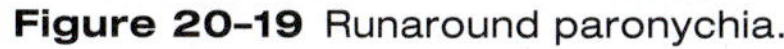

Figure 20-19 Runaround paronychia.

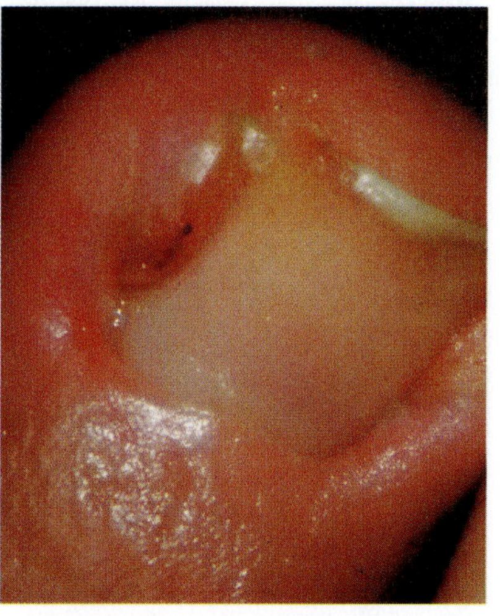

Figure 20-20 Chronic paronychia.

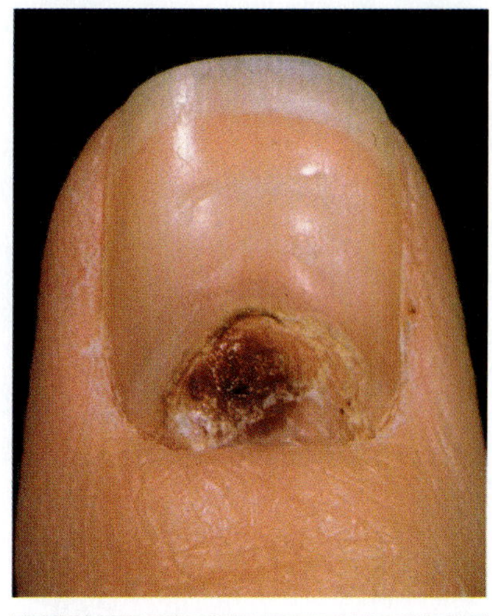

Figure 20-21 Pyrogenic granuloma.

swelling, and tenderness of the tissue. It can occur at the base of the nail, around the entire nail plate, or on the fingertip. Paronychia around the entire nail is sometimes referred to as "runaround paronychia" (Figure 20–19). Chronic paronychia occurs continually over a long period of time and causes damage to the nail plate (Figure 20–20). It can be caused by the use of unsanitary implements or by aggressive pushing or cutting of the cuticle.

- **Pyrogenic granuloma** (py-roh-JEN-ik gran-yoo-LOH-muh) is a severe inflammation of the nail in which a lump of red tissue grows up from the nail bed to the nail plate (Figure 20–21).
- *Onychomycosis* (ahn-ih-koh-my-KOH-sis), or **tinea unguium** (TIN-ee-uh UN-gwee-um), is ringworm of the nails (Figure 20–22). A common form is whitish patches that can be scraped off the surface. A second form is long, yellowish streaks within the nail substance. The disease invades the free edge and spreads toward the root. The infected portion is thick and discolored. In a third form, the deeper layers of the nail are invaded, causing the superficial layers to appear irregularly thin. These infected layers peel off and expose the diseased parts of the nail bed. 2

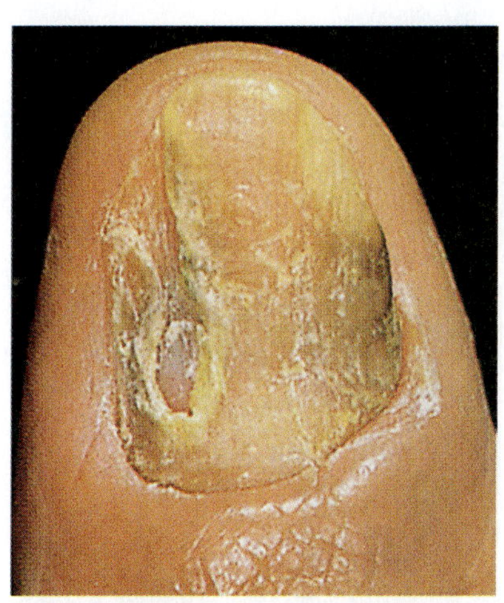

Figure 20-22 Tinea unguium (onychomycosis).

20

INTRODUCTION TO MANICURING

The ancients regarded long, polished, and colored fingernails as a mark of distinction between aristocrats and common laborers. Manicuring, once considered a luxury for the few, is now a service used by many men and women. The word *manicure* is derived from the Latin *manus* (hand) and *cura* (care), which means the care of the hands and nails.

To perform professional manicures, it is important to develop competence when working with nail care tools. Nail care tools consist of equipment, implements, materials, and cosmetics.

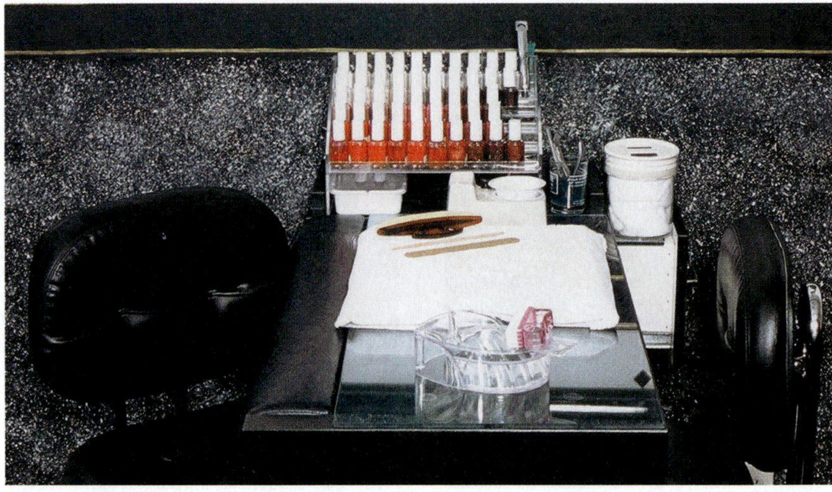

Figure 20-23 Manicure table.

Equipment

Equipment includes the permanent tools and items used to perform nail services. They do not require replacement until they are no longer in good repair.

- *Manicure table with adjustable lamp.* Most standard manicuring tables include a drawer for storing sanitized implements and cosmetics, and an attached, adjustable lamp (Figure 20–23). The lamp should have a 40-watt bulb. The heat from a higher-wattage bulb will interfere with manicuring and sculptured nail procedures. A lower-wattage bulb will not warm a client's nails in a room that is highly air-conditioned. The warmth from the bulb will help to maintain product consistency.
- *Client's chair and nail technician's chair or stool.*
- *Finger bowl.* A plastic, china, or glass bowl that is shaped specifically for soaking the client's fingers in warm water and antibacterial soap (Figure 20–24).
- *Wet sanitizer.* A receptacle large enough to hold the disinfectant solution in which to immerse implements for sanitizing purposes. A cover is provided with most wet sanitizers to prevent contamination of the solution when it is not in use (Figure 20–25).
- *Client's cushion.* The cushion is usually 8 to 12 inches long and especially made for manicuring (a towel that is folded to cushion size can also be used). The cushion or folded towel should be covered with a clean, sanitized towel before each appointment.
- *Sanitized cotton container.* This container will hold clean, absorbent cotton.
- *Supply tray.* The tray holds cosmetics such as polishers, polish removers, and creams.
- *Electric nail-dryer.* A nail-dryer is an optional item used to shorten the length of time necessary for drying the client's nails.

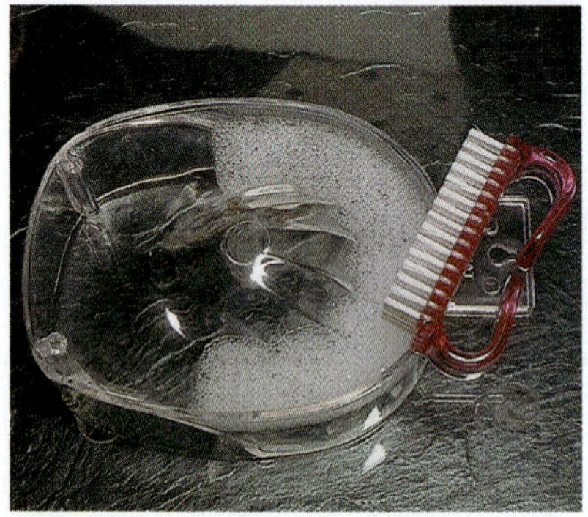

Figure 20-24 Finger bath with soapy water.

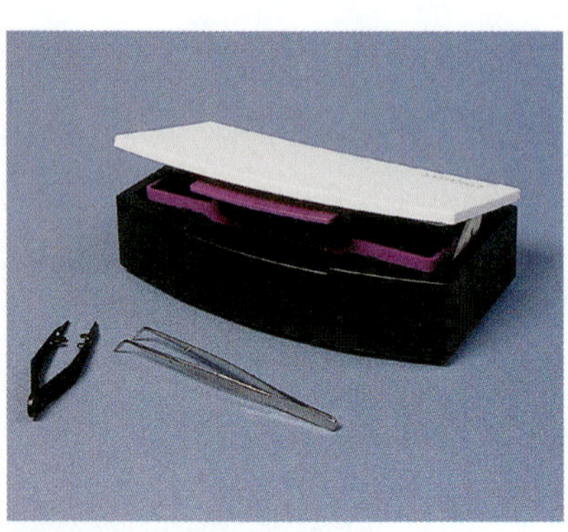

Figure 20-25 Wet sanitizer.

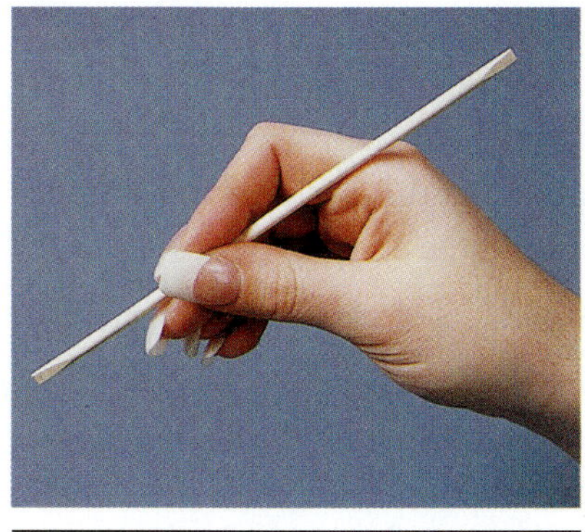

Figure 20-26 Orangewood stick.

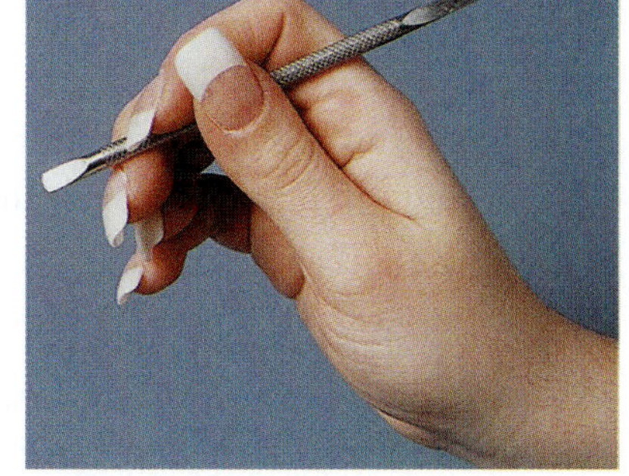

Figure 20-27 Cuticle pusher.

Implements

Implements are tools that must be disinfected, sanitized, or discarded after use with each client. They are small enough to be sanitized in a wet sanitizer.

- *Orangewood stick.* Use the orangewood stick to loosen the cuticle around the base of a nail or clean under the free edge (Figure 20–26). Hold the stick similarly to a pencil. For applying cosmetics, wrap a small piece of cotton around the end.
- *Cuticle pusher.* The steel pusher, also called a cuticle pusher, is used to push back excess cuticle growth (Figure 20–27). Hold the steel pusher in the same way as the orangewood stick. The spoon end is used to loosen and push back the cuticle. If the pusher has rough or sharp edges, use an emery board to dull them. This prevents digging into the nail plate.
- *Metal nail file.* A metal nail file is used to shape the free edge of hard or sculptured nails (Figure 20–28). Most professional nail technicians use 7- or 8-inch nail files because some states do not allow shorter files to be used. Since a nail file is metal and reusable, it must be sanitized after each use. When using a nail file, hold it with the thumb on one side of the handle and four fingers on the other side.
- *Emery board.* Many nail technicians prefer an emery board to a nail file (Figure 20–29). It is also a good choice for filing soft or fragile nails, because it is not as coarse as a nail file. An emery board has two sides, a coarse-grained side and a fine-grained side. The coarse side is used to shape the free edge of the nail, and the fine side is used to bevel the nail or smooth the free edge. Hold the emery board in the same manner as a nail file, with the wider end in your hand so you can file with the narrow end. To bevel, hold the emery board at a 45-degree angle and file, using light pressure, on the top or underside of the nail. Emery boards cannot be sanitized. They may be given to the client or broken in half and discarded after use. It is not a good idea to save an emery board in a plastic bag for each client. Bacteria can grow on the unsanitized implement before the client's next appointment.

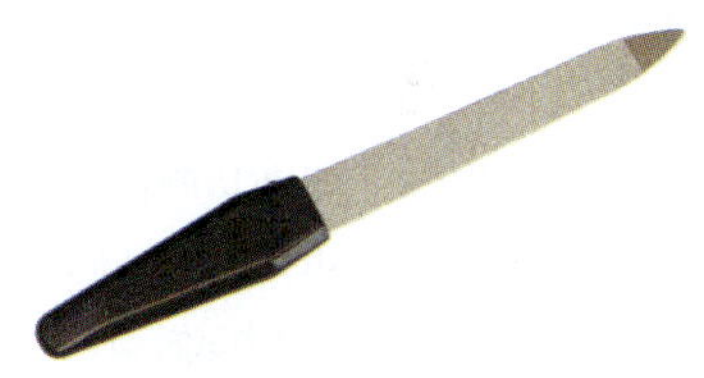

Figure 20-28 Metal nail file.

20

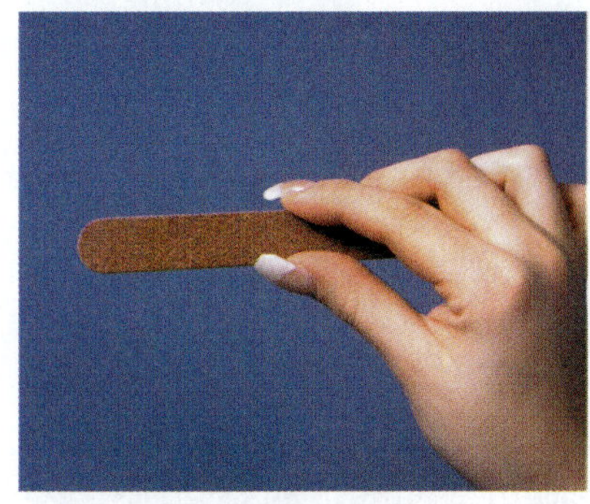

Figure 20-29 Emery board.

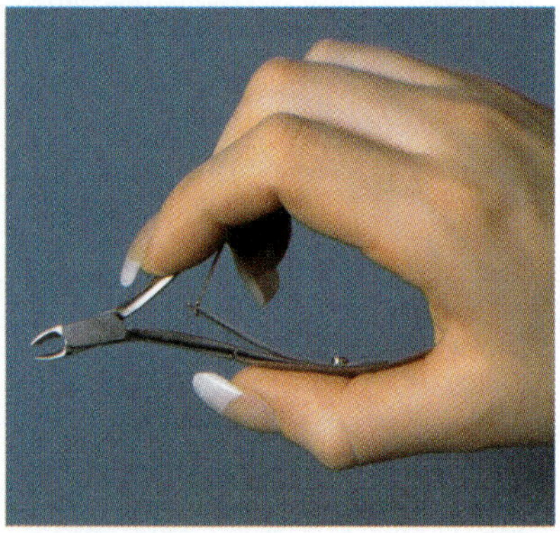

Figure 20-30 Cuticle nipper.

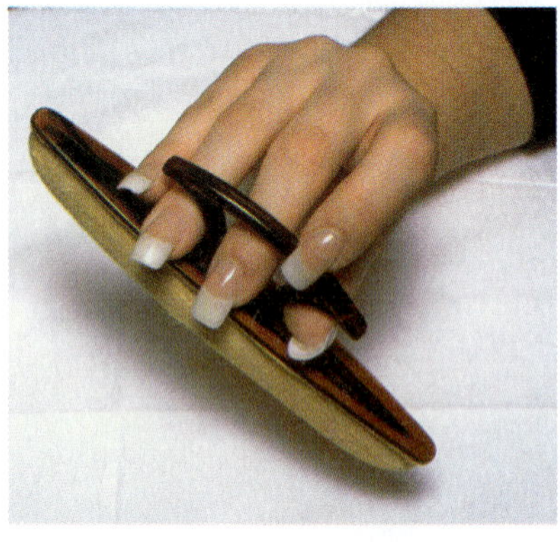

Figure 20-31 Nail buffer.

Follow state regulations for storage of sanitized manicuring implements. They must be stored in sealed containers, sealed plastic bags, or a cabinet sanitizer until they are needed.

- *Cuticle nipper.* A cuticle nipper is used to trim away excess cuticle at the base of the nail (Figure 20–30). To use the nippers, hold them in the palm of the hand with the blades facing the cuticle. Place the thumb on one handle and three fingers on the other handle, with the index finger on the screw to help guide the blade around the cuticle.
- *Tweezers.* Tweezers can be used to lift small bits of cuticle from the nail.
- *Nail brush.* A nail brush is used to clean fingernails and remove bits of cuticle with warm, soapy water. Hold the nail brush with the bristles turned down and away from you. Place the thumb on the handle side of the brush that is facing you, and the fingers on the other side.
- *Nail buffer.* The buffer is made of leather or chamois and is used to add shine to the nail and to smooth out corrugations or wavy ridges (Figure 20–31). There are two types of chamois buffers. The first has an open handle; the second has a closed handle on the top. To use the open-handled buffer, place the fingers around the handle with the thumb on the side of the handle to help guide it. To use the closed-handled type, rest the thumb along the edge of the buffer to guide and support the implement. Another way to hold a closed-handled chamois buffer is to place the middle and ring fingers through the closed-handled buffer if it has an open slot. Be guided by your instructor on how to hold the chamois buffer.
- *Fingernail clippers.* Fingernail clippers are used to shorten nails. For very long nails, clipping reduces filing time.

Sanitation for Implements

It is recommended that you have two complete sets of metal implements so that a complete sanitized set can be ready for each client with no waiting between appointments. If you have only one set of implements, remember that it takes 20 minutes to sanitize implements after each use. Use the following steps to sanitize implements effectively:

- Wash all implements thoroughly with soap and warm water and rinse off all traces of soap with plain water (Figure 20–32). Dry them thoroughly with a sanitized towel.
- Metal implements should be immersed in a wet sanitizer that has cotton at the bottom and has been filled with an approved disinfectant (Figure 20–33). The required sanitation time is usually 20 minutes. Dry the implements with a sanitized towel when they are removed from the wet sanitizer.
- Follow state regulations for the storage of sanitized manicuring implements. They must be stored in sealed containers, sealed plastic bags, or a cabinet sanitizer until needed.

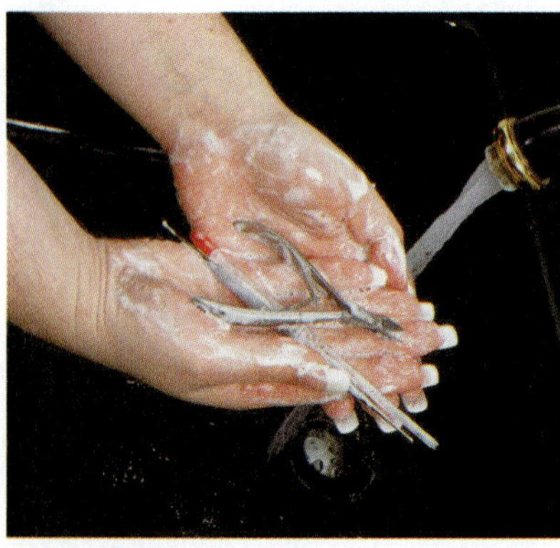

Figure 20-32 Wash implements first.

Materials

Materials are supplies that are used during a manicure and need to be replaced for each client.

- *Disposable towels or terry cloth towels.* A fresh, sanitized terry towel is used to cover the client's cushion before each manicure. Another fresh towel should be used to dry the client's hands after soaking in the finger bowl. Other terry or lint-free disposable towels are used to wipe spills that may occur around the finger bowl.

- *Cotton or cotton balls.* Cotton is used to remove polish, wrap the end of the orangewood stick, and apply nail cosmetics. Some nail technicians prefer to use small, fiber-free squares to remove polish because they don't leave cotton fibers on the nails that might interfere with polish application.
- *Plastic spatula.* The spatula is used to remove nail cosmetics from their containers. Always use a spatula, not the fingers, to remove cosmetics as a closed container of nail cosmetics is a perfect place for bacteria to grow.
- *Plastic bags.* Tape or clip a bag to the side of the manicuring table to hold materials used during a service. Line all trash cans with plastic bags. Be sure to have a generous supply of bags so that they can be changed regularly during the day.
- *Approved solution for jar sanitizer.* Alcohol (99 percent) is sometimes used as a disinfectant for the manicure table and implements. Many other products are also available. Consult your state board or health department for information about the required strength.
- *Powdered alum or styptic powder.* Powdered alum, or styptic powder, is used to contract the skin to stop minor bleeding that may occur during a manicure. To use, blot the cut with powdered alum on a cotton-tipped orangewood stick.

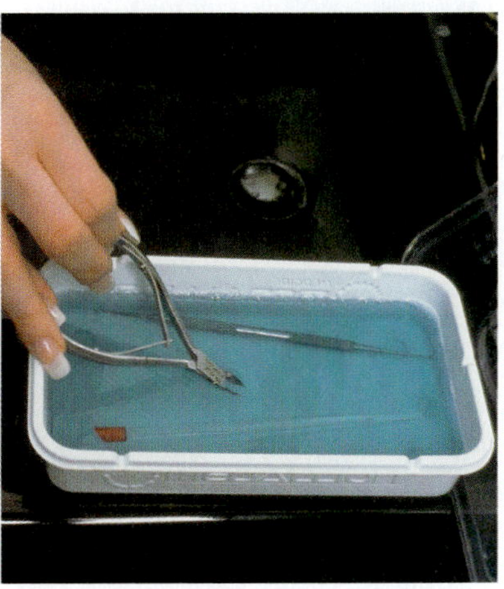

Figure 20-33 Place implements in disinfectant.

Cosmetics

A professional nail technician needs to know how to use each nail cosmetic and what ingredients it contains. It is also important to know when to avoid using a product because of a client's allergies or sensitivities. This section identifies and describes some of the basic nail cosmetics, as well as lists their basic ingredients (Figure 20–34).

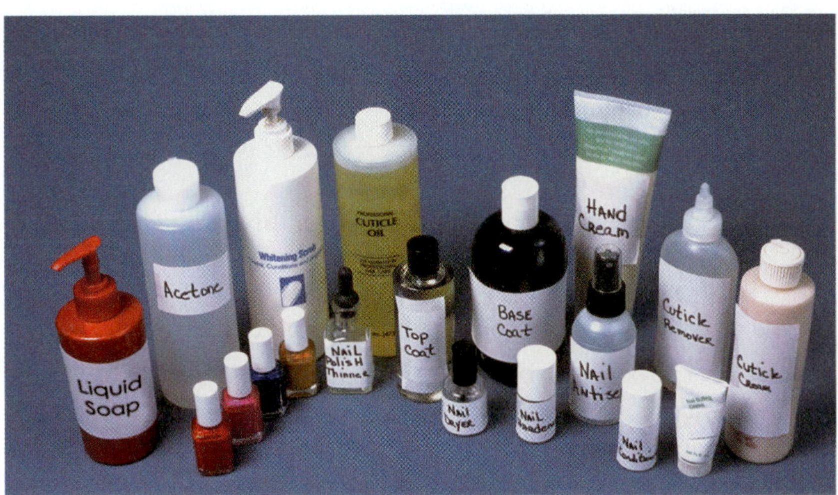

Figure 20-34 Nail cosmetics.

- *Antibacterial soap.* This soap is mixed with warm water and used in the finger bowl. It contains a detergent and an antibacterial agent that is used to sanitize the client's hands. It comes in four forms: flaked, beaded, cake, and liquid.
- *Polish remover.* Polish remover is used to dissolve and remove nail polish. It usually contains organic solvents and acetone. Sometimes oil is added to offset the drying effect of the acetone. Use non-acetone polish remover for clients who have artificial nails, since acetone will weaken or dissolve the tips, wrap glues, and sculptured nail compound.
- *Cuticle cream.* Cuticle cream is used to lubricate and soften dry cuticles and brittle nails. It contains fats and waxes such as lanolin, cocoa butter, petroleum, and beeswax.
- *Cuticle oil.* Cuticle oil keeps the cuticle soft and helps to prevent hangnails or rough cuticles. It gives an added touch to the finish of a manicure. Cuticle oil contains ingredients such as vegetable oil, vitamin E, mineral oil, jojoba, and palm nut oil. Suggest that your clients use it at bedtime to keep their cuticles soft.
- *Cuticle solvent or cuticle remover.* Cuticle solvent makes cuticles easier to remove and minimizes clipping. It contains 2–5 percent sodium or potassium hydroxide, plus glycerin.
- *Nail bleach.* Apply nail bleach to the nail plate and under the free edge to remove yellow stains. Nail bleach contains hydrogen peroxide. If nail bleach cannot be purchased, use 20-volume (6 percent) hydrogen peroxide.
- *Nail whitener.* Nail whiteners are applied under the free edge of a nail to make the nail appear white. They contain zinc oxide or titanium oxide. Nail whiteners are available in paste, cream, coated string, and pencil form.
- *Dry nail polish.* Dry nail polish (pumice powder) is used with the chamois buffer to add shine to the nail. Some clients prefer it to liquid clear polish. Dry nail polish contains mild abrasives that are used for smoothing or sanding, such as tin oxide, talc, silica, and kaolin, and is available in powder and cream form.
- *Nail strengthener/hardener.* Nail strengthener is applied to the nail before the base coat. It prevents splitting and peeling of the nail. There are three types of nail strengthener.
    1. Protein hardener is a combination of clear polish and protein, such as collagen.
    2. Nylon fiber is a combination of clear polish with nylon fibers. It is applied first vertically and then horizontally on the nail plate. It can be hard to cover because the fibers on the nail are visible.
    3. Formaldehyde strengthener contains 5 percent formaldehyde.
- *Base coat.* The base coat is colorless and is applied to the nail before the application of colored polish. It prevents red or dark polish from yellowing or staining the nail plate. Base coat is the first polish applied in the polish procedure, unless a nail strengthener is being used. It contains more resin than colored polish to maintain a tacky surface, so the colored

polish will adhere better. Base coat also contains ethyl acetate, a solvent, isopropyl alcohol, butyl acetate, nitrocellulose, resin, and sometimes formaldehyde.

- *Colored polish, liquid enamel, or lacquer.* Colored polish is used to add color and gloss to the nail. Usually it is applied in two coats. Colored polish contains a solution of nitrocellulose in a volatile solvent such as amyl acetate, and evaporates easily. Manufacturers add castor oil to prevent the polish from drying too rapidly.
- *Top coat or sealer.* The top coat, a colorless polish, is applied over colored polish to prevent chipping and to add a shine to the finished nail. It contains nitrocellulose, toluene, a solvent, isopropyl alcohol, and polyester resins.
- *Liquid nail dry.* Liquid nail dry is used to prevent smudging of the polish. It promotes rapid drying so that the polish is not tacky, and prevents the polish from dulling. It has an alcohol base and is available in brush-on or spray.
- *Hand cream and hand lotion.* Hand lotion and hand cream add a finishing touch to a manicure. Since they soften and smooth the hands, they make the finished manicure as beautiful as possible. Hand cream helps the skin retain moisture. It is thicker than hand lotion and is made of emollients and humectants such as glycerin, cocoa butter, lecithin, and gums. Hand lotion has a thinner consistency than hand cream because it contains more oil. Hand cream or hand lotion can be used as the oil in a conditioning hot-oil manicure.
- *Nail conditioner.* Nail conditioner contains moisturizers. It should be applied at night, before bedtime, to help prevent brittle nails and dry cuticles.

Types of Polish Application

There are five coverage options that may be used in applying polish.

- *Full coverage.* The entire nail plate is polished.
- *Free edge.* The free edge of the nail is unpolished. This helps to prevent the polish from chipping.
- *Hairline tip.* The nail plate is polished and 1⁄16 of an inch is removed from the free edge. This prevents polish from chipping.
- *Slim-line or free walls.* Leave a 1⁄16-inch margin on each side of the nail plate. This makes a wide nail appear narrower.
- *Half-moon or lunula.* The lunula at the base of the nail is left unpolished.

Polish is usually applied in four or five coats. The base coat is applied first, followed by two coats of color and one or two applications of topcoat. Roll the polish bottle in the palms of the hands to mix. Never shake polish. Shaking causes air bubbles to form, which will make the polish application rough. Apply all coats of polish in the following manner.

1. Remove the brush from the bottle and wipe one side on the bottle neck so that a bead of polish remains on the end of the brush. Start in the center of the nail, position the brush 1⁄16 inch away from the cuticle, and brush toward the free edge.

20

Using the same technique, do the left side of nail, then the right side. There should be enough polish on the brush to complete three strokes without having to dip it back into the bottle. The more strokes used the more lines or lumps will show on the client's nail. Small areas missed with the first color coat can be covered with the second coat.

2. Apply two coats of colored polish with the same technique used for the base coat. Complete the first color coat on both hands before starting the second coat. Polish on the cuticle should be removed with a cotton-tipped orangewood stick saturated in polish remover.
3. Apply one or two coats of top coat to prevent chipping and to give nails a glossy look. The use of an instant nail dry spray is optional, but is effective in preventing smudging and dulling.

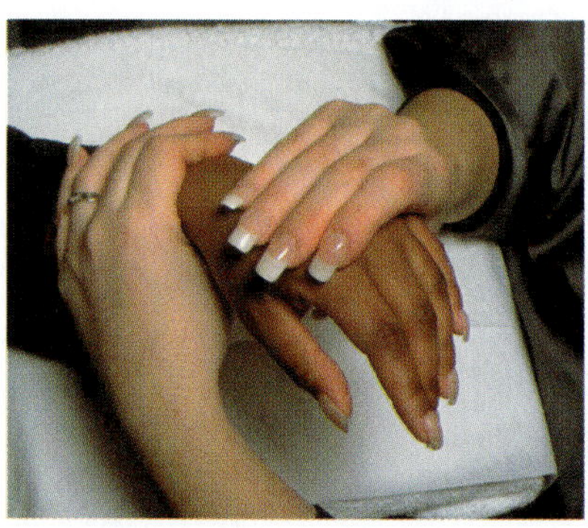

Figure 20-35 Movement to limber the wrist.

HAND AND ARM MASSAGE

A hand and arm massage is a thoroughly relaxing service that should be incorporated into manicure procedures. Use the massage techniques learned in Chapter 12 to perform the following procedures.

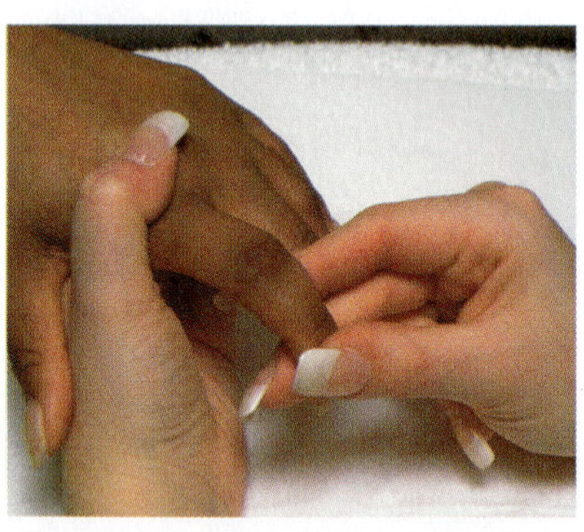

Figure 20-36 Grasp each finger and rotate.

Hand Massage Techniques

1. Relaxation movement. This is a form of massage known as joint movement. Apply hand lotion or cream. Place the client's elbow on a cushion. With one hand, brace the client's arm. With the other hand, hold the client's wrist and bend it back and forth slowly 5 to 10 times, until you feel the client has relaxed (Figure 20–35).
2. Joint movement on fingers. Bring the client's arm down, brace the hand with the left hand, and with the right hand start with the little finger, holding it at the base of the nail. Gently rotate the fingers to form circles. Work toward the thumb, three to five times on each finger (Figure 20–36).
3. Circular movement in palm. Use the effleurage manipulation. Place the client's elbow on the cushion and, with your thumbs in the client's palm, rotate in a circular movement in opposite directions (Figure 20–37).
4. Circular movement on wrist. Hold the client's hand with both of your hands, placing your thumbs on top of client's hand, your fingers below the hand (Figure 20–38). Move the thumbs in a circular motion in opposite directions, from the client's wrist to the knuckle on the back of the client's hand. Move up and down three to five times. At the last rotation, wring the client's wrist by bracing your hands around the wrist and gently twisting in opposite directions.
5. Circular movement on back of the hand and fingers. Now rotate down the back of the client's hand using the thumbs. Rotate down the little finger and the client's thumb, and gently squeeze off at the tips of the client's fingers (Figure 20–39). Go back and rotate down the ring finger and index finger, gently squeezing off. Now do the middle finger and squeeze off at the tip. This tapering to the fingertips helps blood flow.

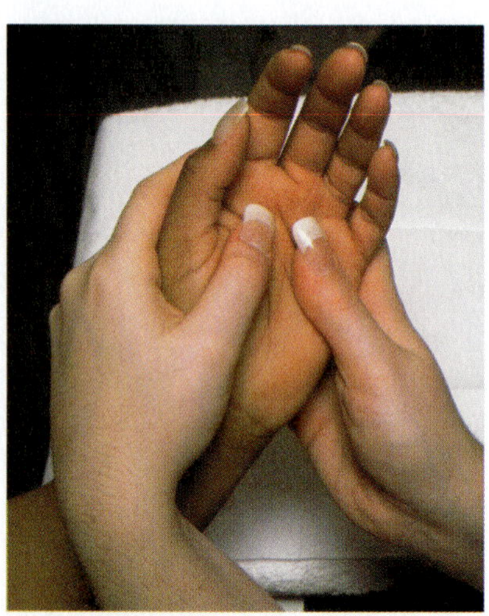

Figure 20-37 Movement to relax the hand.

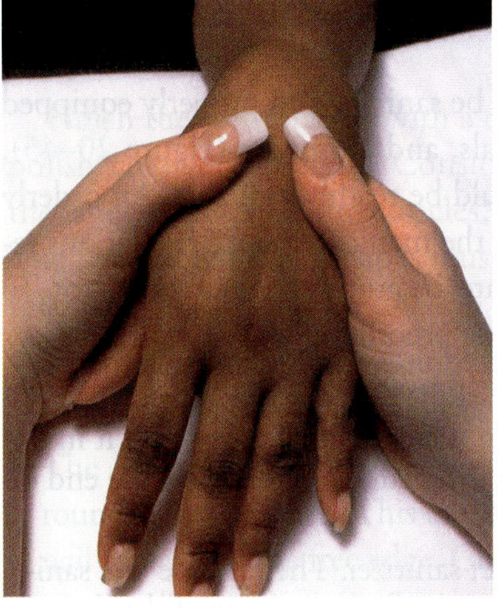
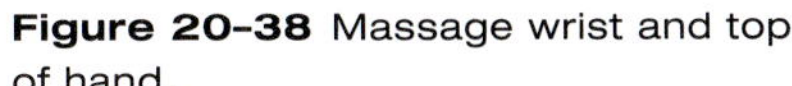

Figure 20-38 Massage wrist and top of hand.

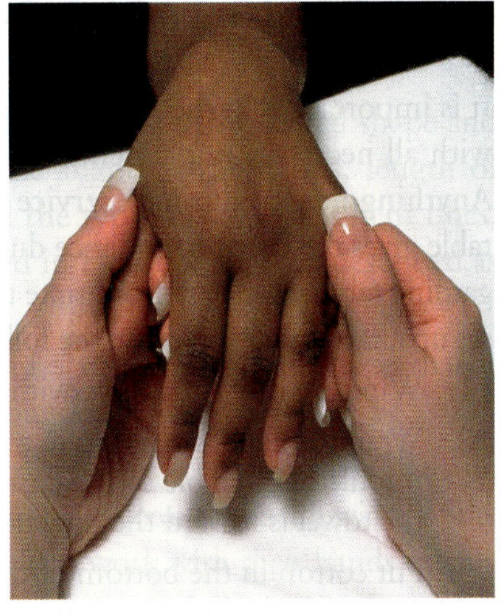

Figure 20-39 Taper each finger.

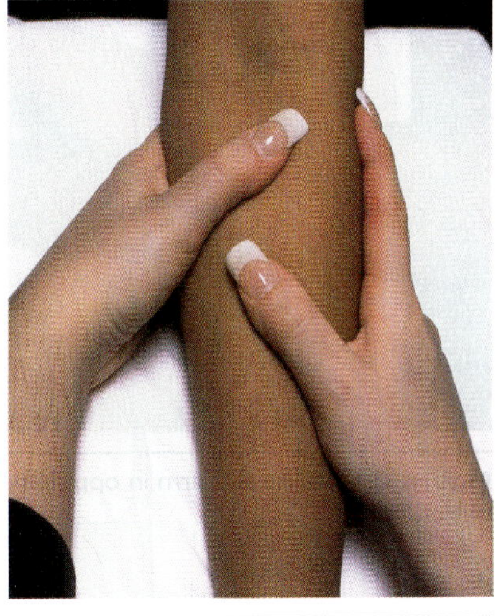

Figure 20-40 Massage arm from wrist to elbow.

Arm Massage Techniques

1. Distribution of cream or lotion. Apply a small amount of cream to the client's arm and work it in (Figure 20–40). Work from the client's wrist toward the elbow, except on the last movement, when work should be from the elbow to the wrist. Finally, squeeze off at the fingertips, as at the end of a hand massage. Apply more cream if necessary.
2. Effleurage on arms. Put the client's arm on the table, bracing the arm with your hands. Hold the client's hand palm up in your hand. Your fingers should be under the client's hand, your thumbs side by side in the client's palm. Rotate your thumbs in opposite directions, starting at the client's wrist and working toward the elbow. When you reach the elbow, slide your hand down the client's arm to the wrist and rotate back up to the elbow three to five times. Turn the arm over and repeat three to five times on the top side of arm (Figures 20–41 and 20–42).
3. Wringing movement on arm, friction massage movement. A friction massage involves deep rubbing to the muscles. Bend the client's elbow so the arm is horizontal in front of you, with the back of the hand facing up. Place your hands around the arm with your fingers facing in the same direction as the arm, and gently twist in opposite directions as you would wring out a washcloth, from wrist to elbow (Figure 20–43). Repeat up and down the forearm three to five times.
4. Kneading movement on the arm. Place your thumbs on the top side of the client's arm so they are horizontal. Move them in opposite directions, from wrist to elbow and back down to wrist. This squeezing motion moves the flesh over the bone and stimulates the arm tissue. Do this three to five times.
5. Rotation of the elbow, friction massage movement. Brace the client's arm with your left hand and apply cream to the elbow. Cup the elbow with your right hand and rotate your hand over the client's elbow (Figure 20–44). Repeat three to five times. To finish the elbow massage, move your left arm to the top of the client's forearm. Gently slide both hands down the forearm from the elbow to the fingertips as if climbing down a rope. Repeat three to five times.

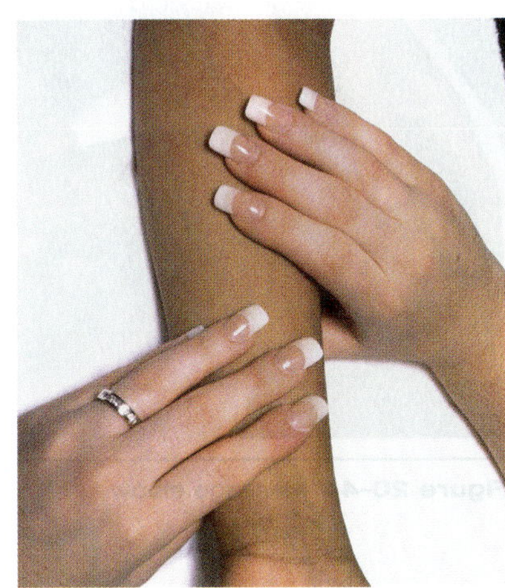

Figure 20-41 Massage under part of arm to elbow.

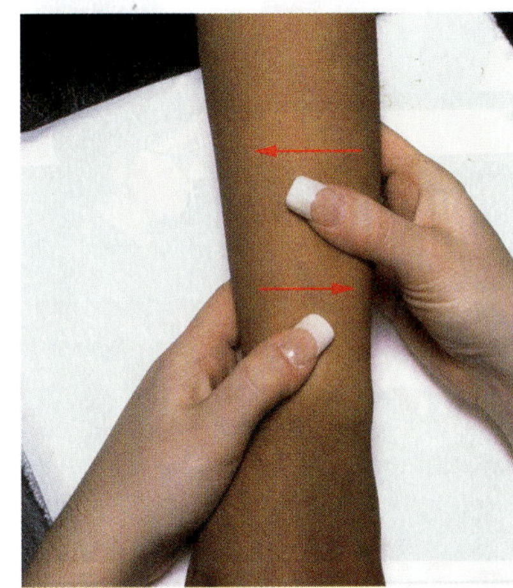

Figure 20-42 Massage top of arm from wrist to elbow.

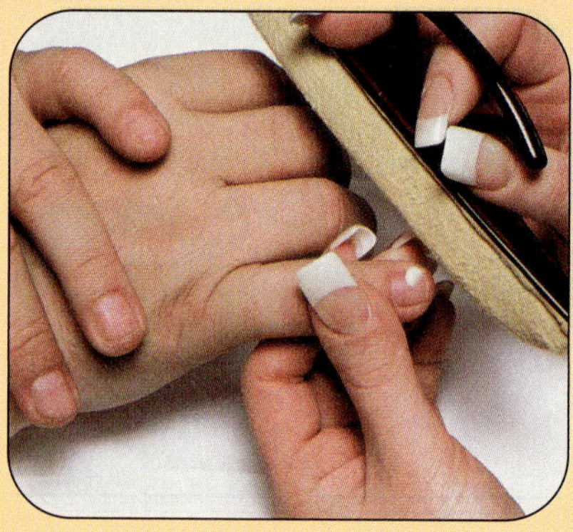

Figure 20-59 Buff nails with chamois buffer.

10. Clean under the free edge. Clean under the free edge with a cotton-tipped orangewood stick, hold the first hand over the soap bath, and brush a last time to remove bits of cuticle and traces of solvent that remain on the nail. Then let the client put the first hand on a sanitized towel.
11. Repeat Steps 5 through 10 on the second hand.
12. Buff with a chamois buffer (Figure 20-59).
13. Apply cuticle oil.
14. Bevel nails if necessary.
15. Apply hand lotion and massage the hands and wrists (Figure 20-60).
16. Polish the nails with a clear matte polish if desired (Figure 20-61).
17. Complete manicure post service procedure.

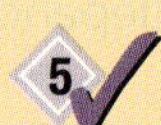

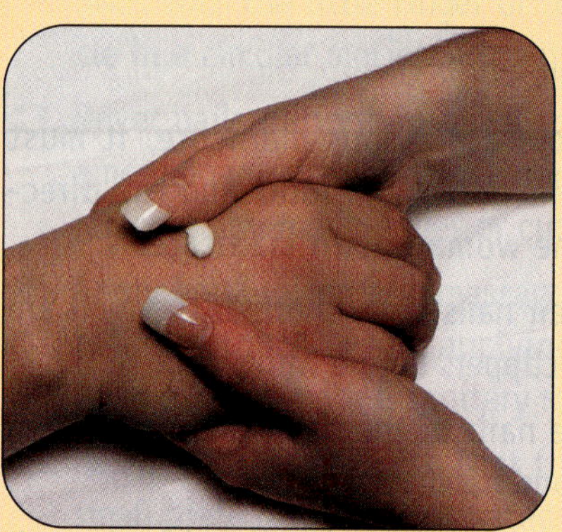

Figure 20-60 Apply hand lotion and massage.

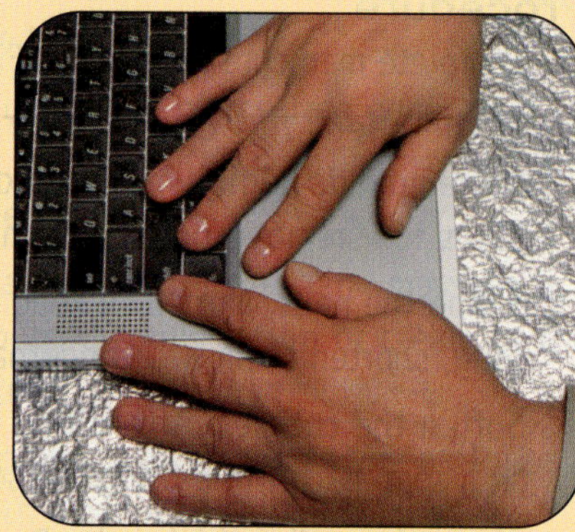

Figure 20-61 Finished man's manicure.

chapter glossary

cuticle	toughened skin around the base of the nail
free edge	part of the nail plate that extends over the tip of the finger
hangnails	condition in which the cuticle splits around the nail
leukonychia	condition of white spots on the nails due to air bubbles, bruising, or injury to the nail
lunula	half-moon shape at the base of the nail
melanonychia	darkening of the nail due to increased and localized pigment in the matrix bed
nail	an appendage of the skin; horny protective plate at the end of the finger or toe
nail bed	portion of the skin on which the nail plate rests
nail folds	folds of normal skin around the nail plate
nail plate	horny plate resting on and attached to the nail bed
nail root or matrix bed	where the nail is formed
onyx	technical term for nail
onychatrophia	wasting away of the nail
onychauxis	thick overgrowth of the nail
onychia	inflammation of the matrix with pus, redness, swelling, and shedding of the nail
onychocryptosis	ingrown nails
onychogryposis	thickening and increased curvature of the nail
onycholysis	loosening of the nail without shedding
onychomadesis	the separation and falling off of the nail from the nail bed
onychophagy	bitten nails
onychoptosis	shedding of one or more nails, in whole or in part
onychorrhexis	abnormal brittleness of the nail plate
onychosis	technical term applied to any deformity or disease of the nail
paronychia	bacterial infection of the tissues surrounding the nail
pterygium	forward growth of the cuticle with adherence to the nail surface
pyrogenic granuloma	severe inflammation of the nail in which a lump of red tissue grows up from the nail bed to the nail plate
tinea unguium	ringworm of the nail

responsibilities are considerably less than those associated with business ownership.

In a **booth rental** arrangement, the barber will generally rent a chair in the barbershop from the shop owner. He or she is solely responsible for his or her own clientele, supplies, record keeping, workstation maintenance, and accounting. Usually, the only obligation to the shop owner is the weekly rent along with other agreed-upon fees such as utilities, laundering services, etc.

With the possible exception of the rent, there are no hard-and-fast rules about the conditions of booth rental. Each shop owner or "landlord" develops a contract or arrangement for compensation of operational expenses or *overhead.* In some cases, stipulations concerning shop behavior, attire, and hours of operation are also included in the agreement. These are all factors that should be discussed and taken into account before signing a booth rental contract.

One of the main advantages to renting a chair or workstation is that you can become virtually self-employed for a relatively small investment. The initial expenses are fairly low and usually limited to the costs incurred with rent, supplies, products, and personal promotion or advertising. For many booth renters, the low overhead can balance equitably with the income generated as a beginning barber with a small clientele. However, the rule is: Make sure that the clientele is large enough to cover the overhead costs. The overhead includes not only the rent, but also the consumable supplies and products that are needed to perform services.

Chair or booth rental may also be ideal for those individuals who are interested in part-time employment, want to supplement another income, or prefer to take a stepping-stone approach to shop ownership. Regardless of the motivation, a booth rental arrangement provides the means for an individual to retain most of the control and decision making as it applies to work schedules and professional goals.

Booth rental also has its share of obligations and responsibilities, and some individuals may not feel ready to assume them. For example, booth rental necessitates that detailed and accurate records be maintained for income tax purposes. In addition, the procurement of an individual business or operational license may be required, along with malpractice and health insurance coverage and expenses. Be sure to familiarize yourself with applicable state and federal laws. Renting a booth also means that paid holidays or vacation benefits are nonexistent. Instead, you will have to plan ahead and set aside savings for such times when you are not working or an emergency arises.

1

Barbershop Ownership

Business ownership is a serious step that requires commitment and follow-through. The aspiring barbershop owner should be prepared to research the business idea thoroughly before making any final decisions or signing any contractual documents.

Business *ownership* involves planning; decision making; financial obligations; contractual agreements; policy making; compliance with local, state, and federal laws; insurances; hiring and firing; purchasing; and all other details of business operations. *Management* is associated with production and involves an understanding of the daily operations as applied to the business and the people working within the establishment. In most barbershops, the owner is the manager as well as one of the practicing barbers.

There are 12 initial tasks that need to be performed when the decision to open a barbershop has been reached. The following list represents some key steps associated with establishing a barbershop:

1. Determine the type of ownership: sole proprietorship, partnership, corporation, or franchise. Decide whether you want to buy an existing business, start one from the ground up, or invest in a franchise business.
2. Determine the services to be offered and the market to be reached.
3. Determine the type of shop environment desired, including theme, mood, and décor of the premises. These decisions, along with the intended market, will help to determine the best location for the business.
4. Find a suitable location, research costs, and design a floor plan.
5. Create a **business plan** including financial projections, budgets, sales estimates, start-up costs, etc.
6. Arrange for financing or capital investment.
7. Plan and research equipment, fixtures, and furnishings purchases.
8. Establish a record-keeping system.
9. Establish shop policies, procedures, and protocols.
10. Arrange for advertising and publicity.
11. Recruit, hire, and train employees.
12. Design a plan to establish good public relations within the community.

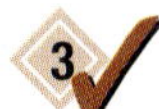

Types of Business Ownership

There are four types of business organizational structures to be considered when planning to open a barbershop: **sole proprietor**, **partnership**, **corporation**, and **franchise**. Thorough research should be done before deciding which type of organizational structure is the most desirable for individual circumstances. A CPA (Certified Public Accountant) should be able to provide all the information necessary to make this decision. In some cases, the type of business chosen will depend on the amount of available capital; in others, personal preference will dictate the choice. Review the characteristics of each type of business ownership as follows.

Sole Proprietor

If the individual has enough money to finance the cost of setting up and operating the barbershop, individual ownership or sole proprietorship should be considered.

A sole proprietorship has certain advantages over a partnership or corporation.

- The owner is the boss and manager.
- The owner determines policies and makes all decisions.
- The owner receives all profits.

Sole proprietorship has the following disadvantages:

- The owner's working capital is limited by the amount of personal or available funds.
- The owner is personally liable for all business debts and bears all losses.
- The owner is personally responsible for all business operations.

Partnership

When two or more individuals share ownership they form a partnership, although not necessarily equally. One reason for forming a partnership arrangement is to generate more capital for investment in the business. This can be facilitated through a "silent partner" arrangement in which an investing partner looks for a financial return on an investment but does not actively take part in the daily operations of the business. Other partnerships are based on the partners working together within the business with like-minded goals and responsibilities.

The advantages that a partnership has over individual ownership are:

- More capital is made available to equip and operate the business.
- Work, responsibilities, and losses are shared.
- Combined abilities and experience assist in the solution of business problems.

The chief disadvantages of a partnership are:

- Each partner is responsible for the business actions of the other.
- Disputes and misunderstandings may arise between partners and become irresolvable.
- Each partner is personally liable for all debts of the business.

There should always be a written agreement defining the duties, responsibilities, and percentage of ownership of each member. Shop policies, procedures, and protocols should be drawn up together and a consensus reached before implementation.

Corporation

When three or more individuals intend to operate a barbershop, a corporation may be a good alternative to a partnership. A corporation has the advantage over a partnership in that its stockholders are not legally responsible in case of loss or bankruptcy. Other factors associated with a corporate organizational structure include:

- The division of profits is proportionate to the number of stocks owned by each individual.
- A charter is required by the state and identifies each individual in the corporation.
- A board of directors governs the management, policies, and decision making in accordance with the corporation's charter.
- The stockholders cannot lose more than their original investment in the corporation.
- The corporation is subject to taxation and regulation by the state. Federal tax laws allow some types of small corporations to be taxed on a partnership basis. This option should be explored since most barbershops would fall into a small-corporation category. An accountant and lawyer should be consulted on all matters.

FRANCHISE

To be successful in today's business market requires a competitive edge. Building name recognition and developing business savvy costs money, time, and hard work. A franchise is a form of a chain organization with a regional or national name, consistent image, and business formula that is used throughout the businesses. Franchises are owned by individuals who have paid a fee to use the name; in turn, they receive a business plan and can take advantage of broadscale marketing campaigns. Decisions such as location, size, décor, and pricing are determined by the parent company and often offer employees the same benefits as corporately owned shops and salons. Franchise ownership may work to your advantage because the systems, knowledge, and expertise are already in place. 4

Purchasing an Established Barbershop

An *established barbershop* is one that is in operation at the time that it is put on the market for sale and has a solid, repeat-clientele base. Empty storefronts that formerly housed a barbershop, or those that were in existence for less than a few years, do not qualify as "established." Each purchase opportunity needs to be well researched and looked at closely before any financial investment is made or contracts signed.

The purchase of an existing barbershop could be a golden opportunity, especially if the owner is retiring. In this type of situation, many of the established customers will probably continue to patronize the shop if they receive equal or better service. There may also be the option of offering the former owner the opportunity to work part-time, even one or two days a week. This can be a win-win situation for both the former owner and the new owner. The former owner adds financially to his or her retirement years with less responsibility and time being required by the business, while the new owner reaps the benefit of a business that maintains some continuity and goodwill for the customers.

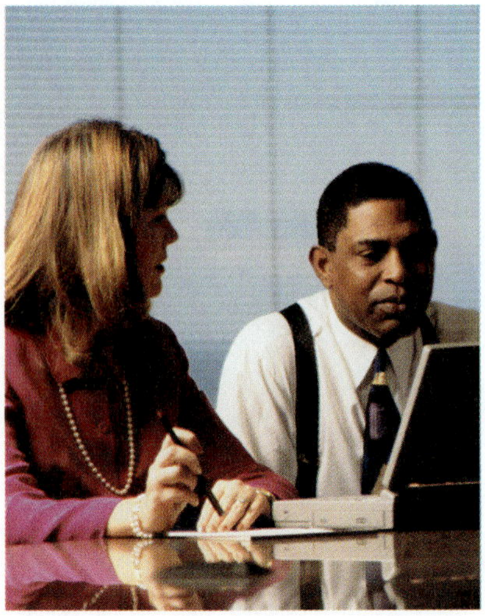

Figure 21–1 Seek professional accounting and legal advice.

While a retiring-owner scenario may provide the best options and opportunities for an aspiring barbershop owner, it is a scenario that may not come along very often. In many cases, the shop space is rental property and what is actually for sale is not much more than fixtures, furnishings, and possibly some equipment. In this type of situation, you would not be buying a business per se, but rather simply taking advantage of the fact that the space was previously set up as the same type of business. It might be worth considering since the plumbing or equipment might already be in place, or because the local populace is familiar with seeing a barbershop in that location. If the location is a good one, and depending on the reasons for the business closure by the former owner, pursuing the purchase of the equipment and signing the lease might prove to be a good opportunity for business ownership.

A third scenario that may present itself is the purchase of an existing barbershop that is operating as a viable enterprise with established employees and their clientele. In any of these scenarios, it is essential to seek the professional assistance of an accountant and a lawyer (Figure 21–1).

Before any sale agreements are signed, an investigation should be made to answer the following questions:

- Is the mortgage, bill of sale, or lease transferable without any liens against it?
- Are there any defaults in the payment of debts?
- Are all the state and federal taxes, including property, Social Security, etc., paid and current?
- Are there lease or current tenant obligations that have to be addressed?

Once the business has been cleared of any financial or ownership obligations, a purchase agreement to buy the barbershop should include the following:

- A written purchase and sale agreement with the names and contact information of both parties.
- A complete and signed statement of inventory, from fixtures to supplies, indicating the value of each item.
- Use of the shop's name and reputation for a definite amount of time (if desired).
- Disclosure of the business's accounts, tax information, and profit-and-loss statements.
- Disclosure of any and all information regarding the shop's clientele and purchasing and service habits.
- A statement that prohibits the seller from competing with the new owner within a specified distance from the present location.

Establishing a Barbershop

Services and Markets

Welcome to the conceptualizing stage of establishing a barbershop (Figure 21–2). When you envision yourself working behind the chair in *your*

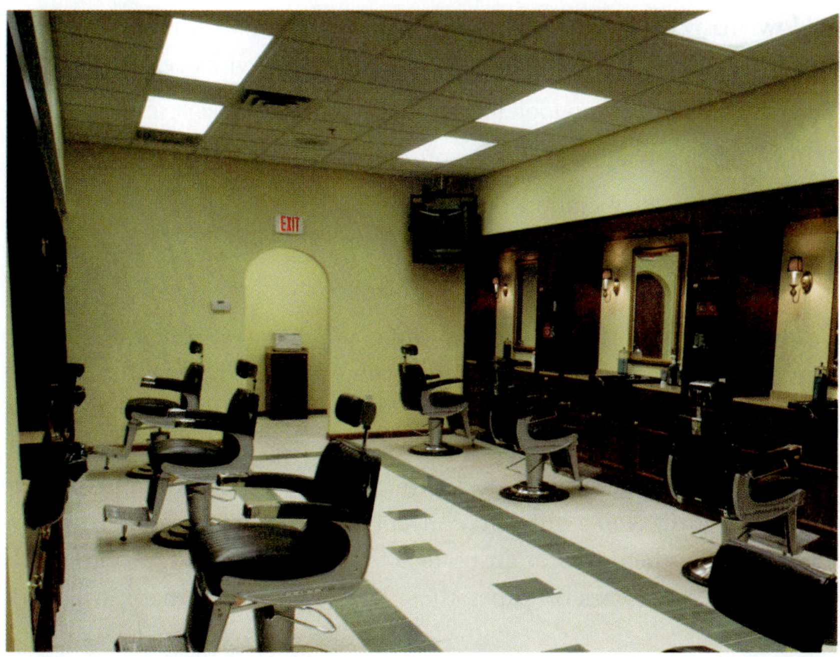

Figure 21-2 Envision your barbershop.

barbershop, what do you see? What does the environment look like? Who is sitting in your chair: a man, woman, teenager, or child? What types of services are you performing: haircuts, shaves, chemical services? Do you think that your barbershop concept has the potential for success based on what you envision?

When it has been decided which services are to be marketed to a specific clientele, a vital starting point has been established from which to develop the barbershop. These decisions will initially serve as a guide when choosing the shop location and design. Next, they will help you to organize your thoughts concerning the equipment, products, and supplies required to service the clientele. This information will then be used to develop the business plan, estimate start-up costs, design a marketing strategy, and secure necessary capital.

It should be clear that the decisions made about services and targeted markets guide important aspects associated with creating the barbershop and help to determine its potential for success. For example, consider a scenario in which male teenagers have been chosen as the targeted market. Explore the following questions that might be asked to help determine the feasibility and potential success of a barbershop that is targeted exclusively to a male teenager clientele base:

- Where is the most ideal shop location to capitalize on this market?
- What is the concentration of male teenagers at the proposed location?
- Is the concentration at the proposed location (near schools, parks, sports fields, etc.) seasonal in nature?
- Is there any direct competition in the area?
- What is the average income or expendable funds of the age group?

- How many haircuts would have to be performed to cover overhead expenses? What is the estimated frequency of shop visits per person?
- What should the shop look like to appeal to male teenagers?
- In what ways would the shop be promoted to this particular group?
- What hours of operation best optimize teenagers' accessibility to the shop?
- Why is targeting this group the best plan for the shop—or is it?

The results you arrive at after exploring, developing, and researching the concept for the barbershop will guide you in making modifications or changes to the general plan. These changes are to be expected and should be handled with a positive problem-solving approach. If your idea does not appear to be viable or realistic after getting all the facts, work through a variation of it or develop a different concept. Take the time to work through ideas and plans before committing to actual contracts and expenditures. If the plan does not work on paper, there is little likelihood that it will work in reality.

The Shop Environment

At this stage, you have a well-thought-out plan, the research to support it has been done, and you are ready to move ahead with creating your barbershop. When you envisioned yourself behind the chair, you may have caught a glimpse of the way your shop would look. Now it is time to take a closer look at that image. What do you see? How big is the space? How many barber chairs do you see? Does every station have a shampoo bowl? What is the color scheme? Is there a reception or retail display area? What style of furniture or cabinetry is used? Is there music playing, and if so, what kind?

The answers to these questions, among others too numerous to mention, will help you make specific decisions about the business environment that you want to create for yourself, clients, and employees. Creating your own barbershop provides a golden opportunity to project your personality, style, and standards into an environment in which you will spend a good portion of your time. Therefore, it should be clean, comfortable, functional, and appealing to yourself and others.

Location

Location, location, location is a mantra sung by many small-business owners, especially those in service industries such as barbering. Visibility, parking, signage, competition, even public transportation access, are just some of the features associated with a good location.

The barbershop must be located in a population area large enough to support it. It should be near other active businesses such as supermarkets, restaurants, banks, etc., that attract walk-by and drive-by traffic. Signage is crucial and should be visible from the roadway.

In general, the shop location should reflect your **target market**, the group that has been identified as the desired clientele and to which marketing and advertising efforts will be directed. Check the local **demographics** concerning the size of the area, population, and average income. Consult with local merchants, banks, and real estate agents to get a feel for the area. This information will assist you in developing shop policies and prices.

When judging the merits of a particular site consider signage, the entrance, the inside area of the space, window placement, water supply, interior and exterior lighting, air-conditioning and heating units, toilet facilities, and parking facilities. Make a list of any structural or plumbing and electrical changes the space will require to facilitate its use as a barbershop and discuss it with the landlord. Although you may be able to negotiate with the landlord, the costs incurred by these changes are usually the tenant's responsibility and should be factored into the start-up costs.

The Lease

In many cases, owning your own business does not mean that you own the building that houses the business. Most of the better business locations, such as strip malls and downtown commercial buildings, are owned by investment property corporations that only lease storefronts and offices.

After the site has been selected, and before signing a lease, check the local zoning ordinances to make certain that the area is zoned to permit the operation of a barbershop.

After all facts have been checked and all obstacles removed, a lease should be negotiated for the premises. A lease protects the barbershop owner against unexpected increases in rent, protects the right of continued occupancy, and clearly sets forth the rights and obligations of both the landlord and the barbershop owner.

Before signing a lease, it should be read carefully and clearly understood by the parties involved. Be sure to have an attorney review the lease to ensure that it contains all the provisions and agreements made between the landlord, and you, the tenant. These agreements may include, but are not limited to, the following:

- An exemption that allows for the removal during renovation of certain fixtures or structures unnecessary to the barbershop, without violation of the lease
- All agreements concerning renovations, repairs, plumbing, painting, fixtures, and electrical installations
- An option that makes provision for you to assign the lease to another person in case a partnership develops or a new owner takes over the business

The Business Plan

A *business plan* is a written description of the proposed business as it appears now and how it will appear in the future. It is a necessary tool to obtain financing and to provide a blueprint for future growth. The business plan should be developed from the information gathered during the preliminary research and should include the following:

- A general description of the business and the services it will provide
- The number of personnel to be hired, their salaries, and other benefits
- An operations plan including the price structure of services offered and monthly expenses such as rent, supplies, repairs, laundry, advertising, taxes, and insurance
- A financial plan that includes a profit-and-loss statement
- A detailed listing of start-up costs including construction, fixtures, furnishings, and equipment

Seek professional guidance if you have any questions about how to develop and write a business plan.

5✓

Finances

One of the results of a good business plan is that it provides an accurate estimate and assessment of the monetary amount necessary to start up and sustain the business for a given length of time. The investment, or *working* **capital**, should be sufficient to cover the rent, wages, and monthly expenditures for a minimum of one year. The number one reason businesses fail is due to undercapitalization! It will take time to build a clientele in a new location, even when an established clientele follows you there, so you must be prepared financially to weather those early lean months.

The shop owner has all the financial responsibility, and a certain percentage of the fees taken in for services will have to be allocated to cover overhead costs. Many times, whatever is left becomes the owner's salary. Obviously, this is not the best way to do business but it happens quite often nevertheless. The best way to avoid this situation is to have enough money set aside to weather the barbershop's clientele-building process.

How much money is enough money? The answer can be determined in part by considering some individual circumstances that may include:

- The clientele and their willingness to move from the previous location
- The availability of other barbers with a following that will work in the shop
- The owner's personal status and financial situation, i.e., single, married, single with dependents, previous debt, etc.
- The availability and type of financing, and its source

As a general rule, no less than one year's worth of operating expenses should be available. If there is no existing clientele, two years of operating capital is not an unrealistic requirement.

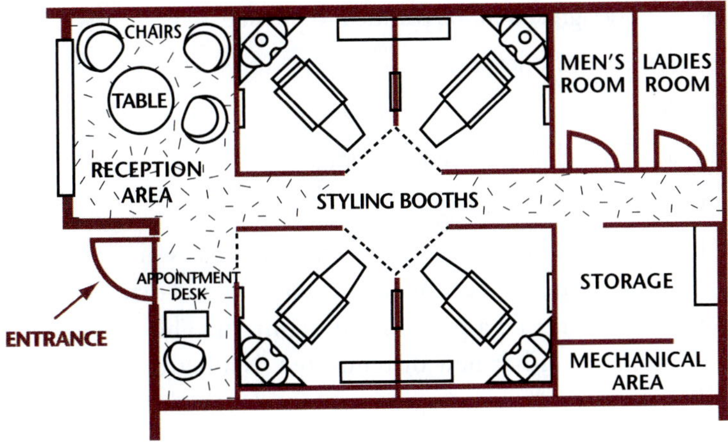

Figure 21-3 Sample floor plans.

Legal Responsibilities

When conducting a business and employing other individuals, it is necessary to comply with local, state, and federal regulations and laws.

- Local regulations may include local building codes, zoning laws, and occupational or business licenses.
- State laws cover sales taxes, professional and business licenses, and workers' compensation.
- State and federal governments govern income tax laws.
- Federal law governs income tax, Social Security, unemployment insurance, cosmetics and luxury tax payments, and OSHA safety and health standards.

Insurances for business establishments include malpractice, premises liability, fire, burglary and theft, and business interruption coverage.

Barbershop Layout

When the location of the shop has been decided and the lease signed, it is time to formalize the layout or *floor plan* of the shop. The shop should be designed to achieve maximum efficiency and economy of space to ensure a smooth operation and traffic pattern (Figures 21–3 and 21–4).

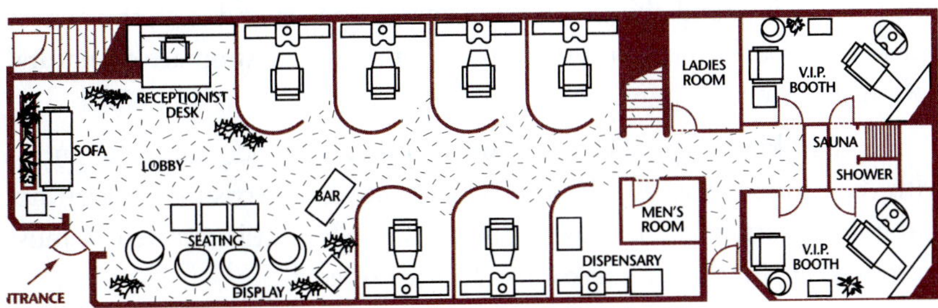

Figure 21-4 Sample floor plans.

The barbershop design should be planned to provide:

- Maximum efficiency of operation
- Adequate aisle space
- Adequate space for each piece of equipment
- Quality mirrors
- Fixtures, furniture, and equipment chosen on the basis of cost, durability, utility, and appearance. (Avoid closeout or odd-sized fixtures or equipment that may be a problem to maintain. The purchase of standard equipment, either new or renovated, is a better investment because it is usually easier to replace or match standard parts and fixtures.)
- Premises that are painted and decorated in colors that are restful and pleasing to the eye
- Adequate restrooms for clients and employees
- Handicap-access facilities and doors
- Good plumbing and sufficient lighting for services
- Proper ventilation, air-conditioning, and heating
- Sufficient electrical outlets and current to adequately service all equipment
- Adequate storage areas
- Sufficient display areas
- An attractive reception or waiting area (This is not to be overlooked. An attractive, adequately furnished, and comfortable waiting area can be one of the barbershop's best promotional devices. It should make the client comfortable and relaxed, and give the impression that the business is really interested in the client's comfort.)

Cleanliness and comfort are two of the most important requisites for a professional-looking barbershop. The equipment should be easily accessible, arranged in an orderly manner, and maintained in good working order. Sanitation procedures must be strictly enforced at all times. *Always consult state barber board regulations in your state when designing the barbershop.*

Advertising

Advertising includes all activities that attract attention to the barbershop. The personalities and abilities of the owner, manager, and staff; the quality of the work performed; and the attractiveness of the shop are all natural advertising assets.

The right kind of publicity is important because it acquaints the public with the various services offered. To be effective, advertising must attract and hold the attention of those individuals to whom it is directed. It must create a desire for the services or merchandise offered.

The choice of an advertising medium is based on the form that will accomplish the desired objective most effectively. For advertising to be effective, it must be repeated. One-time ads or radio spots will produce little return on the investment; conversely, frequent and timely ad placement can make advertising dollars work for the business. Some advertising venues that may be considered for implementation are:

Newspaper advertising

Circulars and flyers

Direct mail

Classified advertising in yellow pages

Promotional giveaways

Radio advertising

TV advertising

Window display

Exterior banners

Client referrals

Contacting clients

Telemarketing

Community outreach and networking

Web site

E-mails

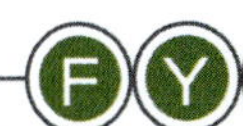

Note: Coupons can be incorporated into all print advertising.

Once clients are attracted to the barbershop, courteous and efficient service will encourage their return and recommendation of the shop to others. Remember that regardless of where advertising dollars are spent, word-of-mouth referrals from a pleased and satisfied client are the best form of advertising.

7

Protection Against Fire, Theft, and Lawsuits

- Keep the premises securely locked.
- Follow safety precautions to prevent fire, injury, and lawsuits.
- Purchase liability, malpractice, fire, and burglary insurance.
- Never violate the medical practice law of your state by attempting to diagnose, treat, or cure disease. Refer the client to a physician.
- Become thoroughly familiar with the barbering laws and sanitation codes of your state.
- Keep accurate records of the number of workers, salaries, length of employment, and Social Security numbers for various state and federal laws affecting the social welfare of employees.

Business Operation

Successful business operation requires an owner or manager who possesses a good business sense, leadership abilities, an understanding of sound business principles, good judgment, and diplomacy. These are all skills that develop over time with experience and application. To jump-start that development, seek out educational opportunities in the form of business seminars or mentoring programs that will help to hone personal management skills that need enhancement. If you are interested in purchasing a franchised shop/salon, utilize all the business operation data the franchise offers.

In addition to efficient and effective management, the success of a business depends on the following factors.

- Sufficient investment capital
- Cooperation between management and employees
- Professional business procedures
- Trained and experienced personnel
- Competitive pricing of services
- Quality customer service

Business problems can be numerous, especially when a new business is just getting started. The first year is the most crucial and every effort should be made by the owner or manager to ensure the shop's success. Some contributing causes to business failure include:

- Inexperience in dealing with the public and employees
- Insufficient capital (undercapitalization) to sustain the business until established
- Poor location
- High cost of operation
- Lack of proper basic training
- Neglect of the business
- Lack of qualified personnel

Record Keeping

Good business operation requires a simple and efficient record system. Records are of value only if they are correct, concise, and complete. *Bookkeeping* means keeping an accurate record of all income and expenses. *Income* is usually classified as the money generated from services and retail sales. *Expenses* include rent, utilities, salaries, advertising, supplies, equipment, and repairs. Retain all check stubs, canceled checks, receipts, and invoices. A professional accountant is recommended to help keep records accurate and processed in a timely manner.

Proper business records are necessary to meet the requirements of local, state, and federal laws regarding taxes and employees. All business transactions must be recorded in order to maintain proper records and are required for:

- efficient operation of the barbershop.
- determining income, expenses, profit, and loss.
- assessing the value of the business for prospective buyers.
- arranging a bank loan.
- providing data on income tax, Social Security, unemployment and disability insurance, wage and hour law, accident compensation, and percentage payments of gross income required in some leases.

One cause for business failure is the lack of complete and systematic records. Business transactions must be recorded in order to judge the condition of the business on an ongoing basis, and simple bookkeeping is usually sufficient for most barbershops. One easy method is to maintain a daily account of the income and expenses of the shop. Daily income receipts can be totaled from the cash register and daily expenditures tracked by keeping receipts, invoices, and canceled checks. It should always be known how much money is coming in and where it is being spent.

The difference between the total income and the total expense is the *net profit.* A profit occurs when the income is greater than the expenses. When the expenses are greater than the income, a loss occurs. An operating budget helps to keep expenditures on track and maximizes the probability of having sufficient income to cover expenses.

Expenses common to operating a barbershop include salaries, insurance, rent, repairs, advertising, utilities, telephone, depreciation, laundry, cleaning, products and supplies, and miscellaneous items.

When transferred to a weekly or monthly summary sheet, daily records enable the owner or manager to evaluate the progress of the business. A summary sheet helps the business owner to:

- make comparisons with other years.
- detect any changes in demand for different services.
- order necessary supplies.
- check on the use of materials according to the type of service rendered.
- control expenses and waste.

Each expense item affects the total gross income. Accurate records show the cost of operation in relation to income. Keep daily sales slips, appointment books, and petty cash books for at least one year. Payroll records, canceled checks, and monthly and yearly records are usually held for seven years. Be guided by your accountant as to how long these documents should be kept.

Purchase and inventory records also are important to keep. An organized inventory system can be used to maintain a perpetual inventory, which prevents overstocking or shortage of supplies. These records also help to establish net worth at the end of the year.

Service Records

Always keep service records or client cards that describe the treatments given and merchandise sold to each client. A card file system or computer-based program kept in a central location can be used for these records. All service records should include the name and address of the client, date of each purchase or service, amount charged, product used, and results obtained. The client's preferences and tastes may also be noted for future reference.

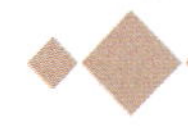

OPERATING A SUCCESSFUL BARBERSHOP

While there are many factors that contribute to the success of the business, the key to a prosperous barbershop is to "*take care of the customer.*" Excellent service, courteous attitudes, and a professional environment promote referrals and repeat business. In order to achieve these standards, the owner or manager must guide employees and the daily operations that contribute to the overall success of the shop.

Personnel

The number of employees will be determined by the barbershop's size and type. For example, a four-chair shop offering basic services such as haircuts and shaves may employ three to four barbers and be successful. The daily maintenance and sanitation duties are usually shared, as are booking appointments and ringing up monetary transactions. Conversely, a larger, higher-end, full-service shop will probably require a full-time receptionist, manicurist, or other staff to keep the operation running smoothly.

21

Since the success of the business depends largely on the quality of the work produced by the staff, consider the following when interviewing prospective employees.

- Personality and attitude
- Image and personal grooming as it relates to the barbershop environment
- Communication skills
- Level of skill
- The clients they will bring with them

Making good hiring decisions is crucial and undoing bad ones is painful to all involved. Develop a system or checklist for hiring that *grades* the job applicant in those categories that are important to the success of the shop. Design objective statements that can be evaluated with yes or no answers and/or that measure statements in terms of satisfactory, needs improvement, or unsatisfactory (Figure 21–5).

Name:			Phone:			Date:
Address:				Zip Code:		
Background Information	Yes	No	Comments	Satisfactory	Needs Improvement	Unsatisfactory
Recent graduate						
Valid Barber License						
Experienced			# of years:			
Personality/Attitude						
Projected self-confidence						
Positive & professional						
Image						
Hair appropriately styled						
Appropriate attire						
Clothing neat/clean						
Shoes neat/clean						
Nails clean/manicured						
Communication Skills						
Maintained eye contact						
Good voice pitch/tone						
Engaged in conversation						
Answered questions						
Asked relevant questions						
Level of Skill						
Performed haircut						
Performed neck shave						
Performed facial shave						
Performs chemical services:						
Permanent waves						
Reformation curls						
Chemical relaxers						
Haircoloring						
Performs women's styling						
Performs other						
Clientele						
Established						
Within range to follow						
Client contact cards viewed						
Totals						

Figure 21-5 Sample Interview Evaluation Inventory.

These distinctions become a tool that can be used in the hiring process because they focus on those areas that need discussion or attention prior to and/or after employment. For example, if a job applicant scores satisfactorily in personality, image, and communication, but is rated as "needs improvement" during the performance of a practical-skill audition, the employer now has a good indication of the assistance that the applicant requires to do the job. Based on the needs of the employer, an educated decision can now be made with a clear understanding and realistic expectations.

The decision to hire should include weighing the positive aspects of the applicant against those that may need improvement. In the preceding example, the employer may decide that since the applicant has the human relations skills so important to the business, coaching the applicant's technical skills would be time well spent for the benefit of the shop. Conversely, if the employer has just lost an employee or has more clients than his or her existing staff can effectively service, he or she may not have the time to mentor the applicant.

The sample Interview Evaluation Inventory in Figure 21–5 should be customized for your own use, but it is recommended that job applicants always perform a practical service that demonstrates their barbering skills as part of the interview process.

Managing Employees

Managing employees effectively can be a challenging experience for many new barbershop owners. As with most other aspects of business ownership, managing people is a skill that can be enhanced with knowledge and experience. Some general guidelines for effective personnel management are as follows:

- *Be honest with employees.* Make clear your expectations of employee behavior and attitude. Let employees know how and when they will be evaluated. Do not wait to give an employee feedback, whether it is positive or negative. Make sure you are both in a private area of the shop and tell him or her what you are thinking or what you have observed.
- *Expect the best.* Always give employees the benefit of the doubt and expect the best intentions from them. Never assume or immediately jump to negative conclusions. Most often, employees are simply trying to be helpful but may not know how to go about accomplishing it.
- *Be a mentor.* As the shop owner you will be viewed as an experienced veteran. Along with this comes the responsibility to help and guide whenever possible. Teach employees what you know and be willing to learn new things from them as well.
- *Share information.* Whenever possible and appropriate, share information regarding shop decisions with employees so that they become part of the process. Share your goals for the shop so that employees can help you attain them.

- *Follow the rules.* If you expect an employee to follow the rules, you must set the example and follow them as well. There should be no evidence or demonstration of double standards in the barbershop.

Benefits

The best business environment is one in which everyone feels appreciated, enjoys working hard, and strives to provide excellent service to the customers. Acknowledge and welcome staff members each day. Show a genuine interest in their well-being. One way to maintain this type of positive work environment is to share the barbershop's success whenever it is financially feasible to do so. Another way is to provide benefit opportunities through thoughtful and careful shop management.

The concept of sharing the shop's success can manifest itself in ways that range from small tokens of appreciation to professional-development opportunities. Supply employees with tickets to trade shows and educational events or schedule group activities. You might sponsor a local team, provide membership to a local gym, or make sure everyone is pictured in the promotional ad. Any method that demonstrates to employees that they are valued and appreciated will enhance the work environment and atmosphere of the barbershop. And don't forget those more simple forms of appreciation such as "thank you," "good job," or "I'm glad you're part of our team."

Employee benefits, such as health insurance or paid vacations, may or may not be financially feasible for some barbershop owners. If the owner's financial situation does not allow for covering the costs of benefits, there are small-group plans that employees may choose to purchase on their own as an alternative to paying for individual coverage.

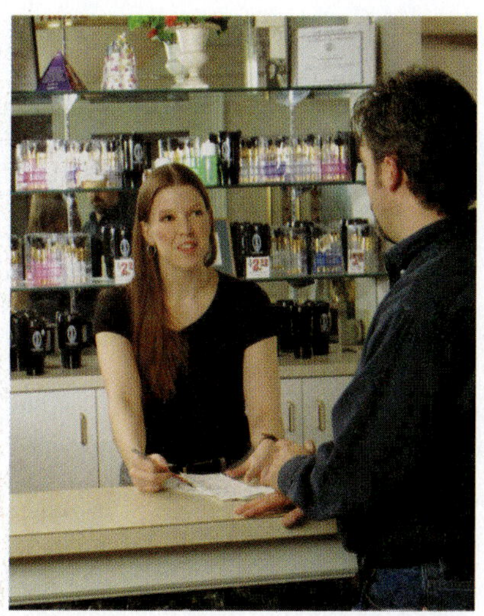

Figure 21-6 Financial transactions are often handled at the reception desk.

Other Business Operations

Pricing of Services

The cost of services is generally established according to the location of the shop and the type of clientele it services. The price list should be posted in a place where it will be seen by clients, such as the reception or checkout desk. Be sure to monitor what the competition is charging for comparable services to remain competitive with pricing.

The Reception Area

First impressions count and since the reception area is the first thing clients see, it should be attractive, appealing, and comfortable. The receptionist, phone system, and retail merchandise may be located in this area. There should be a supply of business cards with the address and phone number of the shop on the reception desk. This is also the place where the client's financial transactions are often handled (Figure 21–6). Be sure to allocate space for a cash register or computer system when designing the shop layout.

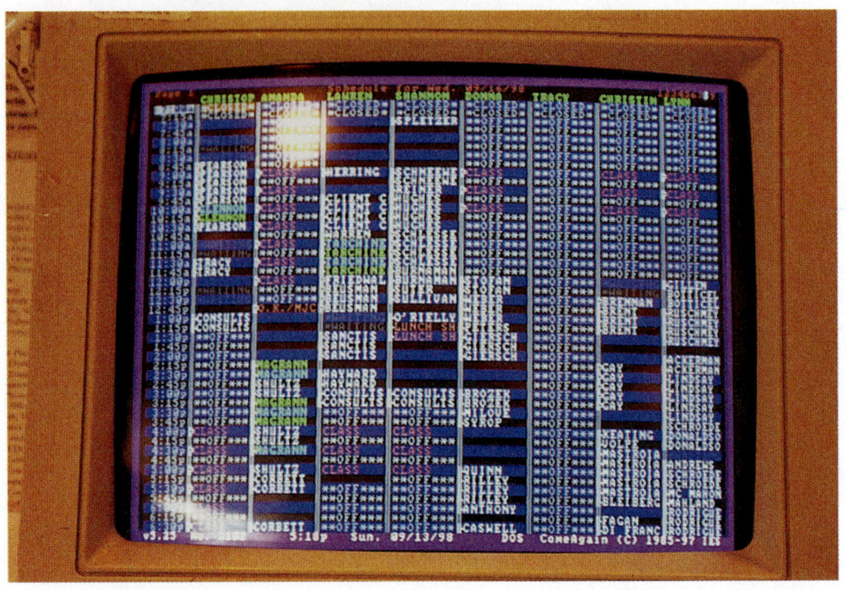

Figure 21-7 A computerized appointment book.

Booking Appointments

Booking appointments must be done with care as services are sold in terms of time on the appointment page. Appointments should be scheduled to make the most efficient use of everyone's time. Under ideal conditions, a client should not have to wait past his appointment time for a service and a barber should not have to wait for the next client. Appointment books are available in traditional heavy stock paper or computer software versions (Figure 21–7).

The size and style of the barbershop usually determines who books the appointments. Large shops often have a receptionist who books the appointments; barbers in smaller shops may book their own appointments depending on the owner's preferred procedure.

Telephone Techniques

The majority of barbershop business is handled over the telephone. Good telephone habits and techniques make it possible for shop owners and barbers to increase business. With each call to the shop, there is opportunity to build on the shop's reputation and clientele base.

During a typical workday in the barbershop, the telephone is used to:

- Make or change appointments.
- Seek new business.
- Remind clients of their appointments.
- Answer questions and render friendly service.
- Handle complaints to the client's satisfaction.
- Receive messages.
- Order equipment and supplies.

- Give directions to clients (post a small map near phones).
- Provide shop hours.
- Determine who is on staff that day.

The phone is usually located at the reception desk or near the cash register. The appointment book should be readily accessible, along with the usual desk supplies. Keep an up-to-date list of frequently called numbers and a recent telephone directory.

The shop's telephone number should be prominently displayed on stationery, advertising circulars, and in newspaper ads. Business cards should be available in the waiting area and at each station.

Good telephone etiquette requires the application of a few basic principles that add up to common sense and common courtesy. When using the telephone, follow these basic rules.

1. Answer all calls as quickly as possible.
2. Express an interested and helpful attitude. Your voice, what you say, and how you say it all make a definite impression on others.
3. Identify yourself and the shop when making or receiving a call. If the requested information is not readily available, ask the client to please hold while you get it.
4. Be tactful. Avoid saying or doing anything that may offend or irritate the caller.
   - Inquire who is calling by saying, "Who is calling, please?"
   - Address people by their last names. Use polite expressions such as *thank you, I'm sorry,* or *I beg your pardon.*
   - Avoid making side remarks or speaking to others during a call.
   - Let the caller end the conversation. Do not hang up loudly at the end of a call.

As a general rule, the most effective speech is that which is correct and at the same time natural. A cheerful, alert, and enthusiastic voice most often comes from a person who has these same personal qualities. A good telephone personality includes clear speech, correct speech patterns, and a pleasing tone of voice.

To make a good impression over the phone, assume a good posture, relax, and then draw in a deep breath before answering the phone. Pronounce words distinctly, use a low-pitched, natural voice, and speak at a moderate pace. Clear voices carry better than loud voices over the phone.

If your listeners sometimes break in with such remarks as "What was that?" or "I'm sorry, I didn't get that," it usually means that your voice is not doing its job well. Try to find out what is wrong and correct it. Some common conditions that cause problems for the person at the other end of the line are:

- Speaking too loudly or too softly
- Speaking too closely or too far away from the mouthpiece

- Speaking in very low or very high pitches
- Using incorrect pronunciation

Booking Appointments by Phone

When booking appointments, take down the client's name, phone number, and the service. You should be familiar with all the services and products available in the shop and their costs. Be fair when making appointment assignments. Do not schedule six appointments for one barber and two for another unless the client requests a particular individual. When a client requests an appointment with a specific barber, every effort should be made to accommodate the request. If the barber is not available, there are several ways to handle the situation.

- Suggest other times the barber is available.
- If the client cannot come in at any of those times, suggest another barber.
- If the client is unwilling to try another barber, offer to call the client if there is a cancellation at the desired time.

Handling Complaints by Telephone

Handling complaints, particularly over the phone, is a difficult task. The caller is probably upset and short-tempered. Respond with self-control, tact, and courtesy, no matter how trying the circumstances may be. This will reassure the client that they are being treated fairly.

Your tone of voice must be sympathetic and reassuring. Your manner of speaking should convince the caller that you are really concerned about the complaint. Do not interrupt the caller. Listen to the entire problem. After hearing the complaint in full, try to resolve the situation quickly and effectively. The following are suggestions for dealing with some problems. If other problems arise, follow the policy of the shop or check with the owner/manager for advice.

- Tell the unhappy client that you are sorry for what happened and explain the reason for the difficulty. Tell the client that the problem will not happen again.
- Sympathize with the client by saying that you understand and that you regret the inconvenience suffered. Express thanks that the person called this matter to your attention.
- Ask the client how the shop can remedy the situation. If the request is fair and reasonable, check with the owner or manager for approval.
- If the client is dissatisfied with the results of a service, suggest a visit to the shop to see what can be done to remedy the problem.
- If a client is dissatisfied with the behavior of a particular barber, call the owner or manager to the phone.

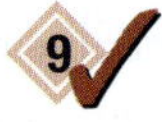

The Business Venture Checklist in Figure 21–8 serves as a basic guideline for aspiring barbershop owners. It is not meant to be completely

CHECKLIST	ACTION	RESULTS	✔
Capital			
Amount available			
Amount required			
Organization			
Individual			
Partnership			
Corporation			
Banking			
Bank Accounts			
Business Plan			
Checks			
Monthly Statements			
Notes and Drafts			
Location			
Area Businesses			
Parking			
Population			
Public Transportation			
Quality of Area			
Signage			
Space Required			
Traffic (drive/walk)			
Zoning			
Layout/Renovation			
Cabinetry			
Design Plan			
Electrical Outlets			
Entrance/Exits			
Exterior Painting			
Floor Covering			
Interior Painting			
Laundry Area (optional)			
Lighting			
Mirrors			
Plumbing			
Reception Area			
Retail Area			
Shampoo Area (optional)			
Shampoo Bowls/Sinks			
Square Footage			
Storage Area			
Telephone Installation			
Toilet Facilities			
Window Placement			
Window Signage			
Workstations			
Equipment/Furnishings			
Barber Chairs			
Coat Rack			
Computer			
Electric Sanitizers			
Fire Extinguisher			
Reception Desk/Counter			
Reception Furniture			
Retail Display			
Trash Receptacles			
Products/Supplies			
Back-bar Products			
Business Cards			
Cleaning Products			

Figure 21-8 Business Venture Checklist.

CHECKLIST	ACTION	RESULTS	✔
Cleaning Tools			
Disinfectants			
Office Supplies			
Paper Goods			
Retail Products			
Services Products			
Record-Keeping System			
Appointment Books			
Computer Software			
Disbursements			
Inventory			
Invoices			
Petty Cash			
Profit and Loss			
Receipts			
Advertising			
Marketing Strategy			
Selection of Media			
Track Coupon Strategies			
Legal			
Business License			
Claims and Liens			
Contracts (other)			
Labor Law Compliance			
Lease/Purchase Contract			
Operational License			
State Board Compliance			
Tax Compliance			
Unemployment			
Wages/Compensation			
Insurance			
Fire, Theft, & Burglary			
Health/Disability			
Liability			
Malpractice			
Management			
Business Reputation			
Community Outreach			
Daily Operations			
Disputes/Complaints			
Employee Hire/Fire			
Ethics/Standards			
Promotions (marketing)			
Monthly Budget			
Advertising			
Depreciation			
Rent/Mortgage			
Repairs			
Services (laundry, etc.)			
Supplies/Products			
Taxes			
Wages			
Methods of Payment			
C.O.D.			
In Advance			
On Account			
Time Payments			

Figure 21-8 (Continued).

inclusive of all the tasks or items that need attention in the start-up of a business, but it should point you in the right direction. The checklist may also serve as a self-assessment instrument that can be used to determine specific areas that require further study before committing to the responsibilities of business ownership.

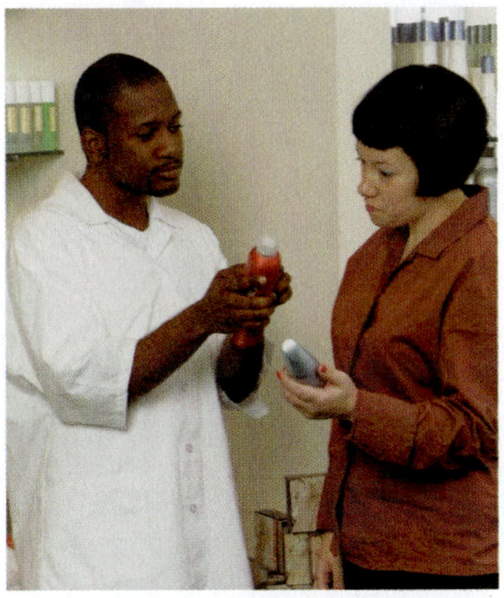

Figure 21-9 Selling retail products benefits everyone.

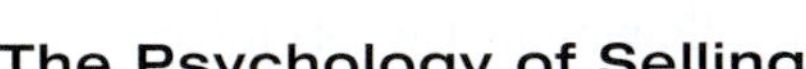

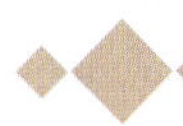

SELLING IN THE BARBERSHOP

The success of any barbershop is based on the professional skill and selling ability of its personnel. Revenue is derived from both the performance of the services offered and the sale of grooming aids. The ability of the professional barber to sell additional services and grooming supplies can greatly influence earnings and enables clients to maintain the look you worked hard to achieve (Figure 21–9).

The Psychology of Selling

Successful selling requires a clear and definite understanding of the client's needs and desires. It does not matter how good a service or a grooming aid may be—unless the client feels a need for it, there will be no sale. To close a sale, the client must perceive the service or product as necessary. Usually this simply requires an explanation of the benefits for clarification and understanding. A hard-sell approach should never be used.

Some motivational factors for purchasing services or products are based on a desire to:

- Improve appearance.
- Improve social relationships.
- Retain one's appearance.
- Get the most value for the money.
- Feel good.

Clients usually resent high-pressure selling tactics and care must be taken to avoid creating antagonism instead of confidence. The approach should be subtle, friendly, honest, and sincere to encourage the client's confidence in the barber's judgment. Remember, barbering services may be obtained in many places, but the personality behind the service is what brings the client back.

21

Selling Services

The barber's professional image can influence and arouse a client's interest in other styling and grooming services. He or she should be a living example of the services and products available in the shop. For example, if the barber wears a hairpiece, his client may feel more confident about trying one as well. If the barber uses a particular shampoo or tonic on the back bar, the client will be more inclined to purchase a bottle from the retail display on his or her way out.

To sell additional services to clients, the barber must be aware of each service, know how to perform it, and be able to explain the benefits to be derived from it.

The client usually considers the barber to be an expert in good grooming and looks to him or her for suggestions and advice. It is the responsibility of the barber to be well informed on all grooming matters so that when advice is asked for, it is correct and appropriate.

Tips on Selling Services

- *New Cuts and Styles:* Tactfully suggest changes that will keep your clients current with modern trends. Have pictures and posters available for easy reference.
- *Facials:* As you cut your client's hair, notice the condition of his or her skin and tactfully suggest one of the following facials: plain facial, dry skin, oily skin, or acne.
- *Mustache and Beard Trims:* If the client wears a mustache and/or beard, the best policy is to ask if he would like a trim. Some clients prefer to trim their own facial hair while others expect the barber to offer the service. This policy should be followed in regards to trimming ear and nose hair as well.
- *Shampoo Service:* Today, most barbershops and salons include a shampoo as part of the haircutting service. Clean hair facilitates greater precision in cutting and styling and helps to maintain sanitation standards in the shop.
- *Scalp Treatments:* A scalp and hair analysis should be performed before every haircut. Treatments for normal maintenance and for dry, oily, dandruff, and alopecia conditions should be available in the barbershop. Explain the benefits of the recommended treatment to the client.
- *Hair Treatments:* Suggest deep conditioning, bluing, temporary color, or dandruff rinses whenever it is appropriate for the condition of the client's hair.
- *Chemical Texture Services:* Permanent waves, reformation curls, texturizers, and chemical hair relaxers can provide clients with minimal to drastic hair texture changes. Educate clients about the advantages, disadvantages, and maintenance requirements of these "permanent" services. Remember, chemical changes to the hair can't be shampooed out. When discussing the option of a permanent wave with a client, offer to "set" the hair on perm rods to help the client envision the finished look. Offer the potential relaxer client a hair-pressing service to envision straight hair or a texturizing process that will gradually ease him or her through the transition of changing from curly to straight hair.

- *Hair Coloring:* Clients with gray hair may welcome the suggestion of a color rinse that would match their client's natural shade and that can be rinsed out if not satisfactory. Mention that there will be a charge only if the rinse is left on. A client liking the temporary rinse may choose a semipermanent or permanent color service for a future appointment.
- *Hairpieces:* Many of the hairpieces available today are so natural looking that even barbers may have a hard time distinguishing between a toupee and a natural head of hair.

For barbers who wear hairpieces, specializing in hairpiece sales is a perfect spin-off of their professional skills and experience with artificial hair. Barbers who do not wear hairpieces, but would like to provide them for their customers nonetheless, can utilize subtle marketing techniques such as displaying a toupee on a mannequin head or advertising posters from the hairpiece supplier.

Selling Grooming Supplies

The sale of grooming aids and supplies should go hand in hand with the sale of services. The purchase of such items as shaving creams, powders, lotions, and styling aids is a natural extension of the barbershop as the center of and source for good grooming.

Shops should maintain an assortment of quality grooming aids to meet the demands and tastes of their clients. When clean, tasteful display cabinets are placed in strategic areas in the shop, little additional effort is required to call a client's attention to the variety of grooming supplies available.

The barber should be able to explain the qualities and benefits of the retail products sold in the shop. Some clients want to know every detail about a product and others just want to know if it works. In either case, barbers need to understand the purpose and contents of the products and their effects on the hair or skin. When barbers provide accurate purchasing advice to clients, the sale of one item inevitably leads to the sale of others on a regular basis.

Display cabinets should always be maintained and well dusted. Update with new items and periodically create more client interest by changing the displays to reflect holidays, sports seasons, or new styling trends.

A well-equipped barbershop with an interest in promoting retail sales should have a variety of grooming supplies available for their clients, such as shaving supplies, lotions and tonics, shampoos, conditioners, styling aids, mustache and beard supplies, hairpiece supplies, and hair supplies.

- *Shaving supplies:* razors, blades, shaving creams, lather brushes and mugs, preshave lotion, and aftershave lotion
- *Lotions and tonics:* facial cleansers, moisturizing lotion, toners, Bay Rum, hair tonics, astringents, and sunscreens

chapter glossary

booth rental	also known as chair rental; renting a booth or station in a barbershop or salon
business plan	a written plan for a business as it is seen in the present and envisioned in the future
capital	the money needed to start a business
corporation	business ownership shared by three or more people called stockholders
demographics	information about the size, population, average income, etc., of a given area
franchise	business ownership in which there is brand name recognition, support, group purchasing, and ongoing training for self and staff
independent contractor	someone who is self-employed and responsible for their own bookkeeping, taxes, insurances, etc.
partnership	business structure in which two or more people share ownership, although not necessarily equally
sole proprietor	single owner and manager of a business
target market	the group that has been identified as the desired clientele and to which marketing and advertising efforts will be directed

chapter review questions

1. Identify two ways a barber may be employed as an independent contractor in the barbershop.
2. Define booth rental.
3. List and define four types of ownership under which a business may operate.
4. List 12 tasks that need to be performed before opening a barbershop.
5. Define established barbershop business.
6. Describe the best location for a barbershop.
7. What is the best form of advertising?
8. Explain the value of summary sheets.
9. Identify two ways in which revenue is generated in the barbershop.
10. Explain why product knowledge is important to successful retail sales.

Learning Objectives

After completing this chapter, you should be able to:

1. **Discuss industry positions available for barbering students.**
2. **Explain the guidelines of goal setting.**
3. **List and discuss personal characteristics important to employment.**
4. **Compare three common wage structures.**
5. **Write a résumé and compile a portfolio.**

Key Terms

commission
pg. 655

cover letter
pg. 657

Model Release Form
pg. 658

portfolio
pg. 657

résumé
pg. 656

This chapter has been provided to assist you in your search for employment in the barbering field. Unlike many other job markets that may have more applicants than positions available, the *need* for barbers and barbershops has actually been on a steady increase since the 1970s. While there may be some who would argue with this statement, a short historical perspective may change their minds and provide you with a context from which to view your own future in barbering.

INDUSTRY TRENDS: THEN AND NOW

Prior to the Vietnam War, the Beatles, and the hippie generation of the 1960s, most average-sized towns had at least one, if not two or three, barbershops. Many of these shops were what might be thought of as the traditional barbershop with 4 to 10 chairs, leather strops hanging at the side, and hair tonics situated in front of the mirror. Some shops did not have shampoo bowls or even offer the service and the majority of haircuts were performed on dry hair. Phrases such as "just a trim" or "a little off the top" were commonly heard instructions from customers.

While there were certainly exceptions to the stereotypical barbershops just described, the majority of high-end barbershops or barbering salons were usually located in cities. It should be understood that 40-plus years ago, today's thriving suburbs, which abut each other and link cities to rural areas in many parts of the country, started out as little more than isolated villages and towns with populations of about 30,000 people. Independently owned businesses, from drugstores and bakeries to banks, butcher shops, and beauty parlors, were the norm. Chain and franchise salons were virtually nonexistent.

Most of the larger corporations and businesses were located in the cities, which had the population to support the higher-end barbershops and salons. Busy executives and professional people were more apt to indulge in shampoo, manicure, facial, or chemical services on a regular basis, in addition to their cuts, shaves, or beard trims. As the suburbs grew, more of these shops could be found in the outlying areas, but they were still few and far between in terms of distance and the inclination to offer a full range of services.

The impact of the long-hair trend generated by musicians and social groups of the 1960s and early 1970s was felt in the traditional barbershops. Some barbers chose not to adapt their skills to the long-hair look and lost customers as a result. While it is true that many young people allowed their hair to grow long without any form or design, there were others who preferred a longer but more controlled look. This look necessitated a different method of cutting and styling, which included preliminary shampoos, more precision cutting of the interior sections of the hair, and blow-drying. At about the same time, unisex salons were introduced and began to capitalize on the longer-hair market. The barbershop's clientele began to dwindle and fewer young people were studying to be barbers. This is also about the time that certain social and industry factions generated the notion that "barbers and barbering are a thing of the past," regardless of whether it was true or not.

Eventually, with fewer young barbers to take their place, some veteran barbers retired and simply closed the doors to their shops. Conversely, younger barbers who enhanced their skills to include new techniques that would satisfy the haircutting needs of their clients are still in business today. As this group now prepares for retirement, new barbers are needed to replace them.

From the 1970s through the 1990s, unisex salons garnered much of the male market and this has resulted in entire generations of males who are more familiar with unisex and beauty salons than with barbershops. Fortunately for the next generation of barbers, of which you are a part, the cycle has gone full circle and men are again seeking out barbershops for their personal grooming services.

The male baby boomer, who is now in his 50s or 60s, craves a return to the shops he knew while growing up. He does not want to be surrounded by the smell of acrylics or chemicals. He wants to feel comfortable and secure in a male domain when he has a haircut or manicure. Young men are wearing shorter styles to the point of fades, military cuts, and shaved heads. These styles require the expertise of a barber and the industry knows it. Barbers are in demand in barbershops, unisex salons, and even in some beauty shops. Check the classifieds from any average-size newspaper and it is likely that you will see a help-wanted ad for a barber or barber-stylist.

The preceding historical perspective should help to explain why it is accurate to say that the *need* for barbers and barbershops has actually been on a steady increase since the 1970s. At that time, the profession needed barbers who could adapt to new trends. The profession needed barbers to maintain and offer an alternative to unisex and beauty salons for men's hair care. The profession now needs barbershops that have been designed to meet the expectations and service requirements of a variety of male preferences, from traditional shops and high-end salons to upbeat and trendy motifs. The profession needs barbers who will pass along their skills and the standards of the profession to others as teachers, state board members, and association leaders. The profession needs skilled artisans who challenge the skill of others in friendly competition at hair and trade shows. The profession needs lobbyists to protect the barbering profession and its future. The profession has needed new and young barbers to replace retiring practitioners all along.

The need is there. How you choose to fulfill that need is your future.

PREPARING FOR EMPLOYMENT

At this stage in your barbering education you probably have some ideas as to where you would like to work upon graduation and licensure. Depending on the state barber board regulations in your state, some students in the class may already be working in a barbershop or styling salon as a receptionist, assistant, or manicurist. When students take advantage of opportunities to work in a barbershop while still in school, they are engaging in valuable learning experiences that will prove beneficial when entering the profession full-time. Participation in the actual day-to-day operations of a shop or salon benefits students by providing the following:

- Exposure to the overall duties, responsibilities, and services of the shop
- Understanding of individual tasks and responsibilities of shop personnel
- Experience in communicating with clients and coworkers
- Experience in perfecting customer service skills
- Observation of advanced services, techniques, and skills
- Familiarity with shop procedures and standards
- Opportunity to lay the foundation for future employment
- Financial gain

If you are not quite sure where you will be working in the near future, think about what you really want out of your career, the services you prefer to perform, and the work environment in which you see yourself as most comfortable. Visit area shops and salons with the intention of finding the right atmosphere and environment for your personality and skills. This journey should not be considered solely as a job hunt, but rather as an exploration of available options. At this stage you should simply explore those options and decide which are the most suitable for you.

Preparing for employment also includes other practical applications such as goal setting, participation in professional activities, résumé writing, and the development of a portfolio. 1

Goal Setting

The topic of goal setting was discussed in Chapter 1. Now it is time to put those plans into motion to achieve your goals in the barbering profession. Review the following guidelines in preparation for this professional journey.

- *Be realistic.* Too often expectations are set so high that regardless of the outcome, the reality is a disappointment. For example, it is unrealistic to expect that a newly licensed barber will be booked solid during his or her first week of employment. Be realistic when planning goals.
- *"Look before you leap"* is an old but accurate expression. Apply this principle whenever a major decision has to be made. Be cautious in business dealings and always seek legal counsel when contracts are involved.

- *Keep an open mind.* Doing so can create more opportunities and probable successes. Personal and professional growth can be the result of keeping an open mind in a field that is technically and professionally advancing each year. There is always something new to learn, new interests to develop, and new roads to explore.
- *Be flexible.* Timing can be extremely important and being flexible will help you to adjust to the circumstances of life. Time and timing, combined with realistic goals and expectations, may produce a very workable plan that allows you to realize your full potential in a steady progression of insight, experience, and skill.
- *Believe in yourself.* Realize that with a realistic approach, flexibility, and an open mind, goals can be achieved. 

Participation

There will be many opportunities while still in school to attend special events relating to barbering that can help prepare you for employment. Attendance at trade shows and educational seminars enhances a student's product knowledge, technical skill, and overall understanding of the industry. In addition, trade shows are fun, stimulating, and a good way to get a feel for the profession. Seminars are offered on a myriad of subjects and topics and platform demonstrations educate in the hands-on arena.

Becoming a member of an industry association or organization on a student level is one of the best ways of getting involved. Trade organizations are usually involved in all aspects of the profession, including the hosting of trade shows and the representation of the industry in legislative circles. The benefits to a student of membership in such groups may include discounted trade show and educational tickets, student competitions, leadership training, and other related interests.

Student competitions offer yet another opportunity for students to experience a thrilling aspect of the profession. Competitions may be sponsored by barber schools, vocational or professional organizations; distributors, manufacturers, and suppliers; or other educational groups. Participation in competition hones the student's professional image, skills, and sense of self-esteem while laying the foundation for future professional performance.

Your school also may offer other opportunities for self-growth and industry awareness. Many instructors use students as teachers' aides. The duties vary and may include office or classroom assistance, either of which will be noted and appreciated by the instructor and create a learning experience for the student. If your school does not have such a program, consider approaching your instructor with the idea.

Participation in any of the preceding or similar activities is of value to a potential employer. It indicates a student's initiative and interest in the profession. Such activities also may indicate a student's willingness to be a team player, the ability to be a leader, or the drive of an achiever. Keep a record of the dates and descriptions of all your participation activities to include on your résumé.

Personal Characteristics

There are several key personal characteristics that will help you get the job you want and keep it. Review the following characteristics and make a mental note of your personal strengths and those that may need enhancement.

- *Motivation* is the drive necessary to take action to achieve a goal. Externally motivated goals may produce results, but internally driven motivation is the most fulfilling and long-lasting.
- *Integrity* is a strong commitment to a code of morals and values. It is the compass that guides you in everything you say and do.
- *Technical and communication skills* must be developed to reach the level of desired success. About 80 percent of your success will depend on communication and people skills; the remaining 20 percent will be based on technical skills.
- *Strong work ethics* are demonstrated by a belief that work is good and by a commitment to delivering quality service for the value received from your employer.
- *Enthusiasm* demonstrates your passion for what you are doing and is contagious in a very positive way.
- *Your attitude* is one of the strongest marketing tools you possess. The other is your personality. Your attitude affects other people and the way in which you view life in general. A positive attitude generates a positive response in those you meet and is easily seen by potential employers (Figure 22–1). 3

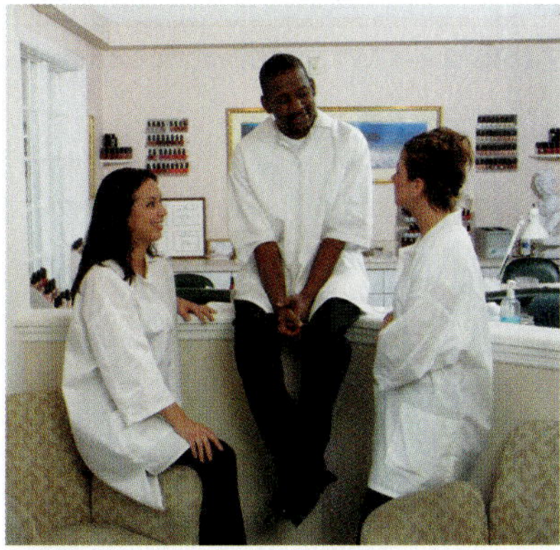

Figure 22-1 A positive attitude is contagious.

Wages and Salaries

The way in which you will be paid for services performed in the barbershop depends on whether you rent a chair (booth rental) or are paid on commission. As discussed in Chapter 21, booth or chair rental involves paying the shop owner a fixed amount of rent for the space. All the fees brought in from the performance of services are basically yours after paying for the rent and supplies. **Commission** wages may be paid as a straight percentage of the total fees taken in for services or may begin with a base salary (also known as a *guarantee*) with a percentage of the amount over the base added to it for a total wage. Using Table 22–1, compare the differences between booth rental, commission only, and a guarantee with commission wage structure based on total service fees of $500. Although commission percentages vary from shop to shop (40 percent to 70 percent), the 70 percent commission rate that was once a union barber's standard commission may still be available in some barbershops.

Booth rental		Commission only @ 70%		Guarantee w/ 70% Commission	
Wage	$500.00	Wage	$500.00	Wage	$500.00
Rent	−125.00		× 70%	Guarantee	−125.00
Supplies/Taxes	−50.00		= $350.00		= $375.00
	= $325.00				× 70%
					= $262.50
					+125.00
Total wage	$325.00	Total wage	$350.00	Total wage	$387.50

Table 22-1 Wage Structure Comparison

The Résumé

A **résumé** is a written summary of your education, work experience, and achievements. While there are many different types of résumé formats that can be customized to suit your needs (Figure 22–2), some basic guidelines are as follows:

- Include your name, address, phone number, and e-mail address on both the résumé and the cover letter.
- List work experience and education information in chronological order from the most recent activities to the past.
- State your objective. Make sure it is relevant to the job.
- Limit the résumé to one page whenever possible and print on high-quality paper.
- Correct grammar, punctuation, and indentation should always be used.
- Include the name of educational institutions from which you have graduated.
- List your abilities and accomplishments.
- Focus on information that is relevant to the position you are seeking.
- Add numbers and percentages when appropriate to expand on your accomplishments.
- List awards, special commendations, and honors.
- Use action verbs such as *achieved, designed, developed,* etc., to begin accomplishment statements.

Name
Address
Phone Number E-Mail

Objective:

Experience:

Accomplishments:

Special Projects:

Honors & Awards:

Education:

Figure 22-2 Sample résumé format.

- Make it easy to read using clear, concise sentences.
- Emphasize transferable skills mastered at other jobs that can be used in a new position.

The **cover letter** should be used to introduce yourself to the employer and to reference the position you are seeking. It also provides an opportunity to expand on specific accomplishments that were only briefly mentioned in the résumé.

The Portfolio

A **portfolio** is a collection of photographs depicting your ability to provide hair care services. The concept of creating a portfolio for the purpose of marketing a skill or talent is not new to individuals in the fields of art, photography, and modeling. Until recently, however, its application to the barber's job search has been almost nonexistent.

The presentation of a portfolio is a graphic way to demonstrate your full range of talent, creativity, and skill to a prospective employer. Therefore, it should contain before-and-after photos of your work (Figure 22–3).

As a marketing tool, a portfolio should represent a barber's best work. Consider keeping an inexpensive camera and film in your kit. After

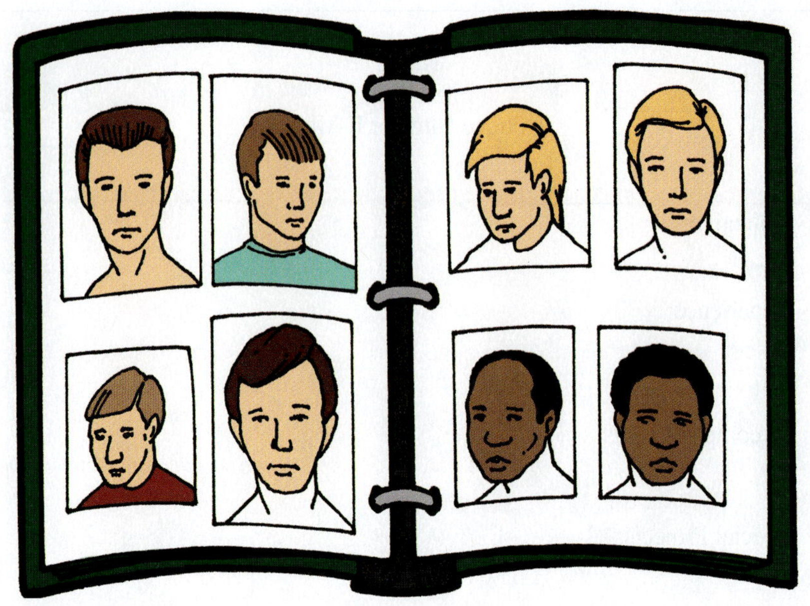

Figure 22-3 Before-and-after photos in a portfolio.

obtaining the client's permission, take before-and-after photographs of your work. Keep a log of the dates, names, and services performed so that the pictures can be labeled. To avoid the possibility of any future complaints or conflicts, ask the client to sign a **Model Release Form** or waiver (Figure 22–4).

5

Where To Look

Your school is one of the best places to begin a job search. Most barber schools maintain contact with shops and salons and post openings at a central location in the school.

Use all the resources available to locate shops and salons in your area, including:

- Fellow students and instructors
- Suppliers who visit the school
- Distributor seminars and classes
- Trade shows

22

MODEL RELEASE FORM

I, ________________, hereby grant permission to ________________, student barber, to photograph the hair services rendered to me on ________________ for the purpose of creating a portfolio of his/her work.

Figure 22-4 Sample Model Release Form.

- Newspaper classified section
- Telephone book (yellow pages)

Field Research

Field research should actually be used for several purposes: first, to become familiar with the types of barbershops that are in the area; next, to help you determine the type of shop that you would like to work in; and lastly, to search for a position as a barber.

Once you have targeted several shops to visit, contact the owners or managers by telephone. Introduce yourself and explain that you are preparing to graduate from barber school and that you would appreciate being allowed to visit the shop. Any mutual contacts you have can also be mentioned at this time. For example, if good old Uncle Charlie is one of the shop's customers, explain that he suggested you visit the shop because he always gets a good haircut there. This puts networking on a very personal level and you'll probably end up with an open invitation to visit.

Field research can also lead to a job that you might not have known was available. Many times there will be a simple "Barber Wanted" sign in the window that would have been missed if you had relied solely on printed ads in the newspaper.

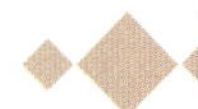

THE EMPLOYMENT INTERVIEW

Arranging the Interview

After you have passed your state board examinations, you will be ready to pursue a position in the barbershops targeted in the field research. The next step is to contact the establishments that you are interested in by sending them a résumé with a cover letter that requests an interview. Make sure that you offer to bring a model so that the owner can observe your technical skills.

In the event that you do not get a response from sending out a résumé, you may have to make some cold-call visits to barbershops. Although this may not seem to be the most desirable way to seek a position, it can work. Remember to have your résumé and barber's license with you, just in case.

Interview Preparation

Job hunting and interviewing is a familiar exercise for most people. The unfamiliar element is that you are seeking a position as a barber. A review of the material on professional image in Chapter 3 should serve as a reminder of the qualities that a shop owner or manager is looking for in an employee. Many employers require job applicants to perform a haircut or other services on a live model. This is a standard practice so don't feel intimidated by it.

Another way in which you can prepare for the interview is to have all your support materials in one place. This includes identification, licensing information, the résumé, your portfolio, and the employment application if available (Figures 22–5 and 22–6). Be prepared to answer questions about your skills and abilities, including how you might handle a difficult client or provide excellent customer service. Think about the questions you would like answered before making the decision to work there.

The Interview

On the day of the interview, dress for success and make sure that your attire is clean, pressed, and appropriate for an interview. Be aware that there are certain behaviors that should be demonstrated during the interview itself.

- Be prompt.
- Carry yourself with good posture.
- Be courteous, be polite, and smile.
- Speak clearly.
- Answer questions honestly.
- Do not bring food or drinks to the interview.
- Never criticize former employers.
- Remember to say *thank you* at the end of the interview.

When you are invited to ask questions of the interviewer, consider the following:

- Does the shop advertise regularly?
- What form of compensation is used?
- What is the procedure for walk-in customers?
- Is there customer overflow and will they be directed to my chair?
- Shall I call you or will you contact me with your decision?

Other factors that an applicant needs to consider are as follows:

- Wage percentage scale
- Pay schedule
- Percentage scale for retail sales
- Benefits (health, life, and dental insurance)
- Sick leave/vacation policies
- Dress code
- Equipment and supplies provided by the shop
- Hours of operation
- New-client policies

EMPLOYMENT APPLICATION

Applicants are considered for all positions, and employees are treated during employment without regard to race, color, religion, sex, national origin, age, marital or veteran status, medical condition, or handicap.

PERSONAL INFORMATION

SS#__________ Phone __________ Date __________

Last name __________ First __________ Middle __________

Present street address City State Zip

Permanent street address City State Zip

If related to anyone employed here, state name: __________

Referred to barbershop by: __________

EMPLOYMENT DESIRED

Position __________

Date you can start __________ Salary Desired __________

Current Employer __________

May we contact? __________

Ever applied with this company before? __________ Where? __________ When? __________

EDUCATION

Name/location of School	Years Completed	Subjects Studied

Subject of special study or research work:

What foreign languages do you speak fluently?

Read fluently: __________

Write fluently: __________

US Military Service Rank Present Membership

In Nat'l Guard/Reserve

Figure 22-5 Employment application form.

Activities (other than religious): Civic, Athletic, Fraternal, etc. (Exclude organizations for which the name or character might indicate race, creed, color, or national origin of its members.)

FORMER EMPLOYMENT

List below last four employers, beginning with the most recent one first.

DATE: Month/Year	Name, Address of Employer	Salary	Position	Reason for Leaving
From: To:				
From: To:				
From: To:				
From: To:				

REFERENCES

Give below the names of three persons not related to you whom you have known at least one year.

Name	Address	Business	Years Known

PHYSICAL RECORD

Please list any defects in hearing, vision, or speech that might affect your job performance.

In case of emergency, please notify:

Name Address Telephone

I authorize investigation of all statements contained in this application. I understand that misrepresentation or omission of facts called for is cause for dismissal if hired.

Signature ______________________ Date ______________

Figure 22-6 Employment application form, continued.

22

Legal Aspects of the Interview

Questions that *may not* be included in an employment application or interview include:

- Race, religion, and national origin
- Citizenship status
- Disabilities or physical traits
- Marital status
- Height and weight
- Arrest record
- Sexual orientation

Questions that *may* be asked include those related to drug use, convictions for a crime, or smoking. Age is usually avoided in an interview unless it is needed to verify that the candidate meets the minimum age requirement for the job. Employers are permitted to ask whether an applicant is over the age of 18 and, if not, whether they can provide work papers. To find out more information, check with your state and federal employment law offices or the *Equal Employment Opportunity Commission* (EEOC).

It is hoped that this chapter has provided you with some innovative ideas and useful suggestions for your job search in the field of barbering. Good luck and happy job hunting!

chapter glossary

commission	a certain percentage of the fees charged for services that become the employee's wages
cover letter	a letter attached to a résumé that introduces the person to the employer and references the position being sought
Model Release Form	form used to permit the use of a model's pictures for print or exposure
portfolio	collection of photographs depicting the barber's work
résumé	written summary of a person's education and work experience

chapter review questions

1. List the textbook guidelines for setting personal and professional goals.
2. List potential shop or salon positions available to student barbers.
3. List three common wage structures.
4. Identify two marketing tools that require preparation.
5. Define résumé, cover letter, and portfolio.

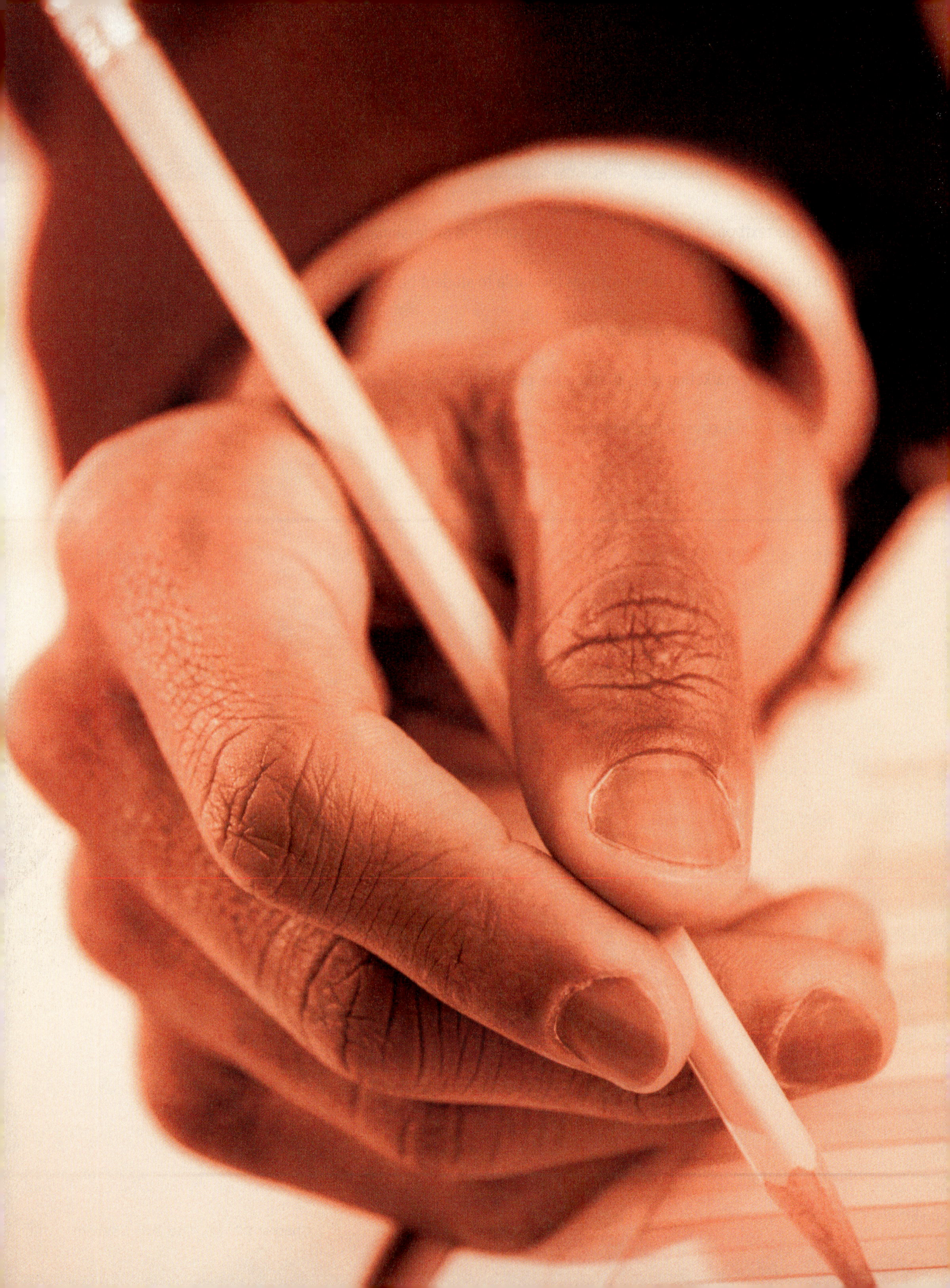

STATE BOARD PREPARATION AND LICENSING LAWS

Chapter Outline

Preparing for State Board Exams

State Barber Board Rules and Regulations

Question 4: What should the hair from the nape to the occipital area look like when projected at 90 degrees from a vertical parting?

a) Longer at the nape; shorter at the occipital
b) A 45-degree angle from nape to occipital; shorter at the nape, longer at the occipital
c) Uniform layers
d) Increased layers

Answer: B, because the hair will be shorter at the hairline and gradually increase in length as the occipital area is reached. In order to hold a vertical parting of hair at 90 degrees in this scenario, the finger placement will be angled at 45 degrees from the longer occipital area to the shorter hair at the nape.

Practical Exams

After completing the barber school curriculum, examination candidates should be competent in their technical skills and ready for state board **practical exams.** Although performance criteria for practical examinations vary from state to state, the basic skills or procedures that are usually evaluated are: haircutting, shaving, shampooing, sanitation, and possibly a chemical service. A fairly standard testing protocol requires candidates to demonstrate competence with the comb, shears, razor, and clippers. Safety precautions, proper draping procedures, and the safe handling of tools are also common performance standards.

Practical exams require a different approach than written exams because you have to perform the procedures. After all, performing services is what barbering is all about and practical exams are the best way to evaluate a person's competency in barbering techniques.

Basic preparation for practical exams should always include practice on the model who you will be taking to the examination. To feel confident about your performance, you must be familiar with the model's hair texture and the haircut that you will be performing. Many states require a taper hair cut (Figure 23–3) and knowing the characteristics of your model's hair and the best techniques for cutting it will help to eliminate some nervousness and stress during the practical exam. When practicing for practical exams, make sure to:

- set up your station as if you were at the state board examinations.
- ensure that all tools and implements are sanitary and in good working order.
- practice all sanitation procedures, including hand washing.
- time yourself.
- request feedback from instructors and the model.
- be clear about what examiners will check and look for in the performance of procedures.

23

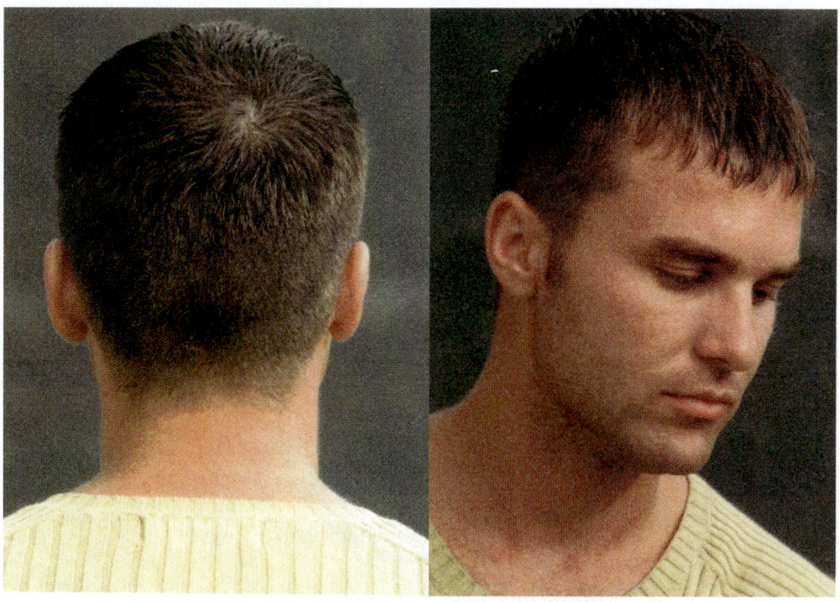

Figure 23-3 One variation of a taper cut.

- read your state board rules and regulations to find specific exam information.
- review the candidate information booklet for specifics about practical testing.

If the correct procedures for performing the services of your state's practical exam are not already second nature to you, it is time for some honest reflection and self-assessment.

Begin by envisioning yourself at the test site. Your model is in place and the lead examiner has given the signal to begin. What do you do first? Next? Think through all the steps of all the procedures and then write each step down on a piece of paper (Figure 23–4). During the next haircut or other practice exam procedure that you perform, use the list for reference. Pretend that you are at the exam and follow as many of the procedures as the situation allows, for example, washing your hands, draping procedures, sanitizing tools, or deciding at what section of the head you will begin the haircut. Refer to your list and make notes as necessary. Revise the list as you notice steps that were left out or overlooked.

23

Preliminary Planning for Practical Exams

Model

In addition to studying and practicing for state board examinations, most barbering test candidates will have to arrange to bring a model for their practical exams. This is not an arrangement that can be left to the last minute and, ideally, you should have been practicing on this model for several months. Several weeks before the test date, confirm the date, time, and travel arrangements with your model. Turn the trip to the examinations into a shared adventure and schedule time to have a celebration breakfast, lunch,

Practical Exam–Haircut Procedure Plan

After given the signal to begin, I will:

Set up tools and linens
Sanitize tools
Wash hands
Drape model for shampoo
Perform shampoo and towel dry the hair
Store soiled linen
Remove shampoo cape and store
Drape model for haircut
Wash hands
Rinse sanitized comb
Start haircut at the top
Proceed with haircut
Shake off cape and remove neckstrip
Drape for outline shave
Perform outline shave
Store soiled linen
Comb model's hair
Wash tools and return to sanitizer
Wash hands and indicate completion of test

Figure 23–4 Sample procedure plan.

or dinner. Plan to see some local attractions after the exams. Reward yourself. You've earned it!

Travel

Arrange any travel plans that need to be made if you are testing in a city other than your own. If you have to travel out of town, consider arriving the day before your exams and staying overnight. This will give you the opportunity to find the location of the test site and reduce the risk of arriving late or getting lost. It should also avail you of a good night's sleep since you won't have a great distance to travel the day of your exams.

Packing

Create a checklist of tools, implements, and equipment that you will need for the practical exams. Have your instructor review the list to make sure it is complete or compare it to the **candidate information booklet** that most states send out when application for examination is made. Make sure that all of your tools are thoroughly cleaned and sanitized. If the written exams are paper tests, bring several sharpened pencils.

Health

Make a conscious effort to eat well and get sufficient rest several days before and up to the examination date. Vitamin supplements can help to give you a nutritional edge when nervous or under stress. Relax. Trust in yourself and do your best. 1

STATE BARBER BOARD RULES AND REGULATIONS

Although state barber board rules and regulations may vary from state to state, the basic concept and functions of state barber boards remain the same: to protect the health, safety, and welfare of the public as it relates to the practice of barbering (Table 23–1). Be guided by your instructor and the specific rules and regulations of your state. The following statements are designed to review these general concepts and functions.

1. The governing body that is responsible for the efficient and orderly administration of barbering rules and regulations is the *state barber board or other board that governs the profession.*
2. The authority to *conduct disciplinary hearings* rests with the state barber board.
3. Additional authority that is given to the state barber board in order to properly administer barber license law is the *power to issue rules and regulations.*
4. The primary objective of the barber license law is to *protect the health, safety, and welfare of the public* as it relates to the practice of babering.
5. The *governor* of the state appoints barber board members.
6. The *state senate* confirms the appointment of barber board members.
7. The state barber board regulates *educational requirements, testing, licensing, inspections, investigations, and disciplinary action.*
8. The objective of barber license examinations is to evaluate a license applicant's *competency.*
9. State barber board rules and regulations *may not* be used to limit the number of licenses or licensees.
10. An important personal requirement for a barber license applicant is to be of *good moral character.*
11. Barbers may be forbidden to perform services on clients when the barber is suffering from a *communicable disease.*
12. State barber boards may discipline a barber by *revocation or suspension of the barber's license.*
13. Licensed barbers are *protected* by the laws of the state against unlawful action by the state barber board.
14. Licensed barbers must be granted a *hearing* before the state barber board can take action to revoke or suspend a license.
15. A licensee who violates the provisions of the barber license law can be cited for *disciplinary action.*
16. Persons who act as a barber without obtaining a license are guilty of practicing in an *unlawful* manner.
17. A barber who has his or her license suspended or revoked has the *right to appeal* to the courts.
18. A person convicted of violating any of the provisions of the license law is guilty of a *misdemeanor.*
19. The purpose of periodic inspections of barbershops is to ascertain compliance with *sanitation regulations and licensure compliance.*

20. A licensee who willfully fails to display a license or certificate is guilty of a *violation* of the barber law.
21. Barber law requires that suspended or revoked licenses must be *surrendered to the state barber board.*
22. The state barber board may suspend or revoke the license of a licensee who is guilty of *gross malpractice.*
23. The *barbershop owner* is responsible for posting sanitation rules, barber law, and/or the state board rules and regulations in the barbershop.
24. The state barber board may suspend or revoke the license of a licensee who is guilty of *immoral behavior.*
25. An apprentice practices barbering under the *constant and direct supervision* of a *licensed* barber.

Alabama – Alabama has no barber laws

Alaska State Board of Barbers & Hairdressers
333 Willoghby, 9th Floor, State Office Bldg.
Occupational Licensing, Juneau AK
Mailing Address: PO Box 110806,
Juneau, AK 99811-0806
907-465-2547 (ph)
907-465-2974 (fx)
license@dced.state.ak.us

Arizona Board of Barbers
1400 West Washington, Rm. 220
Phoenix, AZ 85007
602-542-4498

Arkansas State Board of Barber Examiners
103 E. 7th, No. 212
Little Rock, AR 72201-4512
501-682-4035 (ph)
501-682-5073 (fx)

California State Board of Barbering & Cosmetology
400 R St., Suite 5100
Sacramento, CA 94244-2260
916-323-1101 (ph)
916-445-8893 (fx)

Colorado Office of Barber & Cosmetology Licensure
1560 Broadway, Suite 1340
Denver, CO 80202
303-894-7772 (ph)
303-894-7764 (fx)

Connecticut Examining Board for Barbers, Hairdressers, & Cosmeticians
Dept. of Public Health
410 Capitol Ave., MS 13 App. St.
PO Box 340308
Hartford, CT 06134
860-509-7569 (ph)
860-509-8457 (fx)

Delaware Board of Cosmetology & Barbering
861 Silver Lake Blvd., Suite 203
Dover, DE 19904
302-744-4518 (ph)
302-739-2711 (fx)

District of Columbia Barber and Cosmetology Board
941 North Capitol St., NE, Mail Room 2200
Washington, DC 20002
202-442-4320 (ph)
202-442-4528 (fx)

Table 23-1 State Barber Board Contact Information

Florida Barbers' Board
1940 N. Monroe St., Suite 60
Tallahassee, FL 32399-0790
850-487-1395 (ph)
850-921-2321 (fx)

Georgia State Board of Barbers
237 Coliseum Dr.
Macon, GA 31217
478-207-1430 (ph)
478-207-1442 (fx)

Hawaii Board of Barbering and Cosmetology
1010 Richards St.
Honolulu, HI 96813
Mailing Address: PO Box 3469, Honolulu, HI 96801
808-586-2696 (ph)
808-586-2689 (fx)

Idaho State Board of Barber Examiners
Owyhee Plaza, 1109 Main St., Suite 220
Boise, ID 83702
208-334-3233 (ph)
208-334-3945 (fx)

Illinois Barber, Cosmetology, Esthetics, and Nail Technology
Dept. of Professional Regulation
320 W. Washington St., 3rd Floor
Springfield, IL 62786
217-785-0800 (ph)
217-782-7645 (fx)

Indiana State Board of Barber Examiners
302 West Washington St., Room E034
Indianapolis, IN 46204
317-234-1951 (ph)
317-233-5559 (fx)

Iowa Board of Barber Examiners
Iowa Dept. of Public Health
Lucas State Office Bldg., 5th Floor
Des Moines, IA 50319-0075
515-281-4416 (ph)
515-281-3121 (fx)

Kansas State Barber Board
Jayhawk Tower
700 SW Jackson St., Suite 1002
Topeka, KS 66603-3758
785-296-2211 (ph)
785-368-7071 (fx)

Kentucky Board of Barbering
9114 Leesgate Rd., Suite 6
Louisville, KY 40222-5055
502-429-8841 (ph)
502-429-5223 (fx)

Louisiana State Board of Barber Examiners
4626 Jamestown Ave., Suite I
Baton Rouge, LA 70898-4029
225-925-1701 (ph)
225-925-1702 (ph2)
225-925-1703 (fx)

Maine State Board of Barber Examiners
Dept. of Professional & Financial Regulation
122 Northern Ave.
Gardiner, ME 04345
Mailing Address: State House Station, Augusta, ME, 04333
207-624-8603 (ph)
207-624-8637 (fx)

Maryland State Board of Barber Examiners
500 N. Calvert., Room 307
Baltimore, MD 21201-3651
410-230-8603 (ph)
410-333-6314 (fx)

Massachusetts State Board of Barbers
239 Causeway St., 5th Floor
Boston, MA
Mailing Address: PO Box 9004, Boston, MA 02114
617-727-7367 (ph)
617-727-1627 (fx)

Michigan Board of Barber Examiners
2501 Woodlake Circle
Okemos, MI 48864
Mailing Address: PO Box 30018, Lansing, MI 48909
517-241-9201 (ph)
517-241-9280 (fx)

Table 23-1 (continued)

Minnesota Board of Barber Examiners
1885 University Ave. West, Suite 355
St. Paul, MN 55104-3403
651-642-0489 (ph)
651-649-5997 (fx)

Mississippi State Board of Barber Examiners
510 George St., Room 240
Jackson, MS 39205
Mailing Address: PO Box 603, Jackson, MS 39205-0603
601-359-1015 (ph)
601-359-1050 (fx)

Missouri State Board of Barber Examiners
3605 Missouri Blvd.
PO Box 1335
Jefferson City, MO 65102
573-751-0805 (ph)
573-751-8167 (fx)

Montana Board of Barbers
PO Box 200516
301 South Park
Helena, MT 59620-0513
406-841-2335 (ph)
406-841-2305 (fx)

Nebraska Board of Barber Examiners
State Office Bldg.
301 Centennial Mall South, 6th Floor
Lincoln, NE 68509
402-471-2051 (ph)
402-471-2025 (fx)

Nevada State Barbers Health & Sanitation Board
4710 East Flamingo Rd.
Las Vegas, NV 89121
702-399-9041 (ph)
702-456-4769 (ph2)
702-456-1948 (fx)

New Hampshire Board of Barbering & Cosmetology & Esthetics
2 Industrial Park Drive
Concord, NH 03301
603-271-3608 (ph)
603-271-8889 (fx)

New Jersey Board of Cosmetology & Cosmetologists
124 Halsey St., 6th Floor
Newark, NJ 07101
Mailing Address: PO Box 45003, Newark, NJ 07101
973-504-6400 (ph)
973-648-3536 (fx)

New Mexico Board of Barbers & Cosmetologists
2055 Pacheco St., Suite 400
Santa Fe, NM 87505
Mailing Address: PO Box 25101, Santa Fe, NM 87504
505-476-7110 (ph)
505-476-7118 (fx)

New York State Barber Board - Dept. of State
84 Holland Ave.
Albany, NY 12208
505-476-7110 (ph)
505-476-7118 (fx)

North Carolina State Board of Barber Examiners
5809-102 Departure Dr.
Raleigh, NC 27616
919-981-5210 (ph)
919-981-5068 (fx)

North Dakota State Board of Barber Examiners
PO Box 885
Bowman, ND 58623
701-523-3327

Ohio State Barber Board
77 S. High St., 16th Floor
Columbus, OH 43215-6108
614-466-5003 (ph)
614-387-1694 (fx)

Oklahoma State Barber Board
1000 NE 10th St.
Oklahoma City, OK 73117-1299
405-271-5288 (ph)
405-271-5286 (fx)

Table 23-1 (continued)

Oregon Board of Barbers & Cosmetology
700 Summer St. NE, Suite 320
Salem, OR 97301-1287
503-378-8667 (ph)
503-585-9114 (fx)

Pennsylvania State Board of Barber Examiners
124 Pine St.
Harrisburg, PA 17101
Mailing Address: PO Box 2649, Harrisburg, PA 17105-2649
717-783-3402 (ph)
717-705-5540 (fx)

Rhode Island Board of Examiners in Barbering
3 Capitol Hill, Room 104
Providence, RI 02908-5097
401-222-2827 (ph)
401-222-1272 (fx)

South Carolina State Board of Barber Examiners
PO Box 11329
Columbia, SC 29211
803-896-4491 (ph)
803-896-4484 (fx)

South Dakota Board of Barber Examiners
135 E. Illinois, Suite 214
Spearfish, SD 57783
605-642-1600 (ph)
605-642-1756 (fx)

Tennessee State Board of Barber Examiners
500 James Robertson Pkwy, Rm. 130
Nashville, TN 37243-1148
615-741-2294 (ph)
615-741-1310 (fx)

Texas State Board of Barber Examiners
5717 Balcones Dr., Suite 217
Austin, TX 78731
512-458-0111 (ph)
512-458-4901 (fx)

Utah Cosmetology/ Barber Board
160 E. 300 South
PO Box 146741
Salt Lake City, UT 84144-6741
801-530-6628 (ph)
801-530-6511 (fx)

Vermont Board of Barbers & Cosmetologists
26 Terrace St
Office of Professional Relation, Drawer 09
Montpelier, VT 05609-1106
802-828-2837 (ph)
802-828-2465 (fx)

Virginia Board of Barbers & Cosmetologists
3600 West Board St.
Richmond, VA 23230-4917
804-367-8590 (ph)
804-367-6295 (fx)

Washington Cosmetology, Manicurist, Barber & Esthetician Advisory Board
405 Black Lake Blvd.
Olympia, WA 98507
Mailing Address: PO Box 9026 Olympia, WA 98507
360-753-3834

West Virginia Board of Barbers & Cosmetologists
1716 Pennsylvania Ave., Suite 7
Charleston, WV 25302
304-558-2924 (ph)
304-558-3450 (fx)

Wisconsin Barber & Cosmetology Board
1400 E. Washington, Bureau of Business & Design Professions
Madison, WI 53708
Mailing Address: PO Box 8935, Madison, WI 53708-8935
608-266-5511 (ph)
608-267-3816 (fx)

Wyoming State Board of Barber Examiners
2515 Warren Ave, Suite 302
Cheyenne, WY 82002
Mailing Address: PO Box 9889, Cheyenne, WY 82003
307-754-5580 (ph)

Table 23-1 (continued)

chapter glossary

candidate information booklet	packet of information sent by the barber board to examination candidates upon application for testing and licensure
practical exams	hands-on tests on a live model
written exam	paper-and-pencil or computer-based testing, usually covering theory subjects related to barbering

chapter review questions

1. List the ways in which a student can prepare for written-theory state board exams.
2. List at least five methods for preparing for practical examinations.
3. List the practical-exam procedures you will have to perform in your state.
4. Explain the primary purpose of barber law.
5. Identify the name of the barber licensing board in your state.

GLOSSARY/INDEX

A

D

E

I

J

K

L

M

N

O

P